Springer
Tokyo
Berlin
Heidelberg
New York
Barcelona
Budapest
Hong Kong
London
Milan
Paris
Santa Clara
Singapore

M. Inaba, Y. Inaba

Androgenetic Alopecia

Modern Concepts of Pathogenesis and Treatment

With 425 Illustrations, with 92 in Color

Springer

Masumi Inaba, M.D.
Inaba Clinic
Department of Aesthetic Plastic Surgery
3-31-13 Asagaya-minami,
Suginami-ku, Tokyo, 166 Japan

Yoshikata Inaba, M.D.
Department of Dermatology
The Jikei University School of Medicine
3-25-8 Nishi-shinbashi,
Minato-ku, Tokyo, 105 Japan

and

Department of Dermatology
Inaba Aesthetic Plastic Surgery
3-31-13 Asagaya-minami,
Suginami-ku, Tokyo, 166 Japan

ISBN 978-4-431-70158-3 Springer-Verlag Tokyo Berlin Heidelberg New York

Printed on acid-free paper

Typesetting: Best-set Typesetter Ltd., Hong Kong

Foreword

Until now, the general belief has been that premature baldness (male pattern baldness: M.P.B., or androgenetic alopecia) is a hereditary condition that progresses with age and for which there is no cure. If the father is bald, it is assumed that the child may also be destined to be bald sometime in the future.

The existing theory throughout the world is that the central portion of the hair follicle is the hair root, and hair can never regrow if the hair root has been removed. Dr. Inaba has introduced a new theory that the central portion of the hair follicle is not only the hair root but the upper isthmal portion close to the duct opening of the sebaceous gland. This is a totally new understanding of the hair growth mechanism and the hair cycle. In his experience in the surgical removal of the sweat glands, which also removes the hair root, Dr. Inaba has found increasing evidence that hair regrows if the sebaceous gland is left intact.

The prevailing belief is that the male hormone acts directly on the hair root to cause male pattern baldness. However, Dr. Inaba has found that the male hormone is affected by an enzyme in the sebaceous gland which exercises a secondary effect on the hair root. An important factor in baldness is the size of the sebaceous gland; the relative size of the gland is influenced by diet and animal fats. Thus, baldness is not primarily a hereditary condition but rather a result of the combination of the hereditary strength of the hormone and individual dietary habits.

This new theory helped Dr. Inaba to develop a treatment for baldness based on the prevention of the enlargement of the sebaceous gland. The treatment includes appropriate diet, the use of a shampoo containing an enzyme-suppression agent, and trichogenous agents. We sincerely hope that this book will help many people to overcome or retard their premature baldness.

Robert M. Nakamura, M.D.
Chairman Emeritus
Department of Pathology
Scripps Clinic and Research Foundation
La Jolla, CA 92037, USA

Foreword

Studies in the physiology and pathology of hair, especially clinical research concerned with the growth of hair, have been minimal compared with studies carried out in other fields of medical science. Only a small number of scientists at a few research centers in the United States and Europe have done studies on the growth of hair.

Recently, however, alopecia has emerged as a concern of young people, mainly in Europe, the United States, and Japan, where a high standard of living is enjoyed. Consequently, there has been a sudden rush of studies of hair in the fields of dermatology, plastic surgery, and cosmetic surgery.

As a practitioner and as director of a small hair research center in Tokyo, Dr. Masumi Inaba, the principal author of this book, has carried out numerous studies of the physiology of hair. The regular observation of hair growth by means of a unique operative technique for relief from bromidrosis, which Dr. Inaba developed, well deserves acclaim as a landmark in the field.

Dr. Inaba has now published the result of his work on androgenetic alopecia, an endeavor that he has taken on as a lifetime study. I pay my deep respect to his arduous efforts resulting from reading a wide range of literature, profound observational practice, and knowledge derived from practical clinical work. I am reminded of the famous phrase, "Gradual approach to truth." I am convinced that Dr. Inaba's work published here will serve as an excellent basic reference text for medical practitioners and students in this field in the years to come.

Tai Ho Chung, M.D., Ph.D.
Director and Professor
Biomedical Research Laboratory
School of Medicine
Kyungpook National University
Taegu, Korea

Preface

The recent progress of medicine is, in a word, remarkable. However, the stubborn problems of cancer and pathological human hair loss still elude the search for a final cure. The research that establishes such cures, it could be said, would merit a Nobel Prize.

The complexities of cancer continue to baffle dedicated research teams, but we all look forward fervently to an eventual end to this fearful disease. On the other hand, little attention is paid to the phenomenon of human baldness. Its onset in middle age, or sometimes much earlier, seems to provoke a certain sense of idle resignation, much as if to say that it is just one of the unavoidable hazards of growing older. And, after all, it does no actual harm in other than a cosmetic sense. In some societies a bald head is even considered a symbol of wisdom or virility.

However we elect to perceive it, the phenomenon of androgenetic alopecia, in particular, has been treated rather lightly by much of the medical profession. Any explanation of its causation, spun out by any researcher regarded as an expert, has been thoughtlessly accepted even if it is later found to be quite false. Erroneous notions about the causes of baldness have perhaps been among the leading reasons why basic research and treatment procedures have been delayed for so long. It is only quite recently that serious attention has been brought to bear on the problem.

The authors have conducted basic research studies on the phenomenon of baldness and have developed new treatment techniques over the past 20 years. One conclusion is that the common explanation of the human hair cycle is, in some respects, inaccurate and misleading. This conclusion has been made on the basis of some 10,000 clinical cases and a growing body of histological studies. Much of the histological research work was done with original thick-tissue specimens which provided three-dimensional views of hair generation and regeneration.

As a result, the authors have formulated a new hypothesis to elucidate the phenomenon of human hair loss and regeneration. Research papers that led to this hypothesis have been published in a number of leading medical journals, both in Japan and in other countries. The key feature of the hypothesis is the major role played by the sebaceous gland in the complex process of hair loss and regeneration. Most recently, this hypothesis was presented in the authors' *Human Body Odor* published by Springer-Verlag.

The lifelong process of human hair generation and recession includes the phenomenon of baldness. Recent studies have indicated new treatment approaches to retard or prevent loss of hair which are quite different from those methods attempted in the past. Modern-day medical advances make it seem preposterous that men of less than 100 years of age should continue to lose their hair. It strikes the authors as strange indeed that the onset of baldness at 40 to 50 years of age is accepted by most men as regrettably inevitable. Some men, in fact, begin to grow bald as soon as their early 20s. This seems even more unnatural.

In light of anticipated future advances in medicine, this present book may be no more than a small first step toward the goal of a cure for baldness. It is, however, a step that is fully based on scientific studies, and we wish to commend the contents not only to men (and to some women) who fall victim to baldness but to anyone who has a serious interest in research within the field of dermatology.

Chapters 1–16 have been written with the basic research related to androgenetic alopecia very much in mind. Chapters 17–32 are intended to present in-depth research in the subject matter.

It is the authors' hope that the material presented herein will indeed inspire a renewed determination to conduct further research and development studies that will fully clarify the causative mechanism of male pattern baldness and other types of pathological hair loss and lead to permanent, fully effective remedies for prevention and cure.

Masumi Inaba, M.D.
Yoshikata Inaba, M.D.

Contents

Foreword V
Preface VII

1. Structure of Skin and Hair Follicles 1
1.1 Structure of the Skin 1
1.2 Structure of the Hair Follicle 1
1.3 The Sebaceous Gland 5
1.4 Connective Tissue Sheath 7
1.5 Dermal Papilla 8
1.6 Regional Anatomy of the Scalp 13

2. Preparation of Thick Tissue Specimens 17
2.1 Development of Cellotape Method 17
2.2 Development of Cellophane Sheet Method 18
2.3 Detailed Observations of Thick Tissue Specimens—Preparation of Microscopic and Electron Microscopic Specimens from Thick Tissue Specimen Using Cellophane Sheet 20

3. Generation and Growth of Human Hair 23
3.1 Stages of Hair Growth 23
3.2 The Hair Canal 32

4. Pigmentation of Hair 33
4.1 Hair Color 33
4.2 Embryonic Development of Melanocytes in Human Hair 33
4.3 Generation of Melanin Pigmentation 34
4.4 Regeneration of Melanin Pigmentation 35
4.5 New Growth of Melanin Pigmentation 37

5. Blood Vessel System in Hair Follicles 39
5.1 Vascular System for the Pilosebaceous Unit 39
5.2 Experimental Research 40
5.3 Mechanism Underlying Formation of Vascular System in the Hair Follicle 43

6. Changes in Hair: Causative Factors 45
6.1 Hormonal Control of the Hair Follicle 45
6.2 Hormonal Control of the Sebaceous Gland 45
6.3 Interaction Between the Sebaceous Gland and the Hair Follicle 46
6.4 Development of Axillary Hair 47

7. Hair Regeneration 63
7.1 Hair Cycles 63
7.2 Mechanisms of Regulation of the Hair Cycle 67
7.3 New Concept of Hair Generation and Regeneration 67

8. Regeneration After Subcutaneous Tissue Shaving Procedure 69
8.1 Common Hair Cycle Theory Reconsidered 69
8.2 Bromidrosis 69
8.3 Histological Findings 73
8.4 Relationship of Development Stage of New Hair Follicle and Size of Sebaceous Gland 81
8.5 Relationship Between New Hair Follicle and Time Elapsed After Surgery 81
8.6 Evidence of New Hair Regeneration 81

9. Regeneration After Plucking 85
9.1 Process of Hair Regeneration After Plucking 85
9.2 Summary of Our Findings 96
9.3 Process of Hair Follicle Formation After Subcutaneous Tissue Shaving and Hair Plucking 96

10. Regeneration After Electrical Epilation of the Hair 99
10.1 Basic Principles of Electrolysis and Electrocoagulation 99
10.2 Supportive Findings for Basic Principles of Epilation Treatment 100

11. Regeneration of Scalp Hair 103
11.1 Hair Stages 103
11.2 Supporting Findings 107

12. Hair Regeneration in the Mouse After Application of Anti-Cancer Agent, Particularly in Terms of Epithelial-Mesenchymal Interaction 109
12.1 Anti-Cancer Agents and Hair Loss 109
12.2 Regeneration of Hair Follicle After Application of Anti-Cancer Agent 109
12.3 Regeneration from Remaining Bundle Telogen Hair Follicles 113
12.4 Regeneration from the Upper Isthmal Portion After the Plucking of Telogen Hair 116
12.5 Regeneration After Destruction of the Sebaceous Gland 116
12.6 Hair Regeneration in the Mouse 117

13. New Concept of the Hair Cycle (Sebaceous Gland Hypothesis) 119
13.1 Common Hair Cycle Theory Subject to Revision 119
13.2 New Concept of the Hair Cycle in Humans 119
13.3 Essential Hair Cycle Hypothesis and Supportive Findings 121

14. Other Important Findings in the Hair Follicle 123
14.1 Location of the Central Portion of Hair Regeneration 123
14.2 Mechanism of the Descending Hair Follicle 130
14.3 How Is the Hair Matrix Formed? 133
14.4 Comparison of Epidermal and Follicular Cells 135
14.5 Why the Growth (Anagen) Stage and Regressive (Catagen) Stage Are Confused 137

15. Hormones Classified According to Secretory Organ of Origin 143
15.1 Male Hormones 143
15.2 Estrogens 152
15.3 Progesterone 153
15.4 Distribution of Estrogen and Progesterone Receptors in Scalp Tissue 153
15.5 Adrenal Steroid Hormones 155
15.6 Thyroid Hormone 156
15.7 Anterior Pituitary Gonadotropins 156

16. Neuronal and Other Factors That Influence the Hair Follicle 159

17. Androgenetic Alopecia 161
17.1 Definition of Androgenetic Alopecia 161
17.2 Occurrence and Frequency 162
17.3 Incidence of Baldness in Japanese 163
17.4 Hair Density in the Scalp 165
17.5 Factors Affecting the Hair Cycle 165
17.6 Various Signs of Scalp Hair Loss 166

18. Etiologic Factors in Male Pattern Baldness 169
18.1 Seborrhea and Dandruff 169
18.2 Dietary Factors 169
18.3 Genetic Predisposition Theory 170
18.4 Aging 170
18.5 Insufficient Blood Circulation 170
18.6 Scalp Tension 171
18.7 Nervous Stress 171
18.8 Hair Conditioners 171
18.9 Hormonal Factors 172

19. Sebaceous Gland Hypothesis of Androgenetic Alopecia (Inaba 1985; Inaba and Inaba 1992a) 175
19.1 Review of Hormonal Mechanisms in Hair Regeneration 175
19.2 Development of the Sebaceous Gland Hypothesis 175
19.3 Mechanism of the Development of Androgenetic Alopecia 176
19.4 Hair Follicles and Sebaceous Glands Relative to 5α-DHT Production 176
19.5 Sebaceous Gland Hypothesis for Male Pattern Baldness; Supportive Findings 177

20. Histological Findings in Androgenetic Alopecia 179
20.1 Histological Findings 179
20.2 Histochemical Findings 183

21. Causal Mechanism of Progressive Androgenetic Alopecia 185
21.1 Fetal Period 185
21.2 Neonatal Period 185
21.3 Childhood Period 186
21.4 Adult Period 188
21.5 Balding Period (Solitary Coarse Hairs) 188
21.6 Complete Baldness 189

22. Differential Diagnosis (Types of Baldness Other than Male Pattern Baldness) 191
22.1 Alopecia Areata 191
22.2 Alopecia Cicatrisata 195
22.3 Alopecia Gradus Induced by Hairstyling 195
22.4 Baldness Due to Syphilis 196
22.5 Other Contributory Diseases in Baldness 196

23. Relationship of Diet to Androgenetic Alopecia 197
23.1 Malnutrition and Androgenetic Alopecia 197
23.2 Relationship of Animal Fat Intake to Androgenetic Alopecia 197
23.3 Japanese Diet 199
23.4 Relationship of Diet to Baldness and Hircismus (Offensive Body Odor) 200
23.5 Diet Therapy for Androgenetic Alopecia 201

24. General Measures for Prevention of Baldness 205
24.1 Prevention of Baldness by Measures That Promote Healthy Scalp Hygiene 205

25. Therapy for Androgenetic Alopecia ... 209
25.1 Increased Massage and Circulation ... 209
25.2 Diet Therapy ... 210
25.3 Conventional Treatment ... 210

26. Agents Used for the Treatment of Androgenetic Alopecia ... 211
26.1 Background and Historical Aspects of Agents Used for the Treatment of Androgenetic Alopecia ... 211
26.2 Treatment of Androgenetic Alopecia with Steroidal Antiandrogens ... 211

27. Other Products Being Developed by Pharmaceutical and Cosmetic Companies ... 215
27.1 Treatment of Androgenetic Alopecia with Chemical Products ... 215
27.2 Chemical Structure of These Products ... 216
27.3 Mechanism of Hair Growth in Relation to New Drugs ... 216
27.4 Mechanism of Action of New Drugs on Target Tissue ... 217
27.5 Viprostol ... 217
27.6 Other Products in Development ... 217

28. Trial Treatment of Androgenetic Alopecia with Oxidizing Agents (Inaba and Inaba 1984) ... 221
28.1 The Hair Growth-Stimulating (Trichogenous) Effect of Cold Wave Hair Styling ... 221
28.2 The Cold Wave Principle ... 221
28.3 Basis of Hair Regeneration ... 221
28.4 Discovery of an Effective Trichogen ... 222
28.5 Development of New Tonic Formulation ... 223
28.6 Treatment of Androgenetic Alopecia with Stabilized Chlorine Dioxide (Inaba 1985) ... 224
28.7 Supporting Findings ... 225
28.8 Individual Case Reports of Patients with Androgenetic Alopecia Treated with the Inaba Reagent ... 226
28.9 Classification of Active Principles of Hair Tonics by Mechanism of Action (Reviewed by Imada 1983) ... 229
28.10 Future Aspects of Hair Care Products ... 232
28.11 Trichogenous Agents in the United States ... 232

29. Operative Treatment for Androgenetic Alopecia ... 233
29.1 Punch Graft Method ... 233
29.2 Minigrafts ... 237
29.3 Single Hair Graft Transplantation ... 238
29.4 Multiple Strip Composite Graft ... 244
29.5 Histological Findings After Transplantation of Single Hair-Bearing Graft or Micrograft ... 244
29.6 Flap Procedures ... 251
29.7 Scalp Reduction Procedures ... 262
29.8 Scalp Skin Elongation Method ... 264
29.9 Signs of Disturbed Circulation with Juri Flap Methods ... 267
29.10 Advantage and Disadvantages of Juri and Partial Flaps ... 267
29.11 Free Flaps ... 267
29.12 Histological Study of Free Coarse Hair-Bearing Graft Transplantation ... 268
29.13 Marechal Operation (Bilateral Ligation Method) ... 275

30. Artificial Hair Implantation ... 277
30.1 Artificial Hair Implantation ... 277
30.2 Our Experience of Artificial Hair Implantation ... 278
30.3 Artificial Hair Newly Developed by Nido Ltd. ... 280
30.4 Percutaneous Implantation ... 282
30.5 Histological Findings ... 282

16. Neuronal and Other Factors That Influence the Hair Follicle 159

17. Androgenetic Alopecia 161
17.1 Definition of Androgenetic Alopecia 161
17.2 Occurrence and Frequency 162
17.3 Incidence of Baldness in Japanese 163
17.4 Hair Density in the Scalp 165
17.5 Factors Affecting the Hair Cycle 165
17.6 Various Signs of Scalp Hair Loss 166

18. Etiologic Factors in Male Pattern Baldness 169
18.1 Seborrhea and Dandruff 169
18.2 Dietary Factors 169
18.3 Genetic Predisposition Theory 170
18.4 Aging 170
18.5 Insufficient Blood Circulation 170
18.6 Scalp Tension 171
18.7 Nervous Stress 171
18.8 Hair Conditioners 171
18.9 Hormonal Factors 172

19. Sebaceous Gland Hypothesis of Androgenetic Alopecia (Inaba 1985; Inaba and Inaba 1992a) 175
19.1 Review of Hormonal Mechanisms in Hair Regeneration 175
19.2 Development of the Sebaceous Gland Hypothesis 175
19.3 Mechanism of the Development of Androgenetic Alopecia 176
19.4 Hair Follicles and Sebaceous Glands Relative to 5α-DHT Production 176
19.5 Sebaceous Gland Hypothesis for Male Pattern Baldness; Supportive Findings 177

20. Histological Findings in Androgenetic Alopecia 179
20.1 Histological Findings 179
20.2 Histochemical Findings 183

21. Causal Mechanism of Progressive Androgenetic Alopecia 185
21.1 Fetal Period 185
21.2 Neonatal Period 185
21.3 Childhood Period 186
21.4 Adult Period 188
21.5 Balding Period (Solitary Coarse Hairs) 188
21.6 Complete Baldness 189

22. Differential Diagnosis (Types of Baldness Other than Male Pattern Baldness) 191
22.1 Alopecia Areata 191
22.2 Alopecia Cicatrisata 195
22.3 Alopecia Gradus Induced by Hairstyling 195
22.4 Baldness Due to Syphilis 196
22.5 Other Contributory Diseases in Baldness 196

23. Relationship of Diet to Androgenetic Alopecia 197
23.1 Malnutrition and Androgenetic Alopecia 197
23.2 Relationship of Animal Fat Intake to Androgenetic Alopecia 197
23.3 Japanese Diet 199
23.4 Relationship of Diet to Baldness and Hircismus (Offensive Body Odor) 200
23.5 Diet Therapy for Androgenetic Alopecia 201

24. General Measures for Prevention of Baldness 205
24.1 Prevention of Baldness by Measures That Promote Healthy Scalp Hygiene 205

25. Therapy for Androgenetic Alopecia ... 209
25.1 Increased Massage and Circulation ... 209
25.2 Diet Therapy ... 210
25.3 Conventional Treatment ... 210

26. Agents Used for the Treatment of Androgenetic Alopecia ... 211
26.1 Background and Historical Aspects of Agents Used for the Treatment of Androgenetic Alopecia ... 211
26.2 Treatment of Androgenetic Alopecia with Steroidal Antiandrogens ... 211

27. Other Products Being Developed by Pharmaceutical and Cosmetic Companies ... 215
27.1 Treatment of Androgenetic Alopecia with Chemical Products ... 215
27.2 Chemical Structure of These Products ... 216
27.3 Mechanism of Hair Growth in Relation to New Drugs ... 216
27.4 Mechanism of Action of New Drugs on Target Tissue ... 217
27.5 Viprostol ... 217
27.6 Other Products in Development ... 217

28. Trial Treatment of Androgenetic Alopecia with Oxidizing Agents (Inaba and Inaba 1984) ... 221
28.1 The Hair Growth-Stimulating (Trichogenous) Effect of Cold Wave Hair Styling ... 221
28.2 The Cold Wave Principle ... 221
28.3 Basis of Hair Regeneration ... 221
28.4 Discovery of an Effective Trichogen ... 222
28.5 Development of New Tonic Formulation ... 223
28.6 Treatment of Androgenetic Alopecia with Stabilized Chlorine Dioxide (Inaba 1985) ... 224
28.7 Supporting Findings ... 225
28.8 Individual Case Reports of Patients with Androgenetic Alopecia Treated with the Inaba Reagent ... 226
28.9 Classification of Active Principles of Hair Tonics by Mechanism of Action (Reviewed by Imada 1983) ... 229
28.10 Future Aspects of Hair Care Products ... 232
28.11 Trichogenous Agents in the United States ... 232

29. Operative Treatment for Androgenetic Alopecia ... 233
29.1 Punch Graft Method ... 233
29.2 Minigrafts ... 237
29.3 Single Hair Graft Transplantation ... 238
29.4 Multiple Strip Composite Graft ... 244
29.5 Histological Findings After Transplantation of Single Hair-Bearing Graft or Micrograft ... 244
29.6 Flap Procedures ... 251
29.7 Scalp Reduction Procedures ... 262
29.8 Scalp Skin Elongation Method ... 264
29.9 Signs of Disturbed Circulation with Juri Flap Methods ... 267
29.10 Advantage and Disadvantages of Juri and Partial Flaps ... 267
29.11 Free Flaps ... 267
29.12 Histological Study of Free Coarse Hair-Bearing Graft Transplantation ... 268
29.13 Marechal Operation (Bilateral Ligation Method) ... 275

30. Artificial Hair Implantation ... 277
30.1 Artificial Hair Implantation ... 277
30.2 Our Experience of Artificial Hair Implantation ... 278
30.3 Artificial Hair Newly Developed by Nido Ltd. ... 280
30.4 Percutaneous Implantation ... 282
30.5 Histological Findings ... 282

30.6 Case Reports ... 283
30.7 Mechanism of Epilation After Implantation of Artificial Hair ... 284
30.8 Advantages of Artificial Hair Implantation ... 285
30.9 Drawbacks of Artificial Hair ... 286
30.10 Other Problems Related to Artificial Hair ... 286

31. Another Solution: Hairpieces (Wigs) ... 287
31.1 Conventional Wig ... 287
31.2 New Wigs ... 289

32. Mechanism of Linear Scar Formation After Scalp Surgery: Preventive Measures ... 291
32.1 Case Studies ... 291

Afterword ... 299
Acknowledgments ... 300
References ... 301
Index ... 325

Structure of Skin and Hair Follicles 1

1.1 Structure of the Skin

The skin consists of two layers, the epidermis and the dermis. The epidermis is the surface layer, exposed to the outside world. Beneath it is the dermal layer, which lies above the subcutaneous tissue level. Epidermal thickness over the body is 0.1–0.15 mm, quite thin, except for the epidermis of the heel and the palm of the hand, which is a bit thicker. The dermis is generally thicker than the epidermis, measuring 1–2 mm (Fig. 1.1).

The epidermis itself has several sublayers; the basal, spinous, granular, and cornified layers, on the actual surface of the skin. A clear layer is observed between the granular and cornified layers in the epidermis of the palm and heel (Fig. 1.2).

Mitotic activity (cell division) occurs in the basal layer. The divided cells migrate upward to the spinous or granular layers while further dividing and are finally keratinized to form the cornified layer. At length they expire and fall off the skin surface. Their life cycle from cell division to final discard is about 4 weeks.

The dermal layer consists of connective tissue, capillary vessels, and other components. The capillary vessels in the dermis supply nutrients to the epidermis. The upper part of the hair follicle, which lies within the dermis, includes the sebaceous gland, follicular nerve plexus, lymph duct, and eccrine gland.

The lower part of the hair follicle, with the apocrine gland, lies within the subcutaneous tissue beneath the dermal layer.

1.2 Structure of the Hair Follicle

The hair follicle is composed of epithelial components (the matrix and outer root sheath) and dermal components (dermal papilla and connective tissue sheath). A cylindrical depression formed by an invagination of the epidermis penetrates the corium into the connective tissue which contains the hair root. Attached to the follicles are sebaceous glands and the tiny muscles (arrectores pili) which enable the hair to stand upright.

The hair follicle itself, replete with follicle and sebaceous gland, is called a skin appendage. As shown in Fig. 1.3, a microscopic view of the lower portion of the hair follicle shows that is has a characteristic bulb at its lower end. The hair bulb does not function like a plant bulb, in which nutrition for the plant stem is absorbed from the surrounding soil. The hair root does not take in nutrition from the surrounding tissue. Connective tissue, including capillary vessels in the dermal layer, protrudes upward to the bulb and forms the dermal papilla, which nourishes the entire hair follicle. In this respect, the dermal papilla can be said to resemble the root of a plant. The lower half of the hair bulb, shaped to mostly enclose this dermal papilla, is called the bulb matrix.

The connective tissue contained within the hair bulb is the dermal papilla. The sizes of the papilla and surrounding bulb are directly related to the size of the hair produced (Fig. 1.1) (Durward and Rundall 1958). In anagen follicles, the dermal papilla is attached to a basal plate of connective tissue by a narrow stalk.

This matrix, where mitotic activity takes place, is the maker of the hair follicle. The cells which divide here grow to form different types of tissues which are keratinized upward to the skin surface.

The innermost portion of this keratinized tissue is the hair itself, which consists of the medulla, the cortex of the hair root, and the hair cuticle (Fig. 1.4a–c).

Like the hair of other mammals, human hair consists primarily of keratin, a specialized fibrous protein remarkable for its strength, elasticity, and

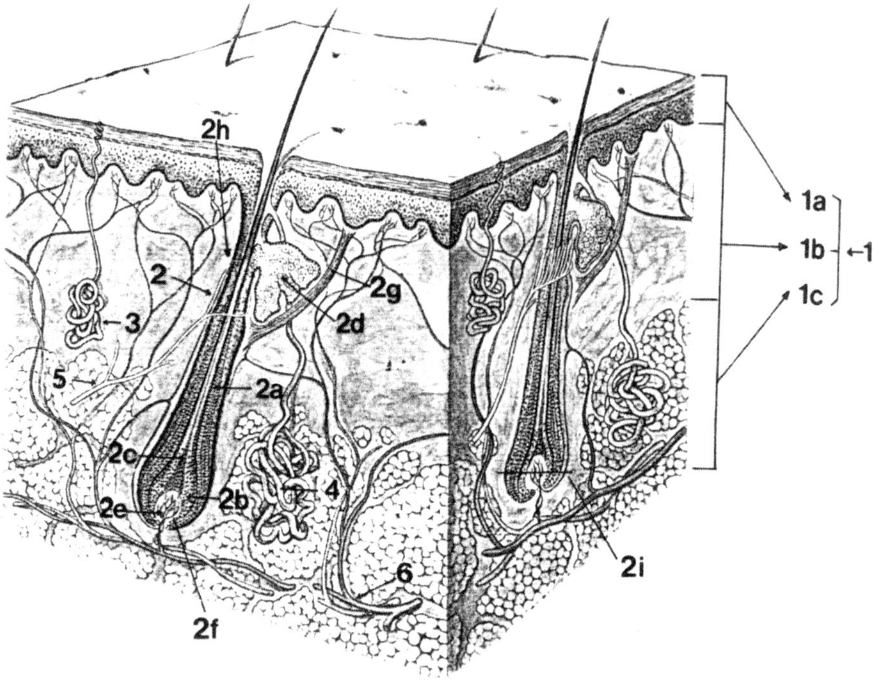

Fig. 1.1. Skin and hair follicle structure. *1*, Skin; *1a*, epidermis; *1b*, dermis; *1c*, subcutaneous tissue. *2*, Pilosebaceous unit; *2a*, outer root sheath; *2b*, inner root sheath (Henle's layer, Huxley's layer, sheath cuticula); *2c*, hair tissue (hair cuticula, cortex, medulla); *2d*, sebaceous gland; *2e*, dermal papilla; *2f*, hair matrix; *2g*, arrector pili muscle; *2h*, upper isthmal portion; *2i*, Auber's critical line; *3*, eccrine gland; *4*, apocrine gland; *5*, nerves; *6*, blood vessel (from Inaba 1981 with permission from Nikkei Science). ×125

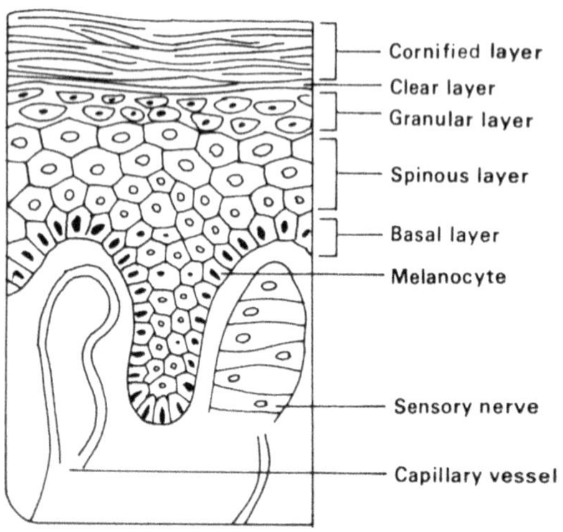

Fig. 1.2. Cross section of the epidermis

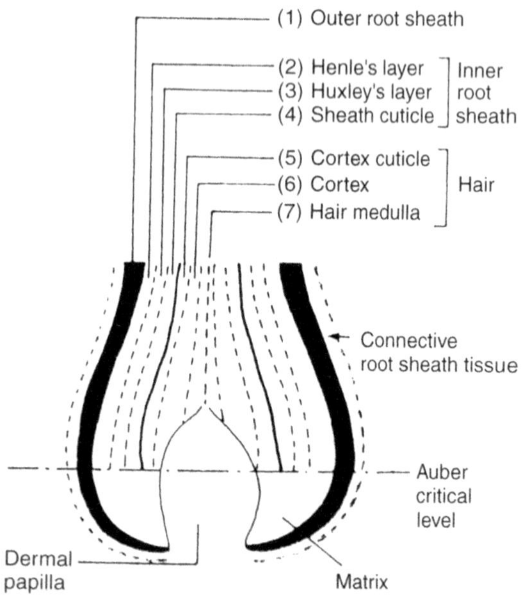

Fig. 1.3. Structure of the hair bulb

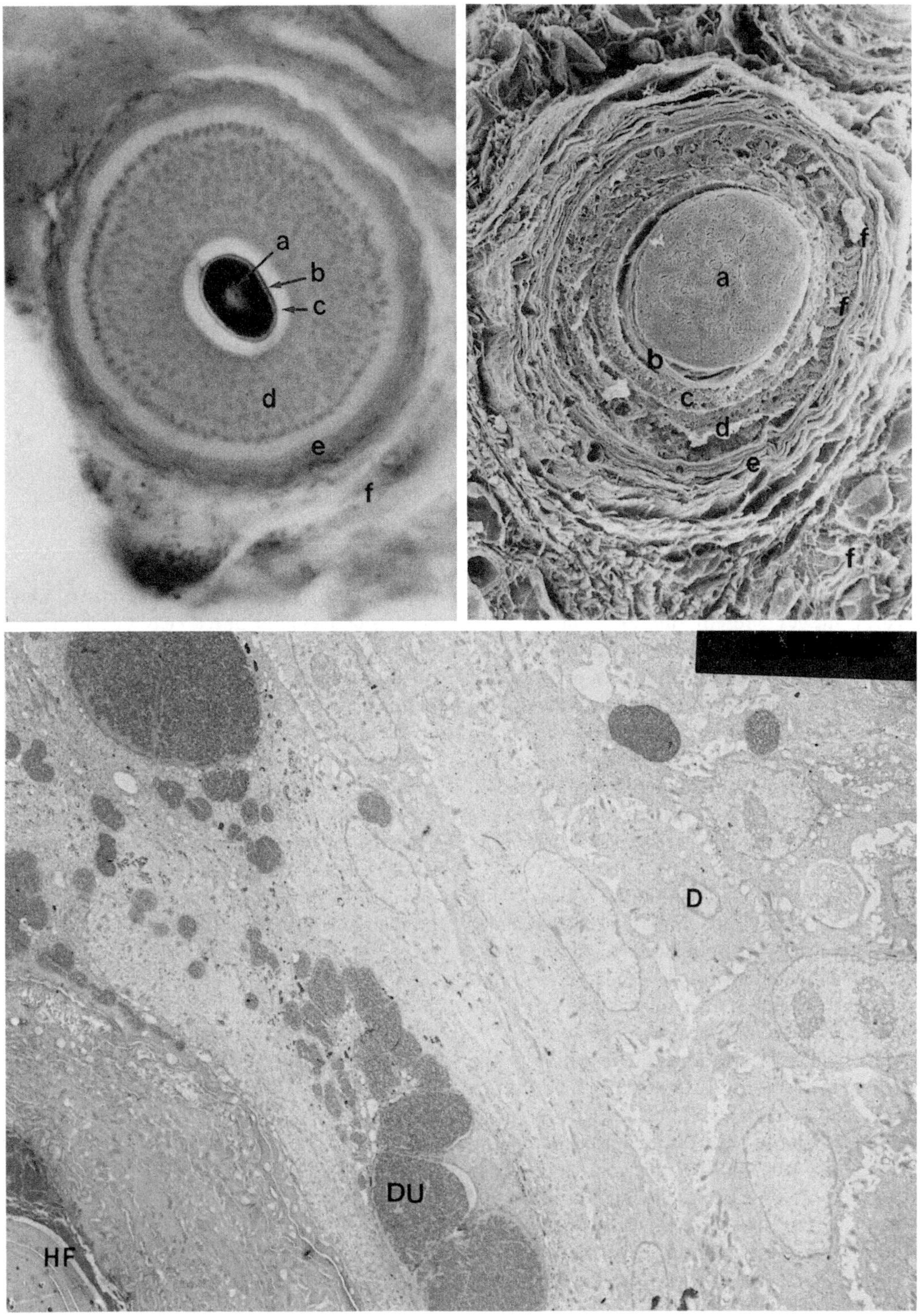

a b c

Fig. 1.4a–c. Cross section of the hair. **a** Histologic and **b** scanning electron microscopic findings. *a*, Hair cortex; *b*, cuticle; *c*, inner root sheath; *d*, outer root sheath; *e*, connective sheath; *f*, dermis ×450. **c** The sebaceous duct between the hair follicle and dermis. *HF*, Hair follicle; *D*, dermis; *DU*, duct. ×7000

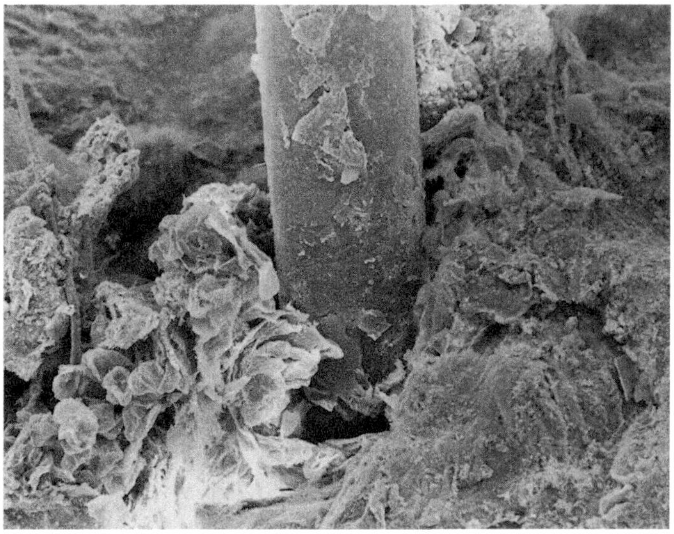

Fig. 1.5. Scanning electron micrograph of skin surface hair protruding from the hair canal can be seen. ×1300

resistance to chemical damage. The visible hair shaft is the dead protein and the product of a dynamic, living structure known as the hair matrix. Living cells in the matrix multiply rapidly. Immediately above this multiplication area is the zone of keratinization, where, by a process of dehydration and chemical change, the new cells die, creating the dense, cohesive mass of keratinized cells called the hair shaft. As cells are added at the base of the follicle, the shaft moves out and hair "grows" (Fig. 1.5).

The hair is enclosed within the follicle by the inner root sheath. This inner sheath terminates close to the follicle's upper isthmal portion (adjacent to the secretory duct opening of the sebaceous gland) (see Fig. 9.8), and has three layers: the cuticle, Huxley's layer, and Henle's layer.

All three layers undergo differentiation in the same sequence, but at different rates; first, Henle's layer, then Huxley's layer, and, finally, the cuticle. It is important to note that complete hardening and differentiation of the inner root sheath occur before the layers of the developing hair keratinize within it. The filamentous structure which is produced from the surrounding germinal layer is compressed by keratinization of the inner root sheath (see Fig. 8.12, Fig. 9.5d).

The hair is surrounded by the cuticle, which is wrapped around the hair as it grows outward from the skin surface (Fig. 1.6). The cuticle consists of flattened, overlapping cuticle cells that show a laminar structure. It has two layers, the outer exocuticle and the inner endocuticle.

The lower portion of the hair bulb is divided into distinct regions by the Auber critical level (Auber 1952), an imaginary line drawn across the widest diameter of the dermal papilla. Below Auber's borderline is the true hair matrix, which consists of undifferentiated cells. Cell differentiation is said to occur above this borderline, forming the hair (medulla, cortex, and cortex cuticle) and the inner root sheath (sheath cuticle and Henle's and Huxley's layers).

These observations indicate that tissues of different morphologies are not generated from the undifferentiated cells (hair matrix) below the Auber borderline, but from the matrix surrounding the dermal papilla. Using autoradiographic methods, Epstein and Maibach (1969) showed that the matrix cells of the different cell layers of the

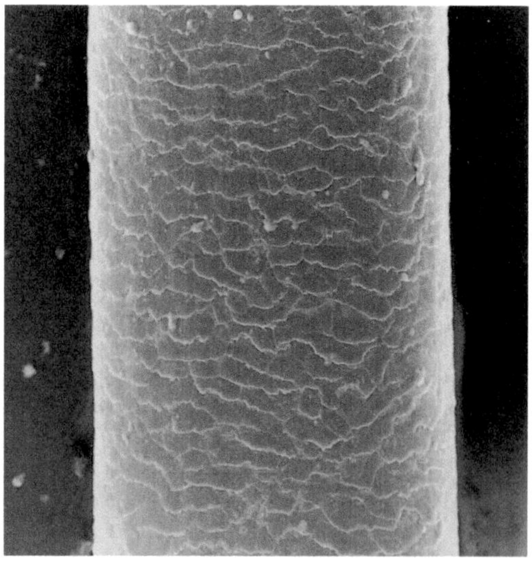

Fig. 1.6. Scanning electron micrograph of normal cuticle. The cuticle of the hair is made up of a series of ring-like overlapping cells that surround the cortex. ×1300

follicle were adherent to the basal lamina. The cells at the top of the dermal papilla produce the cortex part of the follicle structure. Moving downward over the papilla, one encounters the matrix cells of the cuticles, i.e., the cuticle of the hair fiber and the cuticle of the inner root sheath, the matrix cells of Huxley's and Henle's layers, and, finally, the outer root sheath. The connective tissue surrounding the cellular part of the hair follicle is called the connective tissue sheath (see Fig. 1.3).

The outer root sheath consists of certain serial cell groups and an extension of the germinal cell layer of the epidermal cells.

The outer sheaths of follicles are composed of comparatively static cells that store a large amount of glycogen, which is used as an energy source for cellular activities in bulbs (Uno et al. 1968).

From a histological standpoint, the outer root sheath consists of one or two cell layers in the hair bulb portion; its thickness increases as it descends, eventually consisting of more than three cell layers. Ito and Sato (1986) suggested that it consisted of two cell layers in the hair bulb portion, that the cell population increased in the outer layer, and that the cells in the inner layer were flatly placed in a row, exhibiting a peculiar type of keratinization other than that related to trichilemma.

The sebaceous gland connects to the hair follicle close to the skin surface, and has a secretory tract connected to the skin pore. The follicular portion, which lies between the sebaceous gland's secretory duct opening and the attachment of the arrector pili muscle (which holds the hair erect from the central point of the follicle), is called the isthmal portion of the follicle. A considerable number of capillary vessels is concentrated at the upper isthmal portion of the follicle, the sebaceous gland, the dermal papilla, and the lower portion of the follicle. These capillaries are closely connected to the dermis.

This anatomical description of skin and hair follicle structure provides one vantage point for observation. From a morphological standpoint, however, the follicle is an extension of the epidermis and is keratinized by a process quite similar to that which keratinizes the epidermis. The germinal cells within the basal and spinous layers of the epidermis have corresponding counterparts in the germinal cells of the hair matrix. In either instance, cell division takes place, the new cells grow, differentiate, and soon keratinize.

The hair and inner root sheath within the follicle keratinize vertically, while the epidermis keratinizes on a horizontal plane. The resultant structures are quite different. The causative mechanisms of these differences have not yet been clearly identified (see Section 14.5).

The entire epithelial portion of the hair follicle is surrounded and supported by a connective tissue root sheath, which elaborates a basement membrane and the vitreous membrane. This sheath consists of longitudinal and circular layers of collagen, and bears the follicle blood supply. At the lower end of the anagen hair, the connective tissue root sheath inverts into the hollow of the matrix, supplies it with blood, and directs the matrix cells to form the hair and inner root sheath. When the dermal papilla is in the resting stage, the hair matrix involutes, and the hair goes into the catagen and telogen stages. When the dermal papilla dies or is destroyed, hair growth ceases completely and permanently (see Section 1.5).

The follicular unit of the adult scalp is an area circumscribed by coarse reticular dermal collagen; it contains two to four terminal follicles, one (or rarely two) vellus follicles, their associated sebaceous glands, and the insertions of the corresponding arrector pili muscles. In the normal adult scalp, follicular units tend to have a geometric, hexagonal shape (reviewed by Headington 1984; Baden 1987).

1.3 The Sebaceous Gland

1.3.1 Structure of the Sebaceous Gland

In humans, sebaceous glands (Fig. 1.7a,b) are found over the entire body surface, except for the palms, soles, and dorsum of the feet.

The sebaceous glands are an integral part of the pilosebaceous apparatus and empty into the follicular canal through a short duct. However, in the mucous membranes, they open directly to the surface.

Sebaceous glands not associated with hair may also be found in the mucocutaneous junction. In the eyelids, large sebaceous glands, the meibomian glands, are found.

The sebaceous glands are relatively small over most of the body and are usually found at a density of less than 100 per square centimeter of body surface. The glands in certain areas, such as the face, neck, and scalp, however, are much larger and more numerous, with a density of up to 800 glands per square centimeter. These large glands are hormone dependent, being stimulated by androgens, so they make an appearance at the time of puberty, and in elderly individuals they may atrophy. The largest glands occur in specialized pilosebaceous units called sebaceous follicles, which have a small vellus hair and a widely dilated follicular canal.

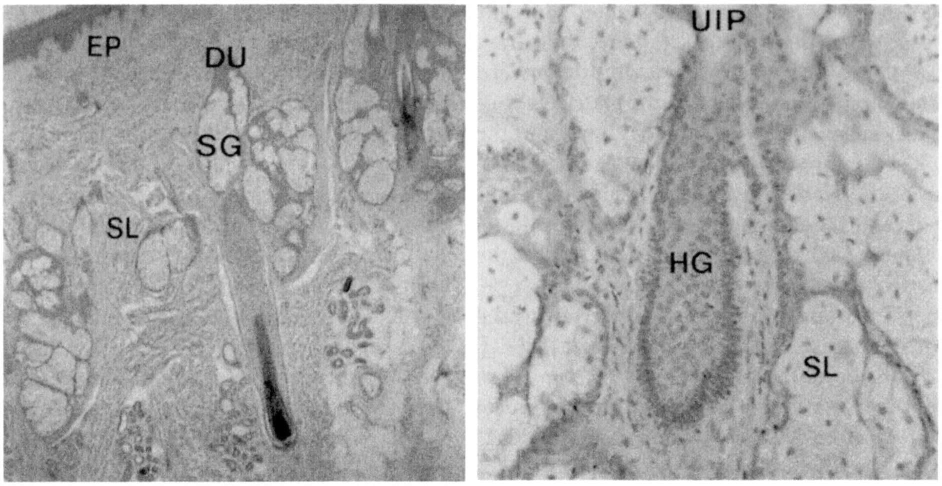

Fig. 1.7a,b. Sebaceous gland structure. The cells surrounding the follicle are analogous to the cells found in the basal epidermis level. *EP*, Epidermis; *HG*, new hair germ; *SL*, sebaceous lobule; *UIP*, upper isthmal portion; *DU*, secretory duct; *SG*, sebaceous gland. **a** H&E, ×75 **b** E&E, ×250

Regardless of size, all sebaceous glands have the same structure. The duct is a transitional zone between the follicular canal and the lipid-producing cells of the individual sebaceous acinus. Therefore, although a granular layer is present at the junction with the follicular canal, it disappears below, and there is an abrupt transformation to lipid-producing cells.

The outermost cells of the acinus, the basal cells, rest on a basal lamina comparable to that of the epidermis. The basal cells are the germinative cells of the gland. They are small, flattened or cuboidal, and densely basophilic. Usually there is only one layer of basal cells. As the cells proceed toward the center of the acinus, there is a progressive accumulation of lipid. The cells become laden with lipid droplets; their basophilic cytoplasm thus becomes compressed into a fine reticulated pattern. The cells enlarge greatly, their nuclei become distorted and disintegrate, and eventually the cells rupture, thus forming sebum, the lipid product of the gland.

Sebum contains glycerides and free fatty acids (57.5%), wax esters (26%), squalene (12%), and a small amount of cholesterol and cholesterol esters (Dawning et al. 1970).

1.3.2 Development of the Sebaceous Gland

When the anlagen of sebaceous glands appear on the posterior surface of the hair pegs, they are solid hemispherical protuberances consisting of columnar or round cells at the periphery, and ovoid or flattened cells at the center.

The size of the anlagen varies according to the region in which the hair follicle is located.

When the gland is larger, it can be divided into a bulbous part, the head, and a narrow part, the neck, connecting it with the infundibulum of the follicle. In the beginning, the gland has no duct. The duct appears first as a ridge-like septum which separates the hair canal from the newly-formed keratinizing sebaceous duct. The early appearance of keratohyalin granules and keratin in the cells of the solid cord that grow upward into the epidermis from the infundibulum plays an important role in the formation of the hair canal. It appears to be an independent formation within the epidermis and is present only in fetal skin, at least in its upper part.

The lower part will participate in the formation of the intraepidermal infundibular unit of the adult skin (Pinkus and Steele 1955).

From their earliest differentiation at 13–15 weeks of fetal life, the sebaceous glands are large and functional. The sebum forms a part of the vernix caseosa. Growth of sebaceous buds takes place from the peripheral layer of cells of all portions of the gland. The gland becomes multiacinar, with great variability in size and shape according to the area in which the follicle is located. In the fetus, the further development and enlargement of the gland depends upon the encroachment or fusion of nearby acini, with the appearance of septa splitting the gland into single units (Montagna and Parakkal 1974).

At times, individual acini seem to have the faculty of undergoing total destruction, once differentiation has started. The mitotic activity in the undifferentiated cells at the periphery of any acinus, according to Montagna and Parakkal (1974), is mainly focal and is indispensable for the formation of new acini. At the end of fetal life, the sebaceous glands are well developed and large and spread over the entire surface of the skin, but particularly in those areas in which, in later adult life, there will be the most glandular activity.

After birth, the size of the sebaceous glands is rapidly reduced and they enlarge and become actively functional again only at puberty [reviewed in Serri and Huber (1963)].

1.3.3 Sebaceous Duct: Histological and Ultrastructural Findings

The stratified squamous epithelium that lines the sebaceous duct is continuous with the peripheral zone of cells that surrounds the acinus and extends into the epithelium of the pilary canal. These cells have been well described by Knutson (1974) and, more recently, by Jenkinson et al. (1985). The normal pilary canal is typical of a well-developed keratinized epithelium, with a stratum granulosum, containing ultrastructural elements, such as keratohyalin granules, lamellar granules, and bundles of tonofilaments, and a stratum corneum. The cells of the sebaceous duct also contain the ultrastructural elements of keratinization, although a distinct stratum granulosum and stratum corneum are absent.

According to Morohashi (1968), the sebaceous duct cells contained not only a number of keratohyalin granules, membrane-coating granules, and tonofibrils, but also lipid vacuoles. Numerous discharged membrane-coating granules were observed in the intercellular spaces. Gap junctions decreased in number after the discharge of membrane-coating granules. The most striking features were seen in those sebaceous ducts proximal to the infundibulum after androgen administration. The sebaceous ducts underwent cohesive hyperkeratinization. A gradual decrease in the number of membrane-coating granules in the cytoplasm was observed.

The study revealed that there were distinct ultrastructural differences in both sebaceous duct keratinization and lipid formation between normal duct cells and those from animals treated with androgen. It was postulated that these ultrastructural changes in the sebaceous duct cells induced by the administration of androgen represented merely a quantitative, rather than qualitative, difference in sebaceous duct function, i.e., sebaceous duct keratinization and lipid formation.

Inaba suggested that when vellus hairs are replaced by coarse hairs (see Section 6.4.2) or when the density of hair follicle increases (see Section 6.4.3) the sebaceous duct area is observed to function as a stem cell.

1.3.4 Relationship Between the Hair Cycle and Sebaceous Gland

It is well known that the human hair follicles go through the cycle of anagen, catagen, and telogen stages. Tanaka et al. (1965) found that the morphological changes in the sebaceous gland were not independent, but were closely related to the hair cycle, and thus stressed the need to study both. Chase and Eaton (1959) reported that the sebaceous gland became swollen during the telogen stage of the hair follicle. According to Parnell (1949), the hair and the sebaceous glands become larger during the growth phase and smaller in catagen and telogen. A similar general reduction in the volume of sebaceous glands occurs during hair loss caused by alopecia areata (Moretti et al. 1963) and pattern alopecia (Rampini et al. 1968).

Sato (1976) removed the hair from the dorsal skin of 53 rats (DD type) and proceeded to take samples of the skin at regular intervals to make histological and histochemical studies. The size of the sebaceous gland was determined by measuring the diameters with a micrometer and calculating the average. The size of the sebaceous gland was found to be largest during the early anagen stage when the hair follicle was starting to grow and the sebaceous gland cells were actively multiplying. There was no evidence of the sebaceous gland increasing in size during the telogen stage. Along with the fluctuation of enzyme activity, there was a cycle of increase and decrease of the sebaceous transformation in relation to the hair cycle. It has been confirmed that the size of the sebaceous gland of the hair follicle of rats is large during the anagen stage and small during the telogen stage. Morohashi (1968) comments that the sebaceous gland changes its function during the different stages of the hair cycle, but that human hair follicles each have different cycles (a mosaic pattern). He states that there are multiple hair follicles and hair groups to consider. The relation between the hair cycle and the function of the sebaceous gland is still not completely evident.

1.4 Connective Tissue Sheath

The connective tissue surrounding the cellular part of the hair follicle is called the connective tissue sheath (Fig. 1.3). This sheath extends from the level of the attachment of the sebaceous gland to the hair bulb, and capillaries are present between the connective tissue sheath and the follicular epithelium below the level of the sebaceous gland.

As described later (Chapter 5), using a fine nylon ligature, above the secretory duct opening of the sebaceous gland and the infundibular portion of hair follicles, the authors found that a microcirculatory system starting from the subpapillary blood plexus below the epidermal layer and surrounding the follicular appendix in the connective tissue sheath was present and that this vascular system was of prime importance, with the principal blood supply coming from the subpapillary blood vessels to form the microcirculation around the pilosebaceous unit.

According to this finding, the connective tissue sheath is related to hair regrowth in single-hair transplantation. If this sheath is not damaged, the transplanted hair regrows soon after transplantation (Section 29.5.4).

According to Urabe et al. (1992), ultrastructurally the connective tissue sheath comprises three layers: (1) the inner collagen layer, composed of collagen fibers running parallel to the hair long axis; the inner layer of this sheath is the vitreous membrane, which is a distinctive basal lamina; (2) the middle collagen layer, composed of transverse collagen fibers and intermingled fibroblasts; and (3) the outer collagen layer, composed of collagen fibers, running in various directions, and cellular constituents such as fibroblasts, blood vessels, and fat cells (Hashimoto 1981; Ito and Sato 1990).

Immunohistochemically, various antibodies have been used to identify the epithelial components of hair follicles, but specific markers for the connective tissue sheath (CTS) have not been found.

Alpha-smooth muscle (α-SM) actin is a differentiation marker of smooth muscle cells and is present in all smooth muscle cells and pericytes (Skalli et al. 1989).

According to Urabe et al. (1992), immunohistochemical and immunoelectron microscopy studies revealed the presence of α-SM actin in fibroblasts located in the CTS of human anagen hair follicles. Immunostaining was positive from the base of the bulb to the upper part of the lower portion of the mature anagen hair follicles. The late catagen hair follicles were not stained. Ultrastructurally, α-SM actin was detected only in the fibroblasts located in the innermost layer of the transverse collagenous fibers. Since α-SM actin is located in cells with contractile potential, it is conceivable that this newly identified layer may play an important role in the morphological changes occurring in the lower portion of the hair follicle during the hair growth cycle.

1.5 Dermal Papilla

Hair follicle buds are induced during embryogenesis from epidermal cells by underlying mesenchyme that becomes encased in the base of the mature follicle as the dermal papilla (Sengel 1976).

Classic heterotopic recombination experiments have demonstrated that dermis from hair-bearing regions can induce follicle formation in glabrous epidermis (Kollar 1966, 1970; Sengel 1976, 1984).

The connective tissue contained within the hair bulb is the dermal papilla. The development and function of the epithelial part of the anagen follicle (epithelial bulb) are critically dependent on interactions with the dermal papilla (Oliver 1967a,b; Pinkus 1978; Jahoda and Oliver 1984; Oliver and Jahoda 1988; Link et al. 1990). The size of the papilla and surrounding bulb are directly related to the size of the hair produced (Durward and Rundall 1958).

In anagen follicles, the dermal papilla is attached to a basal plate of connective tissue by a narrow stalk. In small follicles there may be no visible vasculature, while terminal hair follicles show variable numbers of papillary blood vessels.

The dermal papilla contains relatively few specialized fibroblast cells surrounded by the extracellular matrix, which contains mucopolysaccharides (Montagna et al. 1952a) and interstitial collagen (Couchman et al. 1990; Messenger et al. 1991), all of which is separated from the epithelial part of the follicle by a trilaminar basement membrane. It appears that these cells may regulate the hair follicle by secreting growth factors and/or extracellular matrix components, in view of the constant size ratio of the dermal papilla and the hair follicle (Van Scott and Ekel 1958; Ibrahim and Wright 1982) and in view of differentiation in other tissue (Bernfield et al. 1984; Li et al. 1987). Even in the telogen phase, appreciable cytoplasmic volume is still evident (Fig. 1.8).

At the beginning of anagen, papillary cells show a marked increase in RNA content (Roth 1965). There is a close relationship between the cytological activity of dermal papillary cells and hair bulb matrix cells (Straile 1965); this relationship controls the epidermal matrix and, thus, the physical characteristics of the hair produced (Van Scott and Ekel 1958; Van Scott et al. 1963). The dermal papilla may determine the cyclical rhythm of the follicle (Cohen 1965; Sengel 1976).

Dermal papilla cells are considered to play a fundamental role in the induction and maintenance of hair growth (Geary 1952; Chase 1955; Cohen 1961; Oliver 1967b; Sengel 1976; Jahoda and

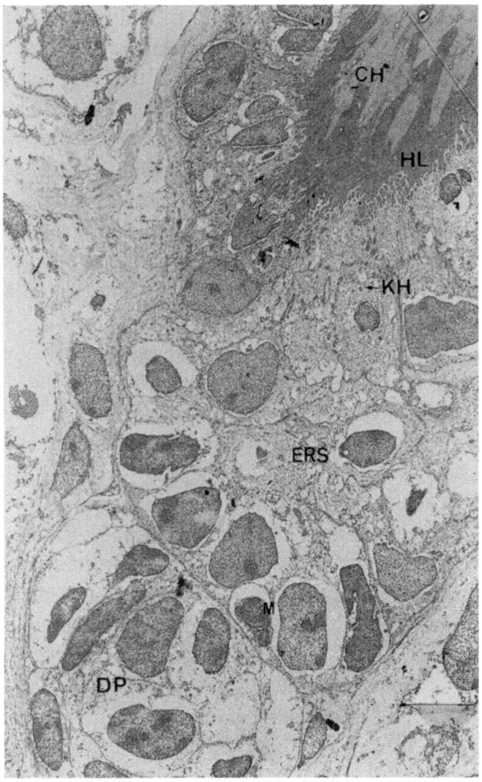

Fig. 1.8. In the telogen phase appreciable cytoplasmic volume in the dermal papilla is still evident. *KH*, Keratohyaline granules; *CH*, club hair; *ERS*, external root sheath (epithelial column); *DP*, dermal papilla; *HL*, horny layer; *M*, melanocyte. ×11700

Oliver 1981; Jahoda et al. 1984; Pisansarakit and Moore 1986). Cohen (1961), who devised microdissection techniques for operating on vibrissa follicles in the rat, transplanted various root components to various ectopic sites.

A specific role of the dermal papilla in the maintenance of hair growth has been demonstrated (Oliver and Jahoda 1981; Butcher 1982; Jahoda and Oliver 1990).

However, studies of the effects on whisker growth of follicles whose various components were removed in situ have shown that, after removal of the dermal papilla alone, and after removal of as much as the lower third of the follicle, regeneration of new dermal papillae and whiskers may occur from the dermal sheath (Oliver 1966a). Follicle wall implants consisting of the inner root sheath, outer root sheath, and mesenchymal layer, dissected from the lower third of the follicle and transplanted to ear skin, produced short whiskers. However, none of the implants obtained from above the lower third of the follicle regenerated dermal papillae or produced whiskers (Oliver 1967a). Other transplantation experiments have shown that freshly dissected papillae can induce hair growth when implanted into vibrissa follicles (Oliver 1967b; Ibrahim and Wright 1977) and can induce the development of new hair follicles when associated with glabrous ear and/or scrotal sac epidermis implanted under ear skin (Oliver 1970).

Rat vibrissa dermal papillae induced the formation of follicles when they were transplanted between the epidermis and dermis of isolated patches of embryonic mouse skin later grafted onto nude mice (Pisansarakit and Moore 1986).

Papilla cells are also believed to direct the reentry of the resting follicle into the active (anagen) growth phase (Cotsarelis et al. 1990; Lavker et al. 1991). Cotsarelis et al. suggested that follicular stem cells reside in the bulge region; thus, they provided new insights into how the hair cycle may be regulated. During late telogen or early anagen, the normally slow cycling stem cells of the bulge area are activated by dermal papilla cells (which Cotsarelis and his colleagues call the bulge activation hypothesis; see Section 14.1.3). However, we reported (Inaba and Inaba 1992a) that a new hair germ begins to regenerate from the sebaceous isthmus, that is, from the upper isthmal portion close to the duct opening of the sebaceous gland (essential hair cycle) as well as from the remaining lower follicle (common hair cycle) (see Section 13.2; for more detail, see stem cell, Section 14.1.2).

Weinberg et al. (1993) reported as follows: All epidermal populations studied, including the total epidermal keratinocyte preparation from trypsin-split skin, developing hair follicle buds isolated from epidermis, and preformed hair follicles isolated from dermis, formed haired skin when grafted with fresh dermal cells. Only preformed hair follicles produced haired skin on grafts without an additional dermal component. Hair follicle buds grafted alone or with cultured dermal cells reconstituted skin, but without appendage formation. In 1984, Jahoda and Oliver succeeded in culturing dermal papillae isolated from the vibrissa follicle of rats, and they were the first to report the morphology and dynamics of the cultured cells.

Subsequently, it was demonstrated that cultured dermal papilla cells of adult rats induced hair growth in situ when associated with the amputated base of follicles whose lower half had been removed (Jahoda and Oliver 1984; Jahoda et al. 1984; Horne et al. 1986). Furthermore, cultured papilla cells were shown to induce follicle formation in the non-hair-bearing rodent foot pad (Reynolds and Jahoda 1991a).

Katsuoka et al. (1986) and Messenger et al. (1986) cultured dermal papillae isolated from the anagen follicles of hair bulbs of human scalp, and reported their biological characteristics. These cells were found to be morphologically and functionally differentiated from reticular dermal fibroblasts.

1.5.1 Mesenchymal-Epithelial Tissue Interaction

There have been numerous studies of mesenchymal-epithelial tissue interaction. Experimental biology and embryology have contributed much to our knowledge of the ectodermal-mesenchymal relationship in hair growth. In epithelial-mesenchymal interaction, the mesenchymal tissue seems to have the role of regulating epithelial growth and conditioning the display of the differentiating capacity of the hair follicle.

The dermal papilla is the permanent inductive growth element in feathers (Lille and Wang 1941); however, this inductive element is not specific in its effects, since regional skin specificity depends on the overlying epidermis (Lille and Wang 1994; Cohen 1969). Studies of the vibrissae and hair follicles of rodents have shown the same thing (Oliver 1966a, 1967a,b, 1969). There is a need to maintain a certain spatial relationship between the mesenchymal and the epithelial structures of hair follicles. The mesenchyme-derived dermal papilla is thought to be important in regulating the growth of hair follicle epithelium (Oliver and Jahoda 1981; Reynolds and Jahoda 1991a).

Wolback (1951) applied the cancer inducers 3,4-benzpyrene and methylcholanthrene on the mouse body surface, and found that as long as the dermal papilla was maintained in a healthy condition, hair growth continued, but once the dermal papilla was destroyed, hair growth stopped. He suggested that this finding indicated that the dermal papilla is a key factor in controlling the hair follicle.

Since the amount of mitotic activity in the ectodermal matrix is proportional to the size of the dermal papilla (Van Scott and Ekel 1958), enlargement of the dermal papilla controls the increase in the growth rate of the epithelium cells above it (Van Scott et al. 1963). Van Scott et al. (1963) also reported that the replacement time of the entire germinative matrix was calculated to be approximately 23 h.

According to Moretti (1965), various developmental, embryological, and anatomical studies have indicated the simultaneous involvement during hair growth and differentiation of both ectodermally and mesodermally derived skin structures. Furthermore, important biochemical changes occur in the mesenchymal structures surrounding the hair during hair growth cycles. Briggaman and Wheeler (1968) cultured human skin after separating it into epidermis and dermis. While the culture of the epidermis degenerated rapidly, culture of the epidermis and dermis recombined showed the characteristics of epidermal structure, this finding indicating that the presence of the dermal layer is essential for maintaining the activity and epidermal structure of the epidermal cell. Autoradiographic localization of 3-testosterone has shown that in the rat dermal papilla, but not in the hair follicle, the epithelium takes up androgens, suggesting that androgens act on hair follicles via the dermal papillae (Stumpf and Sar 1976) .

According to Itami's recent report (1993), the correlation of (epithelial-mesenchymal) interaction between the hair matrix cell (epithelial cell) and the dermal papilla cell (mesenchymal cell) is significant.

The human epithelial follicle vigorously metabolizes the male hormone. But since it metabolizes the male hormone into Δ^4-androstenedione, which is weaker than activated dihydrotestosterone (DHT), the epithelial follicle is not qualified to be the target tissue of male hormone.

To the contrary, the cultured beard dermal papilla cell exhibits several times as high a level of 5α-reductase activity as does the occipital dermal papilla cell. In hair tissue, the anagen target tissue is the dermal papilla, and it may be presumed that the epithelial tissue proliferates due to some factors produced by the dermal papilla.

The above findings substantiate our sebaceous gland hypothesis regarding hormonal influence, i.e., it is important that testosterone is converted to DHT and it influences the dermal papilla through the blood circulation around the hair follicle.

1.5.2 Development of Mesenchymal Cells

The initial appearance and development of the hair follicle is strictly linked to the morphogenesis of the skin in the embryo. The skin is an organ composed of the epidermis and dermis. In the morphogenesis of the hair follicle, both the epidermal and the dermal components play a fundamental role. The crowding of the nuclei in the epidermis seems to be the first event (Pinkus 1958; Serri and Huber 1963; Robins and Breathnach 1979). The subsequent development of the initiated follicles then occurs under the influence of the condensation of dermal cells associated with each of the growing follicular plugs (Davidson and Hardy 1952; Kollar 1970; Sengel 1976). Dhouailly (1977) established that the types of follicles initiated in embryonic skin grafts and their distribution pattern were governed by the regional origin of the dermis. According to Pisansarakit and Moore (1986) the initiation and development of

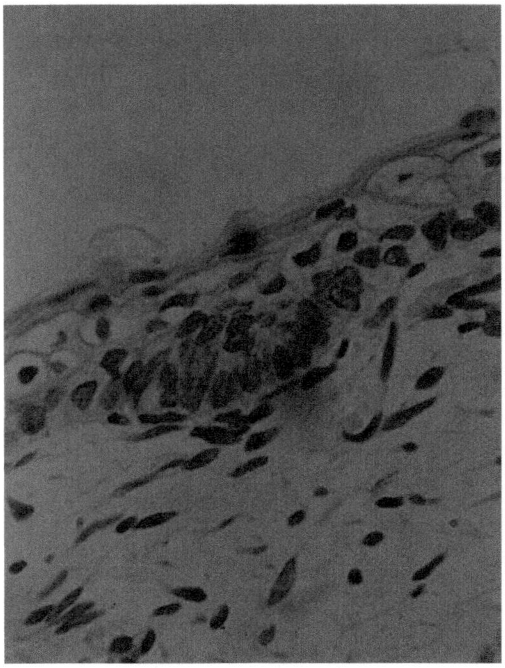

Fig. 1.9. Crowding of nuclei in the epidermis. Primary hair germ is not necessarily accompanied by mesenchymal cells. ×800

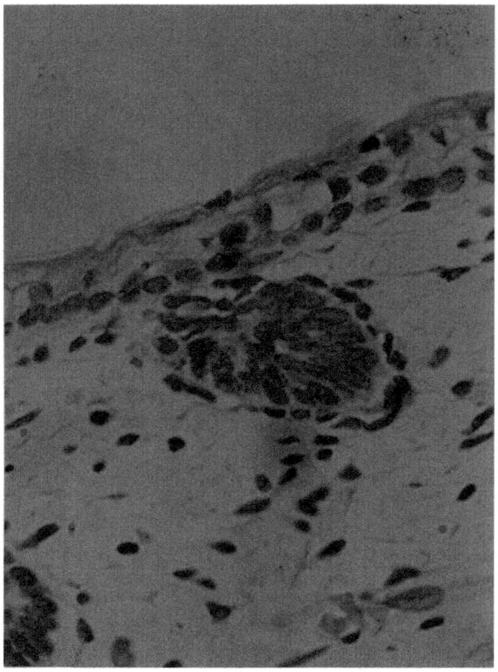

Fig. 1.10. A few mesenchymal cells surround the primary hair germ. No aggregation of mesenchymal cells can be observed in the lower portion of the hair bud. Compare with Fig. 3.2. ×800

hair follicles occur as a consequence of interactions between the epidermis and dermis during fetal life. It may be presumed that the mesenchymal tissue induces the formation of epithelium.

The question of whether epidermal or dermal modification appears first has thus been the subject of discussion in regard to the histogenesis of human hair (Kobayashi 1987). The authors have researched epithelial-mesenchymal tissue interaction related to the generation and regeneration of hair and also to regeneration from the bundle telogen hair follicle (Inaba and Inaba 1994b).

1.5.2.1 Hair Generation

In the generation of human hair (Chapter 3), the crowding of the nuclei (primary hair germ) is not necessarily accompanied by mesenchymal cells, when as observed in thick tissue specimen preparations (Fig. 1.9). As the germ cells within the epidermis become enlarged, a few mesenchymal cells accumulate around the hair germ (Fig. 1.10), afterwards accumulating below the hair germ (Fig. 3.2).

1.5.2.2 Hair Regeneration

The common hair cycle is divided into three stages, namely, anagen, catagen, and telogen (Section 7.1). The dermal papilla atrophies to a point located close to the telogen follicle (remnant dermal papilla). In the regeneration of the hair follicle, the hair bud is formed from the secondary hair germ located at the lower tip of the follicle in the telogen stage. At a certain angle, the bud descends downward to form the hair bulb.

After developing the subcutaneous shaving method for the radical treatment of bromidrosis, the authors proposed a new hypothesis, namely, that the location of the central portion of hair regeneration lies at the sebaceous isthmus, that is, the upper isthmal portion close to the duct opening of the sebaceous gland (stem cell) (Figs. 7.1b, 14.4). Figure 1.11 also shows the epithelial bud regenerating from the duct opening of the sebaceous gland, but no mesenchymal cells (dermal papilla) are observed below the epithelial bud (Fig. 1.11, left panel).

Mesenchymal cells develop afterwards (Fig. 1.11, right panel). The same finding can be seen in Fig. 12.1a.

1.5.2.3 Regeneration of Bundle Telogen Hairs

In the bundle hair regeneration that occurs after the use of anti-cancer agents (Figs. 1.12, 1.13, and Section 12.3), the authors consider that, at first, a single mass of mesenchymal cells is newly formed

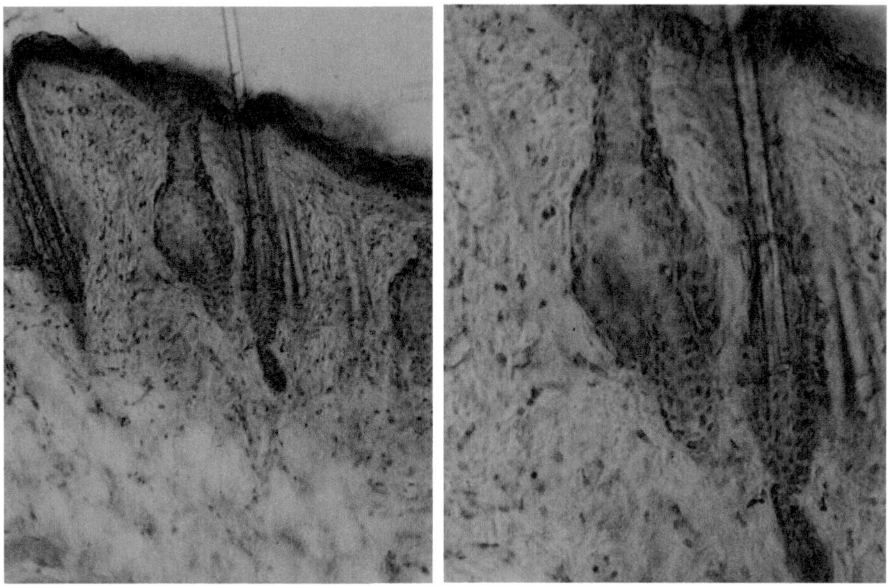

a b

Fig. 1.11. **a** Epithelial-mesenchymal interaction. An epithelial bud regenerates from the upper isthmal portion close to the duct opening of the sebaceous gland (sebaceous isthmus) on the *left side*. Mesenchymal cells are not seen in the lower portion of the hair bud. In the right telogen follicle, an epithelial bud regenerates from the same portion and mesenchymal cells accumulate below the epithelial bud. ×75 **b** High-power view of **a**. ×135

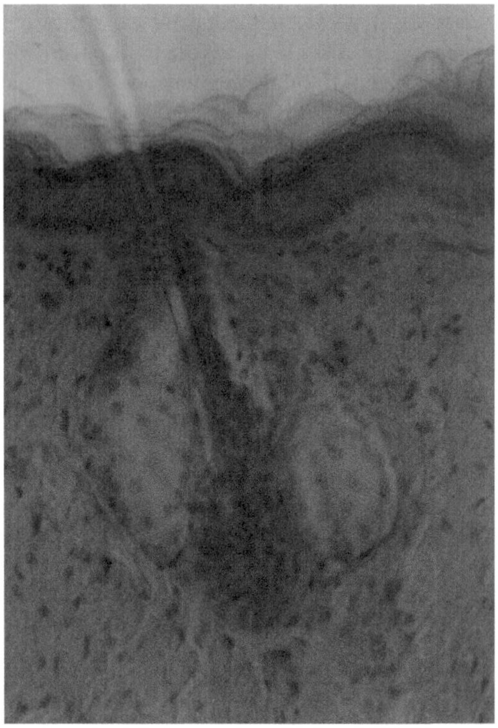

Fig. 1.12. New epithelial cells regenerate from the upper isthmal portion close to the duct opening of the sebaceous gland (sebaceous isthmus) in the bundle hair, but no mass of mesenchymal cells is observed below the new epithelial bud. ×440

in the lower end of the bundle (compound) hair follicles, above which the epithelial cell layer then migrates from the upper isthmal portion (Fig. 12.5). However, in the right side of the compound hair follicles (Fig. 1.13), epithelial cell buds regenerate from the upper isthmal portion close to the duct opening of the sebaceous gland, (sebaceous isthmus) and no mesenchymal cells can be seen below the epithelial sac. A mass of mesenchymal cells develops afterwards (Fig. 1.13a, left).

1.5.2.4 Summary

The above findings indicate that the mesenchymal cells are not a requirement in the generation and regeneration of the hair follicle, but that a new hair germ (epithelial tissue) is generated from the crowding of nuclei in the epidermis or the upper isthmal portion close to the duct opening of the sebaceous gland, as proposed by the authors in their sebaceous gland hypothesis (see Chapter 13). Mesenchymal cells are generated in a later period. The subsequent development of the initiated follicles occurs under the influence of the mesenchymal cells (dermal papilla) associated with each of the growing hair follicles.

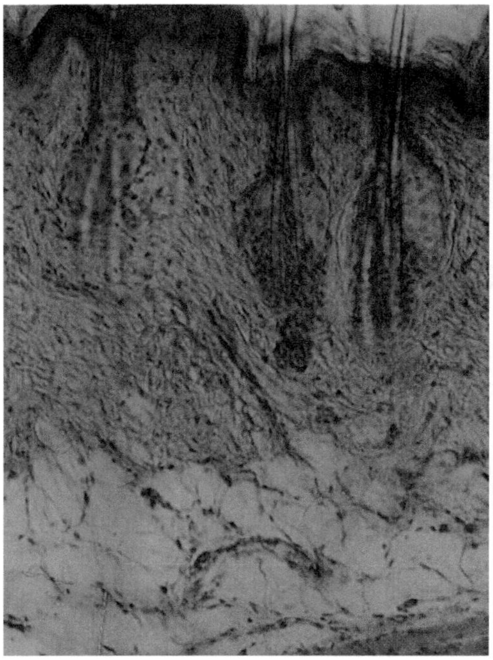

a

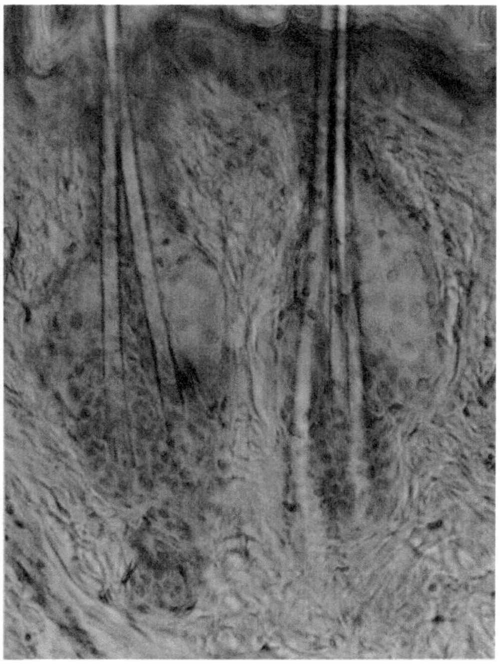

b

Fig. 1.13. **a** On the *left side* of the bundle hair follicles, the epithelial bud cannot be seen. On the *right side* of the bundle hair follicles, the epithelial bud is formed from the sebaceous isthmus, but no mesenchymal cells can be seen below the epithelial bud. ×75 **b** High-power view of **a.** An epithelial bud can be seen, on the *right side* of the bundle hair follicle, but no mesenchymal cells can be observed below the epithelial bud. A single mass of mesenchymal cells has newly formed at the lower end of the bundle hair follicle (*left side*). ×250

1.6 Regional Anatomy of the Scalp

1.6.1 Facial Segments

Normally, the face is divided into three equal segments: hairline to glabella, glabella to columella-labial angle, and columella-labial angle to the skin (Fig. 1.14a,b). In the younger person who has not yet developed temporal recessions, an inverted V or triangular pattern has not yet clearly formed. This frontotemporal triangle is formed by the simultaneous recession of the temporal hairline posteriorly and the frontal hairline superiorly. The hairline of the maturing male recedes uniformly more and more in an inverted V or triangular pattern (Fig. 1.14a).

Hamilton (1951a) studied the pattern of scalp hair generation in Caucasian subjects, ranging from fetuses to subjects in their nineties, reporting on the critical line of alopecia androgenetica. He assumed the presence of a coronal line, connecting both earholes and running over the vertex; recession of the apex 3 cm frontward from this line was regarded as Type IV in his classification of male pattern baldness (Fig. 1.15).

Later, O'tar Norwood (1975) revised Hamilton's findings and suggested that the critical line was 2 cm frontward from the coronal line; this is Type III of Hamilton's classification.

When creating a hairline by the punch or flap method in the treatment of male pattern baldness, the selected hairline should never be so low as to draw attention, but should rather be so natural that it draws no special attention. The hairline may be placed higher than the superior line (line a in Fig. 1.14a) in order to conserve grafts for use more posteriorly, but should never be placed lower than the lower point hairline (Fig. 1.14b). The hairline runs horizontally across the forehead. However, when looked at from above, it forms a crescent shape conforming to the shape of the skull. The lateral point of the reconstructed hairline falls on a line drawn vertically from the outer canthus of the eye (Fig. 1.14a).

The donor region 7.0–8.5 cm from retroauricle is likely to start bleeding due to the presence of the occipital artery (see Section 29.6).

1.6.2 The Layers of the Scalp

The scalp consists of five layers (Fig. 1.16):

1. The skin (epidermis and dermis) is up to 7 mm thick in the occipital area.

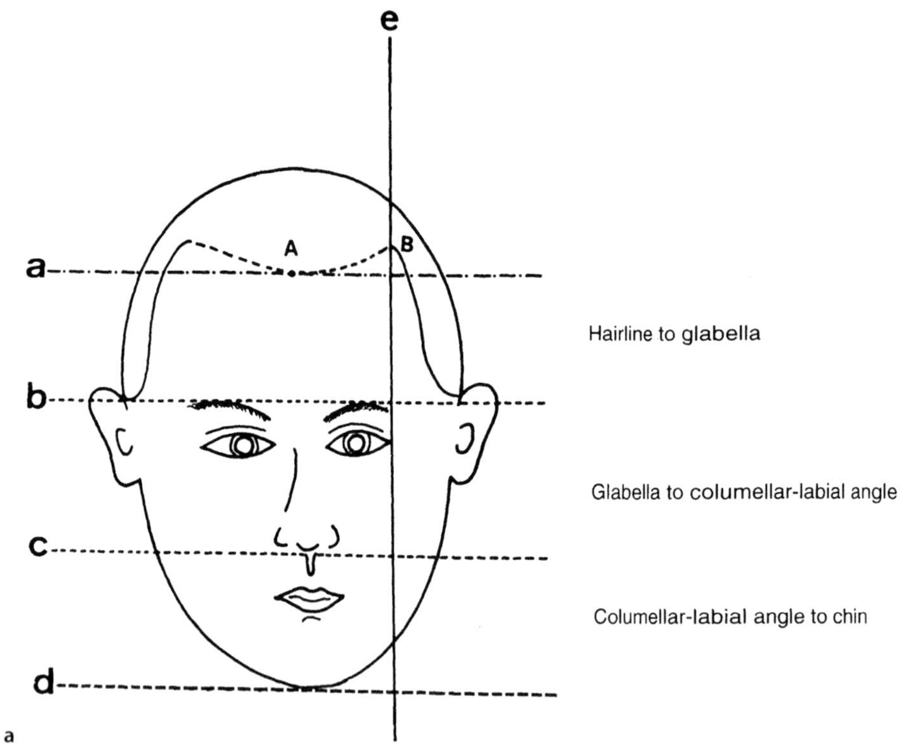

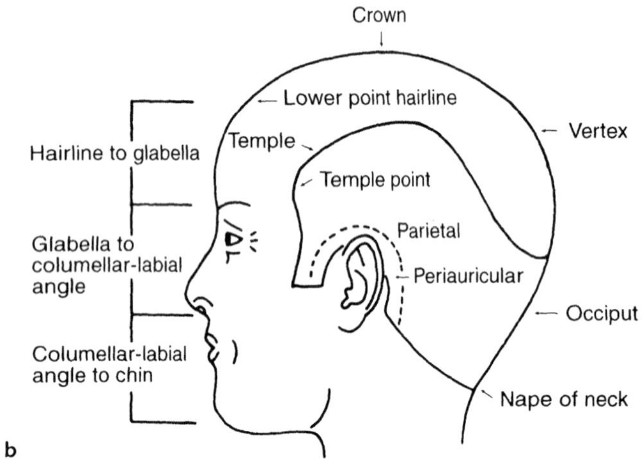

Fig. 1.14. **a** The face (front view) is divided into three equal segments by the horizontal lines *a–d*: hairline to glabella, glabella to columellar-labial angle, and columellar-labial angle to chin. The reconstructed hairline falls on line *e*, drawn vertically from the outer canthus of the eye. The figure demonstrates the importance of placement of the transplanted hairline on the bald scalp. The hairline-to-glabella segment (from *A*) is equal to the glabella-to-columellar-labial angle. The reconstructed lateral hair line (*B*) falls on the line *e* drawn vertically from the outer canthus of the eye. **b** Lateral view of the scalp showing important anatomical sites. **a**, Modified from Unger and Marritt (1988), with permission from Marcel Dekker Inc.; **b**, modified from Norwood and Schiell (1984)

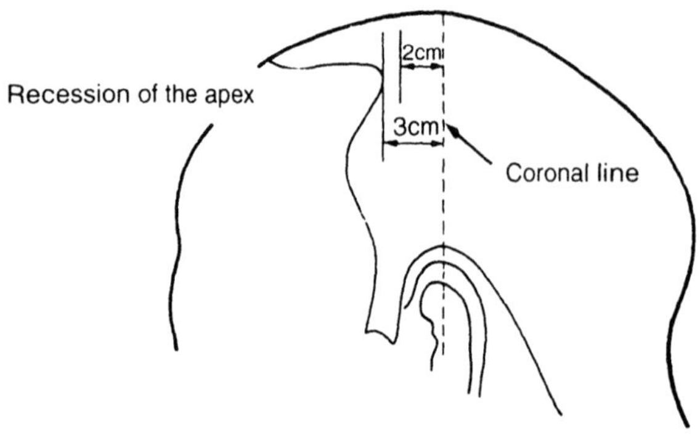

Fig. 1.15. Critical line of alopecia androgenetica (Takashima 1987). Hamilton (1951a) reported this critical line to be 3 cm in front of the coronal line. Norwood (1975) reported the line to be 2 cm in front of the coronal line (modified from Takashima 1987, with permission from Bunkodo Shoten)

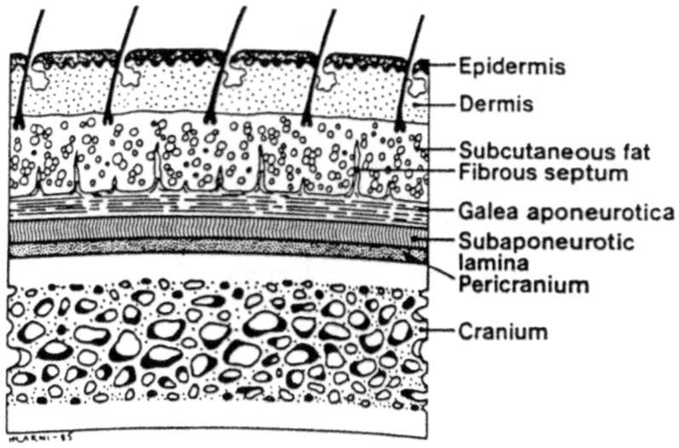

Fig. 1.16. The layers of the scalp (from Nordström 1988a, with permission from Marcel Dekker Inc.)

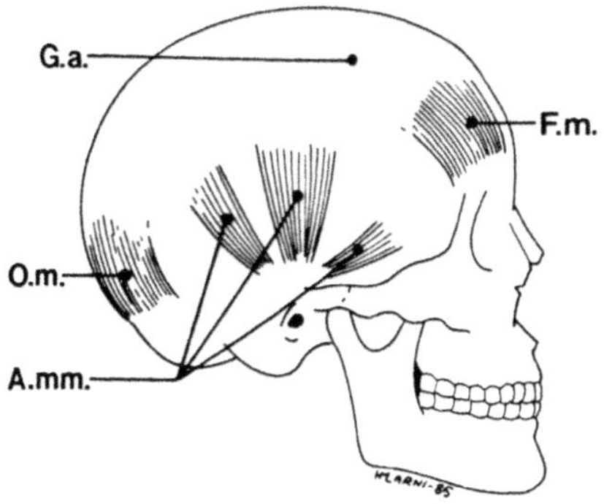

Fig. 1.17. Galea aponeurotica. *G.a.*, Galea aponeurotica; *F.m.*, frontal muscle; *O.m.*, occipital muscle; *A.mm.*, auricular muscles (from Nordström 1988a, with permission from Marcel Dekker Inc.)

2. The subcutaneous layer consists of fat and fibrous tissue firmly connecting the skin with the underlying galea aponeurotica or epicranium. This is the space where the main arteries, veins, and also the lymphatics and nerves travel.

3. The epicranium or galea aponeurotica is a very strong tendon-like structure between the frontal muscle in the forehead and the occipital muscle in the neck. Laterally, the temporoparietal and auricular muscles are in conjunction with the galea aponeurotica (Fig. 1.17).

The occipital muscle inserts into the superior nuchal line and the frontal muscle inserts into the skin in the region of the supraorbital ridge, with the fibers extending into the upper lids and into the subcutaneous tissue at the eyebrows and the nose.

4. The subepicranial layer is a connective tissue layer between the pericranium below and the epicranium above. It is in this very loose, thin, and almost avascular layer that scalping injuries usually occur. Only a few emissary veins cross this layer. It is important to realize that these emissary veins connect the scalp veins with the intracranial venous system.

5. The pericranium is the periosteum of the skull bone and is the deepest layer of the scalp. It is attached to the skull but can accidentally be torn off, for example, during surgery of the scalp; however, it is regenerated if the skull bone is covered with vascular tissue (reviewed from Nordström 1988a).

1.6.3 Blood Circulation in the Scalp

Especially when designing flaps, but also in other surgery of the scalp, it is important to be familiar with the blood supply of the scalp (Fig. 1.18). Of the five arteries to each side of the scalp, three are branches of the external carotid artery. These arteries are (a) the superficial temporal artery with its two main branches, the frontal and the parietal; (b) the retroauricular artery, which is small; and (c) the occipital artery, which is almost as large as

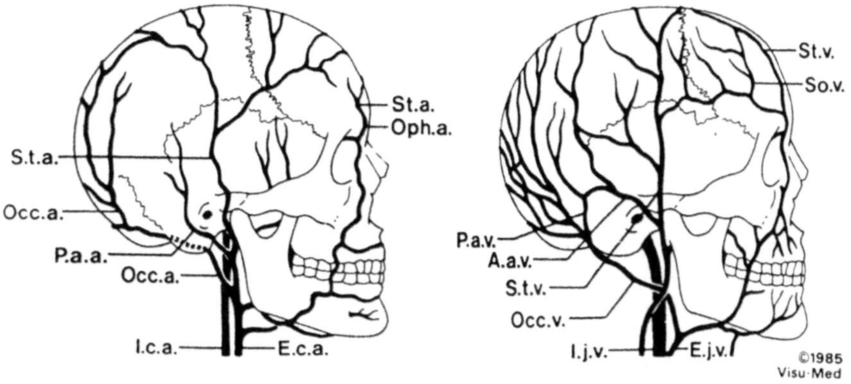

Fig. 1.18. The main arteries and veins to the scalp. *St.a., v.*, Supratrochlear artery and vein; *So.v.*, supraorbital v.; *S.t.a., v.*, superficial temporal artery and vein; *P.a.a., v.*, postauricular a. and v.; *Occ.a., v.*, occipital a. and v.; *E.c.a.*, external carotid a.; *A.a.,v.*, anterior auricular v.; *I.j.v.*, internal jugular v.; *E.j.v.*, external j.v.; *Oph.a*, ophthalmic artery; *I.c.a.*, internal carotid artery (from Nordström 1988a, with permission from Marcel Dekker Inc.)

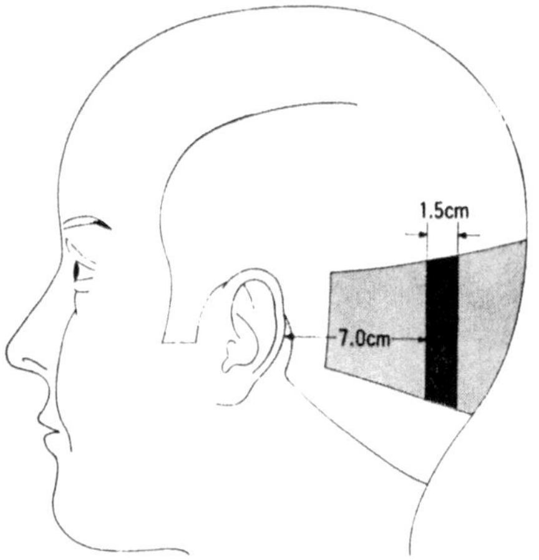

Fig. 1.19. Donor region. The region 7.0–8.5 cm from the retroauricle is likely to start bleeding due to the presence of the occipital artery (reproduced with permission from Ezaki 1990)

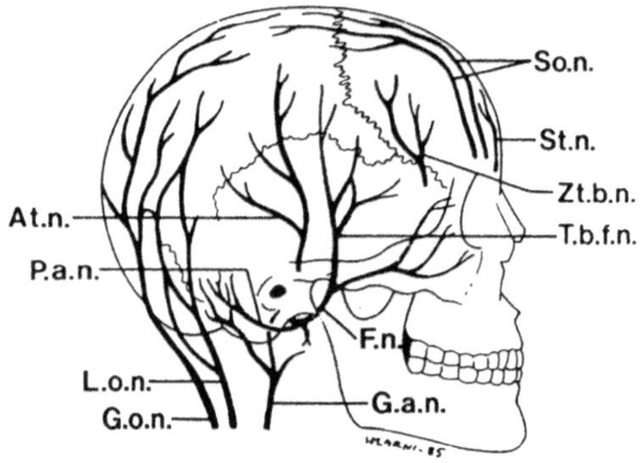

Fig. 1.20. The nerve supply of the scalp. *So.n.*, Supraorbital nerve; *St.n.*, supratrochlear n.; *Zt.b.n.*, zygomaticotemporal branch of the zygomatic n.; *At.n.*, auriculotemporal n.; *T.b.f.n.*, temporal branch of the facial n.; *G.a.n.*, great auricular n.; *L.o.n.*, lesser occipital n.; *G.o.n.*, greater occipital n.; *P.a.n.*, posterior auricular n (from Nordström 1988a, with permission from Marcel Dekker Inc.)

the superficial temporal artery. In the frontal area there are two arteries that arise from the internal carotid artery. These are the end branches of the ophthalmic artery, namely, (d) the supratrochlear and (e) the supraorbital arteries. There are no arteries entering the scalp through the skull bone; all main arteries travel just above the galea in the subcutaneous layer. The course of these main arteries is the reason that scalp flaps survive so well and often make delayed procedures unnecessary (axial pattern flaps).

Veins usually follow the arteries. Most veins drain into the jugular veins, but the emissary veins perforating the skull bone and those following the branches of the ophthalmic artery drain into intracranial veins and thus may carry infections inside the skull (although this seems to be extremely rare) (reviewed from Nordström 1988a).

The occipital artery is located in the region 7.0–8.5 cm from the retroauricular attachment in the hair-bearing temporal region; this may easily lead to bleeding during operation. Although the bleeding itself is not a major problem, it should preferably be avoided because it may disturb the operation procedure (Ezaki 1990) (Fig. 1.19).

1.6.4 Innervation of the Scalp

It is of practical value to know the sensory innervation of the scalp because many surgical procedures can be performed under local anesthesia with nerve blocks. The sensory innervation is directed such that a caudal block creates a field of anesthesia cranially (Fig. 1.20).

The lateral and medial branch of the supraorbital nerve and the supratrochlear nerve provide sensory innervation to the forehead and the frontal part of the scalp. These are branches of the frontal nerve, that is, the superior branch of the trigeminal nerve.

The zygomaticotemporal branch of the zygomatic nerve gives sensory innervation to the temporal region. It is a lateral branch of the maxillary nerve, which is the middle branch of the trigeminal nerve. The lateral part of the scalp just posterior to this receives its sensory innervation from the auriculotemporal nerve. This is a lateral branch of the mandibular nerve, which is the inferior branch of the trigeminal nerve.

The postauricular area is innervated by the great auricular nerve, which is a branch of the cervical plexus. The area just posterior to this is innervated by the lesser occipital nerve, which also branches from the cervical plexus.

The greater occipital nerve provides the sensory innervation to the occipital and posterior crown area of the scalp. It arises from the posterior ramus of the second cervical nerve. Sometimes the third occipital nerve also provides for a small portion of the sensory innervation close to the midline in a caudal occipital area.

The motor branch to the occipital muscle is the posterior auricular nerve, which is a branch of the facial nerve. The temporal branch of the facial nerve supplies the innervation to the frontalis muscle.

All these nerves travel in the scalp in the subcutaneous layer between the skin and the galea aponeurotica. These nerves are conveniently anesthesized with nerve blocks. The frontal region often needs somewhat more local anesthetic than the other areas.

Preparation of Thick Tissue Specimens 2

The standard thickness of a section of prepared tissue specimen embedded in paraffin blocks is 0.003–0.005 mm. In order to obtain a thick section of 0.1 mm, one would have to "stack" more than 200 of these sections. This is not only troublesome but rather impractical. The cell tissue is so thin that it curls up and shrinks when each section is sliced. In order to flatten and extend it, the section is placed horizontally in warm water, then laid on a glass surface for staining. However, the tissue structure itself is then affected and shifts position. Therefore, when these thin sections are put together to create a thick section, it is not possible to study the tissue in its original condition. True, very fine details can be observed with individual thin sections, but with such three-dimensional sections we could not observe the stages of the hair cycle as a whole.

It was obvious that some new method of preparing thick tissue specimens had to be worked out (Inaba et al. 1978d). We tried a number of possible variations. First, we froze the tissue and then sliced it. Since the slicing had to be done by ice-planing with compressed CO_2 gas, however, the tissue specimen broke apart when we tried to slice it thickly. Next, we tried a cryostat technique, to make preparations 0.04–0.05 mm in thickness. But in this instance, even when we sliced the tissue at a temperature of −70°C, which required an extremely expensive microtome, the desired thickness could not be obtained. The third effort involved the use of celloidin, in which the tissue was permeated and then cut thickly. However, it took 2-3 months for the celluloid substance to fully permeate the tissue. Although the specimen was then easy to slice, the details were unclear, because, over this long period, the tissue had solidified with the celluloid and staining was inadequate. Each of these methods had its respective advantages and drawbacks, and we eventually came back full circle to the paraffin block, once again attempting thick slicing. When we did this forcefully, the tissue specimen, as usual, curled or broke into fragments somewhat like the surface of a delicate wood board subjected to rough planing.

2.1 Development of Cellotape Method

We then thought of cellotaping the specimen before slicing. Cellotape was attached to a paraffin-embedded specimen (Fig. 2.1a); with this innovation, the tissue sliced well at 0.2- to 0.3-mm thicknesses (Fig. 2.1b). The thick-section specimen was pressed onto a glass slide by spreading a thin layer of egg albumin-glycerin on the center of the slide to prevent the specimen from peeling off (Fig. 2.2); then, with the cellotape uppermost, it was firmly pressed with the palm onto the slide. Removal of the cellotape without disfiguring the specimen was made simple by using xylene to remove both cellotape and paraffin at the same time (Fig. 2.3).

However, because of the thickness of the specimen, the paraffin remained in the tissue, and staining was still incomplete and left details unclear. To solve that problem, we decided to try immersing the specimen with xylene in warm water, but not by heating, since xylene is flammable. We found that after the cellotape was removed the paraffin could be eluted from the tissue in a xylene-water solution heated at 50°C–60°C. Then, to ensure that paraffin removal was complete, the specimen was placed in fresh xylene for about 60 min. When we stained the tissue at that time with a double-dilution staining solution, the specimen details were quite clear. Putting together four or five of these thick tissue specimens in serial

a
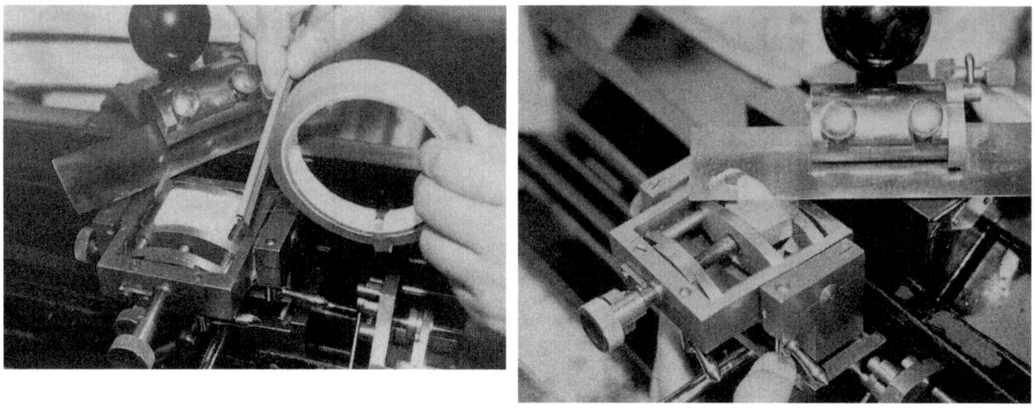
b

Fig. 2.1. **a** Preparation of thick tissue specimens using cellotape. Cellotape is attached to a paraffin-embedded specimen. **b** This specimen is then cut to the required thickness (100–200μm) with a microtome

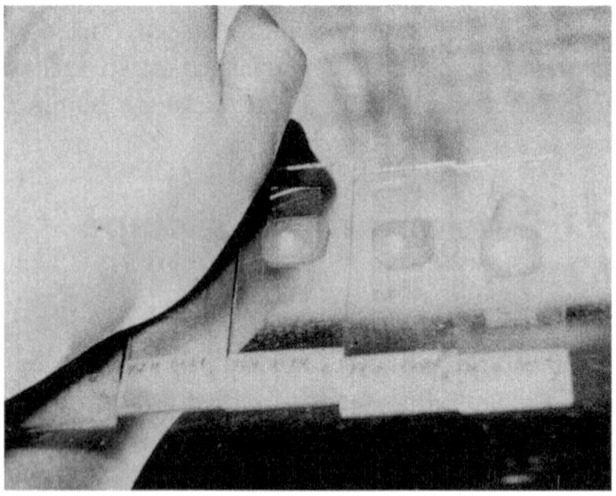

Fig. 2.2. The thick-section specimen is pressed onto a glass slide

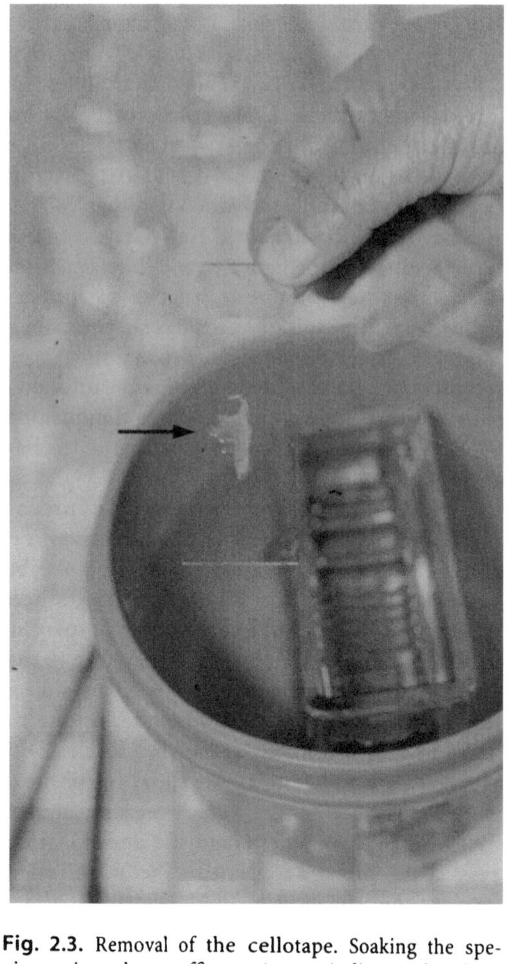

Fig. 2.3. Removal of the cellotape. Soaking the specimen in xylene suffices. *Arrow* indicates the thick specimen

form, we could readily make the three-dimensional observations we wanted (Fig. 2.4). The development of this thick tissue preparation method made it possible to observe the actual process of hair regeneration, as well as the relationship between sweat glands, hair follicles, and sebaceous glands in three-dimensional clarity (Inaba et al. 1979a).

2.2 Development of Cellophane Sheet Method

This method was developed by the basic laboratory at Medical Hair Research Co. (Tokyo, Japan). We discovered that cellotape was not always needed to prepare thick tissue sections from a paraffin-embedded specimen. The authors have re-

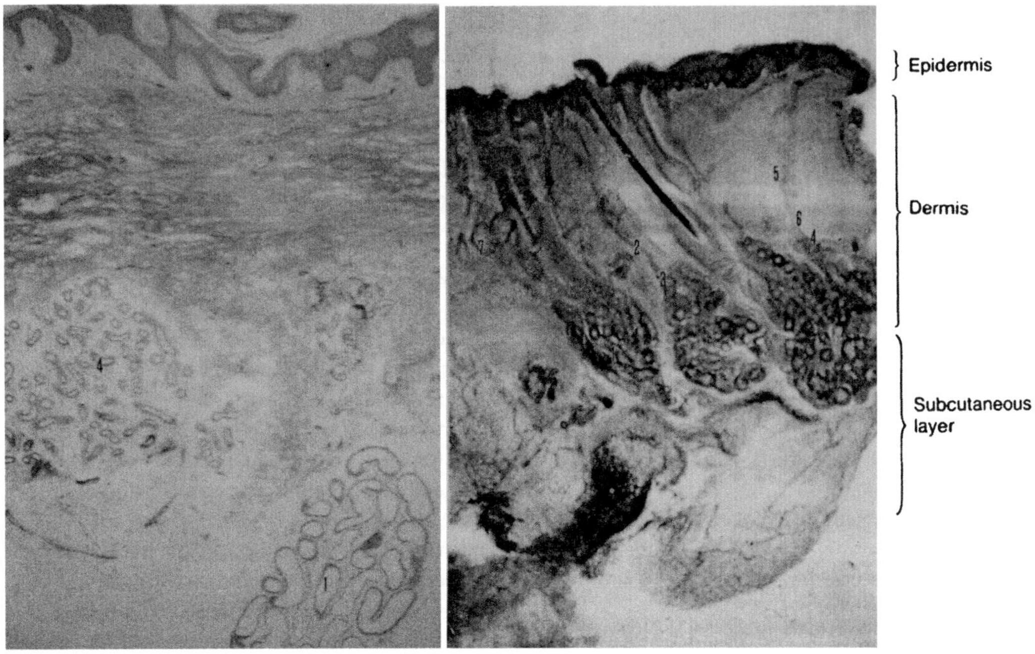

a b

Fig. 2.4a,b. Comparison of conventional and cellulose tape methods of thick tissue preparation. **a** Conventional thin tissue preparation (3- to 5-μm-thick). ×80 **b** Thick tissue preparation (150 μm). Three-dimensional observation is now possible. *1*, Apocrine gland; *2*, apocrine duct; *3*, apocrine coiled duct; *4*, eccrine gland; *5*, eccrine duct; *6*, eccrine coiled duct; *7*, sebaceous gland. ×60

cently developed a cellophane sheet method that is easy and economical (Yamada et al. 1992):

1. Because the paraffin used for embedding is more or less elastic, thick specimens can be sectioned neatly by simply placing a cellophane sheet over the block and pressing it lightly with the fingers (Fig. 2.5).

2. Next, the serial sections of the thick tissue specimen are set in a row (Fig. 2.6b).

3. Excessive paraffin is then removed from each section, leaving the tissue portion intact, i.e., excessive paraffin in the tissue portion is cut off by scissoring as much as possible (Fig. 2.6b).

4. The tissue portions are placed in a row at regular intervals on a glass slide on which egg al-

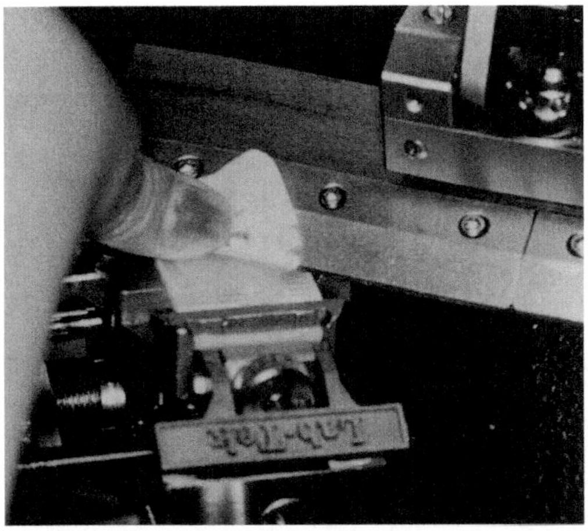

Fig. 2.5. Thick specimens can be sectioned neatly by simply placing a cellophane sheet over the block and pressing it slightly with the fingers

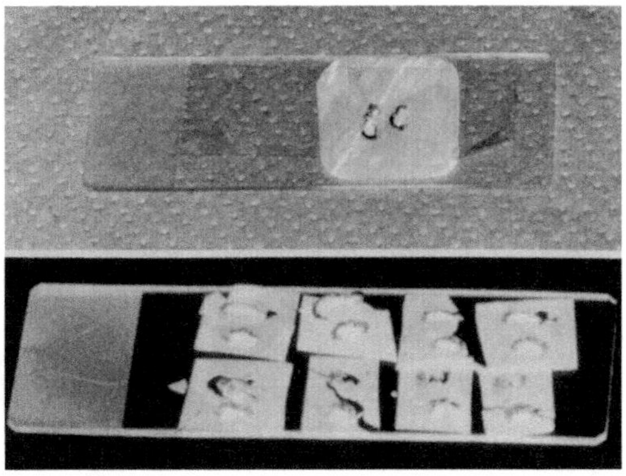

a b

Fig. 2.6. **a** Cellotape method. A paraffin-embedded specimen with cellotape is removed without excessive paraffin. **b** Cellophane sheet method. Serial sections are set in a row. Excessive paraffin is then removed from each section

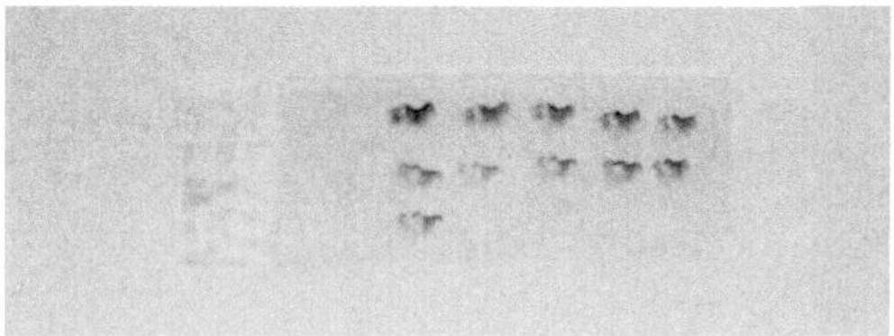

Fig. 2.7. The serial sections, in a row, are stained and enclosed using a double H&E dilution

bumin-glycerin has been spread. Although this depends on the size of the tissue portion, at least ten thick tissue specimens can be placed in two rows (Fig. 2.6b).

5. The specimens are placed over the paraffin-extending apparatus at 40°C for about 1 h to be dried. They are then placed in an incubator overnight at 45°C to be redried.
6. Next, they are placed in a dry heat sterilization apparatus at 60°C to melt the paraffin preliminarily.
7. Excess paraffin is removed with xylol.
8. The specimens are stained and enclosed using a double H&E dilution (Fig. 2.7).

2.3 Detailed Observations of Thick Tissue Specimens—Preparation of Microscopic and Electron Microscopic Specimens from Thick Tissue Specimen Using Cellophane Sheet

Tissue section studies can sometimes be hampered by sections which have initially been cut too thin so that major structural details are not clearly observable. Thick sections, however, can reveal such major details, so that thinner sections can then be cut at areas of particular interest. The cellophane tape and sheet methods of preparing thick tissue sections have enabled three-dimensional observation of such major histological structures. Once these have been closely observed and recorded, thin sections can then be cut with greater precision to study the particular structures in fine detail by electron microscope (Harada et al. 1984).

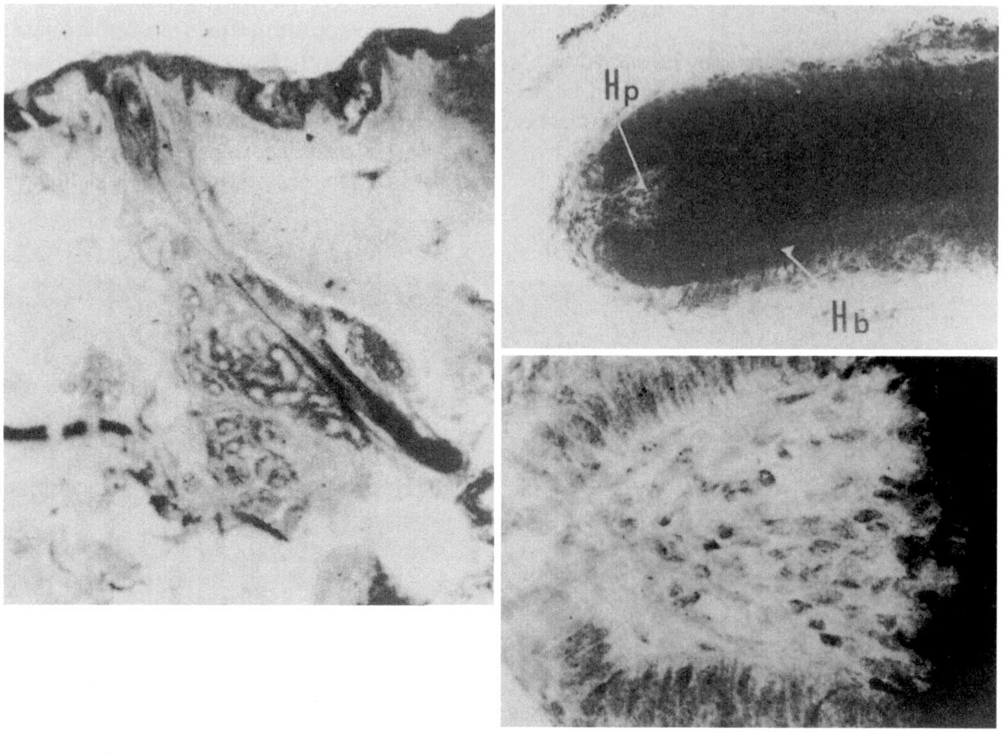

a b c

Fig. 2.8. **a** Thick tissue specimen, 200 μm. ×45 **b** Optical microscopic view of enlarged cross section of the lower hair follicle. *Hp*, Hair (dermal) papilla; *Hb*, hair bulb. ×135 **c** Higher power view of the hair bulb portion. ×1500

2.3.1 Preparation of Thin Tissue Specimen from Thick Tissue Specimen

(a) The glass slide with the tissue fragment affixed to it is first placed in melted soft paraffin, for paraffin infiltration into tissue, at 50°C for 24h, then it is placed in melted hard paraffin at 65°C for 24h. (b) The glass slide is then taken out of the vessel containing the hard paraffin and before it has completely solidified, the tissue is dissected parallel to the glass slide surface with a safety razor. (c) The specimen is then placed in a ceramic dish preheated at 60°C, into which melted hard paraffin is poured. Finally, it is left at room temperature to be cooled. An optical microscope is then used for observation and photography.

2.3.2 Preparation of Electron Microscopic Specimen

(a) The region desired in the thick specimen is confirmed and the glass slide is placed in a xylene solution. The cover glass is taken off to remove the undesired portion. Then the desired region is collected either by natural exfoliation of the tissue slice or by dissecting it with a safety razor. Care must be taken not to press or dry the tissue section. (b) The tissue section is soaked in descending series of ethanols, rinsed lightly with phosphate buffer, and refixed with osmium tetroxide solution. (c) Next, the tissue section is embedded in a resin mixture of epon and araldite, using a flap embedding plate. (d) Slicing is done with a Porter Blum MT-IIB model ultramicrotome (Sorvall, Norwalk, CT, U.S.A.) and the section is picked up on 150-mesh copper grids. (e) Double electron staining is performed with uranyl acetate followed by lead citrate. (f) A JEM-100CXII electron microscope (The Japan Co., Akishima, Tokyo) is used for observation and photography.

2.3.3 Thick Tissue Section Findings

Figure 2.8a shows a thick tissue specimen (200 μm) collected from the axillary skin. There is a three-dimensional view of the lower follicle, and the apocrine and eccrine sweat glands and the sebaceous gland appended to it. Because of this 200-

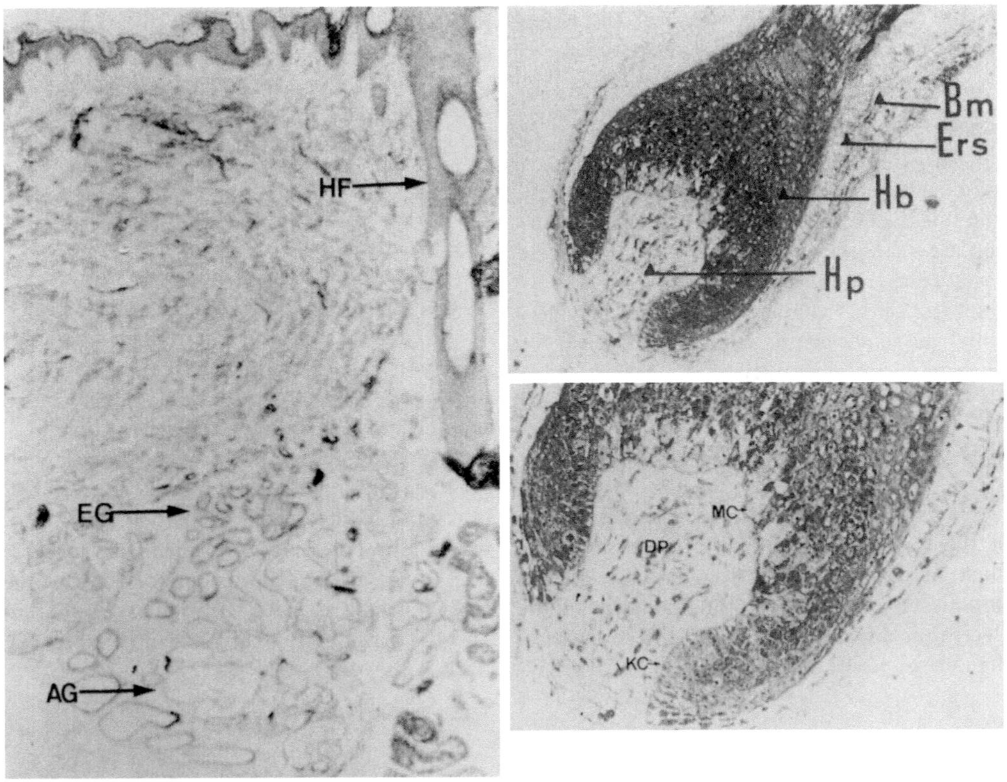

a b c

Fig. 2.9. a Thin tissue specimen produced from thick tissue specimen. *HF*, Hair follicle; *EG*, eccrine gland; *AG*, apocrine gland. ×135 **b** Cross-sectional view of hair bulb prepared for electron microscopic view. *Hp*, Hair (dermal) papilla; *Hb*, hair bulb; *Ers*, external root sheath; *Bm*, basement membrane. ×200 **c** Higher power view of hair bulb portion. *KC*, Keratinocyte; *DP*, dermal papilla; *MC*, melanocyte. ×1500

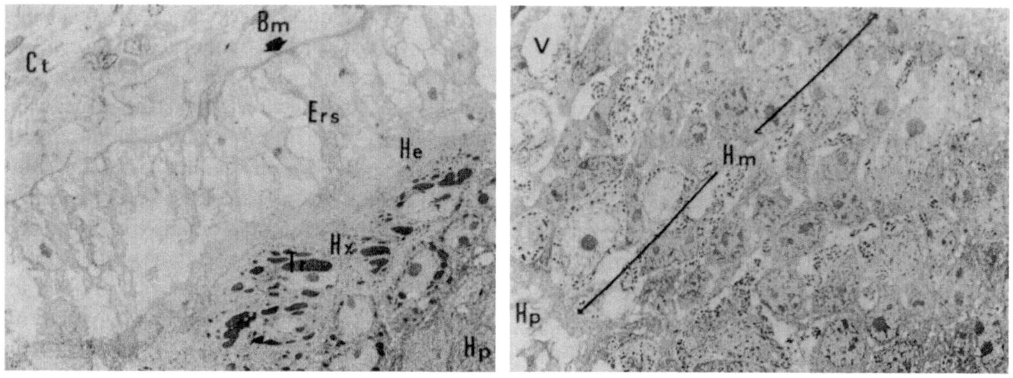

Fig. 2.10. **a** Electron microscopic view of the bulb portion. *Ct*, Connective tissue; *He*, Henle's layer; *Hx*, Huxley's layer; *Tr*, trichohyalin granule; *Bm*, basement membrane; *Ers*, external root sheath. ×7500 **b** Electron microscopic view of the bulb region of the hair matrix surrounding the dermal papilla. *Hm*, Hair matrix; *Hp*, hair papilla; *V*, vacuole. ×7500

μm thickness, a clear view can be obtained by focusing correctly according to its depth. However, when photographed, the picture may not be as clear as in the clinical observations. This specimen is suitable for making the determination of the desired regions.

Figure 2.8b shows an optical microscopic view of the enlarged cross section of only the lower follicle for a study of the hair bulb portion. Figure 2.8c shows a further enlarged view of the hair bulb portion. Tall epithelial cells (germinal cells) enveloping the dermal papilla can be observed.

2.3.4 Thin Tissue Section Findings

We observed the thin tissue specimen produced from the thick tissue specimen. The hair bulb portion was not visible, but the sweat glands were observed clearly on H&E staining (Fig. 2.9a). Figure 2.9b,c shows an optical microscopic cross-sectional view of the hair bulb prepared specially for electron microscopic study.

2.3.5 Electron Microscopic Findings

We carried out electron microscopic observations of the thin tissue specimen prepared from the thick tissue specimen. A toluidine blue-stained thin tissue specimen (1/1000) was used for the electron microscopic study (Fig. 2.9b,c). Nuclei of the dermal papilla cells were recognized. The layers of the outer root sheath, inner root sheath, and hair cortex were observed inwardly from the basal membrane in the hair bulb region.

Figure 2.10 shows the electron microscopic observations. Figure 2.10a shows the findings of the region inward from the connective tissue sheath to dermal papilla. Vacuoles of various sizes can be recognized in the outer root sheath cells. In the inner root sheath, Henle's layer and Huxley's layer containing trichohyalin granules can be observed. Figure 2.10b shows the electron microscopic view of the bulb region of the hair matrix surrounding that dermal papilla. In the middle portion, hair matrix cells and the dermal papilla can be recognized. Also, melanin granules can be clearly seen.

2.3.6 Advantages of Thick Specimen Preparation

As mentioned above, cytologic information can be obtained from the optical microscopic view of sections prepared from a thick tissue specimen much the same as from the conventional electron microscopic view. With this electron microscopic specimen preparation method using the cellophane sheet, satisfactory results can be expected for the obtaining of cytological information, although the formation of artifacts, to some extent (vacuoles etc.), is unavoidable. Comparative studies of other tissue portions, changes with the passage of time, and the use of other fixatives can be expected in the future.

Generation and Growth of Human Hair

3

Detailed observations of the generation of fetal eyebrow hair are the most effective means of studying the process by which the human hair follicle is first formed. To understand the process by which human hair is generated, it is important to review how the hair is generated in the fetus during gestation.

The observations made by Inaba et al. (1981a) and Inaba (1983b) of thick tissue specimens revealed the various stages in the development of original fetal eyebrow hair (Fig. 3.1).

3.1 Stages of Hair Growth

3.1.1 Early Hair Germ Stage

The first indication (primitive hair germ) that a hair follicle is about to form is an aggregation of cells at spaced intervals in the basal layer of the undifferentiated epidermis. The germ cells within the epidermis become noticeably swollen, or enlarged in the shape of a scallop shell, and are referred to collectively as the "primitive hair germ" (Fig. 3.2). This primitive hair germ forms at the end of the 2nd or the beginning of the 3rd month of gestation in the eyebrow region and on the upper lip and the chin. The factors determining the sites of individual hair formations are unknown.

The initiation and development of hair follicles is thought to occur as a consequence of interactions between the epidermis and dermis during fetal life. The question of whether epidermal or dermal modifications appear first has been the subject of discussion.

As the authors indicate, during mesenchymal cell development (see Section 1.5.2) the primitive hair germ, especially in the early fetal eyebrow region (16-week-old fetus), is not necessarily accompanied by mesenchymal cells. Only a few mesenchymal cells can be seen (Fig. 1.9). As the

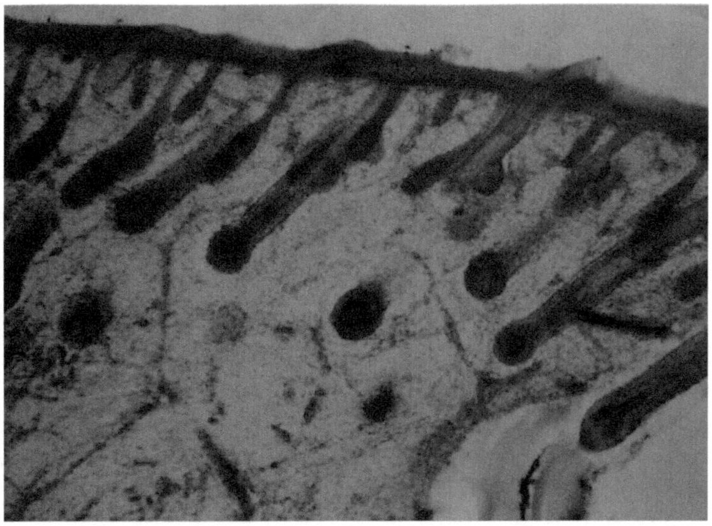
a

Fig. 3.1a,b. Various stages (*st*) in the development of original fetal eyebrow hair, examined in thick tissue specimens. ×100. Hair follicles can be seen in various stages of development. The explanation in the following figure legends is based mainly on this group of follicles

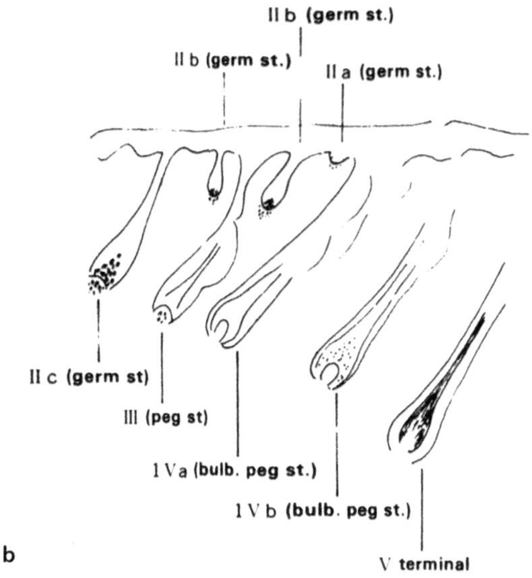

b

Fig. 3.1. *Continued*

germ cells within the epidermis become swollen, a few mesenchymal cells surround the primary hair germ (Fig. 1.10). Mesenchymal cells then gradually accumulate in the lower portion of the bulge (Fig. 3.2).

As shown in Fig. 3.1, germ cells grow gradually as a mass of mesodermal nuclei forms in the bottom of the epithelial sac. The mass of mesenchymal tissue in the bottom of the hair follicle is not yet clear (Fig. 3.3). The primordial sebaceous gland can be seen in the middle of the right side.

During the 4th month, primary hair germs begin to form over the general body surface. As the fetus grows, new primary germs form between the existing ones, and secondary germs develop in relation to the primary germs, so that the follicles are manifested in groups of three (Fig. 3.4).

According to Lyne, the skin forms hair follicles only during fetal life in many mammals. There is much evidence to show that hair follicles are not formed from normal intact epidermis once the adult complement has been established (Hardy and Lyne 1956a; Lyne 1959; Lyne and Heideman

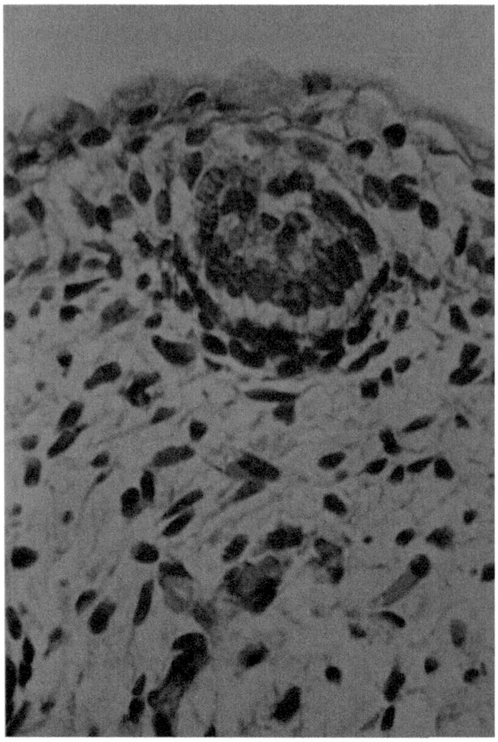

Fig. 3.2 Primitive hair germ. When the crowded basal cells and nuclei (small and darker stained) elongate perpendicularly from the epidermis, the hair germ begins to bulge conspicuously in the dermis. Mesenchymal cells gradually accumulate in the lower portion of the bulge. ×600

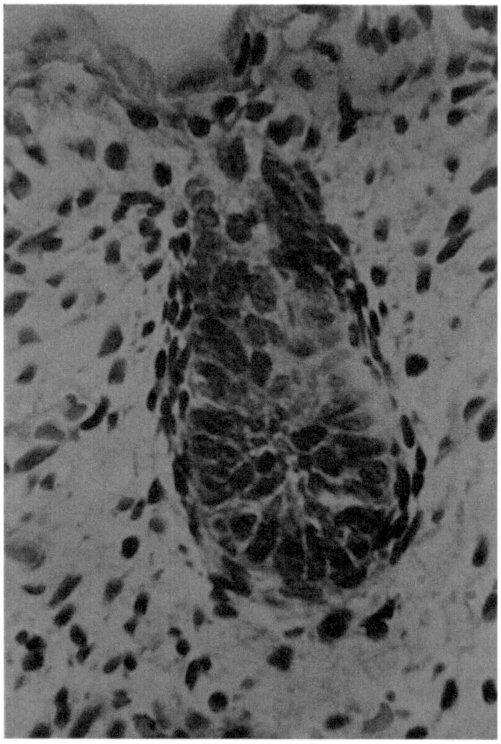

Fig. 3.3. Hair germ stage IIb, as shown in Fig. 3.1a,b. Germ cells grow gradually and a mass of mesodermal nuclei has formed in the bottom of the epithelial sac. The mass of mesenchymal tissue in the bottom of the hair follicle is not yet clear. The primordial sebaceous gland can be seen in the middle of the *right side*. ×600

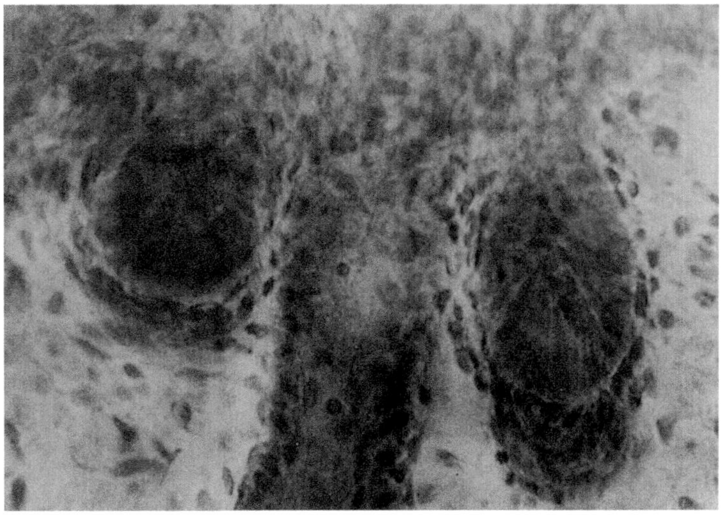

Fig. 3.4. As the fetus grows, new primary germs form between the existing ones, and secondary germs form in relation to the primary germs, so that the follicles are manifested in groups of three. ×600

1959, 1960). An exception to this is the annual new growth of skin and hair covering on the antlers of deer (Billingham 1958).

The hair germ elongates downward at a characteristic angle relative to the epidermis and continues to grow into the dermis to form the original hair follicle. The lower half of the ellipsoid hair germ is enlarged and the germ cell layers are arranged radially (Fig. 3.5a,b). Mitosis takes place, with intermediary cells being observed in the central area. At the "neck" of the forming hair follicle, above the region of intermediary cells, little mi-

a

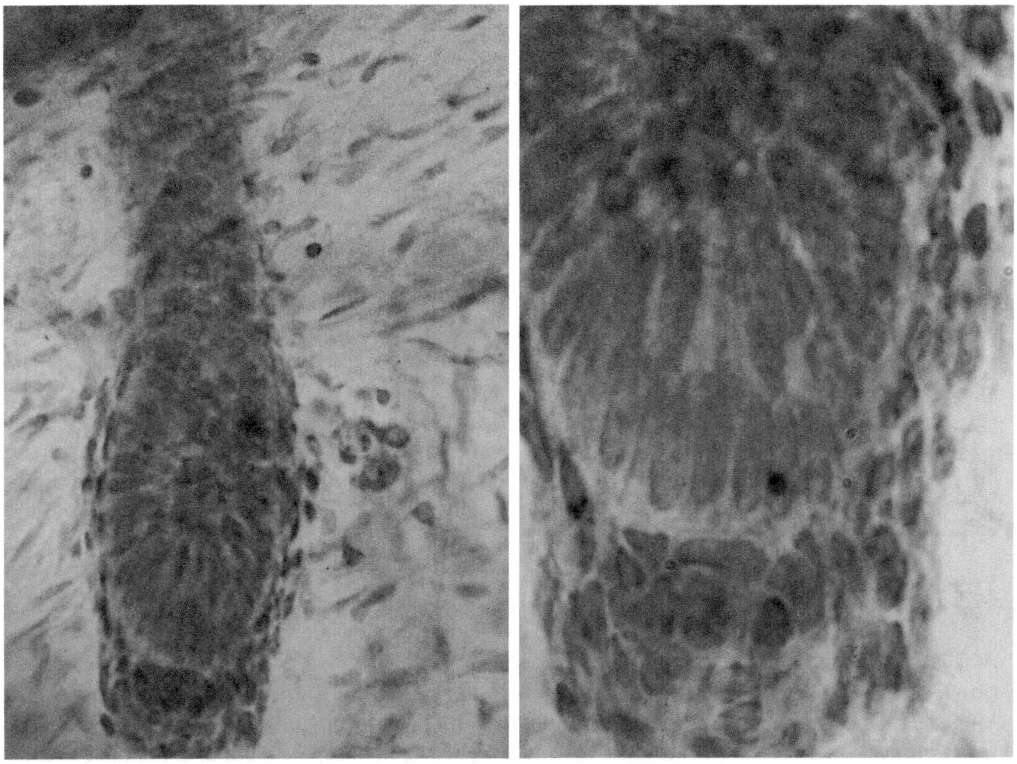

b

Fig. 3.5. **a** Hair germ stage IIb, as shown in Fig. 3.1a,b. The lower half of the hair follicle grows ovally. Cells around it are radiating to the center. The germinal layer in the bottom has grown in height and shows conical formation (early hair cone). ×600 **b** Enlargement of **a**. A club-like mass forms the epithelial sac at the bottom, and mesenchymal tissues have increased and become higher. ×800

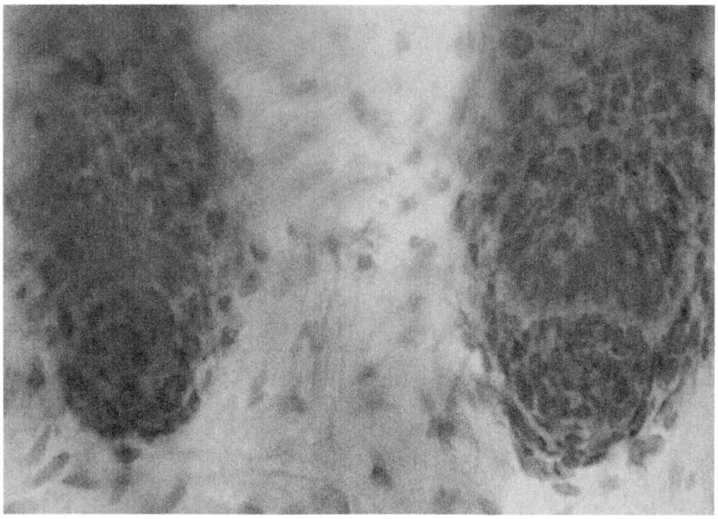

a

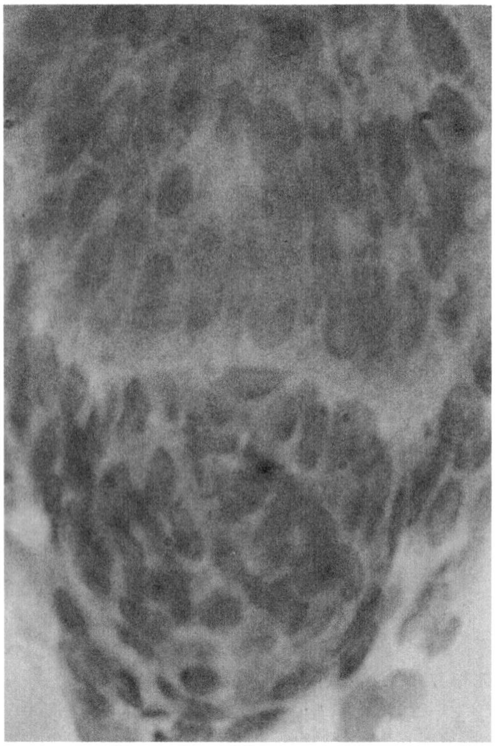

b

Fig. 3.6. a When the length of the entire follicle has increased to approximately twice that seen in Fig. 3.1b, stage IIc, the germ cell layer at the lower tip of the follicle takes on an arc shape. ×600 **b** Enlargement of the lower follicle (corresponds to IIc in Fig. 3.1b). The base of the plug is recognizably concave and can be subdivided according to the shape of the mesenchymal tissue. The mesenchymal tissue has increased in height. ×800

totic activity occurs. The neck remains quite thin (Fig. 3.1b, stage IIb; Fig. 3.5a).

3.1.2 Late Hair Germ Stage

As the forming hair follicle continues to elongate downward, the germinal layer gradually becomes localized in the lower portion of the hair follicle. A mass of mesenchymal cells forms at the tip of the germinal layer to become the future dermal papilla (Fig. 3.6a). The height of the germ cell layer at the bottom of the follicle increases with vigorous mitotic activity. Another major characteristic of this stage is the aggregating of mesenchymal cells. When the length of the entire follicle has increased to approximately twice that seen in Fig. 3.1, the germ cell layer at the lower tip of the follicle takes on an arc (concave) shape (Fig. 3.1b, stage IIc, Fig. 3.6).

The height of the germinal layer at the lower tip increases further, accompanied by increasingly vigorous mitosis. The hair cone, a conical aggregation of cells, is then clearly formed (Fig. 3.6b).

The hair cone, which corresponds to the inner root sheath of the mature hair follicle, begins to form when the nascent hair follicle is still very short.

3.1.3 Hair Peg Stage

The emerging hair follicle continues to elongate downward. The lower portion of the follicle is not yet bulbous, but new young hair can be already formed (Fig. 3.7a) and two solid epithelial swellings begin to appear at its posterior region. The upper swelling is the primordial sebaceous gland (rudiment) (Fig. 3.7b). The arrector pilorum muscle will later become attached to the swelling (bulge) in the lower hemisphere. This lower swelling or bulge of the hair follicle was described as a Wulst by Stöhr (1904). During fetal life, the bulge becomes even larger. At the end of fetal life, the bulge becomes very small.

It is sometimes clear from these thick tissue specimen observations that the rudiment of the sebaceous gland has already appeared in the hair germ and hair peg stage, and that a new hair has begun to develop within the inner root sheath (hair cone), despite the fact that the follicle has not yet formed a hair bulb at its lower tip (Figs. 3.1b, 3.7a, 3.8).

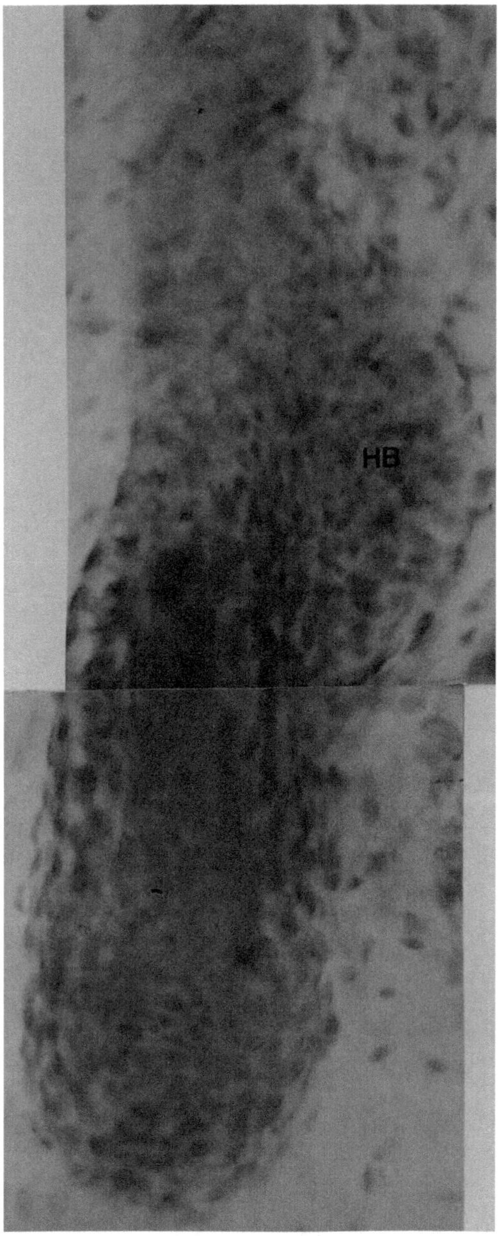

a

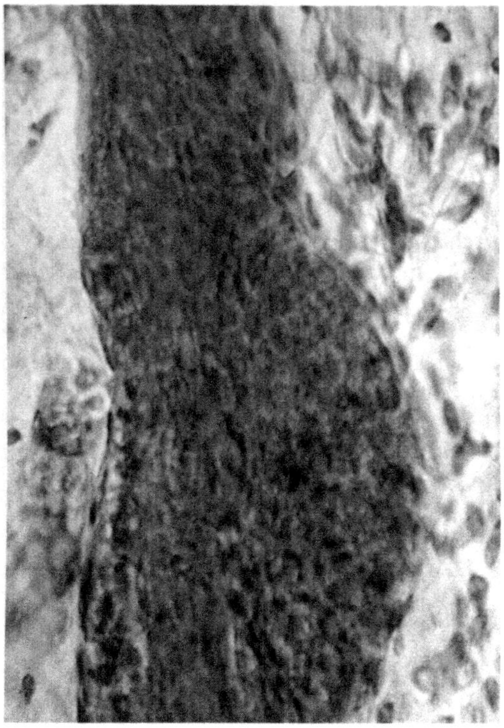

b

Fig. 3.7. a Inside the hair follicle, keratinization takes place in the already formed hair cone, and then a new young hair is formed, despite the fact that the follicle has not yet formed a hair bulb at the lower tip. (See Fig. 3.1b.) *HB*, Hair bulge. ×800 **b** Enlargement of **a**. The swollen bulge can be seen. New young hair extends upward to the upper portion of the bulge. ×800

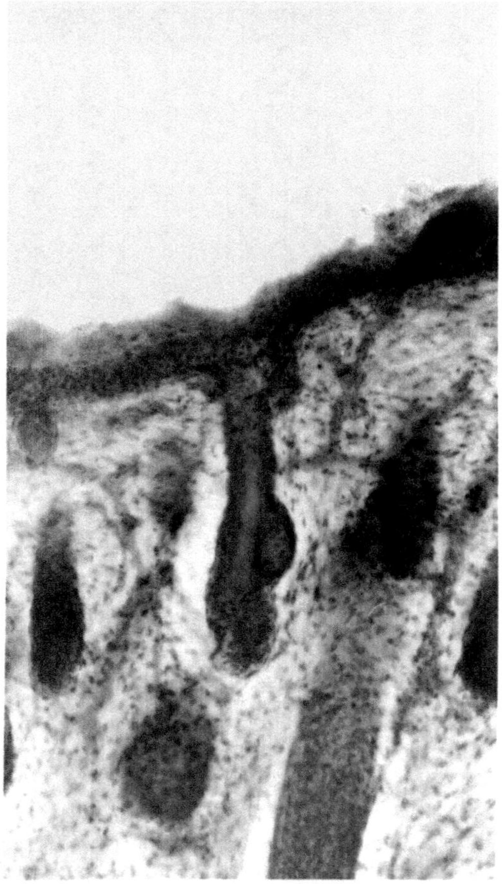

Fig. 3.8. This hair follicle is similar to that shown in Fig. 3.7a. The bulge and sebaceous gland have begun to form in the middle of the right side of the hair follicle. New young hair can already be seen in the follicle. ×150

It is thought that the hair and sebaceous gland differentiate in the bulbous peg stage and that an intraepidermal pathway (hair tract or hair canal) for the hair is organized and hollowed in the hair peg stage (see Section 3.2).

3.1.4 Bulbous Peg Stages

The bulbous peg stage has two major substages, early and late; these deserve description in fine detail.

3.1.4.1 Early Bulbous Peg Stage

In this early stage, a third bud above the sebaceous gland, the rudiment of an apocrine gland, later appears on the posterior surface of the follicular infundibulum in many follicles (Fig. 3.9a). The mesenchymal cells of the dermal papilla in the lower portion of the hair follicle, as shown in Fig. 3.9a,c, are wrapped in the inner and outer root sheaths, as well as the hair tissues of the follicle, to form the dermal papilla. The lower portion of the hair follicle takes on a bulbous shape, but the configuration is incomplete.

As described later, the outer root sheath is compressed by the descending inner root sheath and begins to bulge outward, taking on a characteristic bulbous shape. Meanwhile, the inner root

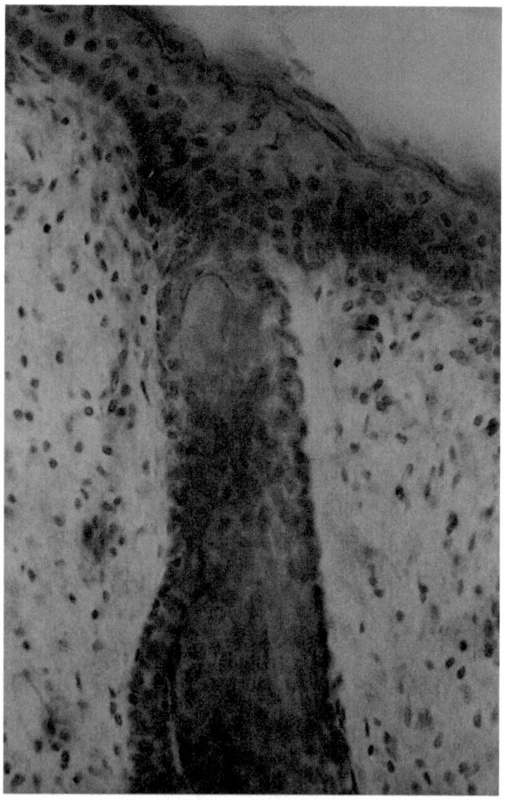
b

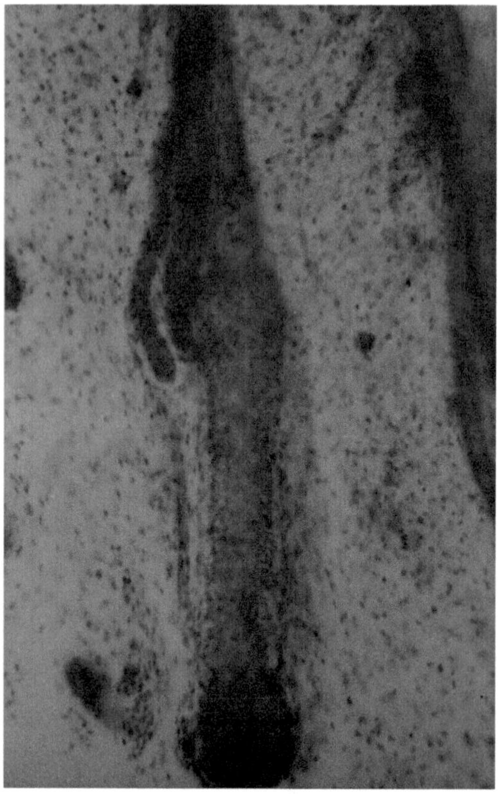
a

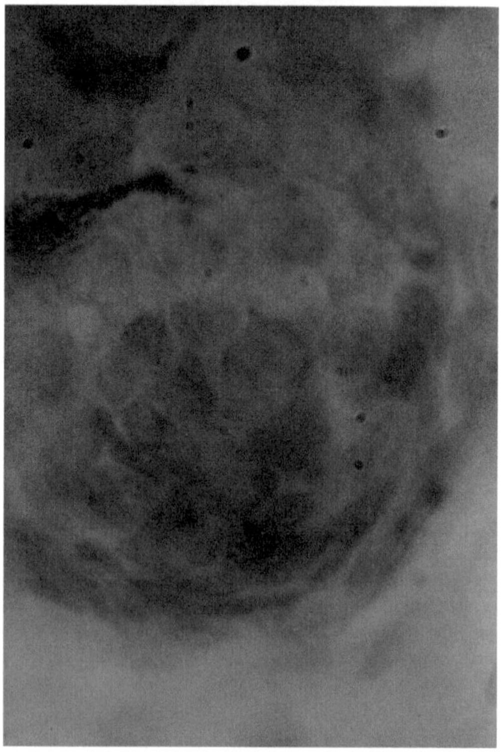
c

Fig. 3.9. a Early bulbous peg stage. Inner root sheath and hair tissue wrap around the dermal papilla and then take on a bulbous shape. A primordial apocrine duct descends from the upper part of the sebaceous gland. ×600. **b** Enlargement of **a**. The formation of sebum in the follicle neck results in the formation of a cyst that subsequently acts as a hair canal. ×600 **c** The lower portion of the hair follicle takes on a bulbous shape, but the formation of the matrix is still incomplete. There is slight formation of the undifferentiated cell layer surrounding the dermal papilla. ×800

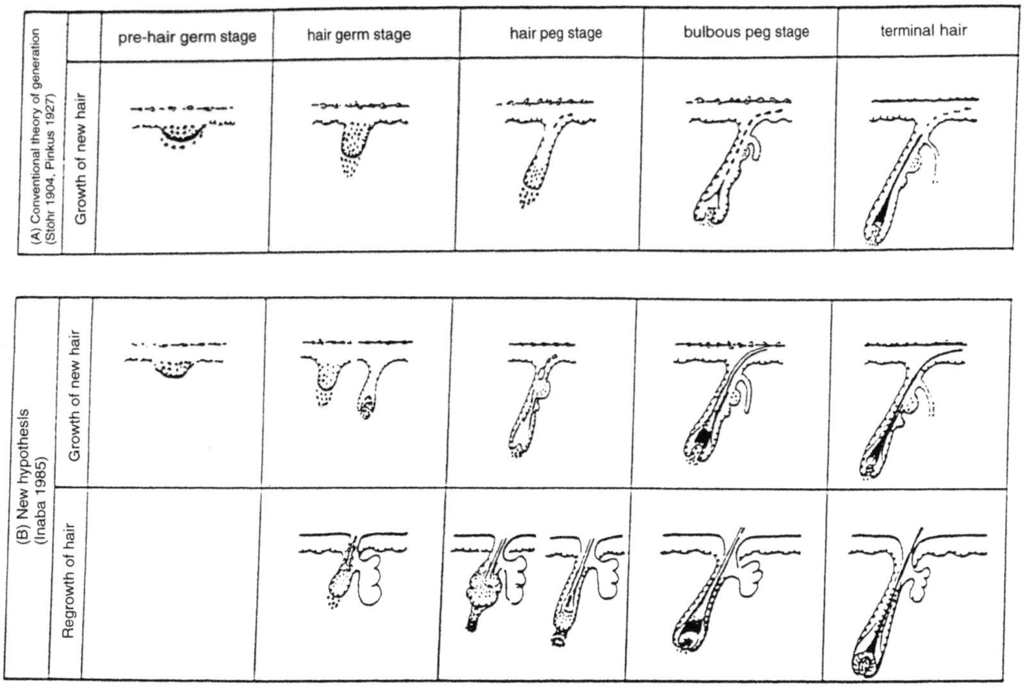

Fig. 3.10. Two hypotheses for the development of human hair follicle (from Inaba 1985)

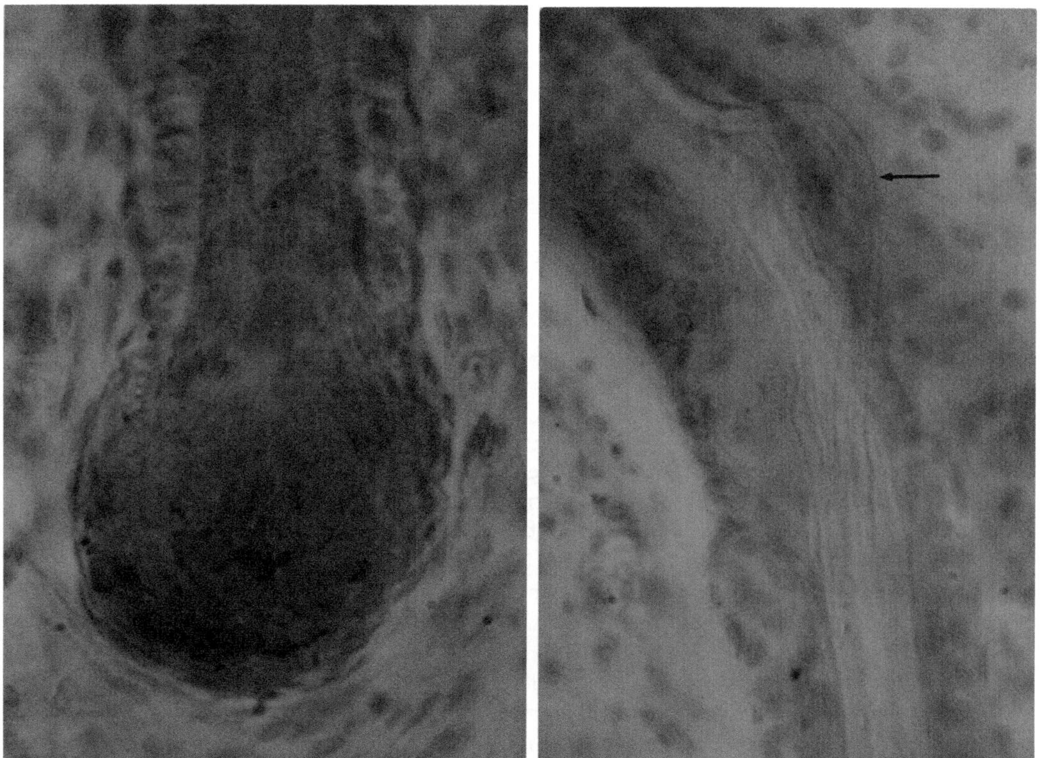

a b

Fig. 3.11. a The bulbous peg stage. The hair follicle in IVa (in Fig. 3.1b) is longer than that in stage III. The lower part of the follicle has formed a hair bulb and is wrapped around the mesenchymal tissue. ×600 **b** The bending phenomenon (*arrow*) is clearly seen. ×600 **c** The new young hair has not emerged on the skin surface. Its apex is protected by cyst formation (hair canal). ×600 **d** The new hair has not yet emerged on the skin surface. It ascends with the development of the matrix. The bending phenomenon is clearly seen

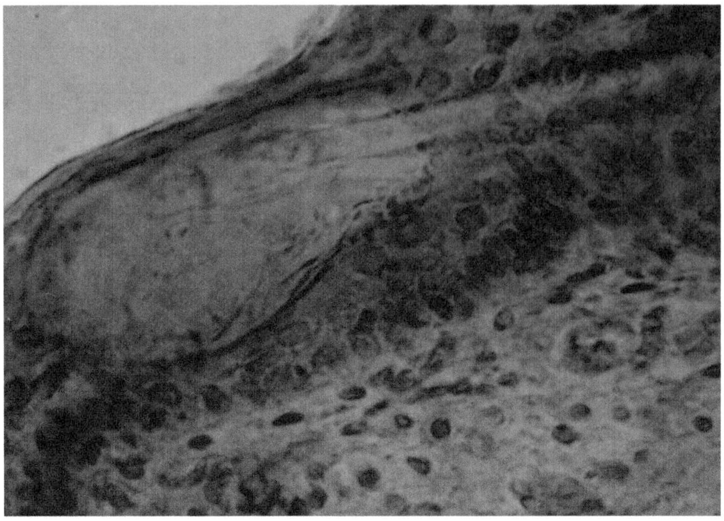

c

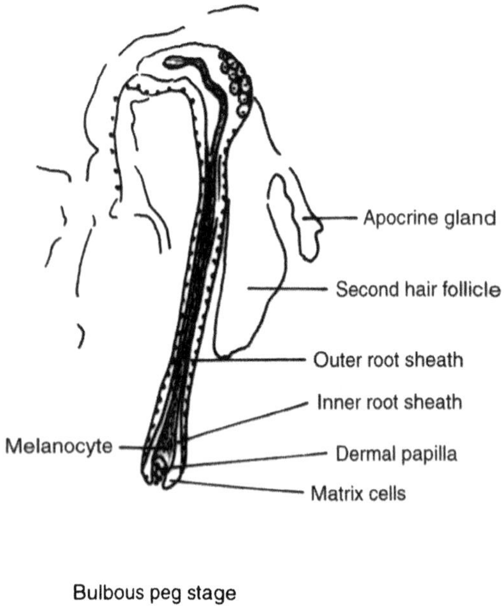

d

Fig. 3.11. *Continued*

sheath is transformed to an undifferentiated cell layer, prior to formation of the hair matrix (Fig. 3.9c). When differentiation of these cells into the various cell types characteristic of the matrix begins, the new hair is prevented from growing upward, toward the skin surface, by a firm interlocking fusion of the inner root sheath and hair sheath cuticle in the upper portion of the follicle. Both the follicle and the hair within it continue to grow downward due to vigorous mitotic activity in the newly formed matrix.

The sebaceous gland, which may already be formed in the hair germ stage (Fig. 3.3), is then clearly differentiated to form sebum in the early hair bulbous peg stage (Fig. 3.9b). This formation of a cyst, which subsequently acts as a hair canal, protects the new young hair apex from damage. When the tip of the new hair, protected by the inner root sheath, reaches the upper isthmal portion, the new young hair starts to grow through the hair canal to be pushed out of the dermis.

In contrast with the conventional theory that the hair canal is formed in the dermis and epidermis prior to generation of the new hair in the hair peg stage (Fig. 3.10, hair peg stage), thick tissue studies reveal that cysts are formed at the tip of the new hair to protect the hair during the formative stage.

3.1.4.2 Later Bulbous Peg Stage

In this stage, the lower portion of the hair follicle becomes clearly bulbous in configuration, but the formation of the matrix is still incomplete; the outer root sheath is not yet compressed as it is in the terminal hair stage. The inner root sheath and new hair continue to form, with a slight precipitation of melanin granules being observed (Fig. 3.11a).

The follicle continues to elongate and develops downward until the formation of the hair matrix is complete. As soon as the matrix is formed, the inner root sheath and hair cortex begin to ascend, growing at the same rate. However, at this stage, the tip of the new hair has not yet emerged on the skin surface (Fig. 11c) and the bending phenomenon can be seen in the region of the infundibulum (Fig. 3.11b).

3.1.5 Terminal Hair Stage

When the matrix within the bulb is fully formed, the lower portion of the hair bulb takes on the characteristic shape of the mature hair follicle. The

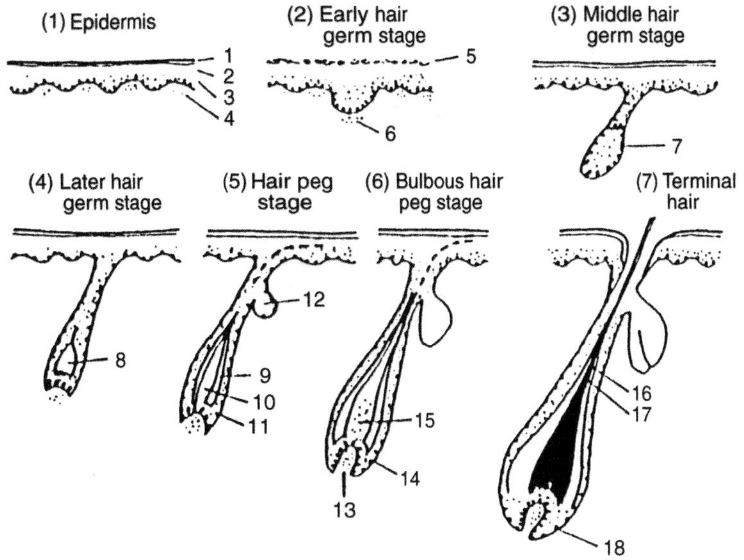

Fig. 3.12. Fetal eyebrow hair generation and growth (Inaba 1985). *1*, Corneal layer; *2*, granular layer; *3*, germinal layer (spinous layer, basal layer); *4*, papillary dermis; *5*, periderm; *6*, mesenchymal cells; *7*, hair germ; *8*, hair cone; *9*, inner root sheath; *10*, hair; *11*, outer root sheath; *12*, sebaceous gland; *13*, dermal papilla; *14*, hair bud; *15*, melanin granule; *16*, hair cuticula; *17*, sheath cuticula; *18*, hair matrix (undifferentiated layer) (from Inaba 1985)

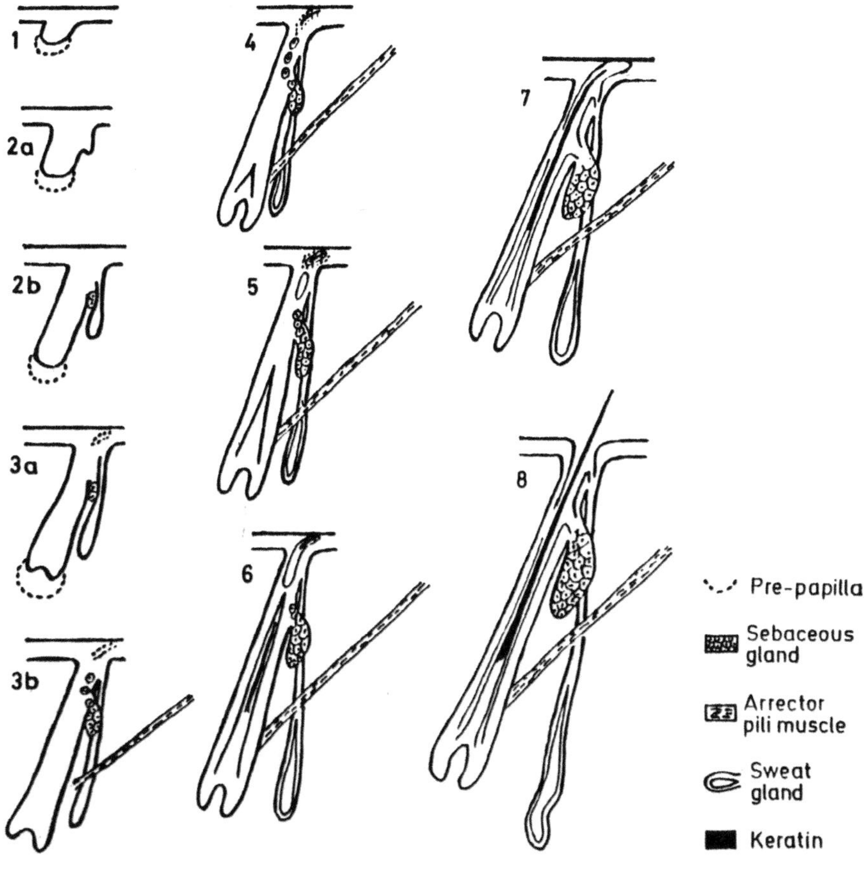

Fig. 3.13. Diagrammatic representation of stages in the development of a primary wool follicle in the skin of a Merino sheep fetus (after Hardy and Lyne 1956a, with permission from Springer-Verlag 1990)

matrix cells then participate in active formation of the inner root sheath, with cell differentiation and further formation of new hair. The hair follicle ceases its downward elongation and the new hair begins to grow upward toward the skin surface at exactly the same speed as the inner root sheath. The prior obstacle of interlocking fusion between hair cuticula and sheath cuticula no longer prevents upward growth. From this moment, the hair grows according to the conventionally accepted concept of the ordinary hair cycle.

3.2 The Hair Canal

The formation of sebum results in the formation of a cyst which subsequently acts as a canal. When the tip of the new hair, protected by the inner root sheath, reaches the upper isthmal portion, the new young hair starts to grow through the hair canal, to be pushed out of the dermis (Fig. 3.9b).

The development of the hair canal has been described in the mouse (Hardy 1949; Davidson and Hardy 1952), in humans (Pinkus 1958), in sheep (Hardy and Lyne 1956a), and in a marsupial (Lyne 1970). In the sheep, the hair canal is formed by the keratinization of cells in the epidermis and by disintegration of sebaceous gland cells that have migrated to the neck of the follicle. Eventually a continuous canal runs from the follicle neck to the upper part of the epidermis. The epidermal stages in the formation of hair canals in mouse pelage hair follicles (Hardy 1949) and mouse vibrissa follicles (Davidson and Hardy 1952) are similar to those described for the bandicoot (Lyne 1957), except that the keratinization process for the vibrissa follicle begins at the surface of the epidermis. No association between sebaceous cells and hair canal formation has been described in the mouse. According to Pinkus (1958), the central cells of this follicular peg undergo degeneration or partial keratinization, so that as the hair grows it appears gradually to push out the plugged end of the canal. This process has been described at the ultrastructural level by Hashimoto (1970) and Holbrook and Odland (1978)(Figs. 3.12, 3.13).

However, the authors have not observed this hair canal in thick tissue specimen observations. The sebaceous gland, which is already formed in the hair peg stage, is then clearly differentiated to form sebum in the bulbous peg stage. This formation of a cyst that subsequently acts as a hair canal protects the new young hair apex (Fig. 3.9b).

Pigmentation of Hair

4

The most important component of human hair (and skin) coloration is the melanosome. This cytoplasmic organelle, on which brown biochrome melanin is synthesized and deposited, is largely responsible for skin color according to its size, type, color, and distribution in the skin. The melanosomes found in human hair, in particular, are the product of melanocytes sited at the interface between the dermal papilla and the matrix of the hair follicle.

Each hair melanocyte is surrounded by 4 or 5 keratinocytes, while in the skin the ratio is 20–25 keratinocytes per melanocyte. The hair melanosomes are two to four times larger than the epidermal melanosome (eumelanin, $0.35 \times 1.0\,\mu m$, phaeomelanin, $0.2 \times 0.7\,\mu m$) and have longer dendrites (Orfanos and Ruska 1968).

Melanocytic proliferation and melanin synthesis are synchronized with hair growth. At the onset of each hair growth cycle, melanocytes initiate melanogenesis and proliferate to produce the population necessary for the particular type of follicle (Silver and Chase 1977; Sugiyama and Kukita 1976).

4.1 Hair Color

Hair color in the human scalp, after birth, depends mostly on the types and amounts of pigmentation present in the medullary and cortical cells of the hair shaft. Hair color also depends on the complement of melanocytes situated at the interface between the dermal papilla and the matrix of the hair follicle. Structural differences in the melanocytes account for black, brown, blond, and red hair. For instance, the melanosomes produced from melanocytes present in black hair (heavily melanized eumelanosomes) are relatively large in size and elliptical in shape, whereas reddish hair contains spherical pheomelanosomes.

The effect of graying hair is, of course, due to a mixture of black, white, and partially pigmented hair. Completely white hair follicles have no melanocytes (or the melanosomes are incompletely melanized). White hairs are the product of a progressive diminution in the production of melanin, as well as the possible final loss of active melanocytes (Montagna and Parakkal 1974) (Fig. 4.1). Whether melanocytes completely expire, or simply go into a dormant stage, has not yet been determined (Fitzpatrick et al. 1958).

There is no basis in demonstrated fact for reports that exceptional stress can turn hair gray "overnight". Nevertheless, even though gradual graying is believed to be an irreversible process, there have been a few reports of eventual repigmentation. The authors have achieved some success with repigmentation through clinical testing of a formula containing an oxidizing agent to accelerate the activity of the tyrosinase enzyme (see Section 28.6).

This tyrosinase enzyme is present in the organelles within the cytoplasm of melanocytes. Melanin is formed only in melanosomes by the action of tyrosinase and is deposited in the structural matrix of melanosomes (Mason 1948).

4.2 Embryonic Development of Melanocytes in Human Hair

The neural crest origin of the melanocytic system (Rawles 1947) is now well established. The first comprehensive work on the embryonic differentiation of hair melanocytes was performed by Mishima and Widlaw (1966) after studies of their epidermal penetration (Zimmermann and Becker

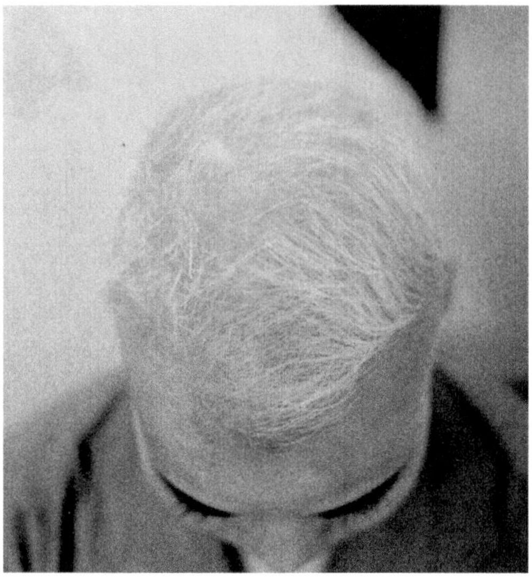

Fig. 4.1. Completely white scalp hair

1959). Mishima (1964) stated that the reaction for premelanin (ammoniated silver nitrate reaction) was specific for nonmelanized melanosomes in albino melanocytes. Mishima believed that the premelanin reaction characterized embryonic melanocytes and may have been related to amelanotic melanocytes. These cells are of importance, since they may play a major role in the repigmentation process in scars, burns, and vitiligo.

4.3 Generation of Melanin Pigmentation

As described above, in the development of fetal eyebrow hairs, the embryonic hair follicle peg descends from the epidermis toward the dermis, and then the germinal layer becomes localized in the lower portion of the hair follicle above the level of the dermal papilla, from hair germ to bulbous peg stage, as shown in Fig. 3.12.

The process of hair pigmentation is quite similar to that of hair generation and does tend to support the author's hypothesis of human hair generation. At the risk of repetition, hair pigmentation depends on the content of melanin granules. Melanocytes sited among the germinative cells in the hair follicle produce the melanin-bearing melanosomes. These melanosomes consist of a structural matrix and a functional melanin-synthesizing enzyme called tyrosinase. Melanin is formed and deposited from the melanosomes as a product of enzyme activity.

According to Mishima and Widlaw (1966), melanocyte differentiation and distribution in human embryonic hair follicles proceed essentially in parallel to that of melanocytes present within the embryonic epidermis (Fig. 4.2). The process can be divided into four steps:

1. Dopa- and premelanin reaction-positive melanocytes manifest their presence in embryonic hair. From the earliest pregerm stage to the end of the hair peg stage, these melanocytes are present without any specific localization or dense concentration at 4 months of fetal age.

At the hair germ stage, the melanocytes are randomly distributed. Dopa- and premelanin-positive cells are distributed throughout the peripheral and inner layers of the follicle at the hair peg stage, corresponding to the penetration of the epithelial cells in the dermis. The pigment matrix appears when embryonic hair development reaches the differentiation stage of infundibulum, bulge, and hair bulb (Pinkus 1958; reviewed in Cesarini 1990).

2. In the bulbous peg stage, prior to 6 months of fetal age, the melanocytes have become mostly localized in the peripheral layer of the outer root sheath of the infundibulum, the lower portion of the bulb, and the pigment matrix, although scant numbers can also be observed in the inner cell layers of the infundibulum and in the middle and upper portions of the bulb.

3. After 6 months of fetal age, the bulbous peg shows a complete localization of melanocytes in the peripheral layer of the outer root sheath of the infundibulum, the lower bulb, and the pigment matrix.

These findings tie in with the authors' findings on the process of development of fetal eyebrow hair. In the hair germ stage, the lower half of the follicle enlarges in an ellipsoid form, with the germinal cell layer being arranged radially.

As the forming follicle continues to peg downward in the hair peg stage, the germinative layer becomes localized in the lower portion of the follicle above the level of the dermal papilla. The inner root sheath cells and new young hair cells are differentiated from the activity of this germinative cell layer.

In the bulbous peg stage, the germinal layer wraps around the dermal papilla to form the matrix and the hair bulb. When matrix formation is complete, the hair follicle is typically bulbous and ceases further descent. The new hair begins to ascend toward the skin surface alone. The formation of keratinocytes in the germinal layer occurs in parallel to the formation of melanocytes (Figs. 4.4, 14.11).

In the terminal hair follicle, melanocytes are formed in the germinal layer, which corresponds

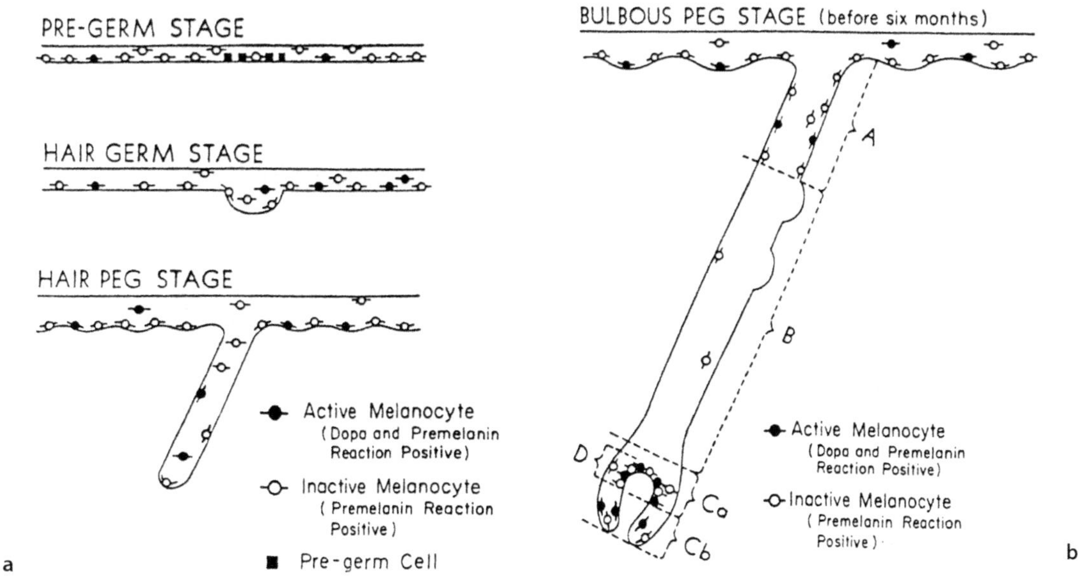

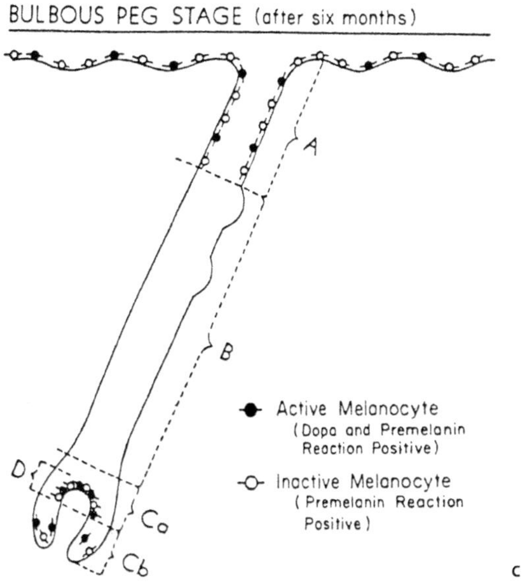

Fig. 4.2. The melanocyte and its melanogenic activity at the pre-germ, hair germ, and hair peg stages (**a**), and at the bulbous peg stage before (**b**) and after (**c**) six months. *A*, infundibulum portion; *B*, middle portion; *Ca*, upper bulb; *Cb*, lower bulb; *D*, pigment matrix (from Mishima and Widlaw 1966, with permission from Mishima)

to the hair cortex and medulla. However, the melanocytes are arranged upward above Auber's borderline. The thickest part of the hair follicle is its onion-shaped bulb. It has been assumed, in the past, that Auber's borderline (1952) delineates the widest diameter of the dermal papilla within the bulb and divides the bulb itself into two distinct regions. The lower part, beneath Auber's borderline, consists of an undifferentiated cell layer, i.e., the hair matrix (Figs. 4.3 and 4.4).

Since it is commonly believed that cell differentiation begins from the activities of the matrix, it is difficult to understand why melanin pigmentation is arranged upward from Auber's borderline. However, this phenomenon can be accounted for by the authors' hypothesis (Figs. 3.12, 14.11).

4.4 Regeneration of Melanin Pigmentation

In human axillary hair, the newly-formed matrix of the regenerating hair acquires a normal complement of melanocytes. It is commonly assumed that a certain number of preexisting melanocytes remain dormant in the dermal papilla, to be reactivated and multiply in numbers during the next anagen stage. During the anagen phase of the hair cycle, the active melanocytes actively synthesize melanin and have well-developed dendrites. Tyrosinase is detected in this phase, whereas no tyrosinase activity can be detected in the telogen phase (Kukita 1957).

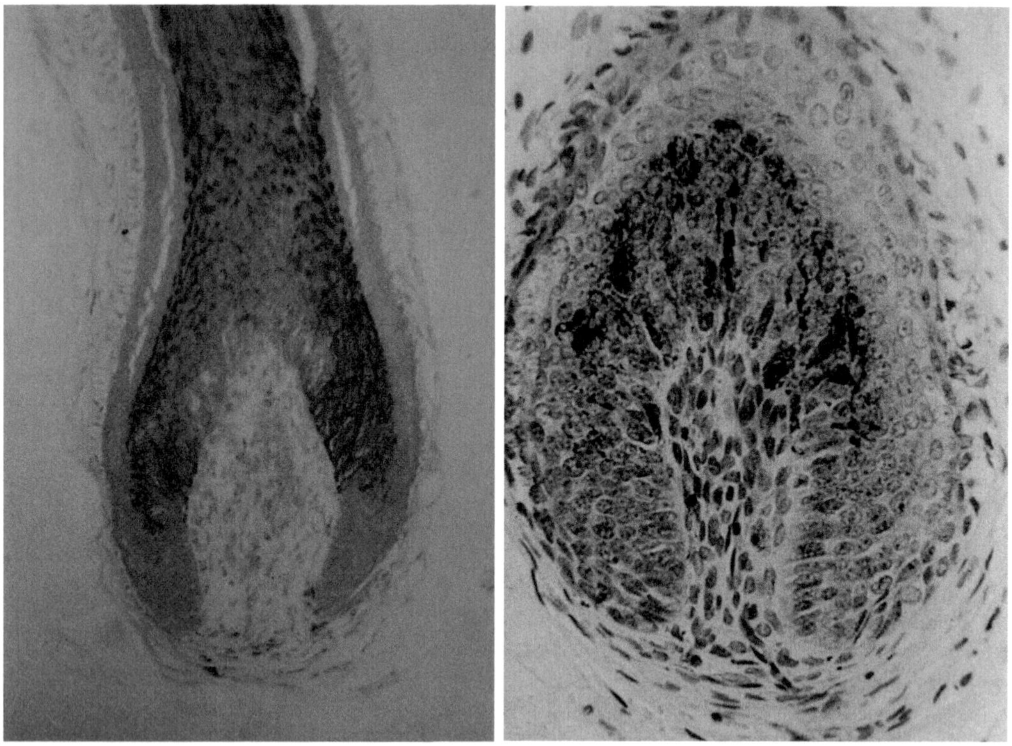

Fig. 4.3. **a** Thick tissue preparation. The hair melanocytes are active in the growing stage of the hair growth cycle and are clearly visible above Auber's critical line. × 400 **b** Thin section derived from thick preparation. × 600

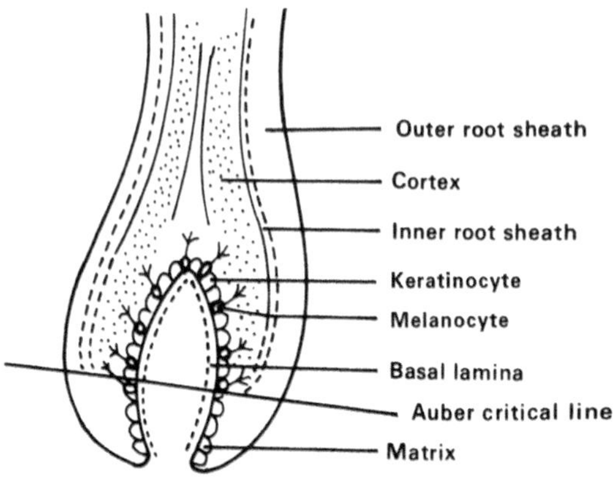

Fig. 4.4. Diagram of an active hair follicle (from Inaba 1985)

Montagna and Parakkal (1974) have reported that when the follicle is in catagen stage, both melanin formation and the formation of the hair medulla cease at exactly the same time. Therefore, the last segment of the hair is white and non-medullated. During early telogen stage, the cells of the hair bulb degenerate and, as a result, the follicle no longer has any true matrix. In the later telogen period, the hair germ, consisting mostly of the outer root sheath, rebuilds a new bulb, which again produces a new hair and inner root sheath. At this time, melanocytes again take their proper place in the follicle. The replacement of hair will activate the hair germ and the dominant melanocytes will be stimulated to divide in the new hair papilla (Taylor 1949; Potten et al. 1971). Silver et al. (1968) have reported that dormant melanocytes rest among the germ cells until the next growth phase takes place, at which time they become dendritic and begin anew to produce and deposit melanin pigment. The results of an ultrastructural study of mouse hair follicles in each stage of the hair cycle suggest that some bulb melanocytes may survive to undergo differentiation in an amelanotic state during catagen and telogen. Thereafter, they may undergo proliferation and differentiation, and repopulate the bulb during early anagen (Silver and Chase 1977; Sugiyama and Kukita 1976).

Starico (1963) observed some dark cells located along the outer root sheath in the middle and the lower part of the follicle in preparations stained with toluidine blue. These cells were dopa-negative and some contained refringent granules; they were not detected in the upper part of the follicle.

4.5 New Growth of Melanin Pigmentation

In the authors' own studies, in which a subcutaneous axillary tissue shaving procedure was used, all matrix-associated melanocytes were removed, along with the hair bulb and almost all of the lower portion of the follicle below the sebaceous gland.

However, when the new hair follicle began to regenerate from the upper isthmal portion, particularly in follicles close to the duct opening of the sebaceous gland, the epithelial matrix cells were fully formed on the interface with the dermal papilla, melanocytes were increased in number, and new deposits of melanin granules were laid down in the hair cortex.

The newly-formed hair matrix of regenerating axillary hair acquires a normal complement of melanocytes. With our subdermal shaving procedure, all matrix-associated melanocytes are removed. Melanocytes of the neogenetic matrix must come from other sources.

The melanocytes of the neogenetic matrix must come from the complement of amelanotic melanocytes that have been shown to exist in the basal layer of the outer root sheath (newly-formed germinal layer) in the newly-formed bud derived from epidermal cells when the epithelial matrix cells are completely formed on the interface with the dermal papilla. In the later bulbous peg stage, the matrix is fully formed; melanocytes increase in number and melanin, and melanin granules are deposited in the hair cortex. This finding is associated with epidermal repigmentation after wound healing.

Blood Vessel System in Hair Follicles

5

5.1 Vascular System for the Pilosebaceous Unit

According to Montagna and Parakkal (1974), there are fewer cross-shunts above the keratogenous zone of the follicle near the hair bulb than in the upper portion of the hair follicle. Cross-shunts also form a network at the location of the sebaceous gland (sebaceous isthmus), which they envelop in tight nets that adhere to sebaceous acini. Above the entrance of the sebaceous duct, parallel vessels form a loose network that rises up to the loops of capillaries in the papillary body. Returning to the base of the follicle, some vessels penetrate the dermal papilla and the tufts.

Each blood vessel, which is thought to form a unit consisting of dermal papilla, sebaceous glands, and hair infundibula, is connected to the subpapillary blood plexus beneath the epidermis.

Jakubovic and Ackerman (1985) have pointed out that the vascular architecture of the dermis consists of a superficial and a deep plexus of arterioles and venules; these superficial and deep dermal plexuses contain many anastomoses. These microcirculatory anastomoses are most abundant in the upper dermis and around the pilosebaceous units and sweat glands.

Up to the present, it was commonly believed that transverse branches of blood vessels in the cutaneous blood plexus and candelabra vessels in the lower blood plexus supplied nutrition to the

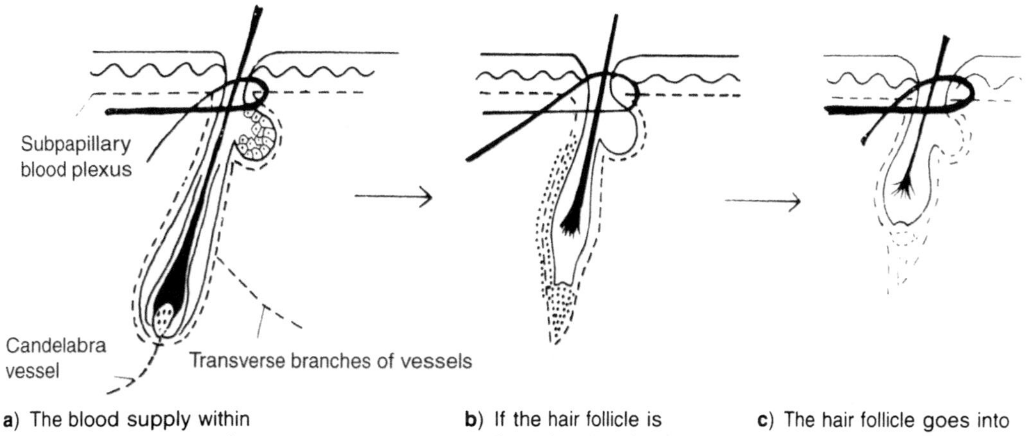

a) The blood supply within the pilosebaceous unit has been considered to form from cutaneous blood plexuses and musculocutaneous arteries.

b) If the hair follicle is ligated at the infundibular portion, the hair follicle becomes a catagen follicle with blood congestion.

c) The hair follicle goes into the telogen stage. This finding indicates that there is a vascular system (microcirculation), forming as a continuous unit from the subpapillary plexuses.

Fig. 5.1a–c. Changes in the hair follicle after ligation of its upper portion (from Inaba et al. 1987, with permission) dermal papilla of the hair follicle. However, the formation of a continuous vascular system for the hair follicle and sebaceous gland appended to it has been observed, and this perifollicular network of blood vessels cross-shunts with the upper dermal vasculature, while blood is supplied originally from the deep dermis, below the subcutaneous adipose tissue (Fig. 5.1a).

Such versatility of blood supply for the hair follicles is observed specifically during various stages of the hair growth cycle (Montagna and Ellis 1957).

5.2 Experimental Research

5.2.1 Experimental Research on Ligating the Upper Portion of the Hair Follicle

In an attempt to observe blood supply in the pilosebaceous unit, we (Inaba et al. 1987) ligated a point above the secretory duct opening of the sebaceous gland and infundibular portion of the hair follicle with a fine nylon ligature. Signs of regressive degeneration and transformation into telogen stage were observed in all hair follicles so treated (Fig. 5.1c).

Although blood was supplied to the follicles from the vascular system in the hypodermal plexus (Fig. 5.1), if the infundibular portion of the hair follicle was ligated (Fig. 5.1a), blood congestion was seen only in the dermal papilla and the connective sheath and not in the candelabra vessel or the transverse branch vessels (Fig. 5.2b). Figure 5.3a–c indicates that if the ligation has been done as described above, the initial catagen stage is induced. Figure 5.4a–d shows the hair follicle in catagen stage. The follicle has shortened and the lower bulb has atrophied. The dermal papilla with remnants of melanin granules can be seen, and the hyaline membrane surrounding the epithelial strand (cord) has thickened (Fig. 5.4d). Beneath the follicle, the vascular system in its growth period can be observed around and inside the invo-

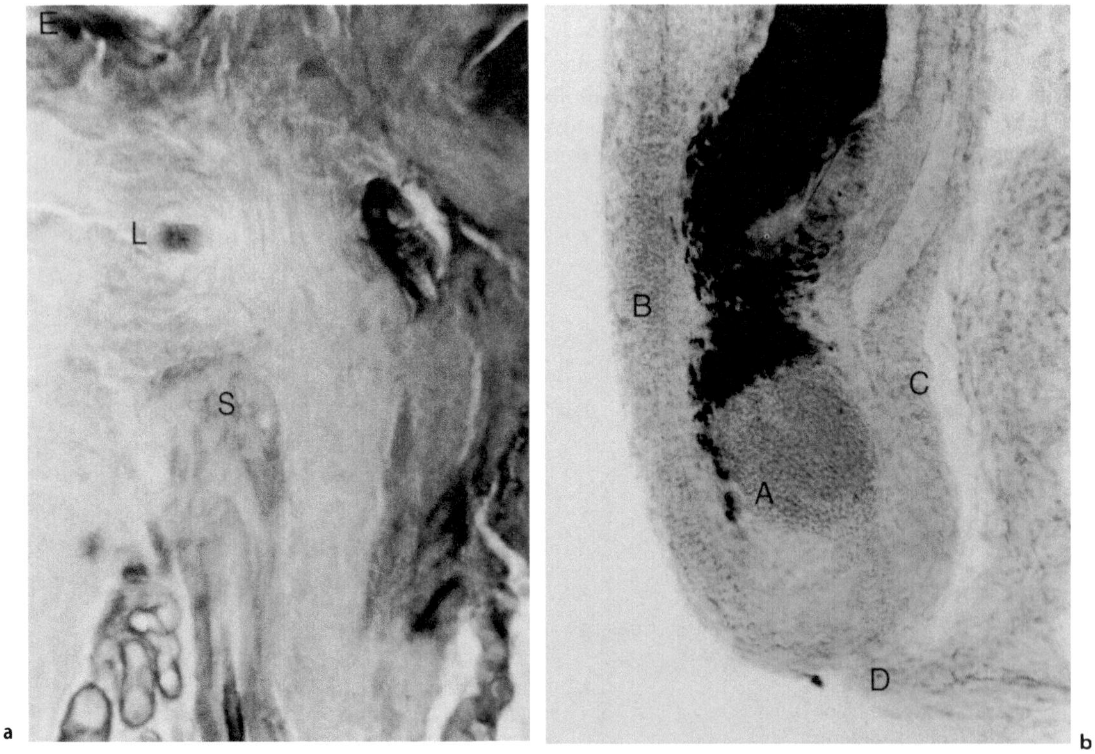

Fig. 5.2. **a** The infundibular portion of the hair follicle is ligated with a fine nylon ligature (*L*). *S*, Atrophied sebaceous gland; *E*, epidermis. **b** The lower portion of the hair follicle with blood congestion. *A*, Blood congestion is observed inside the dermal papilla; *B*, blood congestion is observed inside the left portion of the connective sheath; *C*, less blood congestion is observed inside the right portion of the connective sheath; *D*, no congestion is observed in the candelabra vessel or the transverse branches of vessels. **a** ×250 **b** ×440

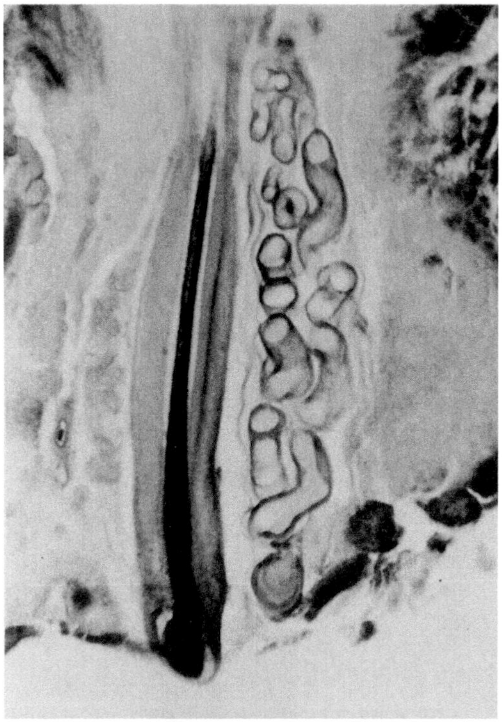

a

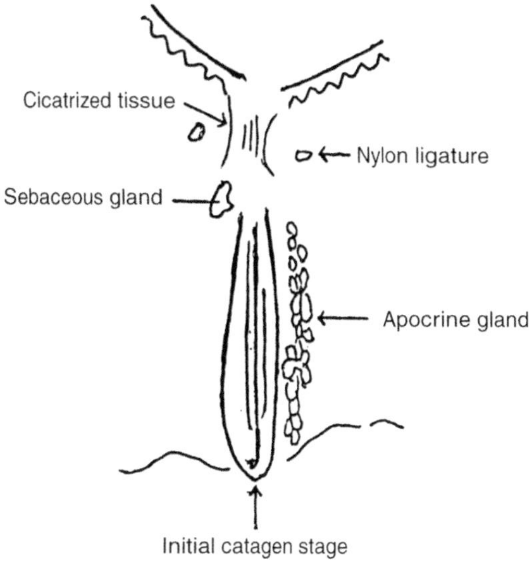

b

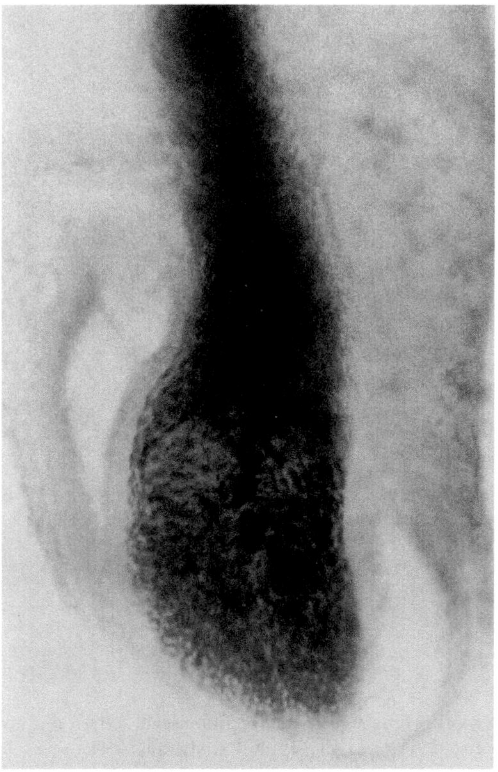

c

Fig. 5.3. **a** Initial catagen stage after ligation at the upper portion of the hair follicle. **b** Diagram of initial catagen stage. **c** Enlarged view of the lower portion of the hair follicle. **a** ×250 **c** ×440

luted epithelial sac (Fig. 5.4d). The sebaceous gland and apocrine gland have atrophied.

These findings indicated both the presence of a microcirculatory system originating from the subpapillary blood plexus below the epidermis and surrounding the follicular appendix and that this vascular system is of prime importance, with the principal blood supply coming from the subpapillary blood to form the microcirculation around the pilosebaceous unit. The blood vessels supplied from the dermal arterial plexus are of only secondary importance. From these findings, it can be surmised that enzyme and hormone activity is continuously taking place in the sebaceous gland.

5.2.2 Experimental Research: Superficial Skin Shaving

We exfoliated the upper epidermal layer above the excretory duct opening of the sebaceous gland of the hair follicle to study the effect on the follicle (Fig. 5.5a). The condition of the hair follicle was typical of telogen stage and the sebaceous gland had atrophied (Fig. 5.5b). In other words, the follicle was involuted and a typical catagen club hair was observed inside it. The dermal papilla at the hair bulb had atrophied but remained attached to the lower tip of the telogen follicle (Fig. 5.5c). These findings indicate that if the epidermis, including the subpapillary blood plexus, is removed, the hair follicle becomes atrophied due to the diminished microcirculation originating from the subpapillary blood plexus.

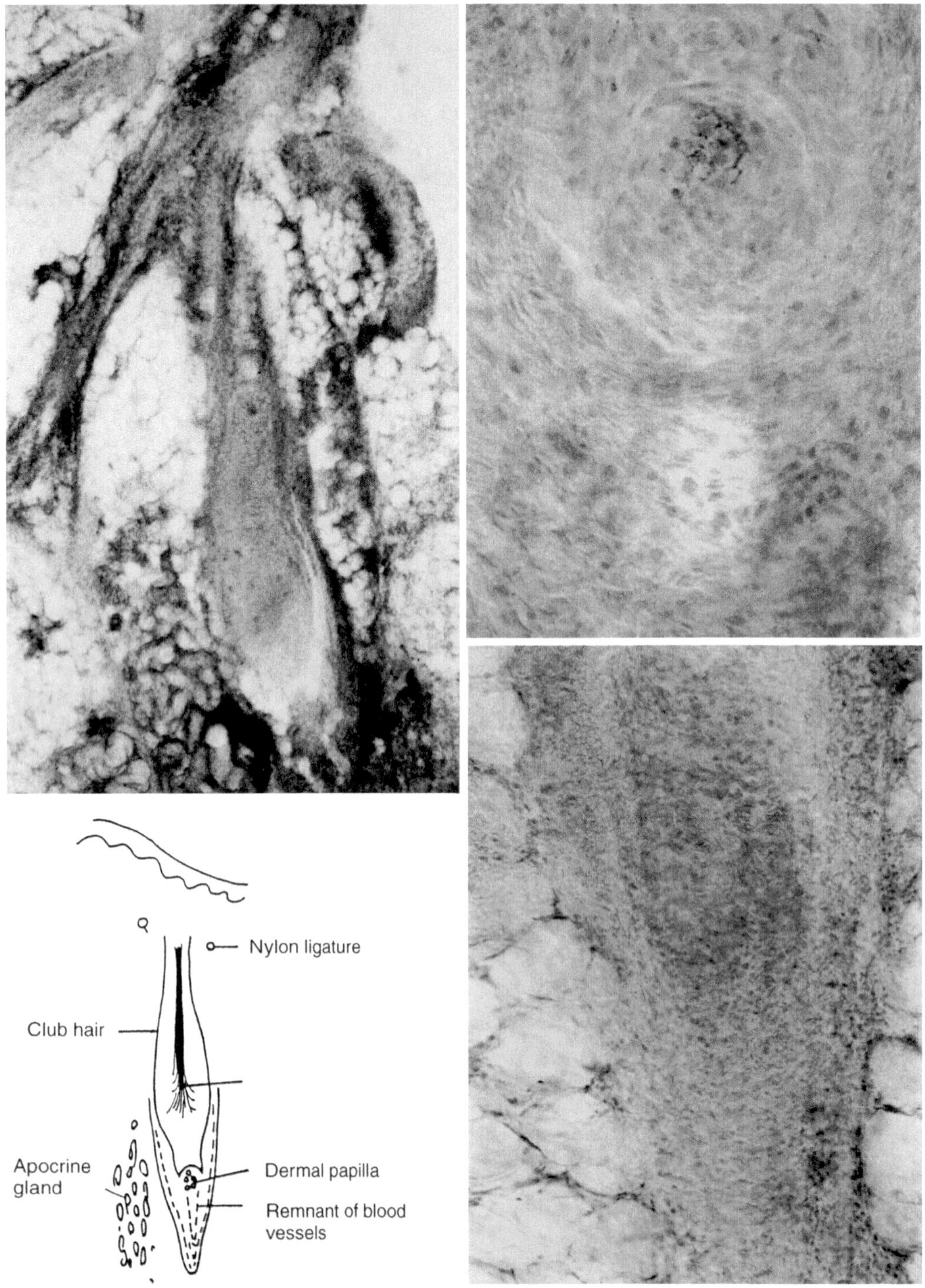

Fig. 5.4. a Catagen stage after ligation at the upper portion of hair follicle. ×250 **b** Diagram of catagen stage. **c** The lower bulb has atrophied. Dermal papilla with remnants of melanin granules can be seen. ×400 **d** The involuted epithelial sac (epithelial strand). ×440

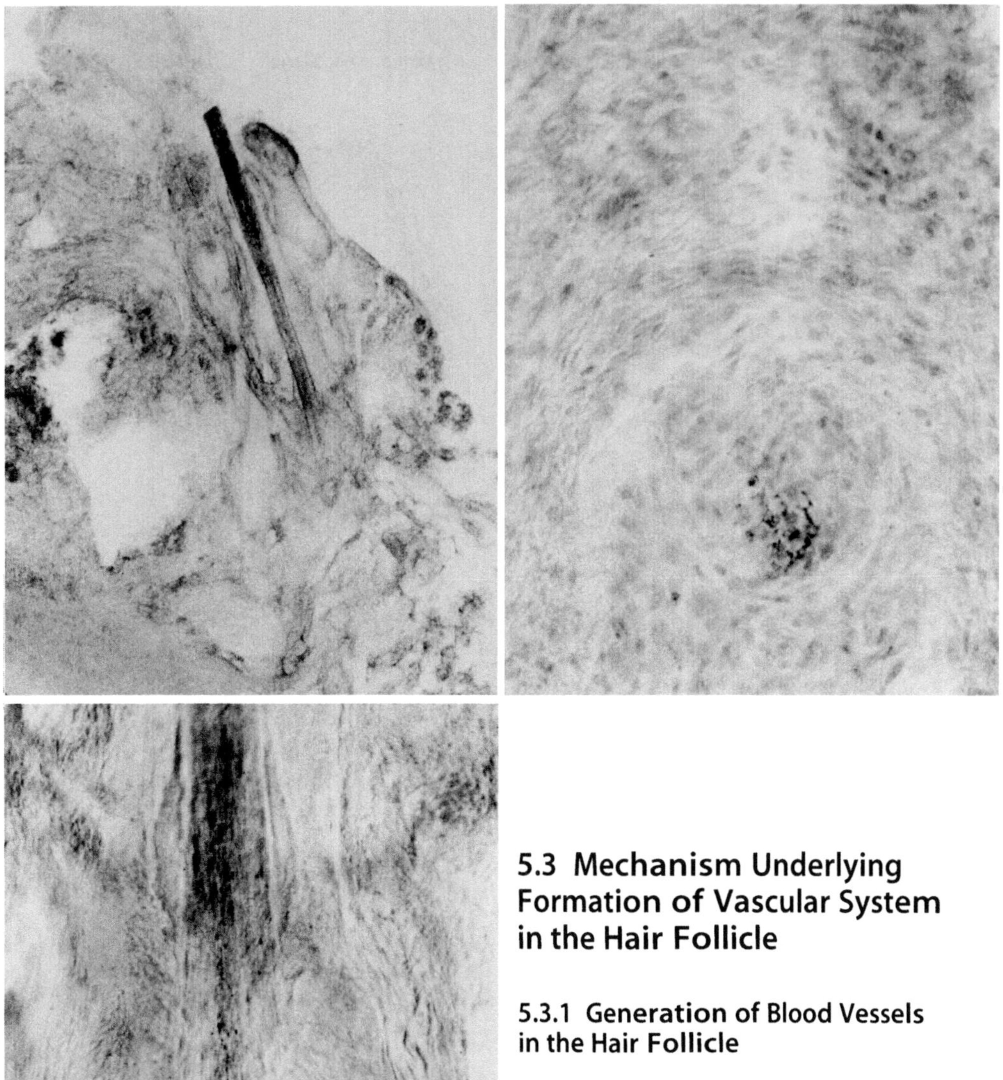
a
c
b

Fig. 5.5a–c. Experimental research involving superficial skin shaving. **a** The upper epidermal layer above the excretory duct opening of the sebaceous gland is exfoliated. ×250 **b** Enlarged view of **a**. The hair follicle shows typical telogen stage. ×440 **c** The dermal papilla (with remnants of melanin granules) at the hair bulb has atrophied, but remains attached to the lower tip of the telogen follicle. ×440

5.3 Mechanism Underlying Formation of Vascular System in the Hair Follicle

5.3.1 Generation of Blood Vessels in the Hair Follicle

The presence of a microcirculatory system originating from the subpapillary plexus can be supported by the following findings in regard to the generation of the hair follicle (Fig. 5.6a). The undifferentiated epithelial cells (hair germ) grow downward, and a mass of mesenchymal tissue (the future dermal papilla) is formed at the bottom of the hair germ. The papillary blood vessels beneath the epidermis and the mass of mesenchymal tissue is then connected by subpapillary blood vessels (hair germ stage) (Fig. 5.6a). New cells are formed by the hair germ cells to become the intermediate cells, and the hair bud then begins to elongate downward. When the hair peg stage begins, the germinal cell layer surrounding the hair germ is limited to the lower portion, and the mass of mesenchymal tissue exists beneath it. Although the hair bulb is yet to be formed at the hair peg stage, the hair cone (future inner root sheath) is formed by the lower germ cells and the hair tissue formed inside it (Inaba 1985) (Fig. 5.6a, hair peg stage).

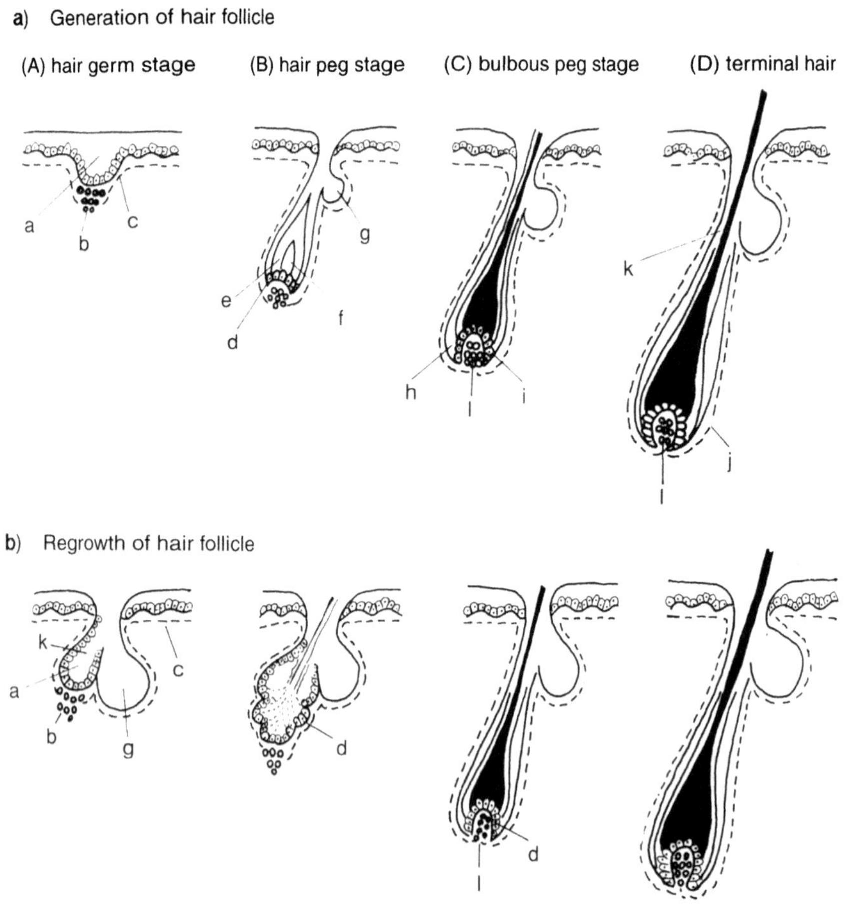

Fig. 5.6a,b. Formation of vascular system in the hair follicle. *a*, Hair germ; *b*, mass of mesenchymal cells; *c*, subpapillary blood plexus; *d*, germinal layer; *e*, inner root sheath; *f*, hair tissue; *g*, sebaceous gland; *h*, hair bulb; *i*, hair matrix; *j*, microcirculation; *k*, isthmal portion; *l*, dermal papilla

As the hair follicle begins to peg downward, it wraps the mass of mesenchymal tissue in bulbous form (bulbous peg stage). Therefore, the vascular system surrounding the hair follicle is formed around the hair follicle as it develops. It is thus understandable that hair follicle microcirculation is generated with the subpapillary blood plexuses.

5.3.2 Regrowth of Blood Vessels in the Hair Follicle

On the basis of the sebaceous gland hypothesis, it can be assumed that regeneration of hair follicles occurs from the isthmal portion adjacent to the duct opening of the sebaceous gland. A mass of mesenchymal tissues is formed at the follicular base. The vascular system appears to be formed as a unit between the sebaceous gland and the budmass of mesenchymal tissue (Fig. 5.6b). The hair follicle pegs downward, with formation of the new hair through the hair peg and bulbous peg stages. When the bulb is completed, the terminal hair grows upward to the skin surface.

Therefore, as in the process of hair generation, a microcirculatory system is formed along with the sebaceous gland and the mesenchymal tissue of the blood vessels beneath the hair germ. After passing through the hair peg stage and the bulbous hair peg stage, the terminal hair is formed, and the microcirculation is formed along with it.

The vascular system can thus be considered to function as one unit between the sebaceous gland and the dermal papilla. The hormones, enzymes, and other substances present in the sebaceous gland have a direct effect on the dermal papilla and the matrix.

Changes in Hair: Causative Factors

6

6.1 Hormonal Control of the Hair Follicle

Much can be learned about the hormonal control of hair growth by studying the sebaceous glands, since the responses of the various components of the pilosebaceous unit are probably similar or identical. Adachi and Kano (1970) have indicated that dihydrotestosterone (DHT) is the active form that testosterone takes in the hair follicle. They showed that glucose-6-phosphate-dehydrogenase (G6PDH), which is stimulated cyclic adenosine monophosphate (AMP), increases considerably during the anagen phase of hair growth (see Section 18.9.3.1). There is a mutual correlation between the degree of progress of alopecia and falling androgen levels. In the skin, evidently, the peripheral metabolite of testosterone, 5α-DHT, and not testosterone itself is responsible for the stimulation of the matrix cells in the hair follicle, e.g., in women with hirsutism (Jenkins and Ash 1973). The same applies to the sebaceous gland in acne (Sansone-Bazzano and Reisner 1971).

According to Schweikert and Wilson (1974a), we now have substantial evidence that there is a complex relation between hair growth in men and the sex hormones.

For instance, the growth of the beard, the hair in the ears, the nasal tip, and upper pubic triangle; and the coarse hair on the trunk and limbs is dependent on adult male levels of circulatory androgens. The occipital region of the scalp is little affected. Growth of hair in the axilla, the lower pubic region, and, at least partly, on the limbs, is stimulated by pubertal changes in both sexes. Certain hair, however, appears to be independent of sex hormones, including lanugo hair, the eyebrows, and the eyelashes. Schweikert and Wilson (1974b) found that isolated hair roots produced mainly androstenedione. In vitro studies, however, cannot establish what happens in vivo, only the capacity of isolated skin to react under artificial conditions. Randall et al. (1982) therefore studied the uptake and metabolism of radioactively labeled testosterone in skin and other organs removed from rats at various intervals after its injection in vivo. They found that, in skin, the major free steroid was unchanged testosterone, with only relatively small quantities of androstenedione, 5α-DHT, androstanediols, and androsterone. After incubating isolated hair roots with androstenedione, Schweikert and Wilson (1974c) found 5α-androstanedione to be the principal metabolite, and suggested that it could be active. On the other hand, androgens may be the paradoxical cause of male pattern baldness in individuals with a genetic predisposition.

Many other studies have addressed the various effects of hormones. In the hair follicle, these effects are not confined only to the matrix, since a hair consists of a complete pilosebaceous unit including the follicle and sebaceous gland. Since cultures of hair follicles have not been successful, hormonal control of the hair follicle has been considered in terms of the entire pilosebaceous unit. Furthermore, the best in vivo conditions for studying androgen metabolism in hair follicles are still not clearly defined.

6.2 Hormonal Control of the Sebaceous Gland

A hair follicle does not exist as an isolated structure; it is part of the whole pilosebaceous unit. The components of the pilosebaceous unit are subject to endocrine control and must be considered in association with one another.

The sebaceous gland plays a most important role in human hair development. This gland has been called an exocrine organ that supplies sebum, which prevents desiccation of skin and hair and bacterial invasion.

According to Inaba et al. (1981b,c), human hair regeneration begins from a point close to the secretory duct opening of the sebaceous gland (the upper isthmal portion of the hair follicle) (Fig. 3.12, regrowth of hair, hair germ stage). A fork-shaped nerve plexus is concentrated at the same site (Ishibashi and Tsuru 1976). These are additional elements of possible interest for any thorough discussion of the structure and function of the sebaceous gland.

Most mammals have sebaceous glands, which vary in number and size in different individuals. They are present all over the human body, except for the palms of the hands and the soles of the feet.

Most sebaceous glands are associated with hair follicles and empty their sebum content through a short duct into the follicular canal, making up one integrated unit, although there are certain exceptions. For instance, in the mucous membranes, the secretory duct opens on the surface of the skin or the mucous membrane itself, independent of the hair follicle.

Sebaceous glands are present in erogenous zones such as the mouth, cheek mucosa, mammary areolas, major and minor pudendal labia, glans penis, preputium, etc. The sebaceous glands in these areas originally coexisted with primordial hair follicles, which have since degenerated. Now only the sebaceous gland remains, and it functions independently.

The lipid product of the sebaceous gland (sebum) is formed by the activity of those cells located on the outermost layer of acini (group of secretory cells) located on the peripheral basement membrane. These particular cells are reproductive (germinal) cells, which rupture and discharge their contents into the secretory outflow in the form of sebum. When lipocyte differentiation occurs, the cellular nucleus shrinks and finally disappears.

With regard to the development of the hair follicle, we can see that the sebaceous gland and its environs are enclosed in connective tissue, as is the hair follicle. This tissue contains a grouping of capillary blood vessels connected to the dermal papilla of the lower hair follicle, integrating both dermal papilla and the sebaceous gland as one unit. This is another indication of the close relationship maintained between the sebaceous gland and the hair follicle. The increase in 5 α-reductase activity is partly a consequence of sebaceous gland enlargement (Dijkstra et al. 1987). DHT is bound to a specific cytosol receptor protein and transferred to the nuclear receptor, and is thus the factor regulating the action of androgens in the periphery. When DHT binding occurs, the mitotic activity of sebocytes is enhanced, resulting in hyperplasia of the sebaceous gland and an increased sebum excretion rate, and the activity of follicular matrix keratinocytes is modulated, being either activated, or inhibited. The endocrine control of the sebaceous gland is reviewed in Section 15.1.2.

6.3 Interaction Between the Sebaceous Gland and the Hair Follicle

In humans, the sebaceous gland is originally formed and begins to function in the fetus. It is quite well developed by the 3rd or 4th fetal month when body hair growth has begun. With maternal androgen stimulation received through placental infusion, the gland begins to develop in the embryonic stage.

Sebum, the product of the sebaceous gland, makes a significant contribution to the vernix caseosa (the sebum coating that covers the fetal body). After birth, these glands become involuted; they remain small throughout childhood until the onset of puberty, at which time they become enlarged. In some cases, this leads to outbreaks of acne vulgaris.

In the rat, the volume of the sebaceous glands also fluctuates in the same way; the hair and the glands are larger in the growth phase and smaller in catagen and telogen (Parnell 1949). A similar general reduction in the volume of sebaceous glands occurs during hair loss in alopecia areata (Moretti 1965) and pattern alopecia (Rampini et al. 1968).

6.3.1 Relationship of Sebum and Hair Growth (Inaba et al. 1981b)

Sebum production appears to be related to hair growth. For example, hair growth is scant and sebum production is decreased in people with panhypopituitarism (Goolamali et al. 1976; Pochi and Strauss 1974, 1977). By contrast, the mean level of sebum production was elevated in women with increased hair growth, in all subjects examined (Pochi and Strauss 1977).

6.4 Development of Axillary Hair

6.4.1 Increase of Axillary Hair Density

Human hair growth begins with fetal lanugo hair, then vellus hair, and finally mature, coarse terminal hair. In the human embryo, hair follicle development begins at the end of the 2nd month of fetal life and comes to an end in the 7th month. It has generally been accepted that there is no true neogenesis of human hair after birth.

Transformation of lanugo hair into vellus hair takes place in the fetal period. Vellus hair during childhood is thin and unmedullated. When puberty begins, these vellus hairs are replaced by coarse hairs that have visible pigmentation, and hair density seems to increase.

In order to examine this question of density, the authors conducted studies of the replacement of vellus hair by coarse hair in the human axilla (Inaba et al. 1981a). Under close examination it was observed that axillary hairs tended to emerge in a linear pattern along visible lines of creasing in the axillary epidermis (Fig. 6.1). Sebaceous glands were also seen in a linear pattern (Fig. 6.2). The number of hairs could be counted after they were trimmed close to the skin surface. With an exact count along a linear distance of 1.5 cm, a mean was determined, and this was used to relate hair density to factors of age and physical type.

Hamilton (1951b) had previously studied the relationship between axillary hair density and such factors as age and hormone levels by measuring the collective weight of axillary hair in various individuals.

In childhood, axillary hair, as well as the hair on the pubis and chin, is all vellus hair. These vellus hairs are all solitary and equidistant from one another. In puberty, they are replaced by coarse hairs. Our own studies (Inaba et al. 1981d) revealed that these coarse hairs replaced solitary vellus hairs in the form of groups of two to three coarse hairs in closely set ostia or in bundles of two more hairs within single ostia. Hairs in groups were more common in women, while bundles were more common in men. This dissimilarity may be due to different hormonal influences and to the greater amount of subcutaneous fatty tissue in the female axilla.

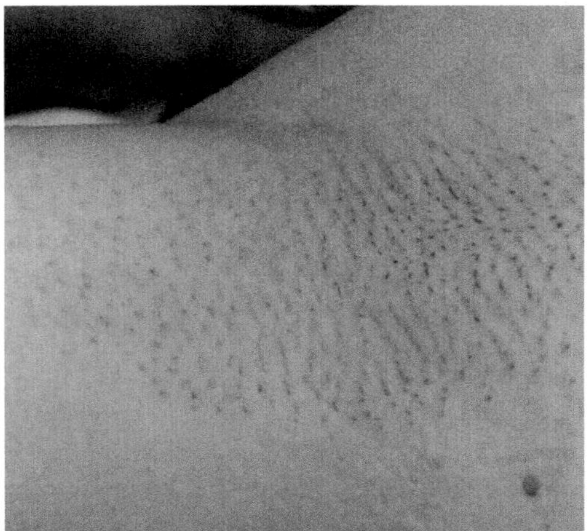

Fig. 6.1. Axillary hairs can be seen in a row

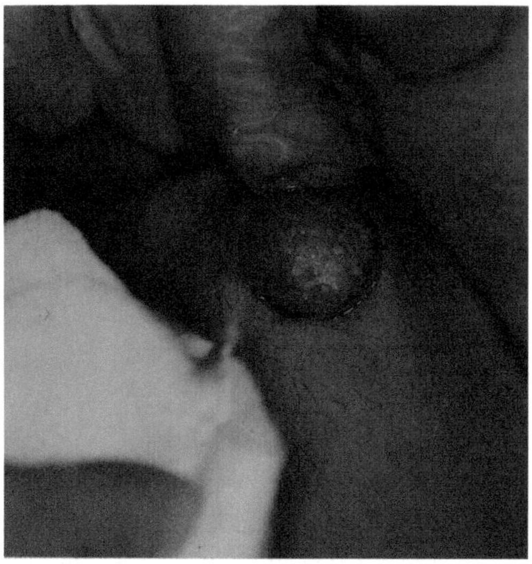

Fig. 6.2. Sebaceous glands can be seen in a row on the undersurface of the skin after tissue shaving

Further studies of axillary hair regeneration revealed that males in their thirties had the greatest numbers of axillary hairs. These numbers decreased in men older than 50 years. The rate of decrease for women over 50 was more remarkable (Inaba et al. 1980b; Inaba 1982a). In the human male, sebum secretion continues until around the age of 80, whereas in the female, it tends to decrease after the age of 50 (Pochi et al. 1963, 1979) (Figs. 6.3, 6.4a).

Women showed little change in the number of axillary hairs between the ages of 20 and 40, but there was a marked decrease after the age of 50 (Figs. 6.3, 6.4b).

An increase in sebaceous gland activity around the age of 8 is an early prepubertal phenomenon that is often the first signal of the onset of maturation (Pochi and Strauss 1977). In an earlier study, Pochi and Strauss (1965) reported data on sebum production throughout human life. At the ages of 6–12 years, the mean sebum production was 0.44 mg lipid/10sq cm/3 h in boys, while no sebum production was discernible in girls.

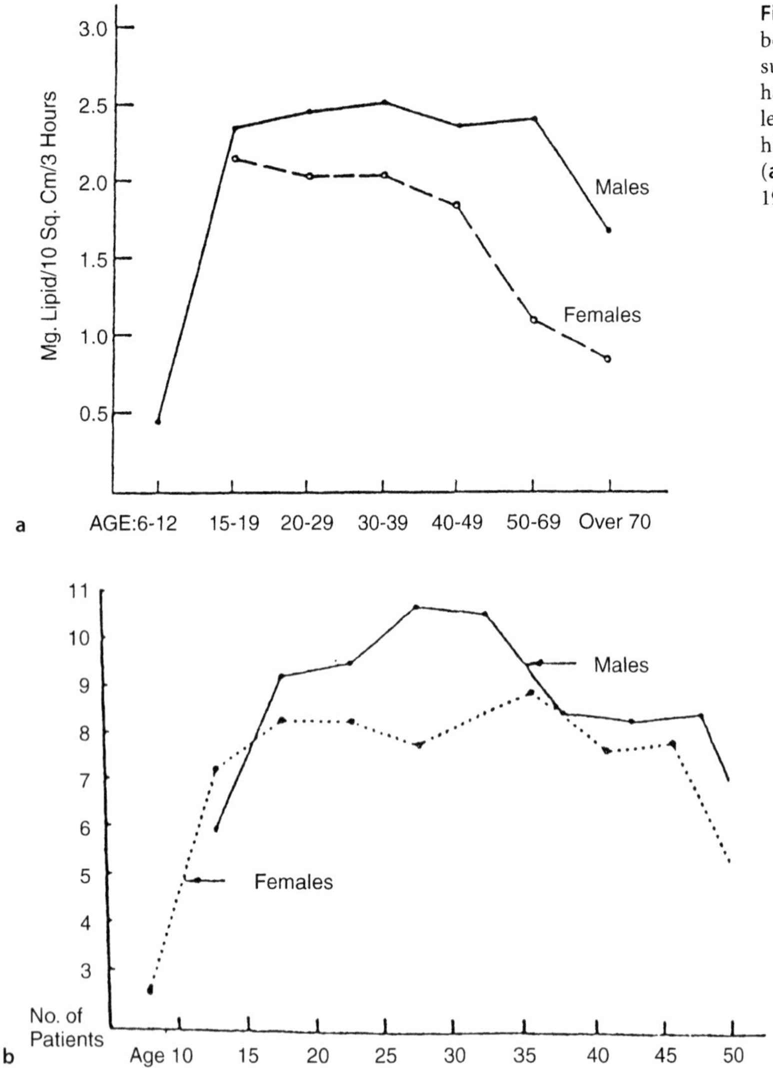

Fig. 6.3a,b. Relationship between age and sex, and **a** skin surface lipid levels. **b** Axillary hair growth. High skin lipid levels by age correspond to high levels of hair growth. (**a** From Pochi and Strauss 1974; **b** from Inaba 1985)

Sebaceous gland activity tends to remain stable for several decades of adult life, and is generally higher in men than in women. Sebum production in women, however, drops significantly in the age bracket of 50–59 years (Cunliffe and Cotterill 1975; Pochi and Strauss 1965; Pochi et al. 1979).

As mentioned above, the authors' findings indicate that sebaceous gland function is clearly and closely related to hair formation. In other words, the sebaceous gland is not a simple exocrine organ but also acts to promote and facilitate hair growth.

6.4.2 How Vellus Hair is Replaced by Coarse Hair (Inaba et al. 1981d)

At birth, the sebaceous glands are quite large and well developed and are distributed over the entire body. They have the same density patterns in various parts of the body that we observe in adults. The sebaceous glands continue to be active in the neonatal period under the lingering, persistent influence of placentally acquired maternal androgens, then become involuted and remain quiescent until the first emerging signs of the eventual onset of puberty (Ramastry et al. 1970; Solomon and Esterly 1970).

The lanugo hair, which is slightly longer than vellus hair, grows on the face, the shoulder, and other areas. In the fetus, both the scalp and forehead are covered by lanugo hair, without a clear scalp-forehead borderline. With the cessation of placental hormone infusion after birth, the enlarged sebaceous glands characteristic of the fetus begin to gradually shrink in size. At the same time,

Fig. 6.5. **a** Sebaceous gland is multilobular. Vellus hair cannot be seen. ×440 **b** High-power view of a sebaceous gland appended to the vellus hair which has become larger; the vellus hair follicle has become multilobular, and the vellus hair itself has died. ×600

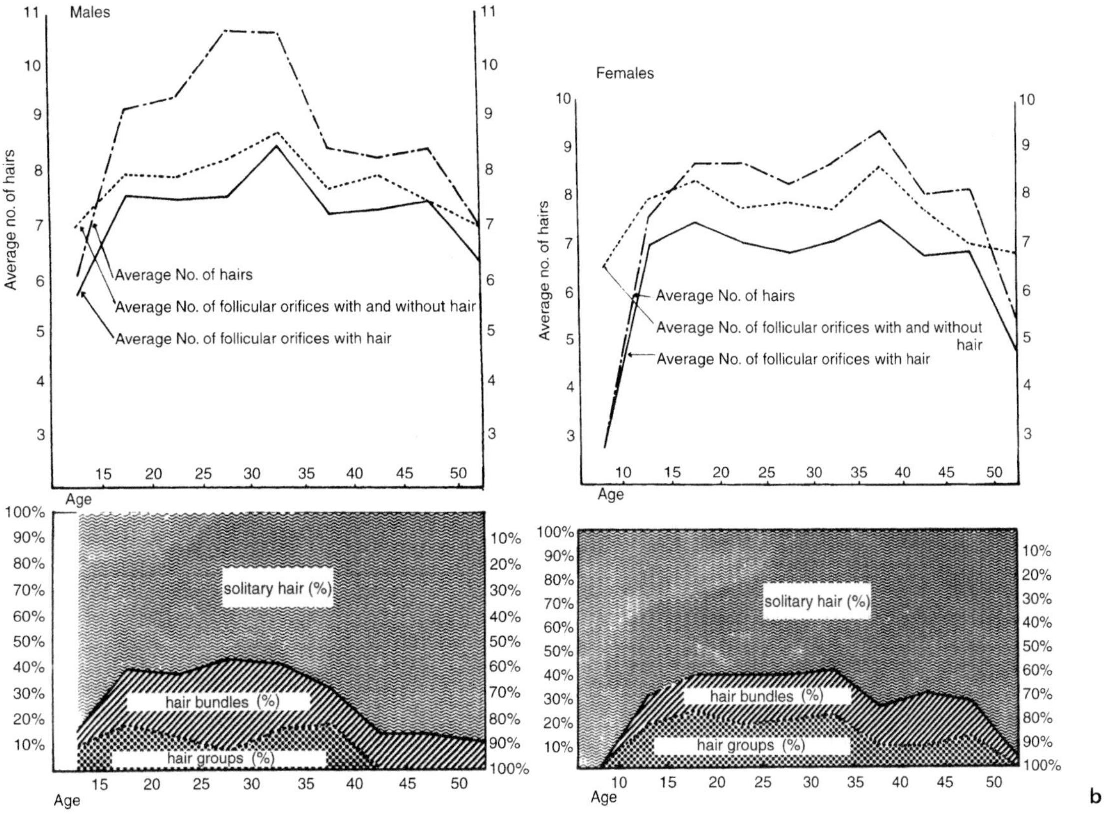

Fig. 6.4a,b. Average numbers of axillary hairs **a** in males, **b** in females. **a** *Upper panel*: in males, the number of axillary hairs is greatest in their thirties. *Lower panel* shows the proportions of solitary hairs, hair bundles, and hair groups. **b** Average number of axillary hairs in females is greatest in their forties. Women show little change in numbers of axillary hairs between the ages of 20 and 40, but there is a marked decrease after the age of 50

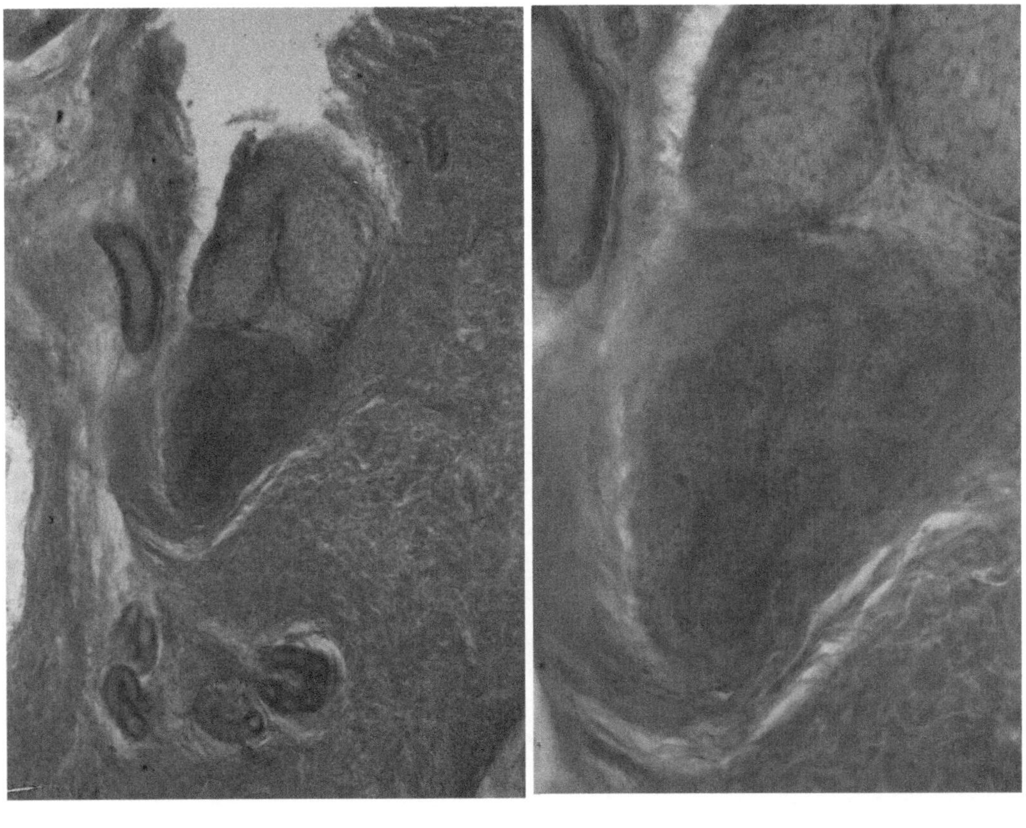

lanugo hair vanishes during infancy and childhood, and the hair borderline above the forehead becomes perfectly distinct. With the onset of puberty the sebaceous glands are once again remarkably enlarged and take on a multilobular shape similar to that of a bell pepper (Fig. 6.5).

At this time, we observe the growth of coarse, androgen-dependent axillary, pubic, beard, and other body hair. It is evident that androgen acts not only on the hair bulb (matrix) but that it also causes this enlargement of the sebaceous gland. Its secondary effect on the matrix prompts the growth of coarse terminal hairs to replace existing vellus hairs.

In a detailed histologic study of the replacement of vellus hair by coarse hair in the axilla, the authors found that, in childhood, all androgen-dependent hair is vellus hair. In puberty, this vellus hair is replaced by coarse hair. As mentioned above, the vellus hairs of childhood are solitary and equidistant from one another. The process by which they are replaced may be related to the increased keratinization in the sebaceous isthmus due to hypertrophy of the sebaceous gland (Morohashi 1968), and this replacement occurs in puberty in a manner thoroughly different from that in the ordinary hair cycle in which expired hairs periodically are replaced by new hairs.

As the sebaceous glands appended to the vellus hair become hypertrophic, the vellus hair follicle becomes multilobular and the vellus hair itself expires. Formation of a new hair bud and a new coarse hair seems to begin from the sebaceous isthmus portion of the follicle adjacent to the opening of the sebaceous duct (Fig. 6.6a), and the new young coarse hair is formed by aggregations of filaments produced from the surrounding germinal layer in the peg stage (Fig. 6.6b). The new hair pegs downward until the formation of a new hair bulb (matrix) is fully completed, and it then grows upward toward the epidermis surface as a coarse terminal hair.

6.4.3 Hair Density Increases After Birth (Inaba et al. 1980b, 1982)

Lanugo hair grows densely during the fetal period, with new primary or secondary hair follicles formed among the first follicles as the infant's skin surface expands. The secondary follicles develop on either side of the preexisting follicles, and usually form groups of three (Fig. 3.4).

In most mammals that have been studied, normal additional hair follicles do not appear to be formed after the complete number of adult follicles has been formed. In humans also, the generally accepted opinion is that true neogenesis of hair does not occur throughout life, but ceases after the 7th month of fetal life. If this is so, what is the mechanism that underlies the remarkable increase in the density of terminal hair during and after the adolescent years?

Axillary, pubic, and some other body hair emerges as a secondary sex characteristic in both human males and females with the beginning of puberty. If no other follicles are formed, the final number of mature terminal hairs, thus spread far apart, would seem quite sparse. But in fact the growth is quite dense. This seems to indicate that new follicles and hairs are formed, but there has been little evidence to support this supposition in the past.

One of the authors and colleagues (Inaba et al. 1981d) have reported that, in childhood, vellus hairs in the axillary region are formed as individual units equidistant from one another. As puberty begins, coarse hairs emerge in bundles and groups to replace the vellus hairs. In the mature individual, solitary hairs account for 65% of all coarse axillary hairs, with hairs in bundles accounting for 17%–22% and those in groups for the remaining 12%–18% (Fig. 6.4a,b).

6.4.4 Development of Hair Bundle

The authors found that, when two or more new hairs form in a single hair canal, the result is a hair bundle. The phenomenon begins at the stage in which there is a common canal in which two or more individual hair follicles are conjoined at the neck of the canal of a primary follicle. We describe two cases below.

6.4.4.1 Case 1

Using thick tissue preparations, we studied the dynamic process by which a bundle follicle is formed in place of a vellus hair follicle; we found the phenomena shown in the micrographs in Fig. 6.7a,b and in the diagram in Fig. 6.7c. The sebaceous gland of a disappearing vellus hair has hypertrophied and has developed three distinct lobes (*a*, *b*, and *c* in Fig. 6.7c) conjoined at a common neck at the excretory duct in the central area. The point where lobes *a* and *b* are conjoined is the site of a disappearing vellus hair; a new primary central original (PCO) coarse hair follicle descends from the neck of the gland between the lobes labeled *a* and *b*. One secondary lateral (SL) follicle has formed in lobe *c* and is pegging downward from the upper isthmal portion. These two new follicles become multilobular. A mass of mesenchymal tissue can be observed at the lower tip of each follicle, which indicates that the bulb has not

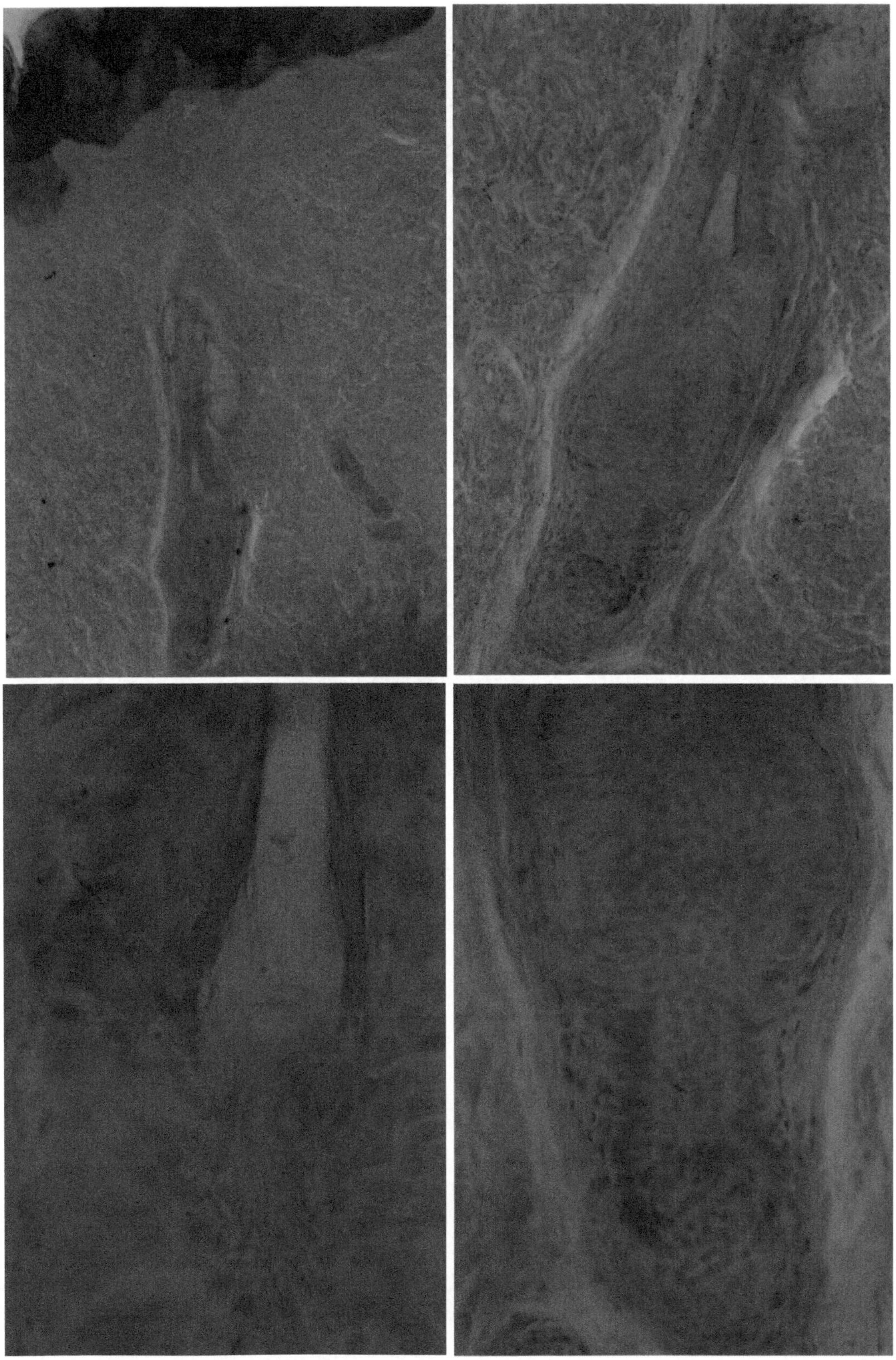

a b c d

Fig. 6.6. **a** Formation of a new hair bud, descending, and a new coarse hair beginning to form from the sebaceous isthmus of the follicle. **b** High-power view of a new young coarse hair formed by the aggregation of filaments produced from the surrounding germinal layer. ×400 **c** Lower portion of new coarse hair. No melanin granules can be seen. This hair is different from the club hair in the catagen stage. **d** Lower portion of the hair follicle. New bud descends downward. The mesenchymal cells can be seen at the lower tip of the bud. No melanin granules can be seen as in the catagen hair follicle. ×400

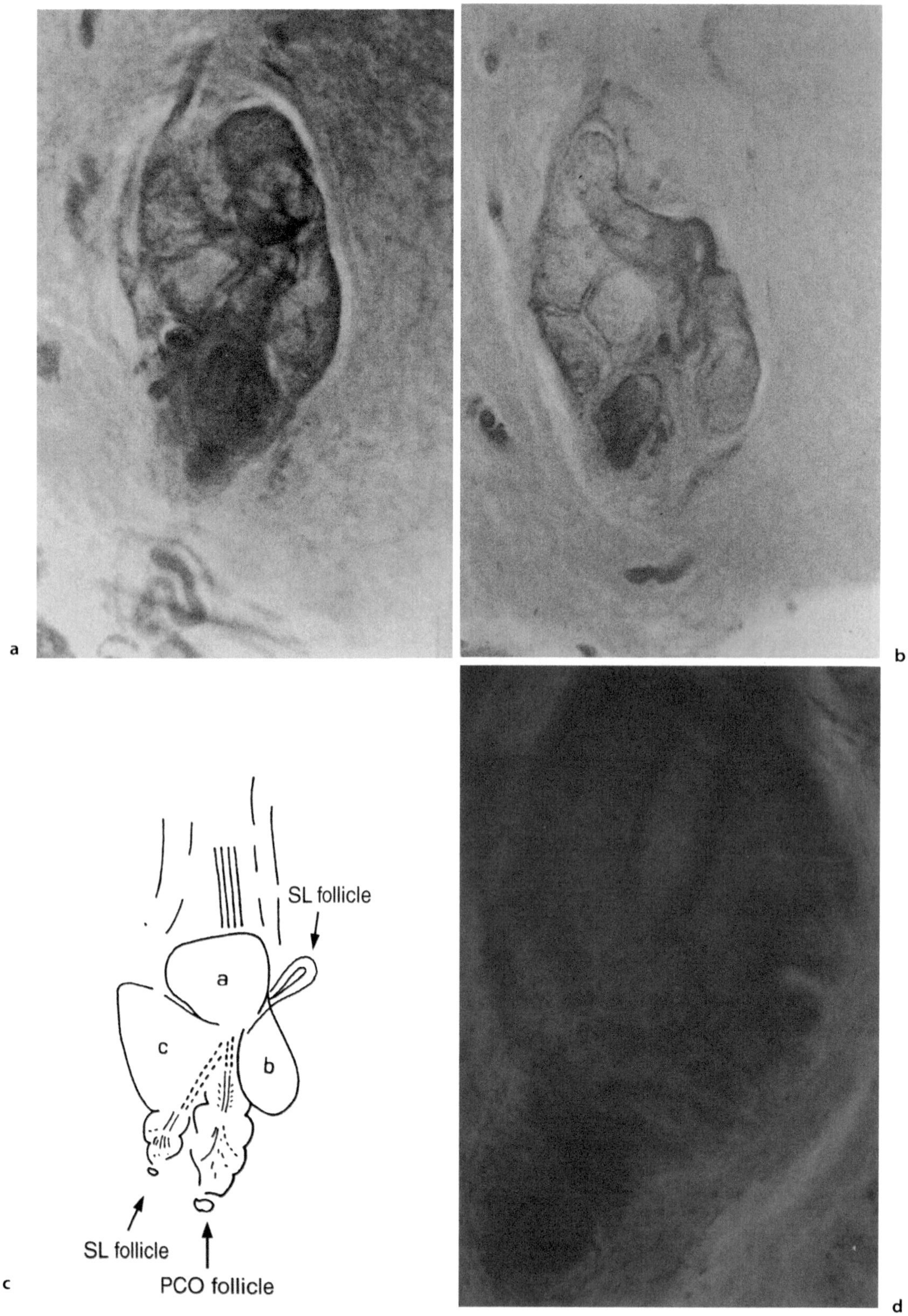

Fig. 6.7. **a** The sebaceous gland of a disappearing vellus hair has become hypertrophied and is divided into three distinct lobes. A new primary central coarse hair follicle is seen descending from the neck of the gland between the lobes labeled *a* and *b* in **c**. **b** A secondary later follicle is shown forming and descending from the sebaceous isthmus of the original follicle. This corresponds to *c* in **c**. ×400 **c** Schematic of development of lobulation of a vellus hair follicle on the way to producing follicles that will bear coarse hairs. *PCO*, Primary central original; *SL*, secondary lateral. **d** High-power view of PCO follicle. A new coarse hair is shown forming within a new epithelial sac. ×400 **e** The new primary and secondary lateral follicles of coarse hairs are shown to share a common canal in the sebaceous isthmus above the sebaceous gland. ×400

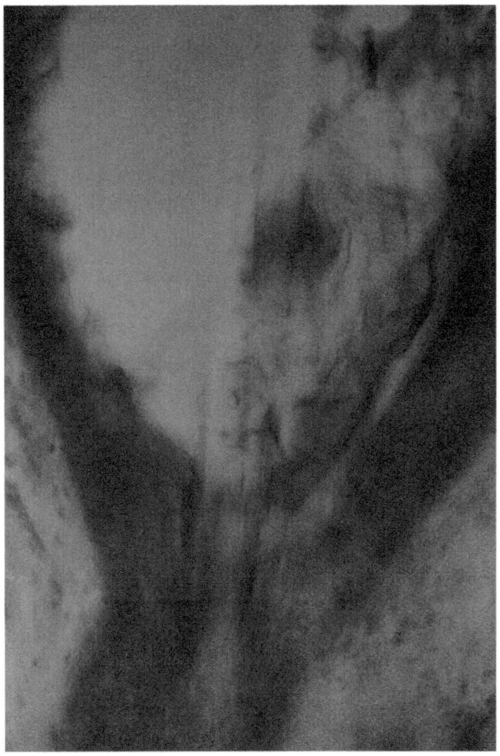

e

Fig. 6.7. *Continued*

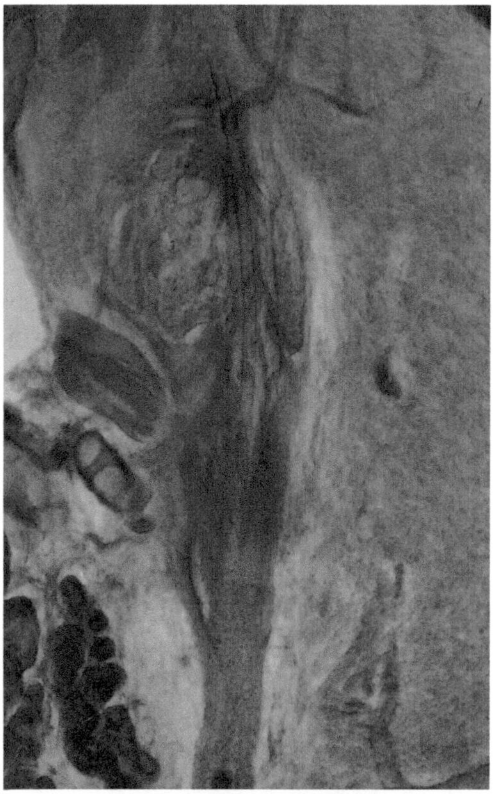

a

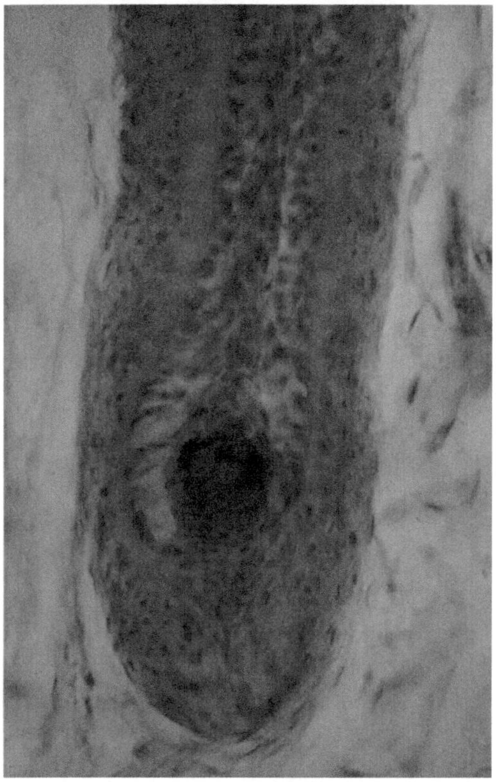

b

Fig. 6.8. **a** The primary central original follicle (*PCO*) is shown in the catagen stage. **b** Lower catagen follicle, showing epithelial strand. **c** A secondary lateral follicle (*SL*) has formed from the sebaceous isthmus of the original central follicle in its descending stage. The follicle shares the neck of the sebaceous gland with the new primary central follicle. **d** The SL also shares the neck of the sebaceous gland with the new primary central follicle. **e** Schematic showing the events shown in **a**, **b**, **c**, and **d**. **f** Nonhuman hair. Stages in the development of an original secondary wool follicle (*O*) in the skin of a merino sheep fetus. Also shown are some derived secondary follicles (*D*) in various stages of development. (After Hardy and Lyne 1956a, 1956b, and Chapman 1990, with permission from Springer-Verlag)

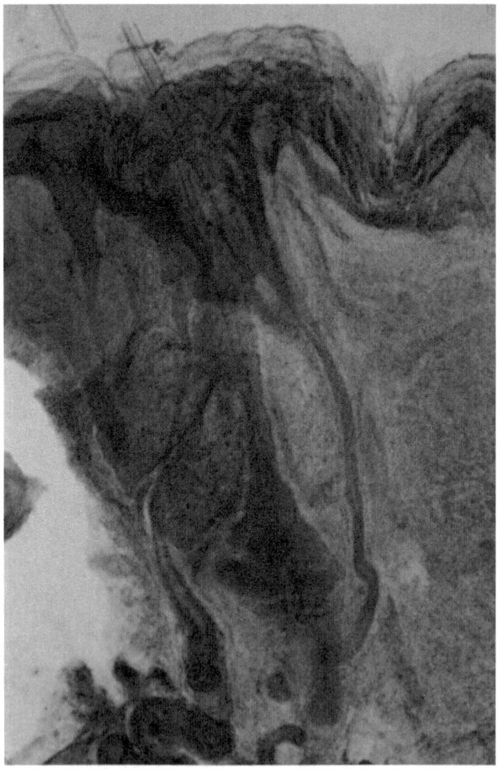

c

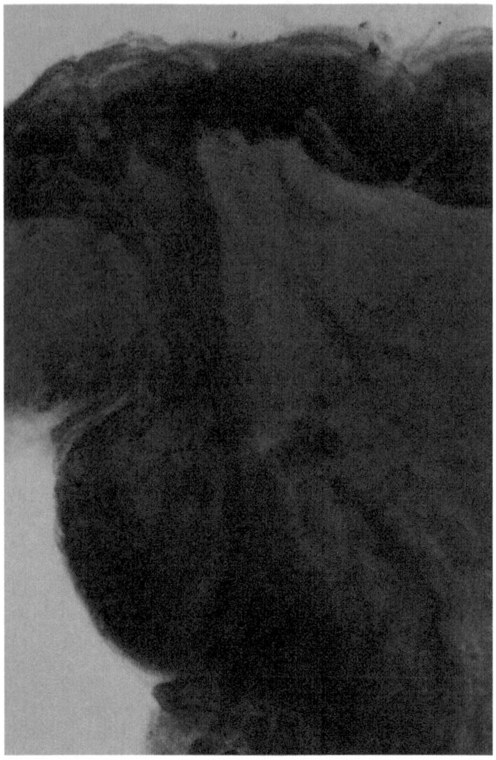

d

Fig. 6.8. *Continued*

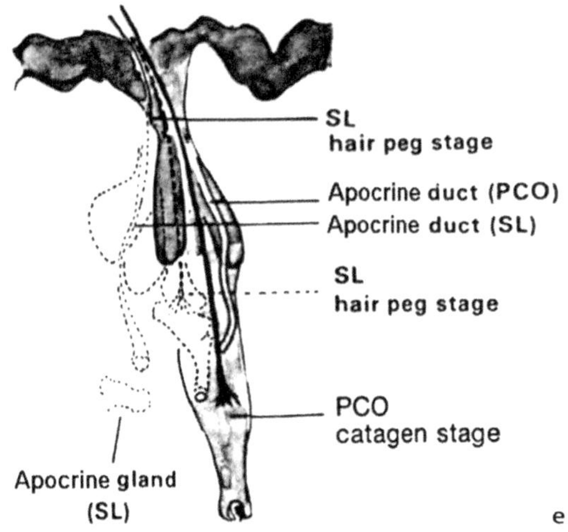

e

yet formed (Fig. 6.7d). A filamentous structure has been formed from the epithelial cells in the lower portion of the follicle. The new coarse hairs (PCO follicle) have already begun to form in the hair follicle (Fig. 6.7d).

In Fig. 6.7e, the two new coarse hairs can be seen to share a common canal in the upper isthmal portion, above the sebaceous gland; no traces of melanin granules were detected in the hair cortex, an indication that this is not the cortex of the former vellus hair or a telogen hair.

6.4.4.2 Case 2

The same phenomena and dynamics are again illustrated in more advanced stages in Fig. 6.8a–d. A schema is shown in Fig. 6.8e.

As in case 1, the sebaceous gland has separated into three lobes. The cervical regions of each lobe have gathered at the upper isthmal portion of the PCO follicle. From each of the lobulized sebaceous glands, a new hair will be formed, by the same mechanism as that described above, and this will be present in the upper isthmal portion of the PCO follicle. In other words, the PCO follicle, as seen in Fig. 6.8a, is in catagen stage. Two hair follicles, SL1 and SL2, have formed from the sebaceous isthmus; that is, the upper isthmal portion of the PCO follicle can be observed at this stage. These follicles have become multilobular, epithelial strands extend in their lower portion, and a mass of mesenchymal cells is recognized in the lower end

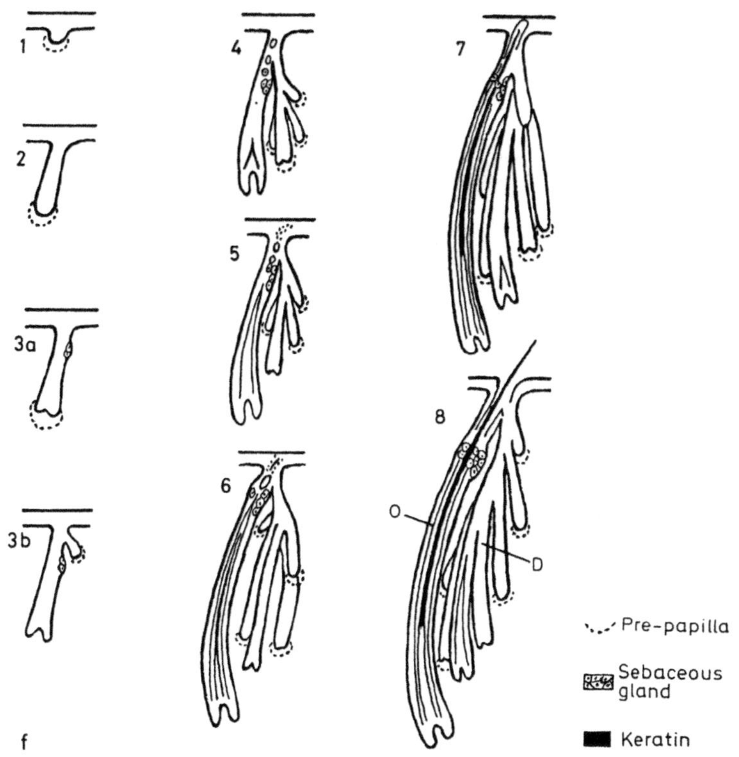

Fig. 6.8. *Continued*

portion. A three-dimensional view is shown in Fig. 6.8e. When the sebaceous gland becomes lobulized, new hairs will be formed according to the number of lobes, and these will be present in the same isthmal portion. In some species, further follicles, known as derived follicles, develop as branches from the outer root sheath of original follicles. The stages of development are the same as for the original follicles except that stage 1 applies to the initial outgrowth from the outer root sheath. When fully developed, the hairs in the derived follicles generally share a common orifice with that in the original follicle. Branching occurs on both primary and secondary follicles in marsupials (Lyne 1957, 1959), on primary follicles in dogs (Lovell and Getty 1957) and on secondary follicles in sheep (Tänzer 1926; Hardy and Lyne 1956a) (reviewed from Chapman 1990). See Section 4.8 in this chapter for further detail.

Figure 6.8f shows the development of secondary follicles in non-human hair.

6.4.5 Hair Grouping

The lobes of the sebaceous gland begin to separate due to the expansion of the skin surface. In this process of lobular separation, the trichilemma also separates. In this early phase, however, the separate hairs still occupy a common orifice at the surface of the skin (Fig. 6.9a,b). The orifice gradually widens, perhaps owing to rapid expansion of the skin surface during puberty. In an upper section at this stage, we found that the lobes of the multilobular sebaceous gland had begun to separate (Fig. 6.9a,b). There was a new hair in the PCO and new hairs in the SL to either side. Photographically in Fig. 6.9c and diagrammatically in Fig. 6.9d, the lower portion of the central follicle is clearly shown to have become multilobular.

From this point on, and with the expansion of the skin surface, the new hair follicles and appendages become separate and independent. Photographically in Fig. 6.10a,d and diagrammatically in Fig. 6.10c, the middle follicle, which corresponds to the PCO, appears to be in the terminal hair stage. Melanin granules can now be seen clearly in the cortex of the new hair. The lower portion of the follicle is a typical bulb. In the cortex of the secondary lateral follicle of Fig. 6.10d, melanin granules, although fewer in number, can also be seen. The lower portion of this follicle is becoming bulb-like. There are not many melanin granules in the cortex above this bulb. The secondary lateral follicle at the left in this figure is still in the hair peg stage.

6.4.6 Development of the Secondary Follicle Group

Development of the secondary follicle group due to the physical expansion of the skin surface during adolescence gradually ceases. The separation of follicles pulled apart by expansion accordingly

a

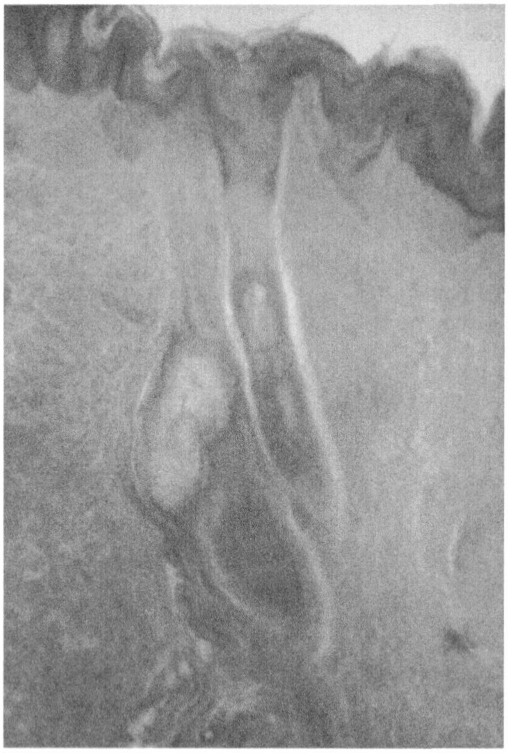

b

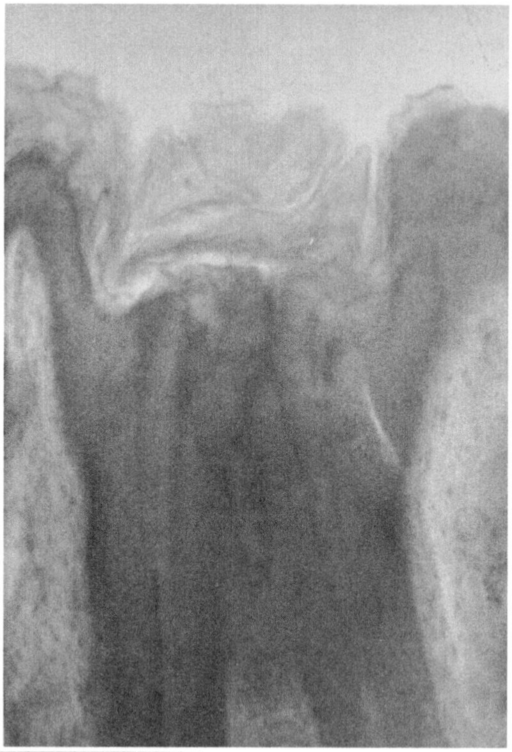

c

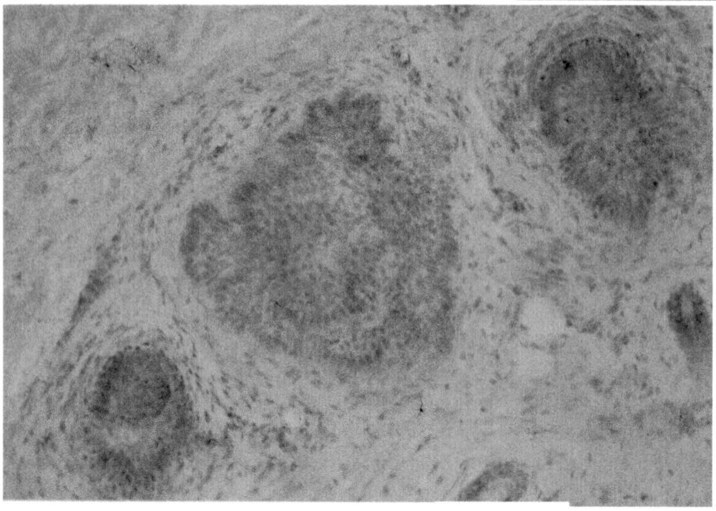

d

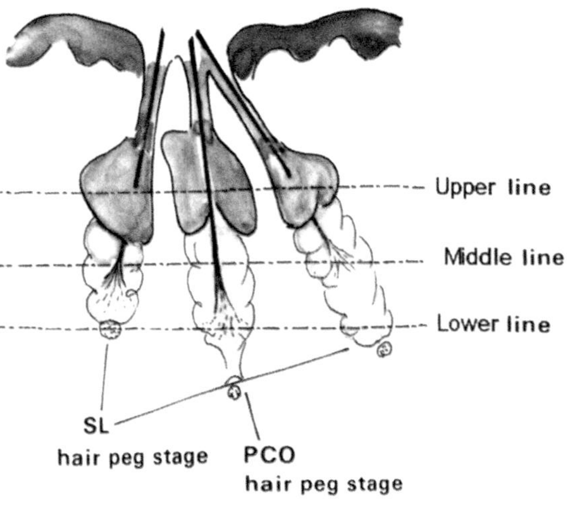

Fig. 6.9. a Lobes of the multilobular sebaceous gland have begun to separate. The common trichilemma has also begun to separate. ×135 **b** Enlargement of the orifice. The orifice itself has expanded and the separation of the trichilemma is clearly shown. ×200 **c** Cross sections of a primary central follicle and secondary lateral follicles are shown at a point of the lower portion of three hairs (**d**, *lower line*). The new young hairs in the peg stage have not yet descended to the level of terminal hairs. ×400 **d** Stage of common orifice but separated trichilemma

a 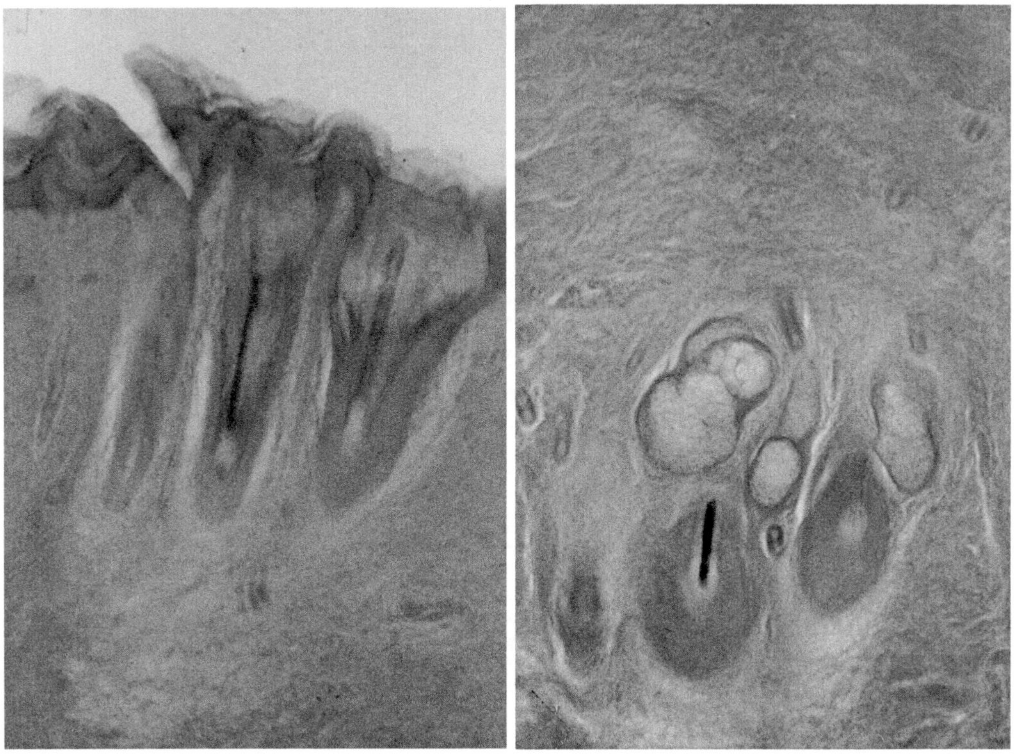 b

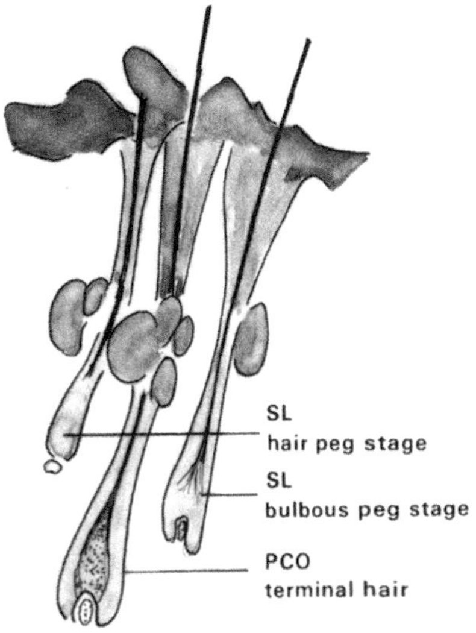

c

Fig. 6.10. **a** The trichilemma has separated at the surface of the skin, and the three follicles have begun to draw apart. ×135 **b** The new hair follicles and the lobes of their sebaceous gland have fully separated. A terminal hair is visible in the primary central follicle. ×135 **c** Stage of separated follicle. A schematic of the events shown in **a** and **b**. **d** Cross section of the lobes of the sebaceous gland showing them starting to separate. This corresponds to the *upper line* in Fig. 6.9d. ×200 **e** High-power view of the lower portion of trio group hair follicles. Cross sections of PCO and two SL are shown. The central PCO follicle is terminal hair. Both SL follicles are in the peg stage. Multilobular findings are clear. ×400

comes to an end. The sebaceous glands of the follicles once again become hypertrophic and multilobular. New hairs may again be formed from the upper isthmal portions of the PCO and the SL follicles, and then from the secondary lateral-derived follicle (SLD).

6.4.6.1 Case 1

A trio group has been formed and three separate hair follicle groups can be observed (Fig. 6.11a). In the central group, the PCO has become terminal hair, the melanin granules are clearly visible, and the secondary central-derived follicle (SCD) can also be observed. It appears to be in the bulbous peg stage. In the hair on the left, the SL can be seen; it appears to be a terminal hair. Above it, the SLD is observed; this is, presumably, in the hair germ stage.

In the hair group on the right side (Fig. 6.11a), the SL and the SLD can be seen. Also, in each trio,

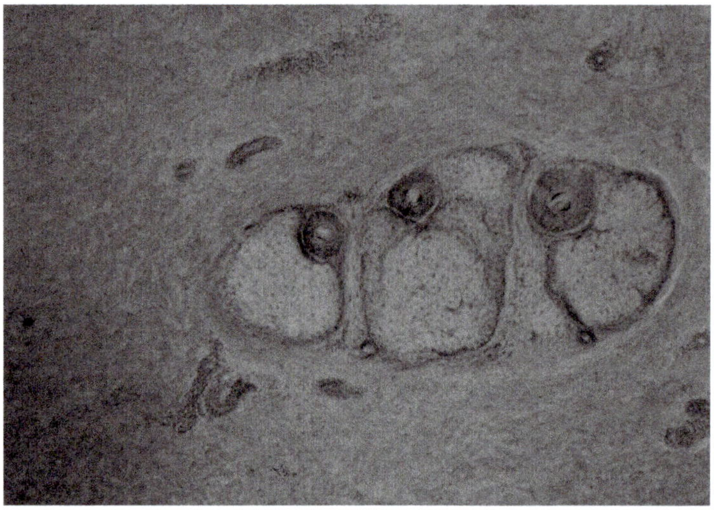

d

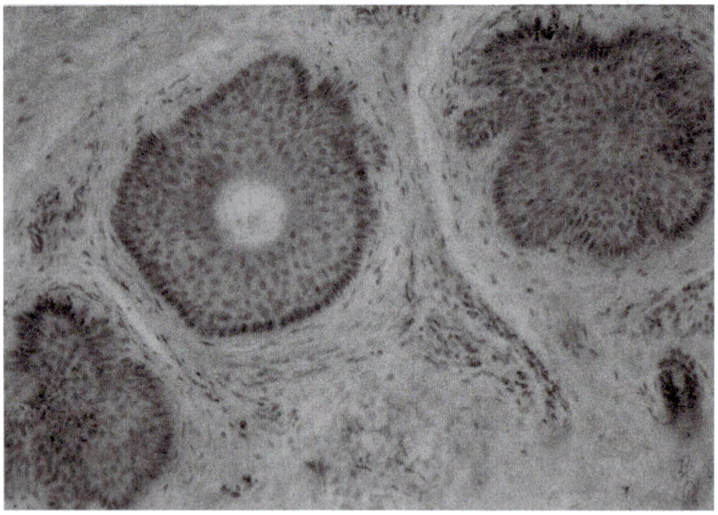

e

Fig. 6.10. *Continued*

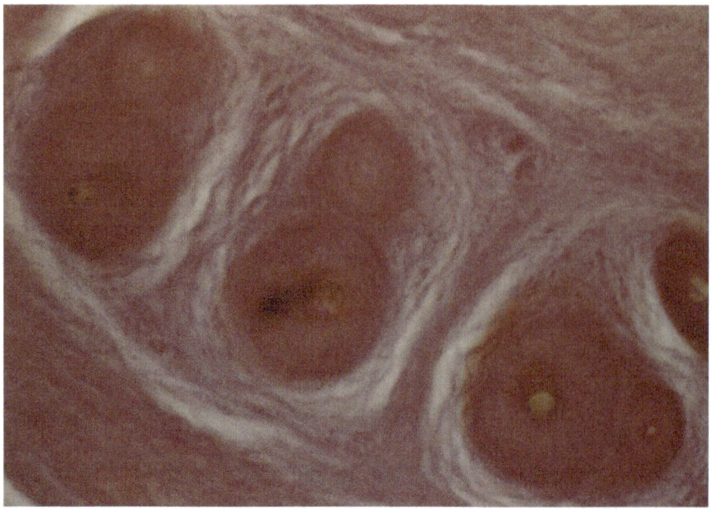

a

Fig. 6.11. **a** Case 1. This micrograph clearly shows the separation of the different follicles as a result of the process shown in Fig. 6.10. ×200 **b** Case 1. High-power view of part of the micrograph shown in **a**, also in cross section. The bundle of three hairs formed in the center of the lower trichilemma (*dark circle*) can be seen. ×400 **c** Stages of development in the secondary follicle group. *SLD*, Secondary lateral-derived follicle; *SCD*, secondary central-derived follicle

Fig. 6.11. *Continued*

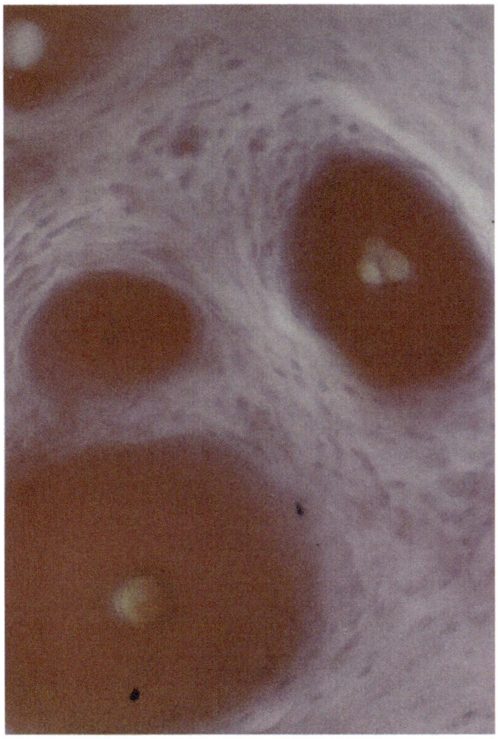

b

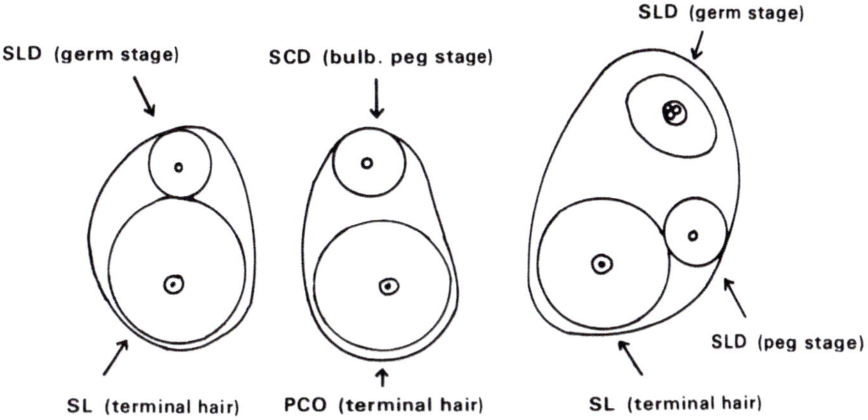

c

a cross section of the apocrine gland can be observed. Figure 6.11b shows an enlarged view of the group of the secondary lateral follicle, in which SLDs can be recognized. In the upper SLD, three germ hairs are observed. A diagrammatic view is shown in Fig. 6.11c.

6.4.6.2 Case 2 (Fig. 6.12a,b)

A trio group has been formed. The trio shown in Fig. 6.12a appears similar to that in case 1.

6.4.6.3 Case 3 (Fig. 6.13)

In secondary follicle groups SL and SLD hairs can clearly be seen.

6.4.7 Increase of Density of Coarse Hair

During puberty, due to hormonal stimulation, the vellus hair of the axillary and pubic areas is replaced by coarse hair. In a previous report (Inaba et al. 1982), we described our clinical findings in regard to the increase of density of coarse hair and identified three types of hair formation: solitary hairs, hair bundles, and hair groups. We suggested that hair grouping occurs after hair bundling, when the bundles are pulled apart by the tension and expansion of the skin as the skin surface is expanded due to the physical growth of the body during adolescence. Some hair bundling, however, persists into maturity in the form of two or more

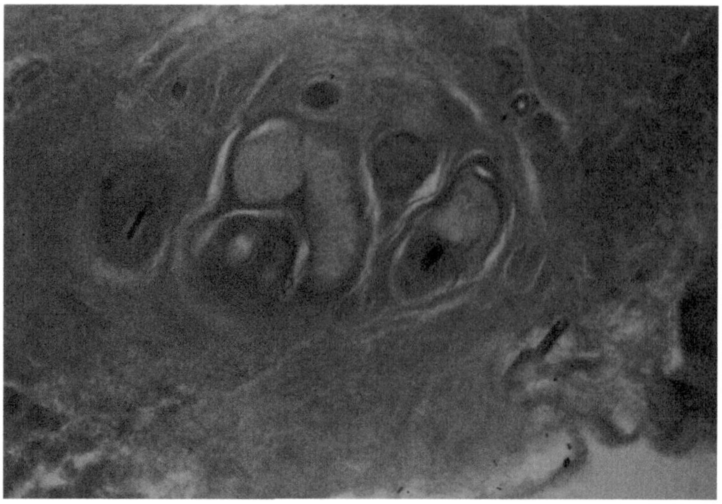

a

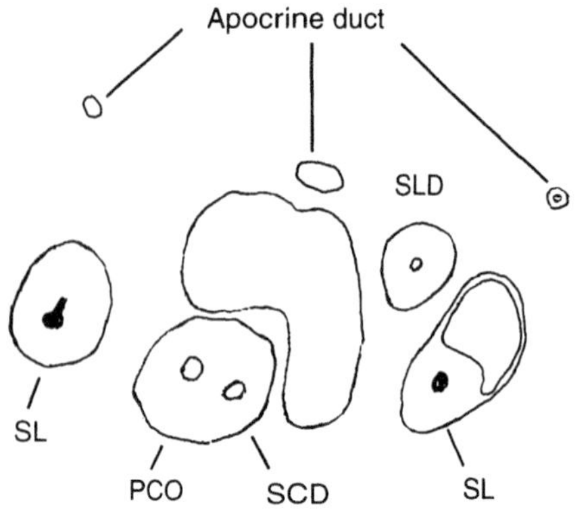

b

Fig. 6.12. **a** Case 2. A secondary follicle grows. SL and SLD hairs can clearly be seen. ×200 **b** Development of secondary follicle group; schematic of events shown in **a**

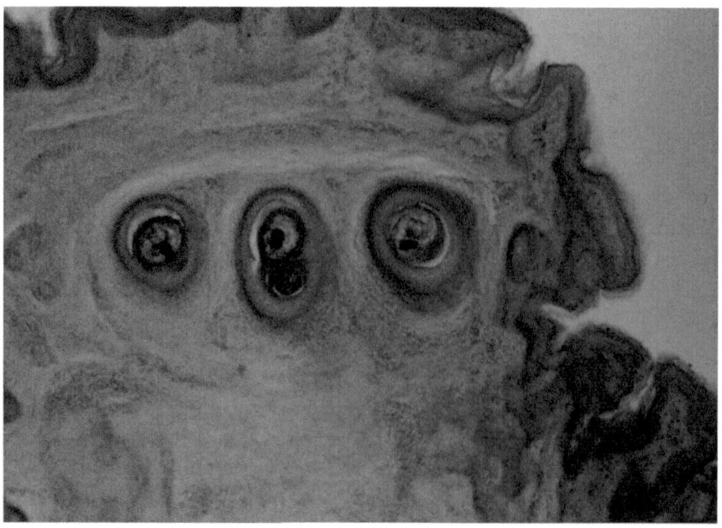

Fig. 6.13. Case 3. A secondary follicle grows. SL and SLD hairs can clearly be seen. ×200

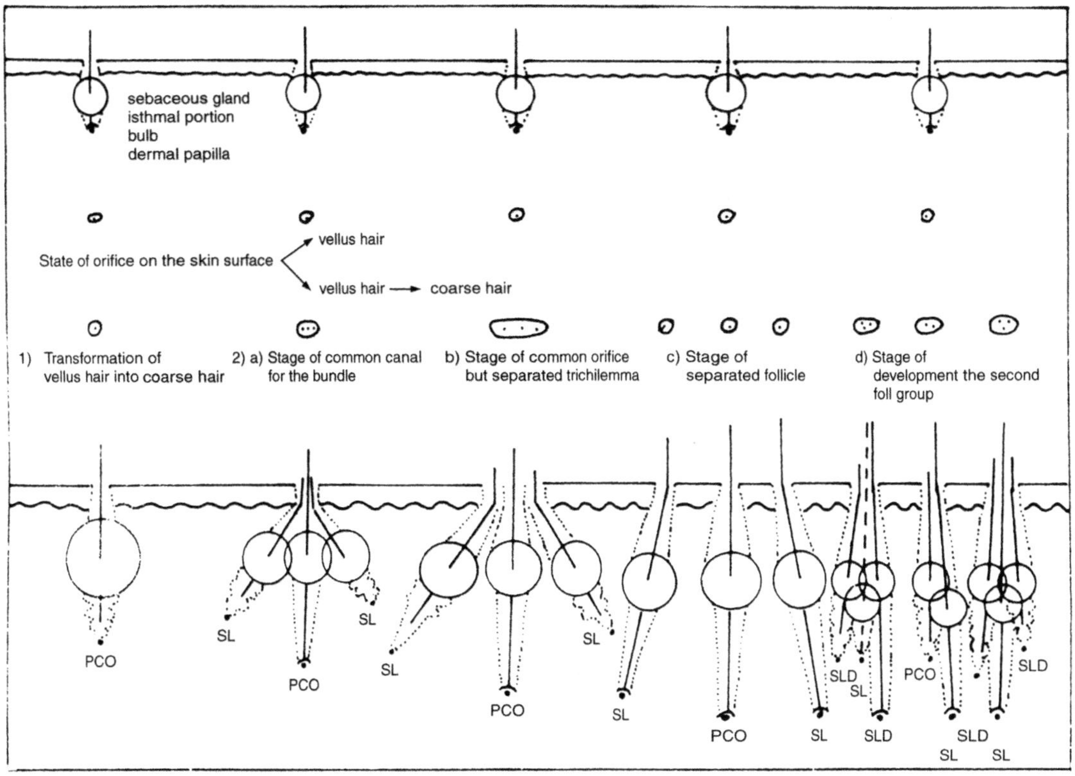

Fig. 6.14. Formation of coarse hair from vellus hair. *PCO*, Primary central original follicle; *SL*, secondary lateral follicle; *SCD*, secondary central-derived follicle; *SLD*, secondary lateral-derived follicle; *St.*, stage. (Reproduced from Inaba 1985)

coarse hairs emerging from a common pillar ostium.

In summary, during puberty and early adulthood, vellus hairs in the axillae disappear and are replaced by coarse hairs in greater density by a series of histologically discernible steps (shown in Fig. 6.14):

1. The vellus hairs of childhood are solitary and equidistant from one another.
2. The sebaceous glands of vellus hair follicles become hypertrophic and sometimes multilobular due to hormonal influence, and the vellus hair itself dies. New coarse hairs spring from the upper isthmal portion, close to the duct opening of simple hypertrophic sebaceous glands.
3. The new coarse hairs from multilobular glands first develop in bundles of two or more that emerge from a common ostium. In time, some bundles of hairs come to have separate ostia from which each coarse hair emerges independently; other bundles of two or more hairs persist in emergence from a common ostium. Individual hairs are also formed from the secondary derived follicles.

The overall effect is the replacement of vellus hair by coarse hair in greater abundance and density.

6.4.8 Review of the Development of Bundle (Compound) Hair Follicles

de Meijere (1894) observed hair grouping in marsupials. Later, Sweet (1907) observed it in *Notaryctes typhlops* Stirling, while Gibbs (1938) reported it in *Trichosurus vulpecula*. Saito et al. (1976) reported that in humans it could be seen in both vellus and coarse hair. Takashima and Kawagishi (1975) reported it in the scalps of Japanese subjects.

Until the present time, the development of bundle (compound) hair follicles has been considered to follow de Meijere's (1894) classification of hair bundles, or compound follicles, into false and real types:

i. False bundles had a short common follicle and branched into separate follicles above the duct opening of the sebaceous glands. de Meijere believed that these bundles were formed by the fusion of follicles which initially were quite separate.

ii. Real bundles originated by budding and a common follicle extended to below the duct opening of the sebaceous glands. Several of the stages in the development of a secondary wool follicle, as described by Hardy and Lyne (1956a,b) and by Chapman (1990), are illustrated in Fig. 6.8f.

These stages are similar to those of a primary follicle, in that no apocrine sweat gland or erector muscle is formed. The first derived secondary follicle appears as a secondary follicle. Branching is usually at or above the sebaceous glands, but may be below them. Observations to date suggest that most of these bundles are formed by the branching of the follicles in the fetus, although, in merino sheep, some of the original secondary follicles, particularly those earliest to develop, never branch. At birth, the branching of secondary follicles is extensive, although many are still immature. In the bandicoot *Perameles nasuta*, these branches arise immediately below the level of the sebaceous gland duct, and develop fairly slowly. The derived follicles then develop rapidly and the original canal becomes the common hair canal for the bundle. More derived follicles arise later by budding, and bundles with from two to five hairs are common (Lyne 1957).

In most species, the hair follicles are arranged in groups. The only comprehensive guide to the arrangement of hair follicles is the study by de Meijere (1894), in which he concluded that there was a basic trio grouping of one larger hair with two smaller ones on either side. In many species, the germs of the first hair follicles appear as isolated structures without any apparent order. However, these follicle primordia are not located at random with respect to one another. In the earliest stages, one follicle apparently inhibits the formation of another. We do not know why two of these follicles, now and then, should not originate close together. Later, each of these first-formed follicles will be the central member of a different hair follicle group.

In sheep, the fibers in the bundles of branching secondary follicles emerge through a common orifice (Hardy and Lyne 1956b), which, however, is separate from those of the associated primary and secondary fibers. This contrasts with the arrangements in the dog and cat (Ellenberger 1906; Strickland and Calhoun 1963). Among adult primates, a variety of follicle arrangements has been observed, some of which have obvious trio groupings (reviewed from Hardy and Lyne 1956a).

How the trio group is formed after the formation of the SL on both sides of the primary PCO remains unclear. The authors have studied the process of the generation of the fetal eyebrow in order to clarify this point (Inaba et al. 1979c), and found that the hair germ from the epidermis would form a trio group. However, the authors suggested at the same time, that in some follicle groups, hair grouping was brought about by hair bundling (Inaba et al. 1980b); i.e., we observed in about 15% of the groups that they had been formed from vellus hairs, and reported that this phenomenon was secondarily caused by the physical expansion of the skin surface with growth. We also found that this phenomenon of grouping gradually ceased and the sebaceous gland became multilobular to form new hairs. This phenomenon of grouping is observed not only in the axillary region but also in the scalp. Also of note, this finding of grouping as a result of bundling explains why, in the early stage of androgenetic alopecia, the scalp becomes visible as single hair groups are formed as a result of bundling (see Chapter 21).

Hair Regeneration

7

7.1 Hair Cycles

Complete replacement of all hairs on the human head with new hairs, through the hair cycle, takes about 5–7 years. The anagen stage lasts several years, the catagen a few weeks, and the telogen several months. Other hair cycles, such as those for the eyelash and the axilla, average 150 and 123 days, respectively (Fig. 7.1).

The number of hairs and their distribution and patterns of growth are the same in men and women. The difference is qualitative. In young adults, regardless of sex, 90% of the 100 000–150 000 scalp hairs are regarded as growing and 10% as resting. This means that 10 000–15 000 follicles are quiescent for about 100 days, and about 100 club hairs would be shed per day (Kligman 1961; Orentreich 1969).

In human hairs, the anagen, catagen, and telogen stages are not simultaneous for all hairs, but occur in a mixed (mosaic) pattern of hair growth which forms combinations at various stages, i.e., a certain number of mature hairs are always present on the scalp or elsewhere. Other mammals which have this pattern include the cat and the guinea pig. Those animals which have almost simultaneous loss and synchronous replacement of all hairs include the mouse, rabbit, and rat. Still other mammals have hair growth without cycle activity. In this case, hairs are not lost but simply continue to grow. Sheep and angora rabbits belong to this class.

Unfortunately, human beings do not belong to this last class and they experience cyclic hair loss. In extreme cases, this hair loss signifies the end of the mature hair cycle itself and the onset of androgenetic alopecia.

7.1.1 Common Hair Cycle (Fig. 7.1a)

7.1.1.1 Anagen Stage

In the active or anagen stage, the dermal papilla, located at the base of the fully differentiated follicle, is almost wholly enclosed by matrix cells which exhibit rapid cell division. Daughter cells migrate upward to differentiate, forming the concentric layers of the hair (medulla, cortex, and cuticle) and of the inner root sheath (cuticle, Huxley's layer, and Henle's layer) (Fig. 7.2a). In the human scalp, the growing phase lasts for more than 5 years (Kligman 1961; Montagna and Parakkal 1974). The end of anagen in the human scalp follicle is characterized by a thinning and lightening of the pigment at the base of the hair shaft, and the melanocytes in the region of the dermal papilla cease producing melanin and resorb their dendrites (Kligman 1961).

7.1.1.2 Catagen Stage

In the catagen stage the hair follicle has ceased to produce new hair. During early catagen, the dermal papilla is condensed and becomes increasingly distant from the regressing matrix. They are still connected, however, by an epithelial column or sheath. The regressed hair assumes a broomlike configuration and becomes a club hair. A characteristic feature of this transition phase is the thickening and corrugation of the vitreous membrane, part of the connective tissue sheath of the follicle. The lower epidermal portion of the hair follicle retreats from the dermal papilla to shorten, and the hair bulb, contracting upward, forms a club hair (Fig. 7.2b,c). This unique process in the hair follicle proceeds quickly, within 2–3 weeks (Kligman 1961; Montagna 1962).

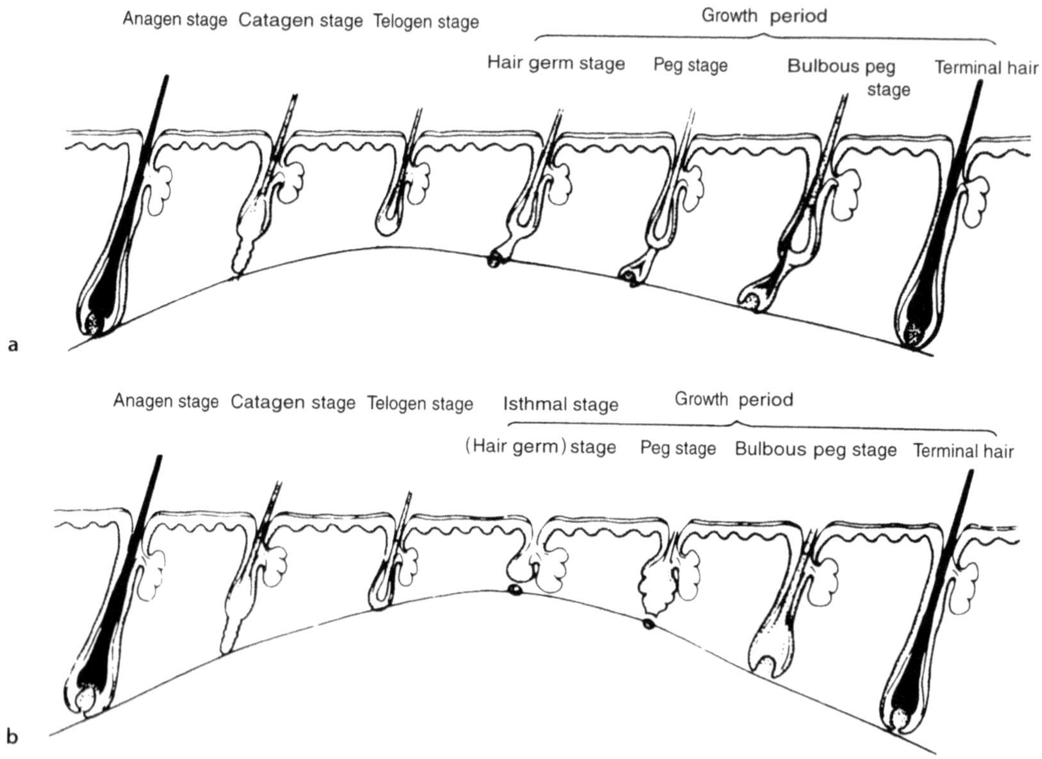

Fig. 7.1a,b. Hair cycle. **a** Common cycle according to Dry (1926) and Segall (1918): The common hair cycle is divided into three stages, anagen, catagen, and telogen. The lower dermal papilla atrophies to a point located close to the telogen follicle. Hair regeneration starts from the secondary hair germ. **b** Essential cycle: The authors (Inaba and Inaba 1992a) suggested that an isthmal stage should be added to the conventional hair cycle, since it was found that when telogen hair was epilated, regeneration was observed from the upper isthmal portion of the hair follicle at the secretory duct opening of the sebaceous gland. (Reproduced with permission from Inaba and Inaba 1989 and from Inaba and Inaba 1992a and Springer-Verlag)

7.1.1.3 Telogen Stage

In telogen or resting stage, the follicle ceases retractive activity, and its length decreases to one-third to one-half of its length in the anagen stage. From this time, the lower portion of the follicle moves upward to a point close to the arrector pili muscle and the hair root becomes superficial, leading to loss of the dying hair (Fig. 7.3a).

The progressive reduction of the epithelial column trails behind it a small nipple of resting cells known as the secondary hair germ.

7.1.2 Regeneration of the Hair Follicle

According to the common theoretical model of the hair cycle (Fig. 7.1a), the lower dermal papilla atrophies to a point located close to the telogen follicle, and the hair bud is then formed at the lower tip of the follicle in telogen stage (secondary hair germ); this subtends the club end and the resting hair (Fig. 7.3a–e). This is the so-called hair germ stage. At a certain angle, the bud descends downward to form the hair bulb. This is the hair peg stage (Fig. 7.3c). After the bulb is formed, new hair fiber is formed from mitotic activity in the matrix. This fiber is formed in the initial hair cone which corresponds later to the inner root sheath. The new hair bulb moves downward to a point which becomes the lower tip of the anagen stage hair follicle (bulbous peg stage) (Fig. 7.3d,e).

Thus, when the new hair begins to grow upward, the prior hair, now in telogen stage, is pushed out and discarded. Previously (Segall 1918; Dry 1926), it was thought that regeneration could not occur without the presence of the secondary hair germ in the telogen follicle; it was also thought that a hair could not be formed unless the hair bulb and matrix were already present. However, we now know that the new hair bud is formed from the secondary hair germ at the lower tip of the telogen follicle, and the hair itself is generated from the matrix after the hair bulb is formed.

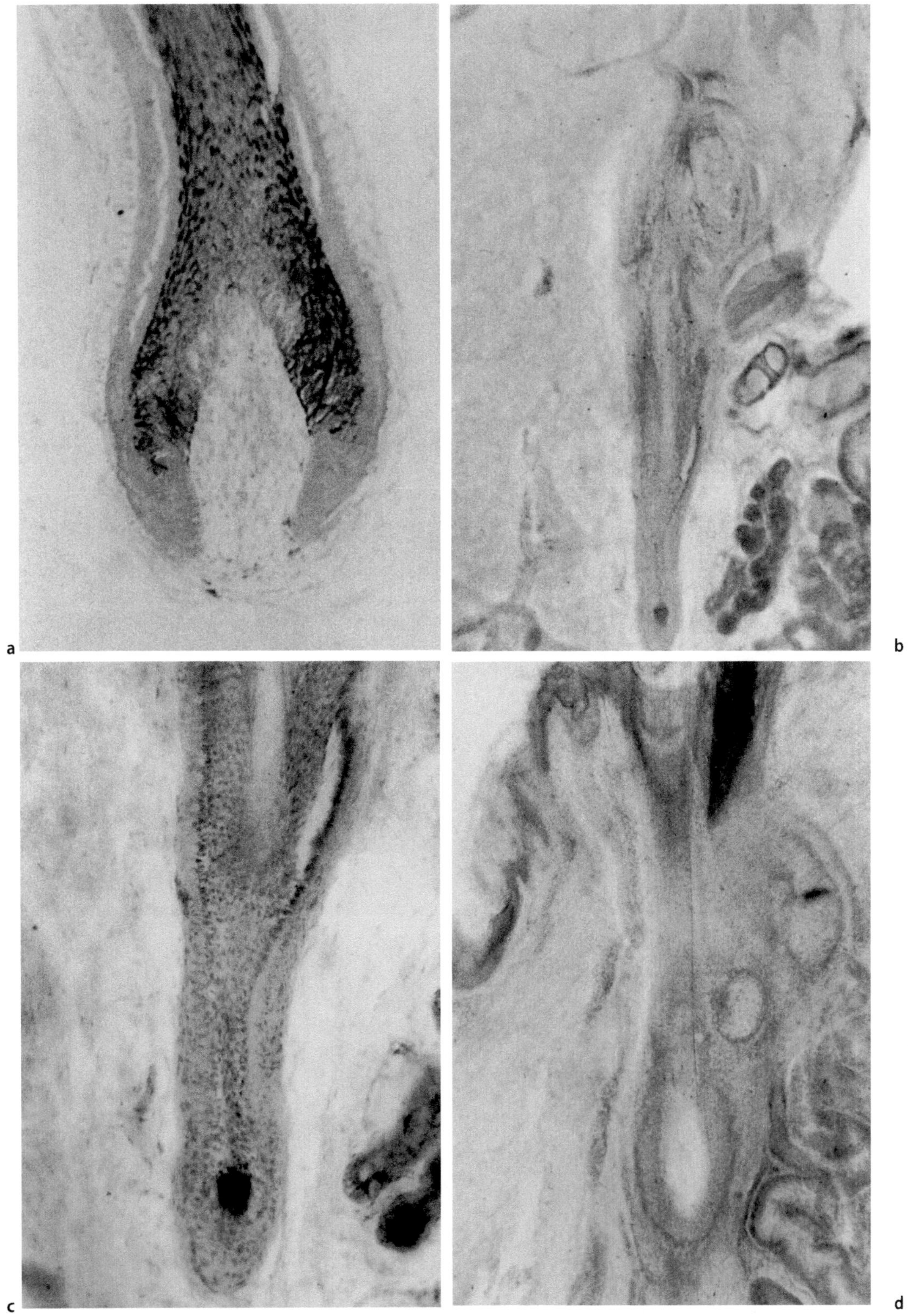

Fig. 7.2. **a** Terminal hair follicle. ×400 **b** Catagen hair follicle. The hair follicle has ceased to produce new hair, and the regressed hair assumes a broomlike configuration and becomes a club hair. ×135 **c** High-power view of the lower portion of catagen hair follicle. Thickening and corrugation of the vitreous membrane can be observed. ×135 **d** Telogen hair follicle. Progressive reduction of the epithelial column trails behind it a small nipple of resting cells (the secondary hair germ). ×135

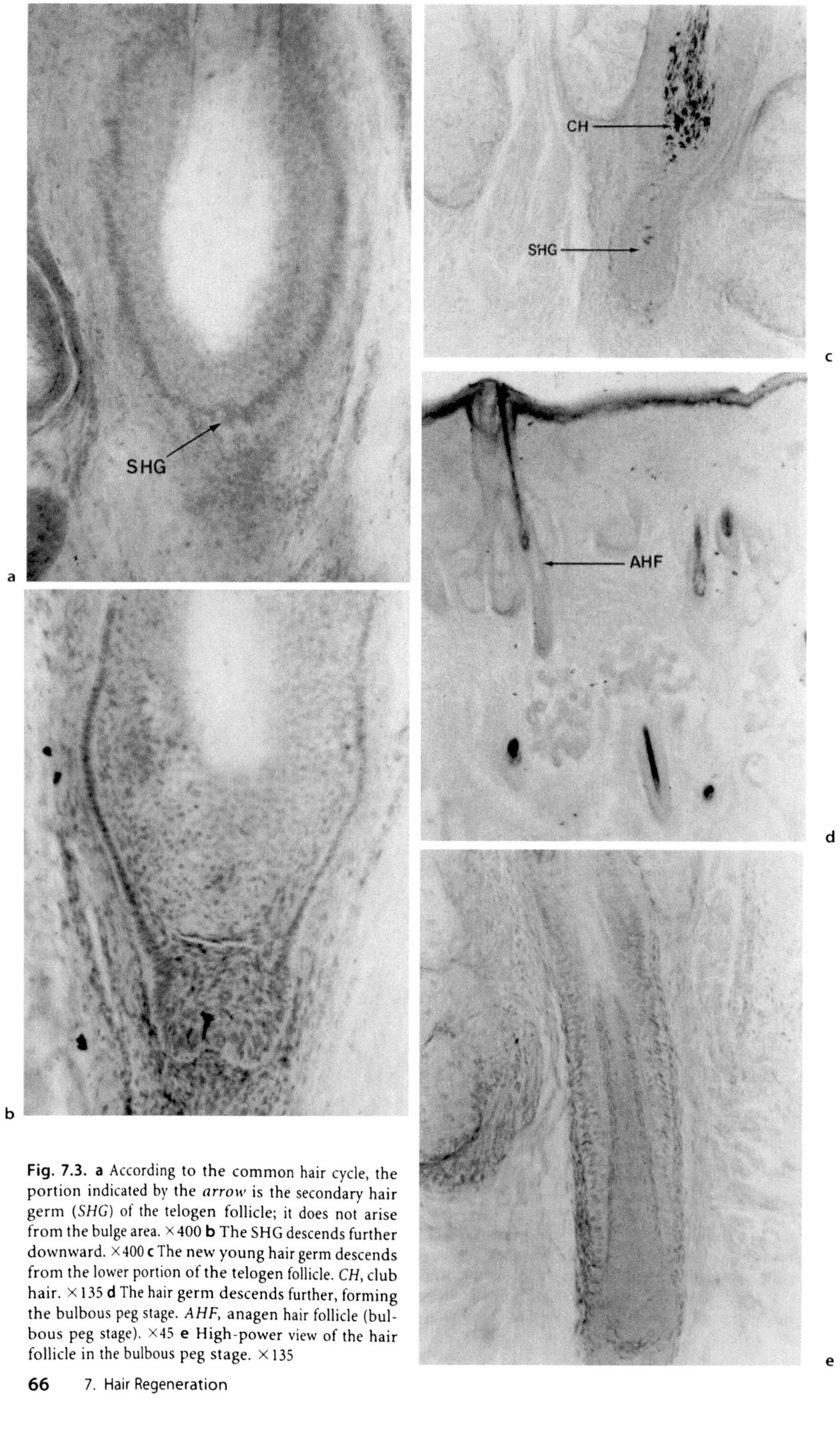

Fig. 7.3. **a** According to the common hair cycle, the portion indicated by the *arrow* is the secondary hair germ (*SHG*) of the telogen follicle; it does not arise from the bulge area. ×400 **b** The SHG descends further downward. ×400 **c** The new young hair germ descends from the lower portion of the telogen follicle. *CH*, club hair. ×135 **d** The hair germ descends further, forming the bulbous peg stage. *AHF*, anagen hair follicle (bulbous peg stage). ×45 **e** High-power view of the hair follicle in the bulbous peg stage. ×135

While the hair cycle of human scalp hair and that of Japanese monkeys accord with the above findings, Moretti (1965) and Sato (1976) state that typical telogen hair follicles are almost never seen in scalp hair. Since the early anagen stage can be observed in the lower portion of telogen hair follicles, the center of hair regeneration was considered to be located at the lower end of the telogen hair follicle. But if this is so, where does regeneration start after a telogen hair containing this presumed hair center is pulled out?

7.2 Mechanisms of Regulation of the Hair Cycle

Our lack of understanding of the regulation of hair growth has been caused, in part, by the lack of good in vitro models (Philpott et al. 1989; Buhl et al. 1989). In the past, a theory of the mechanism of the hair cycle set forth by Caron (Chase and Eaton 1959; Bullough 1975), to the effect that some inhibitor of hair growth accumulates during anagen stage and is then disintegrated during telogen stage, resulting in hair regrowth, gained wide support.

Indeed, a peptide-like inhibitor has been observed in the telogen stage in mouse skin (Pauss et al. 1990). Today such growth factors as transforming growth factor (TGF)-α and -β and epidermal growth factor (EGF) are known to inhibit hair growth (Moore et al. 1985; Hollis and Chapman 1987; Philpott et al. 1990).

The initiation of the anagen stage is presumed to be induced by some sort of signal produced in the dermal papilla.

Philpott et al. (1990) have described the successful growth of human hair in vitro, and have reported the in vitro effects of growth factors and mitogens on the mode of this growth. Those investigators have also shown that EGF and TGF-α are important in the regulation of hair follicle growth, from anagen to a catagen-like state, and differentiation in vitro, and they have suggested a possible mechanism by which TGF-α may act in vivo. TGF-β caused a marked inhibition of hair follicle growth, but no change in morphology (Kealey 1990).

Although EGF receptors are located in the outer root sheath (ORS) (Nanney et al. 1984; Green and Couchman 1984, 1985), the physiological ligand may be TGF-α, which is also a ligand for the EGF receptor (Nanney et al. 1984) and which is known to be produced in the skin (Finzi et al. 1991). Philpott et al. (1990) have now shown that TGF-α elicits the same changes in hair follicle morphology as does human EGF (urogastrone).

The factors that regulate cell division within the hair follicle matrix cells, and which control the hair growth cycle, are still poorly understood, although growth factors (Moore et al. 1981; Green and Couchman 1984, 1985; Panaretto et al. 1984; Nanney et al. 1984; Akhurst et al. 1988; Messenger 1989), steroid hormones (Takayasu and Adachi 1972a; Schweikert and Wilson 1974a; Sultan et al. 1989), dermo-epithelial interactions (Jahoda and Oliver 1984), and the immune system (Sawada et al. 1987; Pauss et al. 1989; Westgate et al. 1991a) have been implicated.

Moore et al. (1991) have reported on the roles played by growth factors. In sheep, EGF receptors are located on skin epithelia. An EGF-like protein was detected by immunochemistry in fetal epidermis, but was not associated with the cells of the developing wool follicles. During subsequent development, this molecule was associated with the sebaceous glands and the outer root sheath. If the ORS is considered as a source of stem cells for the proliferating matrix, EGF may act as a differentiation factor, determining cell fate by cell contact mechanisms similar to those in invertebrates. Fibroblast growth factor (FGF) was found to be localized in the epidermis and basal lamina and in follicle plugs during morphogenesis. At maturity, FGF was found in the ORS and in the region of the basal lamina of the follicle bulb, suggesting a role in bulb proliferation and fiber growth (reviewed from Philpott et al. 1990).

The realization that hair growth stem cells may reside in the bulge area (attachment of arrector pili muscle) in the telogen follicle provides new insights into how the hair cycle may be regulated (Cotsarelis et al. 1990) (see Section 14.1.2, Stem Cells). During late telogen, the normally slow cycling stem cells of the bulge area are activated by dermal papilla cells (bulge activation hypothesis).

7.3 New Concept of Hair Generation and Regeneration

As described in detail in Section 8.2.2, the authors have developed a radical surgical technique, the subcutaneous tissue shaving method, for the treatment of bromidrosis and hyperhidrosis. After applying this procedure, we raised a number of questions about the common concept of the generation and regeneration of hair growth (Inaba 1985; Inaba and Inaba 1990b, 1992a).

These findings indicate that the conventional hair cycle theory is incomplete, and that there is validity in our sebaceous gland hypothesis (Fig. 7.1b), in which we propose that the true hair center is sited in the sebaceous gland and the upper isthmal portion of the follicle. Taking this into account, we suggest that the hair cycle should be divided into four stages: anagen, catagen, telogen, and isthmal.

The formation of early anagen hair from the lower telogen hair follicle, which is consistent with the conventional hair cycle theory, has been observed in the Japanese monkey (Inaba et al. 1992) and in human scalp hair. Since typical telogen hairs were observed in both cases, it would appear that early anagen hair forms from the lower portion of the telogen hair follicle.

It has been thought that the hair follicle was subdivided into transient and permanent portions at the lower end of the telogen follicle or at the point of attachment of the arrector muscle. The conventional hair cycle theory would be valid if regeneration were to start from this remnant dermal papilla. However, telogen hair does not always extend to the site of attachment of the arrector muscle. There are cases in which it retracts within the lobes of the sebaceous gland.

Thus, the hair germ depends on the size of the telogen hair. In particular, when telogen hair is epilated, regeneration has been observed to start from the upper isthmal portion of the hair follicle or from the secretory duct opening of the sebaceous gland (Fig. 12.7). These observations suggest that, while the hair cycle generally proceeds along the lines of the common theory, the essential starting point of regeneration is located in the upper isthmal portion, in particular in the sebaceous isthmus (essential hair cycle) (Fig. 7.1b).

Regeneration After Subcutaneous Tissue Shaving Procedure

8

8.1 Common Hair Cycle Theory Reconsidered

We were compelled to question the generally accepted model of the hair cycle after we developed the subcutaneous tissue shaving method for the treatment of bromidrosis and hyperhidrosis (Inaba and Ezaki 1977; Inaba et al. 1978c; Inaba and Inaba 1986).

Clinical examination of the results of the subcutaneous tissue shaving procedure confirmed that even when the lower part of the hair follicle had been cut off, with only the upper part of the isthmus and the sebaceous glands appended to the follicle remaining, there was regeneration of axillary hair. If we ablated all, or at least some of the sebaceous glands so that little more than the infundibulum was preserved, the axillary hair did not regrow. This finding led us to doubt whether the common hair cycle was an adequate theory and to attempt histological studies.

8.2 Bromidrosis

8.2.1 Etiology of Bromidrosis (Foul-Smelling Perspiration)

The occurrence of bromidrosis depends on the volume of the apocrine glands. A persistent question is why the condition is commonly observed in Caucasians but is rarely seen in Orientals. Apocrine glands are generated from the upper portion of the secretory duct opening of the sebaceous gland. Since Caucasians consume large amounts of animal fat, it is conceivable that, when the metabolic excretion of sebum exceeded the capacity of the sebaceous gland, the apocrine gland developed as a complementary excretory organ. In Orientals, however, whose consumption of animal fat is very low, the sebaceous gland remained small and the apocrine gland atrophied. Bromidrosis is hereditary, and the incidence is about 10% in the Japanese population. Because the condition is relatively rare in the Japanese, those who have it will accept radical treatment (Inaba 1976; Inaba and Inaba 1990b, 1992a).

8.2.2 Surgical Treatment of Bromidrosis

Drug therapy, physical therapy, electrolysis, electrocoagulation, and surgery have been used to treat hircismus without satisfactory long-term results. The subcutaneous tissue shaving method developed by the authors has, thus far, shown very successful results (Fig. 8.1a). A 1-cm incision is made in the axilla and a subcutaneous tissue shaver is inserted. A roller presses down against the surface of the skin, so that when the shaver is moved, sweat glands and hair bulbs appended to the underside of the axillary skin are removed. After the subcutaneous tissue is removed, the sutured axillary skin is held firmly in place with a double tie-over bandage (Fig. 8.1b). This method is ideal, since it gives good cosmetic results and the sweat glands do not regenerate (Inaba 1976; Inaba et al. 1978a,b; Inaba and Inaba 1990b, 1992a). Only a 1-cm scar remains after the procedure (Fig. 8.2).

Because hair roots were removed to the thickness of a split-thickness graft during this procedure, no regeneration of axillary hair was expected to occur. However, postoperative examination revealed that, if the subcutaneous tissue was removed to the level of a thick split-thickness graft, leaving the sebaceous gland intact (Fig. 8.3d), regeneration of axillary hair occurred (Fig. 8.3e). On

a
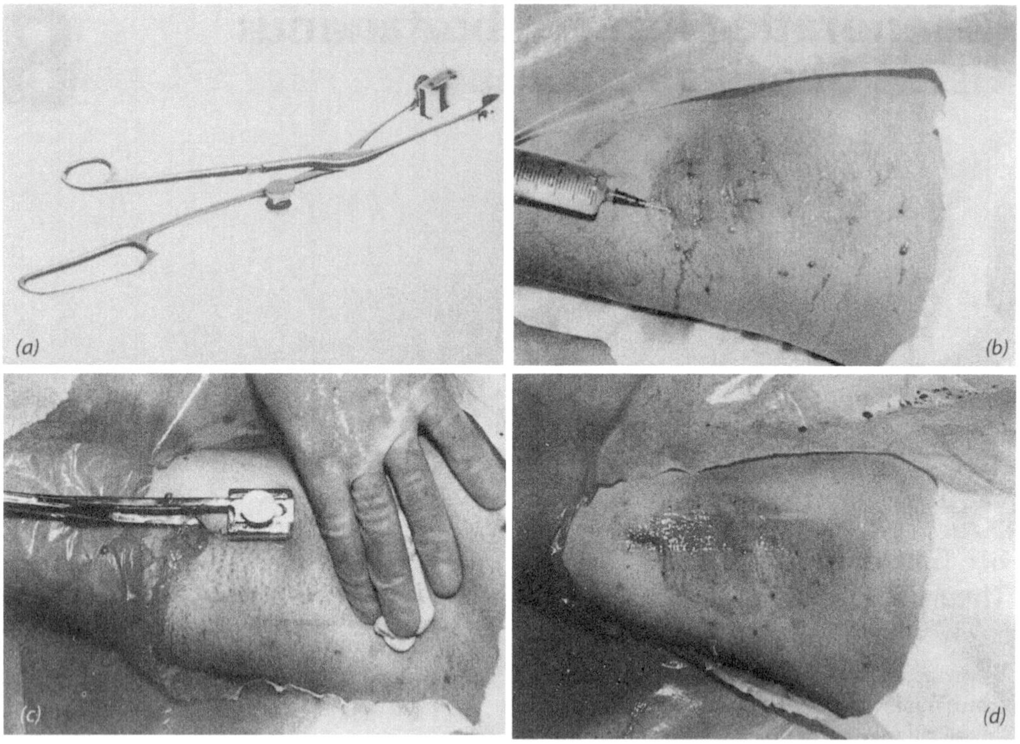

b
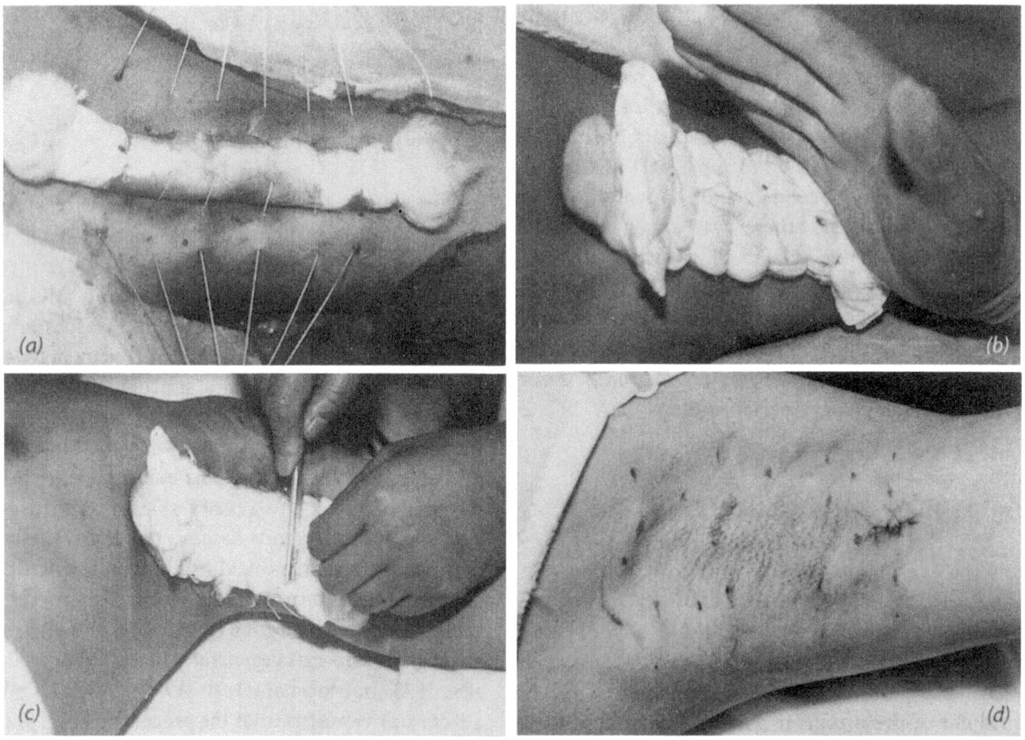

Fig. 8.1. **a** Subcutaneous tissue shaving method. The shaving instrument has a razor and two rollers (*a*). Local anesthetic is administered in a very dilute solution (0.1%) in a total injection volume of 150 ml (*b*). The shaver is inserted through a 1-cm incision (*c*). After shaving to the split-thickness graft level is finished, the shaver is removed from the 1-cm incision (*d*). **b** Double tie-over dressing. To stop bleeding, a double tie-over dressing is applied. Dressing A is sutured into a fixed position; suturing is done through healthy skin. This prevents the dressing from shifting position (*a*). Dressing B is placed over dressing A to enhance fixation (*b*). To improve blood circulation and prevent necrosis, the dressing is partially removed the following day (*c*). Skin surface 7 days postoperatively with the dressing completely removed (*d*)

Fig. 8.2. **a** One year after the subcutaneous tissue shaving treatment. Only a 1-cm scar remains. **b** Scar 1 year after treatment

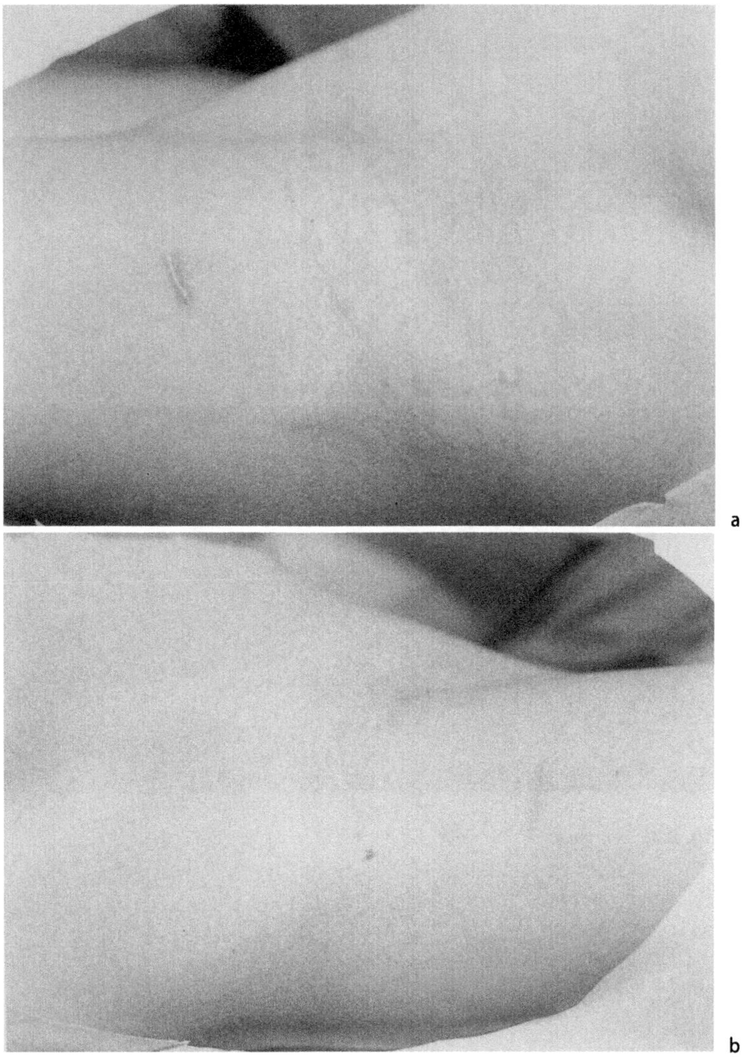

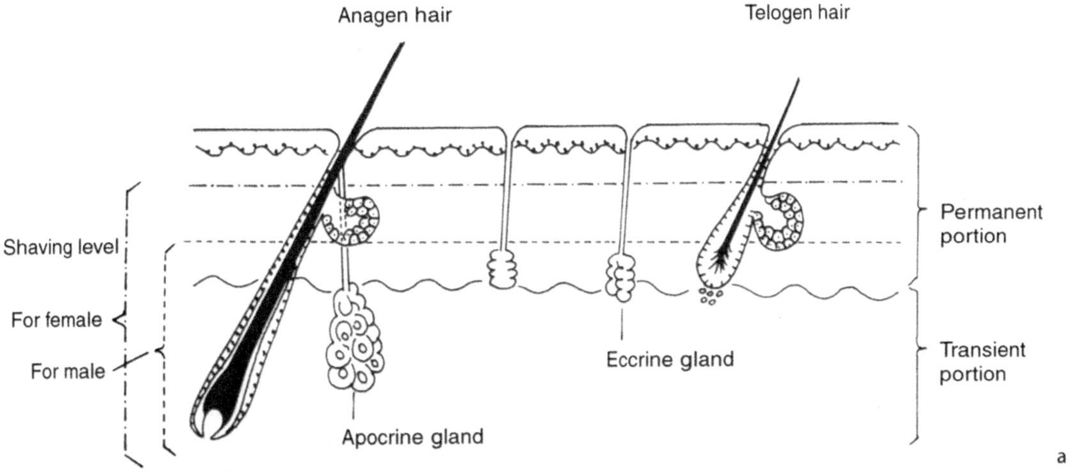

Fig. 8.3. **a** Subcutaneous tissue shaving level. **b** The shaving level for females which removes the sebaceous glands prevents future regrowth of axillary hair (**c**). On the other hand, a lower level setting leaves sebaceous glands and the upper isthmal portion of the follicles intact (**d**) to ensure hair growth (**e**)

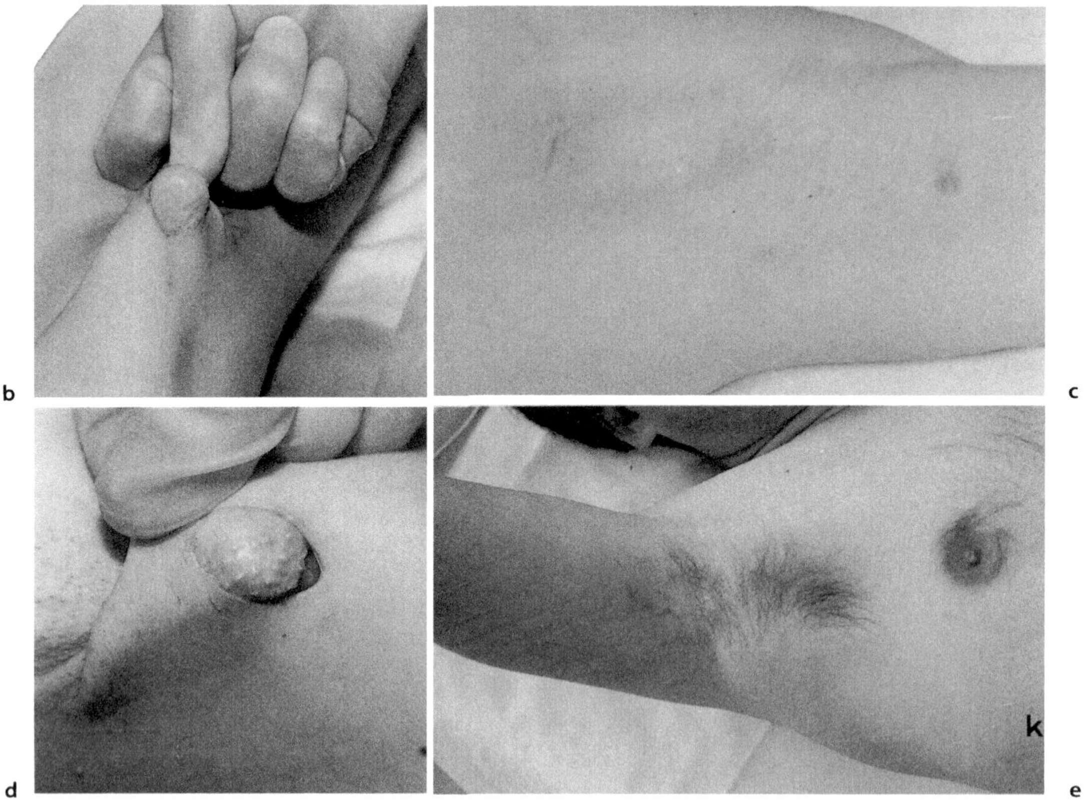

Fig. 8.3. *Continued*

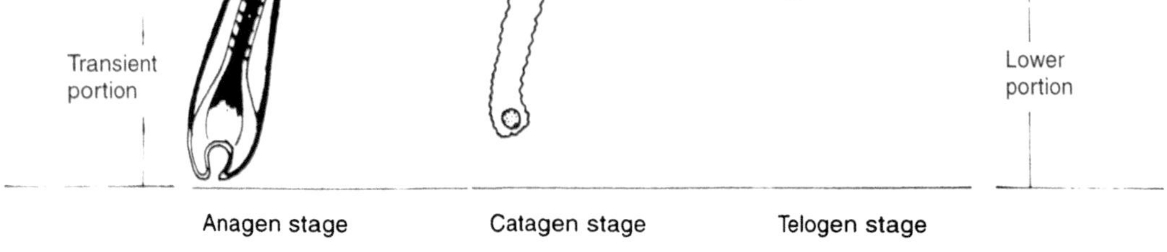

Fig. 8.4. Montagna and Parakkal (1974) divided the hair follicle into transient and permanent portions, the dividing line being drawn at the attachment of the arrector pili muscle. Pinkus (1969) divided the hair follicle into upper, middle, and lower portions, the upper portion extending from the epidermis to the duct opening of the sebaceous gland, the middle portion extending from the duct opening of the sebaceous gland to the attachment of the arrector pili muscle, and the lower portion (corresponding to Montagna and Parakkal's transient portion) extending from the attachment of the arrector pili muscle to the lower tip of the follicle (from Montagna and Parakkal 1974 and Inaba et al. 1979a, with permission from Journal of Investigative Dermatology)

the other hand, if the subcutaneous tissue was removed to the level of a medium split-thickness graft, removing the sebaceous gland (Fig. 8.3b), no regeneration occurred (Fig. 8.3c). In other words, regeneration of hair was observed after the removal of the transient portion and the lower layer of the permanent portion up to, but not including, the sebaceous gland. This finding brought the common hair cycle theory into question (Fig. 8.4).

8.3 Histological Findings

The process of regeneration of axillary hair was examined after the operation for bromidrosis.

8.3.1 Relationship of Hair Formation and Sebaceous Gland (Table 8.1)

If shaving is done just beneath the sebaceous gland (that is, up to medium split-thickness level), then a considerable upper portion of the follicular isthmus (the part between the opening of the sebaceous duct and the bulge that marks the attachment of the arrector muscle) is left intact. The axillary hair regrows. Whether the isthmus has been removed or left behind can be determined by noting the absence or presence of the sebaceous gland (Fig. 8.4). In 30 pilosebaceous complexes (Table 8.1), 53 sebaceous lobes and 48 hair roots were seen. In 17 complexes, 2 or more sebaceous lobes were found, and 13 of these had more than one new hair follicle. Twenty-nine complexes had at least 1 associated hair root; only 1 complex (case No. 9-3) had none. When sebaceous glands had been completely removed, there was no hair follicle formation from the outer root sheath. Regeneration of hair follicles is thus related to the presence of the sebaceous gland and upper isthmus.

8.3.2 Postoperative Regeneration of Axillary Hair [Inaba et al. 1979a (Case 1); Inaba and Inaba 1992a (Case 2)]

8.3.2.1 Case 1

Examination of specimens removed immediately after the shaving surgery showed that the transient

Table 8.1. Axillary hair regeneration in 30 pilosebaceous complexes of 11 patients

A[a]	B[b]	C[c]	D[d]	E[e]
Case 1	1	26	Hair germ	±
	2	17	Peg	+
	3	20	Peg	+
26 yr	4	25	Bulb. peg	+
6 mo	5	15	Peg	+
Case 2	1a	18	Peg	+
	b	20	Peg	+
	c	20	Peg	+
	2a	27	Peg	+
	b	30	Peg	+
	3a	20	Bulb. peg	+
	b	20	Bulb. peg	+
21 yr	4	30	Peg	+
12 mo	5a	18	Peg	+
	b	18	Bulb. peg	+
Case 3	1	20	Peg	+
	2a	43	–	–
	b	17	Bulb. peg	+
	3a	30	–	–
20 yr	b	15	Bulb. peg	+
	4	25	Bulb. peg	+
7 mo				
Case 4	1a	42	Hair germ	–
22 yr	b	25	Hair germ	±
12 mo	c	37	Hair germ	–
Case 5	1a	30	Peg	+
	b	23	Bulb. peg	+
24 yr	c	15	Hair germ	–
10 mo				
Case 6	1a	25	Peg	+
	b	27	Peg	+
	c	23	Peg	+
20 yr	2a	30	Peg	+
8 mo	b	25	Peg	+
Case 7	1a	32	Peg	+
	b	28	Bulb. peg	+
22 yr	c	30	Peg	+
	2a	40	Peg	+
10 mo	b	30	Peg	+
Case 8	1a	25	Peg	+
	b	30	Peg	+
19 yr	2	25	Bulb. peg	+
8 mo	3	15	Peg	+
Case 9	1	20	Bulb. peg	+
	2	20	Peg	+
24 yr	3	35	–	±
6 mo				
Case 10	1a	32	–	–
	b	32	Peg	+
	2a	35	Peg	+
21 yr	b	10	Peg	+
10 mo	c	35	Peg	+
Case 11	3a	30	Peg	+
	b	30	Peg	+
20 yr	4a	36	–	–
9 mo	b	33	Peg	+

[a] Age of patient (years) and time after surgery (months).
[b] Individual follicles and associated sebaceous glands. Numbers indicate sebaceous glands; letters indicate separated sebaceous lobes present in each gland.
[c] Diameter of sebaceous glands in μm.
[d] Stage of hair follicle formation.
[e] Presence or absence of newly formed hair.

a
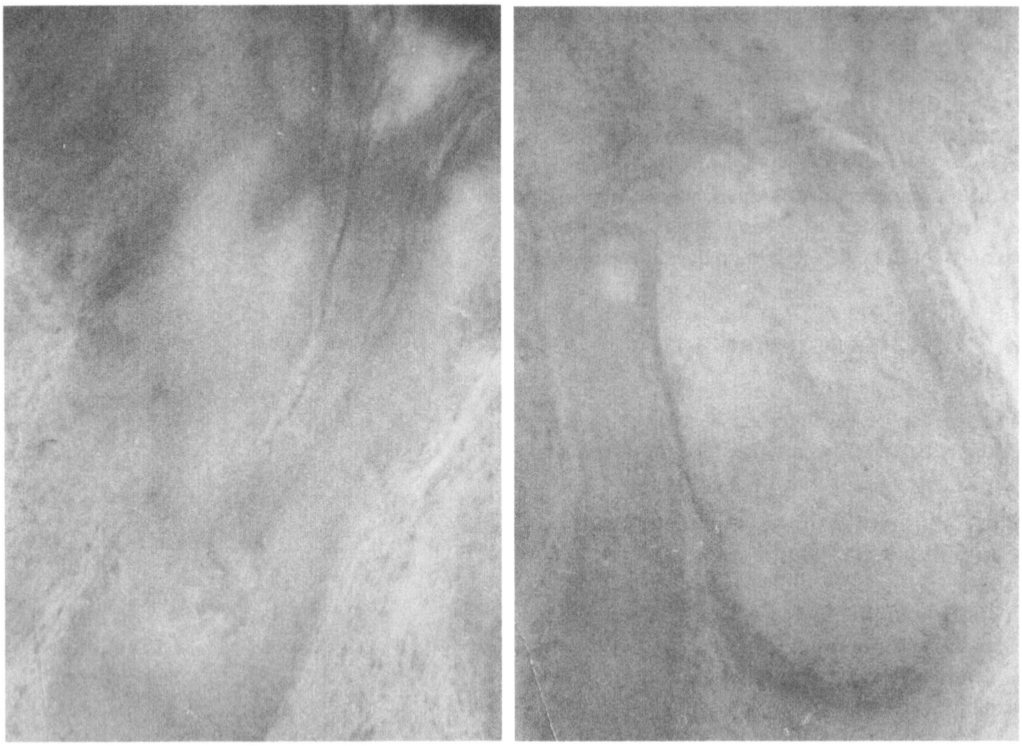
c

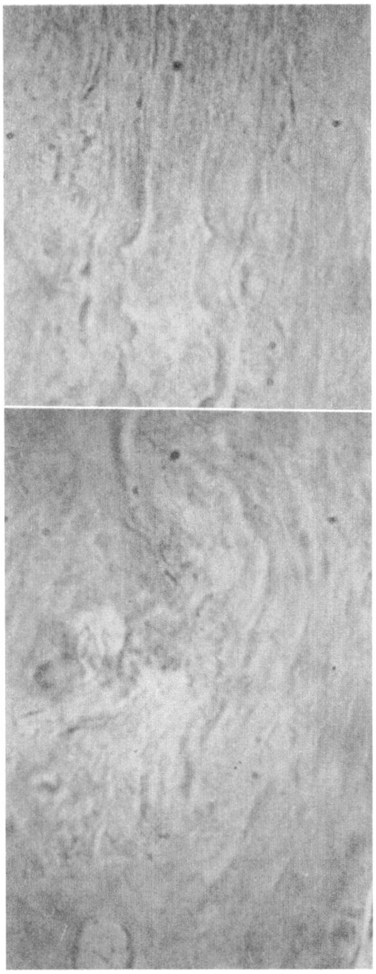
b

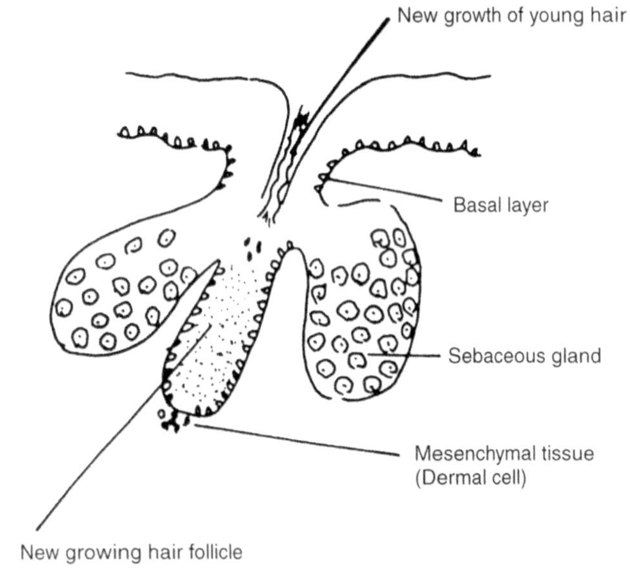

d

Fig. 8.5. Case 1. Hair germ stage. **a** Keratinization suggests a new young hair in the lower portion of the follicle. **b** Higher magnification of middle and lower portions of **a** shows formation of new young hair. ×400 **c** Photomicrograph of thick tissue section corresponding to the drawing in Fig. 8.5d. No hair bulb has formed yet (*Fig. 8.12a, hair germ stage*). Keratinization, suggesting new young hair, is seen in the infundibulum of the follicle shown in **a** and **b**. **d** Pilosebaceous complex, showing early stage of hair regeneration from isthmus of follicle between two sebaceous glands. (**a**, **b**, **c**, Reproduced from Inaba et al. 1979a with permission from Journal of Investigative Dermatology) portion of the follicles (Fig. 8.4) and the lower part of the isthmus, including the bulge area, had been removed. Examination of specimens obtained 6 months after surgery showed that new young hairs were formed from the trichilemma (outer hair root sheath) of the isthmus near the level of the sebaceous duct opening. Postoperative hair follicle formation was different from that in the ordinary hair cycle and must be considered as new hair growth. It shows stages similar but not identical to, fetal hair formation.

8.3.2.2 Case 2

The authors later reexamined the regeneration of axillary hair (case 2) and reconfirmed that the regeneration began from the upper isthmal portion, notably at a point adjacent to the duct opening of the sebaceous gland.

8.3.2.3 Histologic Findings in Each Stage

The development stages of the new follicle are described below.

(a) Hair Germ Stage. The hair follicle in case 1 can be seen between remnant sebaceous glands in the diagram in Fig. 8.5d and the photomicrograph in Fig. 8.5c. The lower end of the hair follicle is situated at the same level as the lower part of the sebaceous gland. No hair bulb has yet formed. Fig. 8.5a,b shows the upper part of the outer root sheath (infundibulum) of the same follicle where keratinization can be seen in the center of the hair sheath. In this specimen, keratinization and vigorous mitotic activity were seen in the isthmus, suggesting the formation of the inner root sheath and young hair, the deepest portion of which was not yet keratinized. In four cases, keratinization was seen in the isthmus without new growth of hair.

In another specimen (from case 2) (Fig. 8.6), when the sebaceous gland was left intact, the new young bud (hair germ) (Fig. 8.6a) began to form at a point adjacent to the duct opening of the sebaceous gland (upper isthmal portion). This hair germ became multilobular and formed a bud (Fig. 8.6c).

This finding suggests that the mesenchymal cells may first be formed at a site adjacent to the duct opening of the sebaceous gland (upper isthmal portion), and that the mesenchymal cells may initiate the epithelial bud.

(b) Hair Peg Stage. As shown in Fig. 8.7a and diagrammatically in Fig. 8.7b, in case 1, two new hair follicles were seen in the dermal layer below the sebaceous gland. In the hair follicle on both sites, the new young hair was already keratinized. Hair cuticula, which was deeply stained, was seen around the hair cortex (Fig. 8.7c). Filamentous structures were seen in the lower part, and these

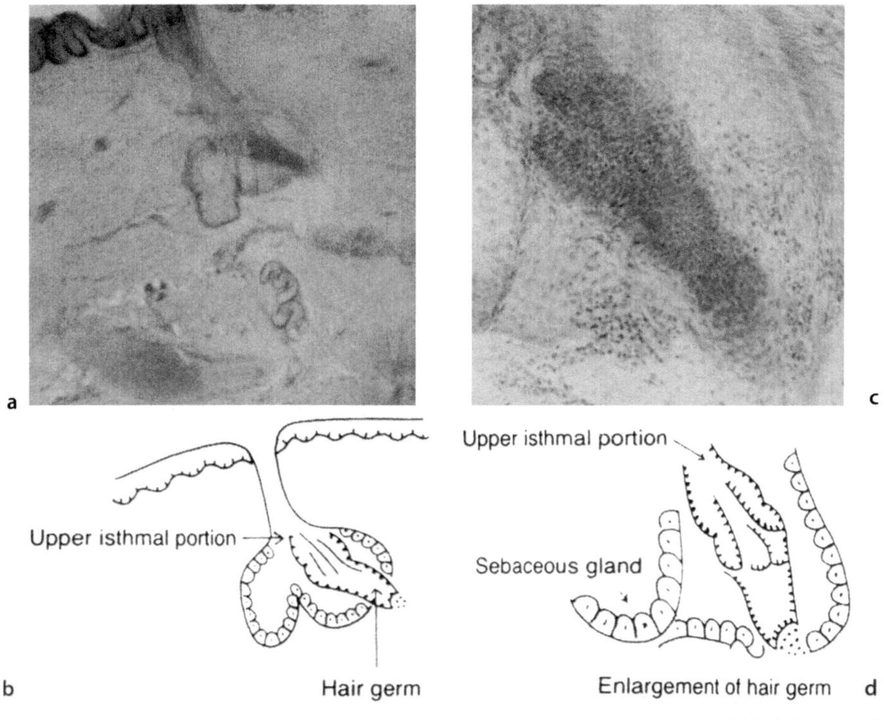

Fig. 8.6a–d. Case 2. Hair germ stage. **a** Formation of a new hair bud .×60 **b** The hair germ begins to form from the duct opening of the sebaceous gland (upper isthmal portion) (hair germ stage). **c** This hair germ becomes multilobular and forms a bud. ×135 **d** Schematic of **c**

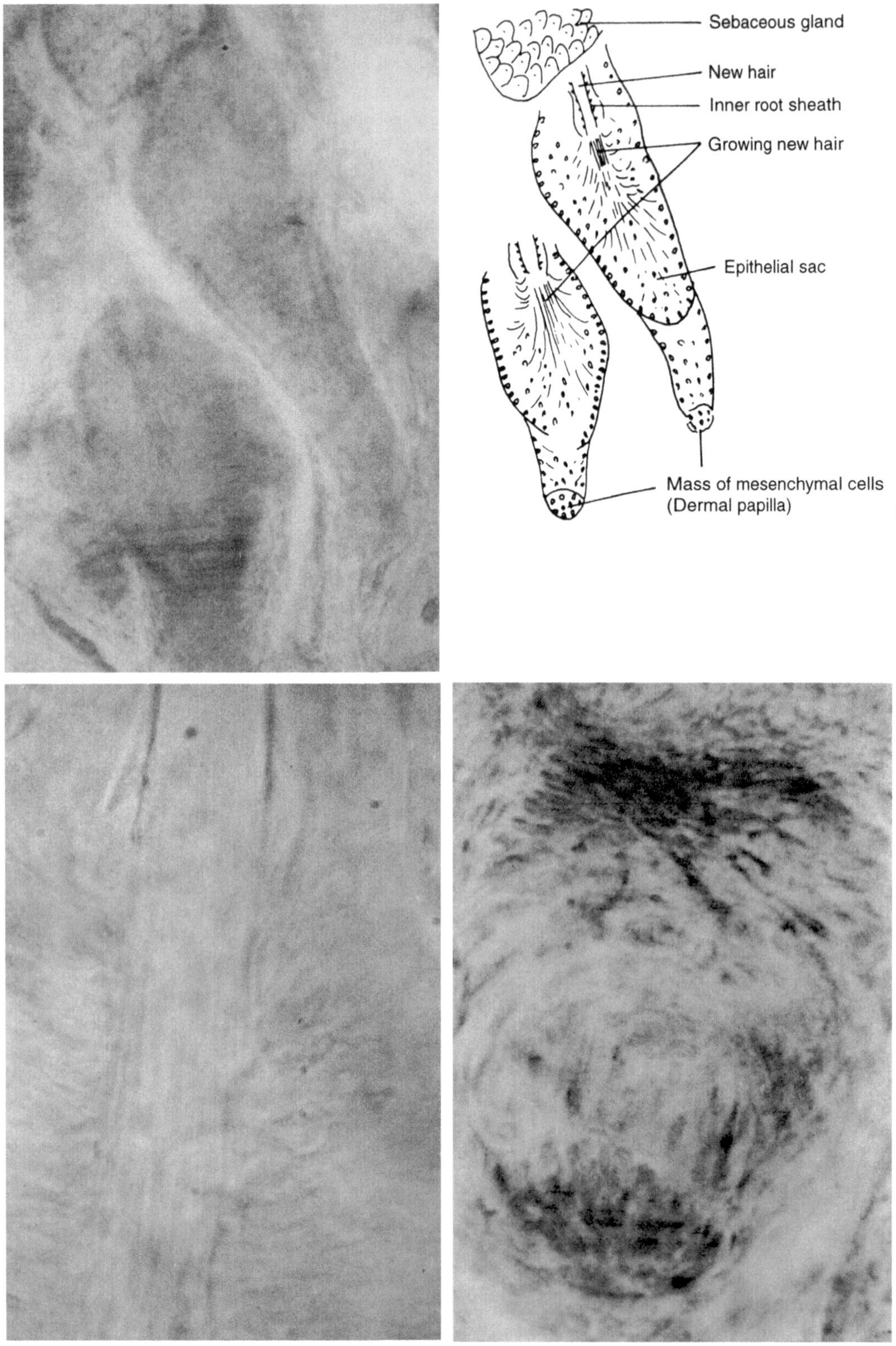

Fig. 8.7. Case 1. Hair peg stage. **a** Micrograph of thick section of pilosebaceous complex shown diagrammatically in **b**. ×135 **b** Pilosebaceous complex with two young hair roots in hair peg stage. **c** New hair in center of budding hair follicle shown in **a**, **b**. **d** Lower part of follicle shown in **a** and **b**. Columnar epithelial cells capping, but not surrounding, a ball of mesenchymal cells (future dermal papilla). ×400

extended downward to cells resembling columnar hair germ cells. The inner hair root sheath appeared to be formed simultaneously and surrounded the hair. (Fig. 8.7c). A mass of mesenchymal tissue (future dermal papilla) was seen at the lower pole but this tissue was not wrapped in the manner of a hair bulb (Fig. 8.7d). At first glance, the picture was similar to the catagen stage, since it suggested the keratinized rootlets seen in the club hair in catagen. However, there was no hyalinization of the inner root sheath, as seen in club hairs. Melanin granules were not present in the epithelial column, and no pigmentation of the upper hair cortex was noted. All these findings suggest a quasifetal anagen stage.

The process of hair pegging occurs as follows. Hair cuticula forms around the newly formed hair cortex and interlocks with the sheath cuticula of the inner root sheath, which, in turn, adheres to the surrounding trichilemmal epithelium. This interlocking fusion prevents the hair from moving upward (Fig. 8.7c). The hair follicle is forced to elongate downward by the active mitotic activity of hair germ cells in the lower part of the epithelial sac.

In the early hair peg stage (shown in case 2 in Fig. 8.8), although the hair bulb (matrix) has not yet developed, the inner root sheath (Henle's layer, Huxley's layer, and sheath cuticle) is first formed from the lower portion of the germinal layer, and following the bud descending inside this hair cone, filamentous structures are produced from the surrounding germinal layer in the hair germ, and then keratinized to form the new young hair (hair cuticle cortex and medulla) (Fig. 8.8c,d, hair peg stage). In this stage, the germinal layer is already divided into six portions (Fig. 8.12, hair germ stage).

In the late hair peg stage (shown in case 2 in Fig. 8.9), as the hair bud elongates downward, this germinal layer becomes localized at the lower portion of the hair follicle above the dermal papilla. Although the hair bulb has not yet been formed at the hair peg stage, the lower germinal layer is already divided into three parts: the outer root

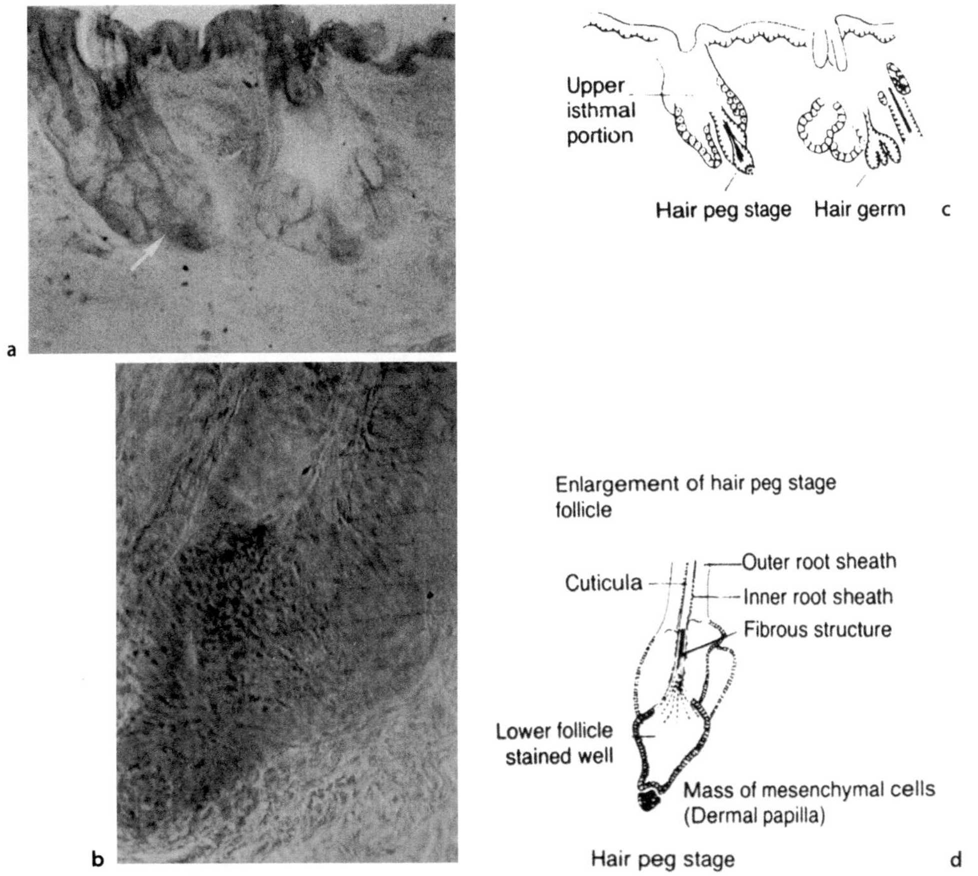

Fig. 8.8a–d. Case 2. **a**, **b** Hair peg stage (*arrow*). Although the hair bulb (matrix) has not yet formed, filamentous structures are formed in the surrounding germinal layer and are then keratinized to form the hair shaft. ×135 **c** Schematic of **a**. **d** Schematic of **b**

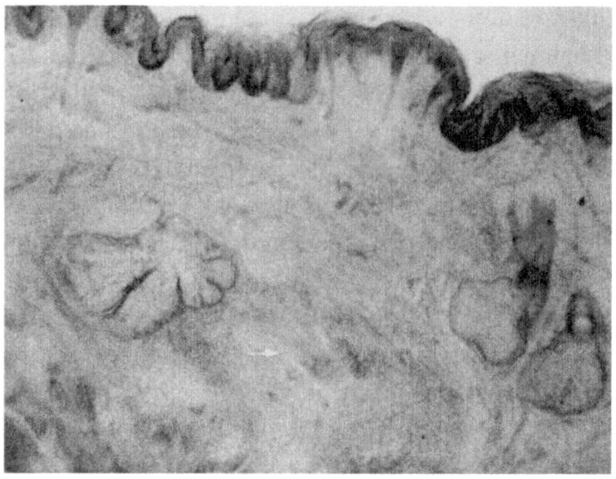

a

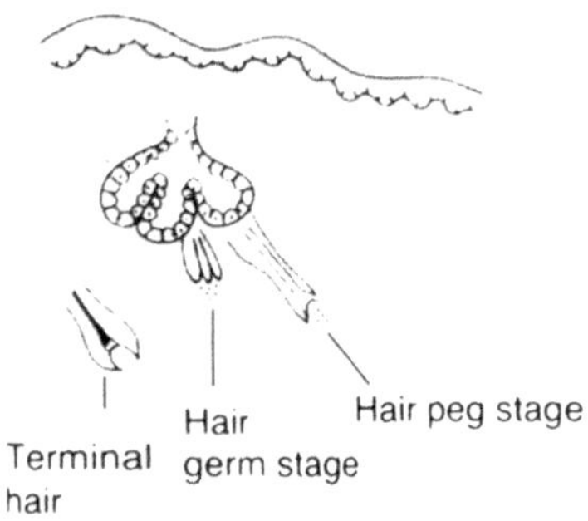

b

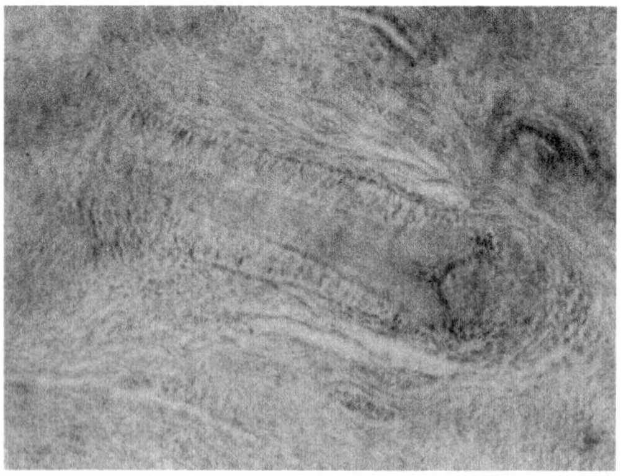

c

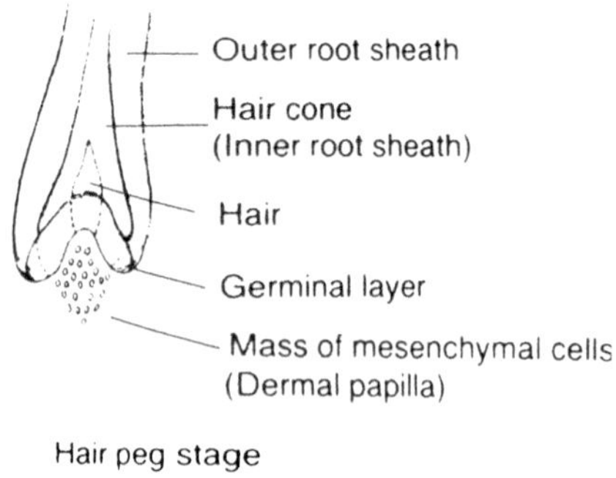

d

Fig. 8.9a–d. Case 2. Late hair peg stage (*arrow*) in **a**. As the hair bud elongates downward, this germinal layer becomes localized at the lower portion of the hair follicle above the dermal papilla. ×60 **b** Schematic of **a**. **c** Enlargement of **a**. ×135 **d** Schematic of **c**

sheath, the inner root sheath, and the hair tissue (late hair peg stage), (see Fig. 8.12).

(c) Bulbous Peg Stage. In case 1, hair follicles are seen descending below two out of three lobes of the sebaceous gland in the diagram (Fig. 8.10b) and in the micrograph (Fig. 8.10a). As seen in Fig. 8.10b,c, the epithelial column has elongated downward in the early bulbous peg stage and the inner root sheath has become thick and long. When the forming hair reaches a level near the permanent site of the dermal papilla, the epithelial cells grow around the mass of mesenchymal tissue, thereby

→

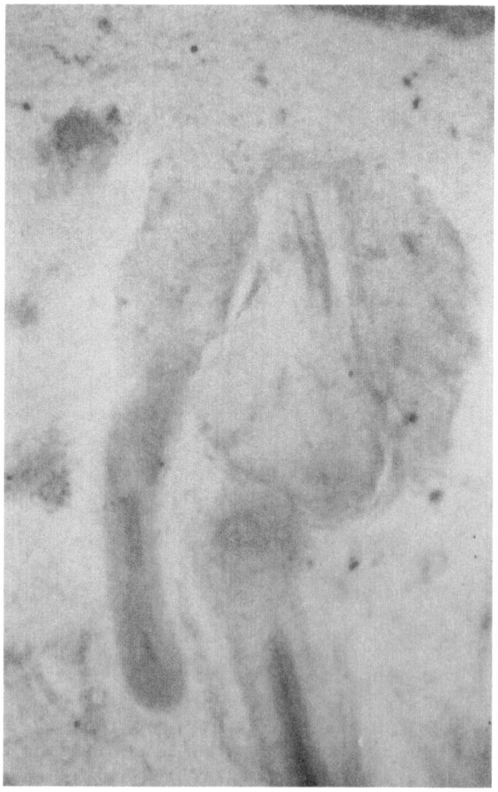

a

Fig. 8.10. Case 1. Bulbous peg stage. **a** Micrograph of thick tissue section of piloseoaceous complex shown in **b**. ×135 **b** Schematic of a pilosebaceous complex showing two new hair roots in bulbous peg stage. **c** Microphotograph of the early bulbous peg stage. There is slight matrix formation and melanocytes have also formed, so that melanin granules are visible. ×400 **d** The follicle on the right is in the terminal hair stage. The matrix has completely formed, and the new hair ascends to the skin surface. ×135 **e** Higher magnification of hair bulb shown in **d**. Melanin granules, which are produced from a melanocyte, have increased and lead to terminal hair with conspicuous pigmentation in the hair cortex. ×400

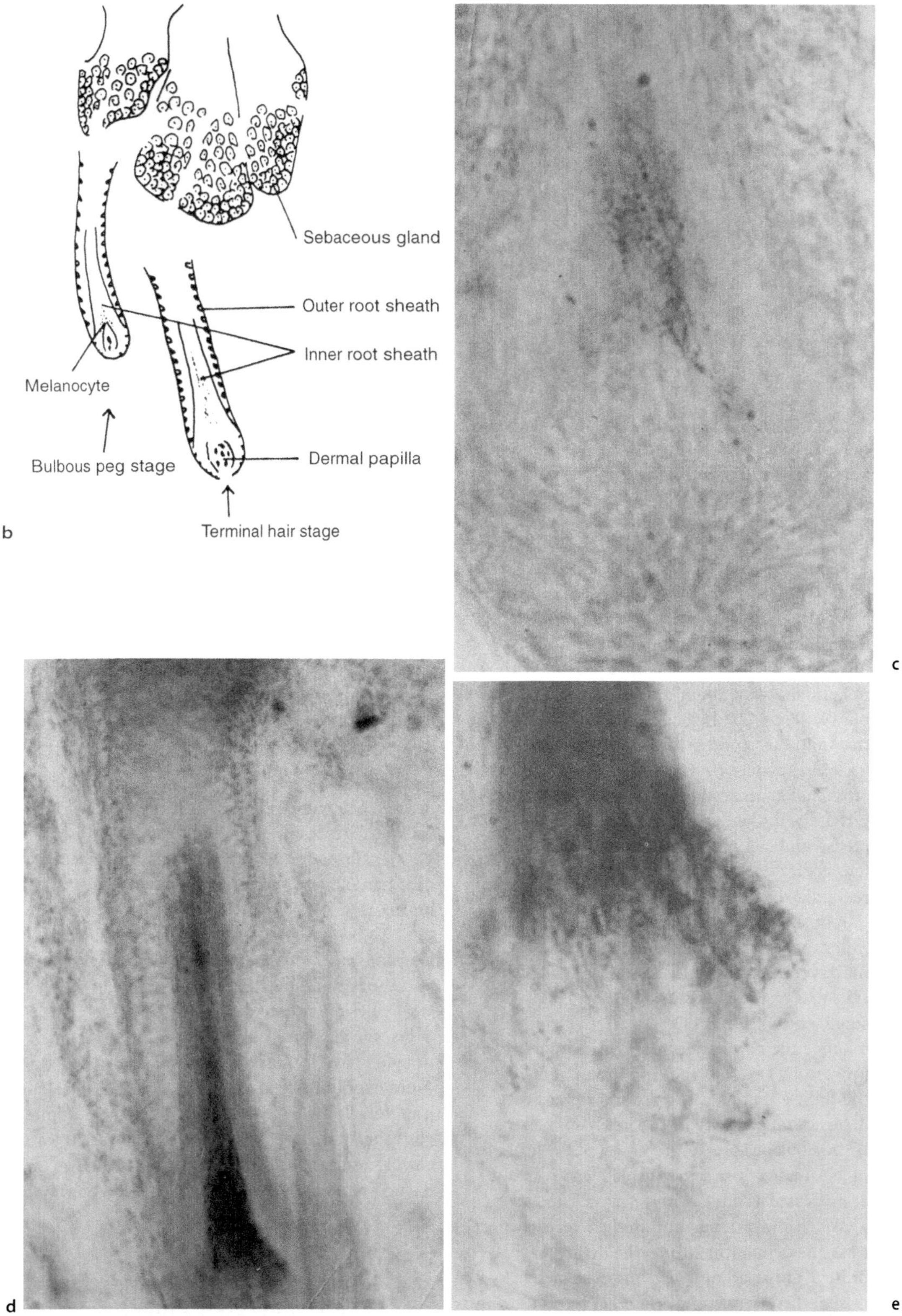

Fig. 8.10. *Continued*

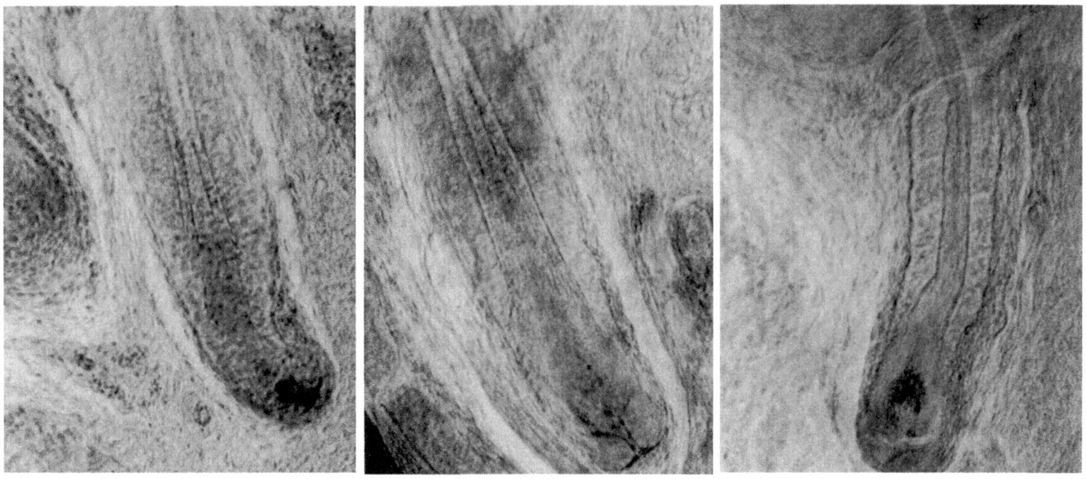

a,b c

Fig. 8.11a–c. Bulbous peg stage. **a** The inner root sheath elongates downward to form the bulb. The germinal layer wraps around a mass of mesenchymal cells to form the matrix. **b** The formation of the bulb is still incomplete and it is not yet compressed as it is in the terminal hair bulb. **c** The matrix grows around the mass of mesenchymal tissue, pressing the outer root sheath outward. Hair grows upward from the matrix. ×135

pressing the outer root sheath outward. Consequently, the outer root sheath becomes thin and the bottom of it has only one to two layers. The hair bulb is formed at this stage. The mass of mesenchymal tissue is wrapped around by the inner and outer root sheath and becomes the dermal papilla (Fig. 8.10b,d). There is slight matrix formation and melanocytes have also formed, so that melanin granules are visible (Fig. 8.10c). When the epithelial matrix cells are fully formed on the interface with the dermal papilla, melanocytes increase and melanin granules are deposited in the hair cortex (Fig. 8.10d,e). Eleven hair follicles were recognized in this bulbous peg stage (Table 8.1).

As the hair follicle begins to peg downward, the inner root sheath elongates downward. The germinal layer wraps around a mass of mesenchymal cells to form the matrix and hair bulb (bulbous peg stage, case 2) (Fig. 8.11).

Since the new hair is prevented from growing upward by firm interlocking fusion of the cuticle, the follicle continues to grow downward with vigorous mitotic activity in the newly-formed matrix. In this bulbous peg stage, however, the formation of the matrix is still incomplete and it is not yet compressed as it is in the terminal hair stage.

When the forming hair follicle reaches a level near the permanent site of the dermal papilla, the matrix grows around the mass of mesenchymal tissue, thereby pressing the outer root sheath outward. Consequently, the outer root sheath is thinned, and has only one or two layers at its bottom. The hair bulb is formed at this stage. The mass of mesenchymal tissue is wrapped by inner and outer root sheaths and becomes the dermal papilla. When the epithelial matrix cells are fully formed on the interface with the dermal papilla, melanocytes increase and melanin granules are deposited in the hair cortex. It is evident that the germinal layer (matrix) surrounding the dermal papilla may be divided into six distinct regions: Henle's layer, Huxley's layer, the sheath cuticle, the hair cuticle, the hair cortex, and the hair medulla (Fig. 8.12).

(d) Terminal Hair. Figure 8.10d shows the fully formed hair bulb with a single layer of tall cylindrical matrix cells covering the dermal papilla (case 1). Dendritic melanocytes have increased in number and size and pigmentation is seen in the hair cortex. The hair follicle stops descending, and the hair begins to ascend toward the skin surface. Hair and inner root sheath grow at the same speed, and the terminal hair grows according to the classical rules of the hair cycle.

As the hair bulb is formed, dendritic melanocytes have increased in number and size and pigmentation is seen in the cortex (case 1). The hair follicle stops descending, the hair and inner root sheath grow at the same speed upward toward the skin surface, and the terminal hair then grows according to the classic theories of the hair cycle (Fig. 8.10e).

8.4 Relationship of Development Stage of New Hair Follicle and Size of Sebaceous Gland

The width of the sebaceous glands was measured with the micrometer of the light microscope (×150). Results are shown in Table 8.2. The seba-

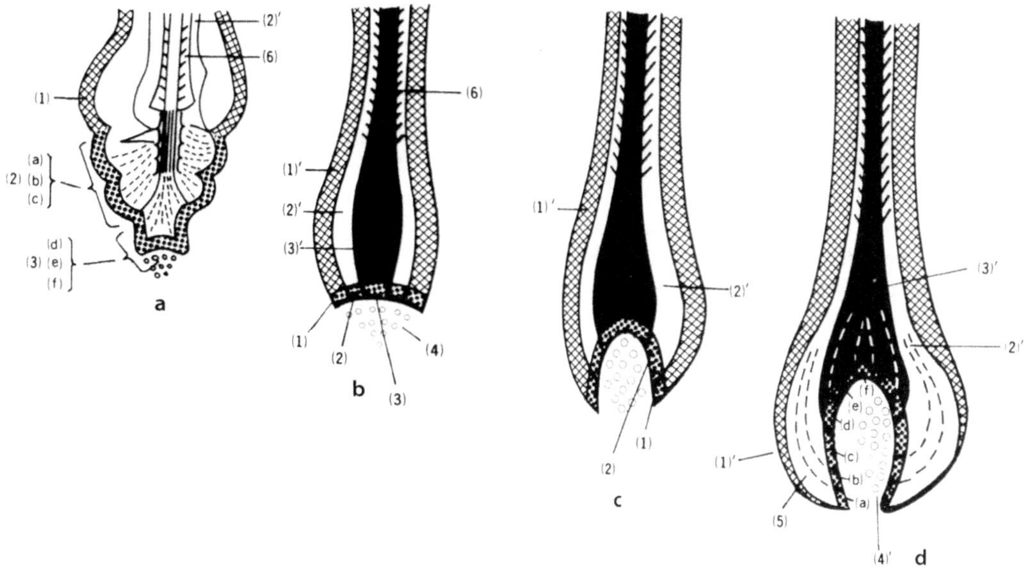

Fig. 8.12. Hair follicle formation after subcutaneous tissue shaving. **a** Hair germ stage. **b** Hair peg stage. **c** Bulbous peg stage. **d** Terminal hair. *(1)* germinal layer of outer root sheath; *(1)'* outer root sheath; *(2)* germinal layer of inner root sheath; *(a)* Henle's layer; *(b)* Huxley's layer; *(c)* sheath cuticle; *(2)'* inner root sheath; *(3)* germinal layer of hair tissue; *(d)* hair cuticle; *(e)* hair cortex; *(f)* medulla; *(3)'* hair tissue; *(4)* mesenchymal cells; *(4)'* dermal papilla; *(5)* matrix; *(6)* cuticula

Table 8.2. Number and size of sebaceous glands during hair regeneration

Stage of hair formation	Number of sebaceous glands	Average width of sebaceous gland
Hair germ stage	5	33.8 μm
Hair peg stage	23	28.2 μm
Bulbous peg stage	31	25.0 μm

ceous gland tends to become smaller as the new hair develops.

8.5 Relationship Between New Hair Follicle and Time Elapsed After Surgery

In regard to the relationship between new hair follicle and passage of time after removal of tissue: No consistent relation was found between the stage of hair development and time elapsed after surgery. Regrowth seemed to depend more on how much the tissue had been damaged by shaving.

Examination of normal axillary skin obtained from other types of operation revealed the ordinary distribution and arrangement of hair follicles and of sebaceous and apocrine glands as described in the textbooks. There never was any budding of accessory hair roots from the region of the upper isthmus. Each follicle was unbranched and ended in one matrix-papilla complex.

8.6 Evidence of New Hair Regeneration

Initiation of new hair follicles begins in human fetal life by the end of the 2nd month and comes to an end in the 7th month. There is little evidence of hair neogenesis in postnatal life, and it is a general rule that scars in human skin will not grow hairs, unless living hair roots, including epithelial matrix and dermal papilla, have been preserved in the deeper tissue. Conversely, the practice of permanent epilation is based on the thesis that destruction of the dermal papilla by surgical, electrical, or chemical means prevents regrowth of hair, even if the upper portions of the hair root are preserved (Oliver 1969). If we disregard benign cutaneous neoplasms, in which rudimentary or more or less functional hair roots may be observed, there is very little evidence for neogenesis of hairs in human skin, and not much evidence in other mammalian skin.

In humans, Kligman and Strauss (1956) described what they considered new formation of vellus hair follicles from the reconstituted epidermis of an abraded area of facial skin. Abnormally directed accessory hair roots are occasionally observed in scalp biopsy material, suggesting that these follicles have sprouted from the upper isthmus area of scalp hairs. This area, which corresponds to the level of origin of sebaceous glands, has also been implicated as the preferred site for the formation of milia and the epithelial collar of mantle hairs (Epstein and Kligman 1956). Ishibashi and Tsuru (1976) called attention to the rich innervation of this region and to the presence of a mantle-like epithelial collar surrounding many hair follicles just below the branching point of the sebaceous duct.

Breedis (1954) described the formation of large numbers of new hair follicles from the epidermis of healing wounds on the back of the rabbit. Although his conclusions were later contradicted by Straile (1959), similar observations to those of Breedis (Hallmans and Stenstrom 1974) have been reported in the immobile skin of the rabbit ear (Joseph and Townsend 1961). Lyne and Brook (1964) favored the occurrence of hair neogenesis in healing wounds in sheep. The formation of many new hairs in the antler skin of deer (Billingham et al. 1959) is not pertinent to our problem, since, in this annual event, completely new skin is grown.

There are, however, two directly applicable observations. In Oliver's studies (1966a, 1969) of rat's whiskers, a new dermal papilla and hair of normal size were formed despite the removal of the hair bulb. Oliver concluded that hair could be regrown from the outer root sheath. He also recognized that the size and length of the new hair was related to the volume of the hair follicle left behind. Hair does not grow if more than one-third of the vibrissa follicle is removed. The other pertinent observation is that of Lyne (1957, 1970) who found that, in certain marsupials, the hair cycle in the classical sense was the exception. In most cases, when the old hair has completed its growth, a new hair follicle buds and grows down from the level of the sebaceous duct.

Our histologic studies demonstrated that human axillary hair regenerates even when the transient portion and a considerable part of the permanent portion of the hair root is removed. Clinically, the absence or presence of the sebaceous gland predicts the state of hair regeneration (Inaba et al. 1978c) and histologically, regeneration depends on the presence of at least part of the isthmus. A new young hair forms when the new follicular bud is in the hair peg stage; the hair keratinizes while the peg grows downward until the formation of hair bulb and matrix are completed. After completion of the bulb, the hair grows in the reverse direction toward the skin surface. In this respect, axillary hair appears to be different from other hairs of the human skin and from the pelage hairs of most mammals. Its behavior resembles that of the sinus hairs (vibrissae) of rodents and perhaps of other species. Our observations, coupled with the clinical findings of Fukuda and Ezaki (1975) that hair may grow from split-thickness scalp skin transplanted in reconstructive surgery for microtia, should encourage additional studies on specialized types of human hair. Observations of the growth of fetal eyebrows have suggested to us a replacement mechanism similar to that found by Lyne in marsupials.

The stereohistologic details of our axillary hair studies also suggest that the hair cortex, cuticle, and inner root sheath are formed and begin to keratinize in the center of the elongating epithelial column, which descends from the cut lower border of the preexisting follicular isthmus, before this epithelial outer root sheath material has united with the underlying mass of mesodermal cells to form a hair bulb with organized matrix and papilla. This means that the tip of the new hair and the surrounding upper end of the inner root sheath remain stationary, while the mitotic activity of trichilemmal cells forces the hair peg downward until it has reached the level of the future bulb. Only then does the hair grow upward through the upper follicle. In this respect, the replacement follicle recapitulates early fetal events as described by Pinkus (1958), who pointed out that, in embryonic skin, the first cells of the inner sheath form when the follicle is very short. It is more appropriate to say that the matrix moves away from the tip of the root sheath and burrows deeper, rather than that the tip pushes upward from the bulb.

Differently from fetal hair, which, according to the classical description, originates below the follicular bulge, the regenerating axillary hair begins to form at the level of the sebaceous gland, far above the bulge area that has been removed by surgery. As shown in Table 8.2, the number of newgrown hairs is related to the number of sebaceous glands. If a follicle possesses more than one sebaceous gland, it usually regenerates more than one new hair root. This finding confirms our contention that there is new formation of hairs at the sebaceous duct level. This occurrence cannot be explained by short telogen hair roots having been left behind during surgery.

Montagna and Parakkal (1974) divided the hair follicle into two parts, i.e., permanent and transient portions. However, it should be separated into upper, middle, and lower portions, as reported by Pinkus (1969) (Fig. 8.4).

Baldness bears some relationship to the size of the sebaceous gland, and it is well known that the bigger the sebaceous gland, the more widespread the baldness. We have found that the sebaceous gland gradually becomes smaller when hair reaches completion in the hair cycle.

It is also remarkable that the newly-formed hair matrix of regenerating axillary hair acquires a normal complement of melanocytes. It is thought

(Montagna and Parakkal 1974) that in the normal hair cycle, some preexisting melanocytes remain dormant in the dormant papilla and become reactivated and multiply during the next anagen. With our subdermal shaving procedure, all matrix-associated melanocytes are removed. Thus, melanocytes of the neogenetic matrix must come from other sources, perhaps from the amelanotic melanocytes that have been shown to exist in the basal layer of the outer root sheath (Starico 1961), and they contribute to the epidermal repigmentation that occurs after wound healing (see Chapter 4).

Regeneration After Plucking

9

The effect of plucking upon hair follicles has been studied in animals. It has been shown that the plucking of telogen hairs initiates new hair growth (Chase 1958; Kligman 1961).

The plucking of growing hairs has conflicting results (Johnson 1975; Ibrahim and Wright 1978). In the rat, plucking does not induce the telogen phase. In short, spontaneous anagen is not identical with the anagen induced by plucking. In the spontaneous process, only the germ cells are activated in early anagen. The artificial induction of catagen or a new cycle has been successful only after an appropriate dose of X-radiation (Uno 1970). Observations indicate that plucking does not have the same effects in humans. Kligman (1961) observed that when a small area with a high percentage of telogen hairs was completely denuded by plucking, hairs did not emerge for several weeks. The resting follicles evidently remained quiescent.

Myers and Hamilton (1951) plucked growing hairs and found the average number of days required for regeneration of hairs in 90% of follicles to be 129 in the crown of the scalp and 117 in the supra-auricular region. The relatively long interval between epilation and regeneration suggests that, in humans, follicles respond to the trauma associated with plucking by temporary regression. Van Scott et al. (1957) reported that, in hair follicles isolated by plucking, in general, the dermal papilla and a large part of the hair follicle bulb was left behind in the skin; yet the dermal papilla regulates hair growth, and the matrix cells at the base of the bulb are essential for this growth (Oliver 1967b). On the other hand, axillary and beard hairs begin to regrow within a short time, despite plucking.

In cases in which it takes a long time for the hair to regenerate, as in the scalp, plucking of hair will result in no hair regrowth for some time. Beard hair regrows very soon after plucking. However, it remains to be discussed why regeneration occurs immediately after plucking.

9.1 Process of Hair Regeneration After Plucking

The authors have reported the regeneration of axillary hair after plucking. In the process of regeneration and growth after the plucking of axillary hair, it was found that, 1 day after plucking, thick tissue had formed around the plucked follicle (Fig. 9.1a). The remains of melanin granules were clustered within the trichilemma in the upper region of the isthmal portion and in the remnant of the dermal papilla. Higher magnification of the remnant of the dermal papilla (Fig. 9.1b) clearly showed the remnants of the melanin granules; Fig. 9.1c showed that the atrophied epithelial layer was situated above the remnant of the dermal papilla. On the 2nd day after plucking, the follicles had shrunk to the level of the arrector pili muscle (Fig. 9.2a). The sebaceous glands and dermal papilla had become smaller in size. The boundary of the epithelial sac was not well defined and the lower portion of the trichilemma was clearly atrophied. The bottom of the follicle was covered with thick connective tissue. Stratified keratinization and projection were observed in the trichilemma of the upper isthmal portion of the follicle, just below the opening of the sebaceous duct (Fig. 9.2b,d).

On the 3rd day after plucking, thick connective tissue had formed around the atrophied hair follicles (Fig. 9.3a). The remains of melanin granules were clustered within the trichilemma in the upper region of the isthmal portion. The trichilemma also showed corrugation below the duct opening

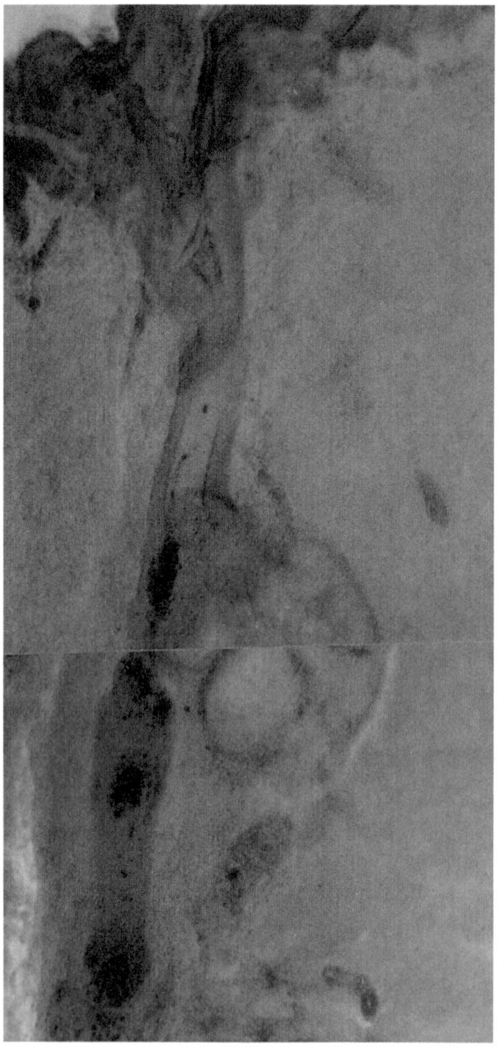
a

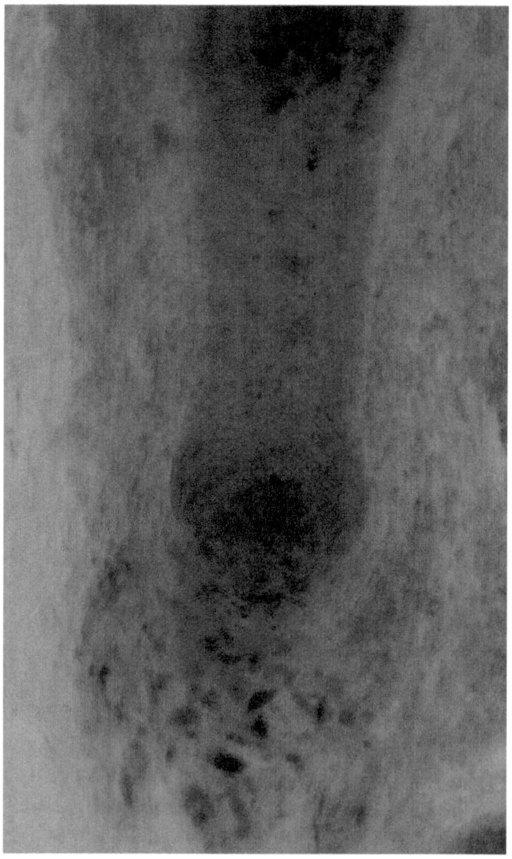
b

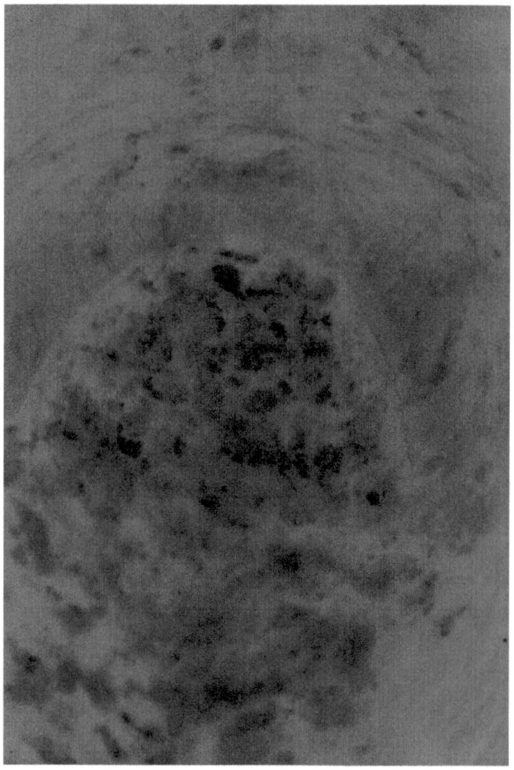
c

Fig. 9.1. **a** One day after the plucking of a hair, thick connective tissue has formed around an atrophied hair follicle; the remains of melanin granules are seen inside the follicle and in the dermal papilla. ×75 **b** Remains of melanin granules are clustered within. ×125 **c** Higher magnification of the lower portion in **b** shows the atrophied epithelial layer surrounding the dermal papilla; remains of melanin granules are seen within the dermal papilla. ×225

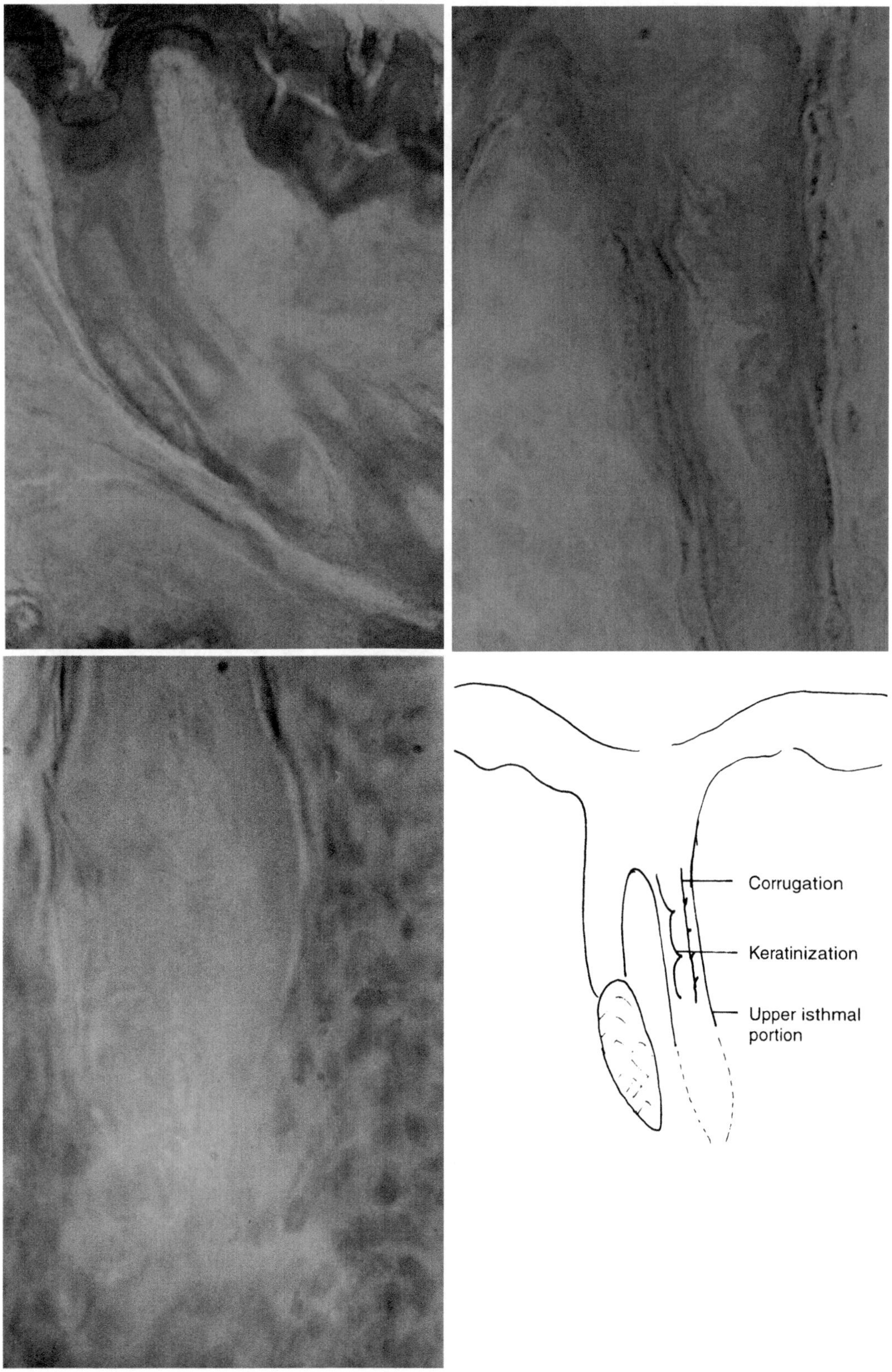

Fig. 9.2. a Two days after plucking. The follicle has shrunk to the level of the arrector pili muscle. The sebaceous gland and lower portion of the hair follicle have become smaller. ×75 **b** Higher magnification of **a**; keratinization and projection are seen in the upper part of the isthmus directly below the secretory duct of the sebaceous gland. ×125 **c** Higher magnification of **a**; the lower part of the hair is seen to have atrophied. ×125 **d** Events 2 days after the plucking of a hair (germ stage)

a

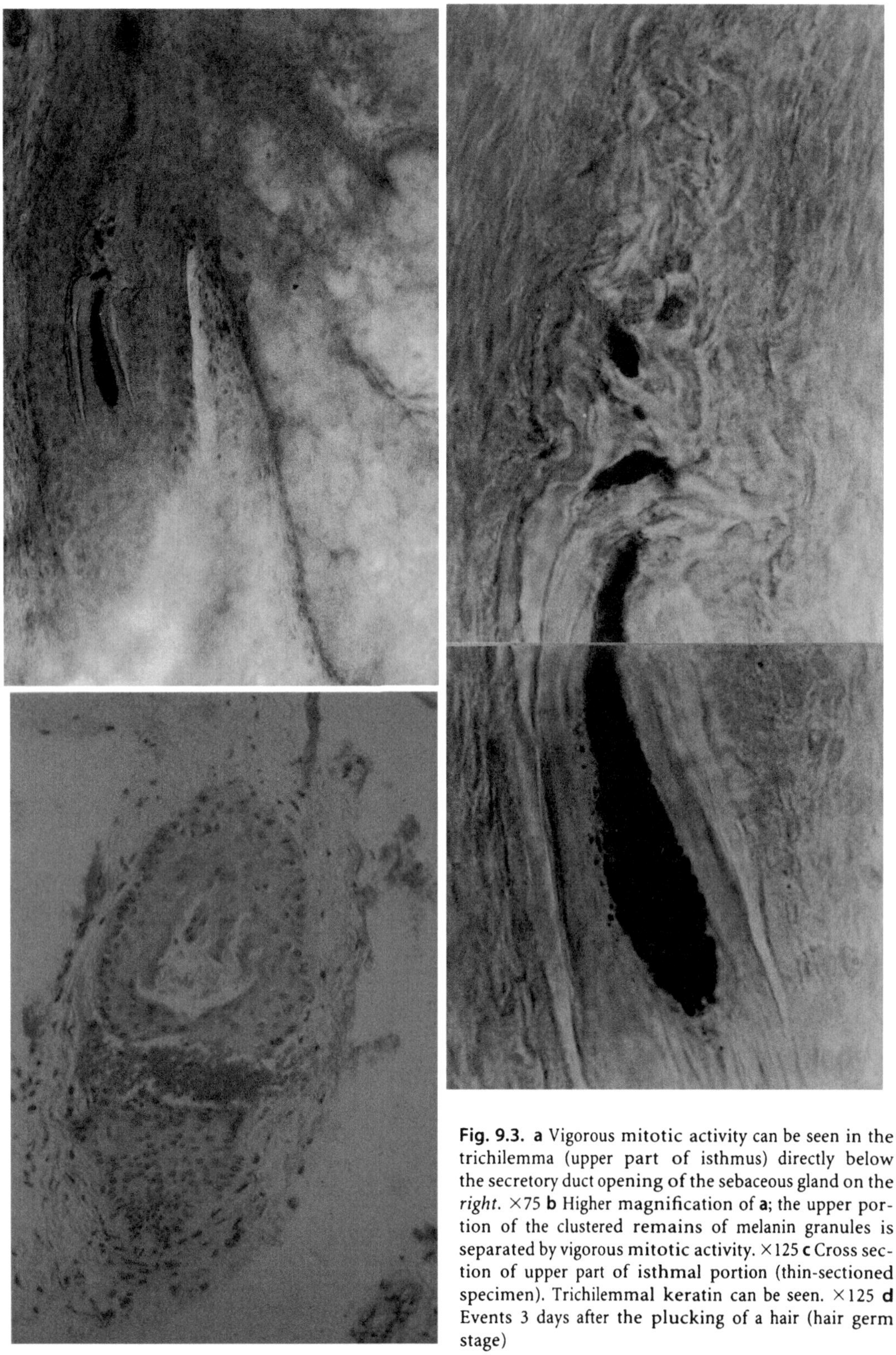

b

c

Fig. 9.3. **a** Vigorous mitotic activity can be seen in the trichilemma (upper part of isthmus) directly below the secretory duct opening of the sebaceous gland on the *right*. ×75 **b** Higher magnification of **a**; the upper portion of the clustered remains of melanin granules is separated by vigorous mitotic activity. ×125 **c** Cross section of upper part of isthmal portion (thin-sectioned specimen). Trichilemmal keratin can be seen. ×125 **d** Events 3 days after the plucking of a hair (hair germ stage)

Fig. 9.4. **a** Six days after the plucking of a hair, a cystic bud is seen in the upper part of the isthmus. ×75 **b** Higher magnification of **a**; filamentous structures, formed in the bottom of the epithelial sac, are seen to have become fibrous and a new young hair has formed in the upper portion of the fibrous structure. ×125 **c** Lower portion of **b** as seen from a different angle clearly shows a mass of mesenchymal cells (future dermal papilla) at the tip of the follicle. ×125 **d** Events 6 days after the plucking of a hair (germ stage)

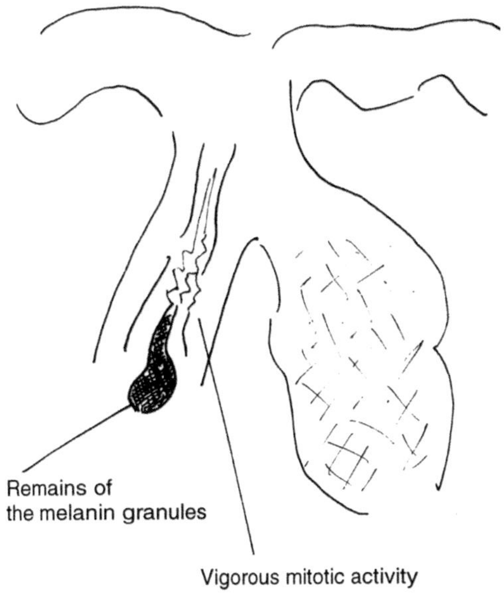

d

Fig. 9.3. *Continued*

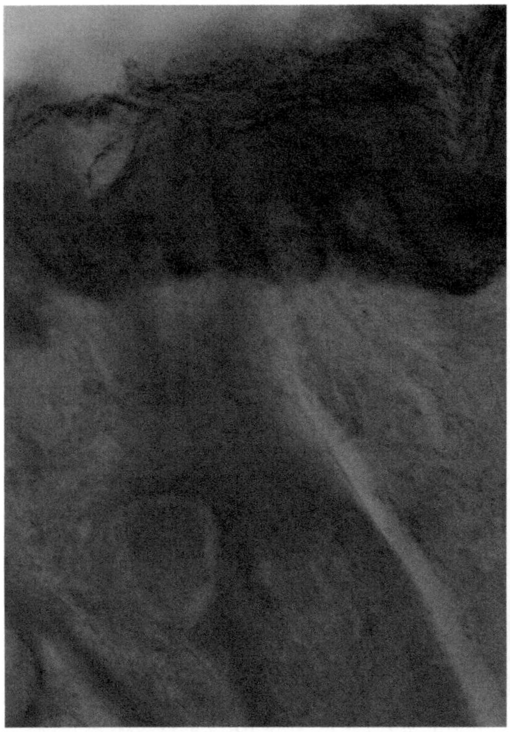

a

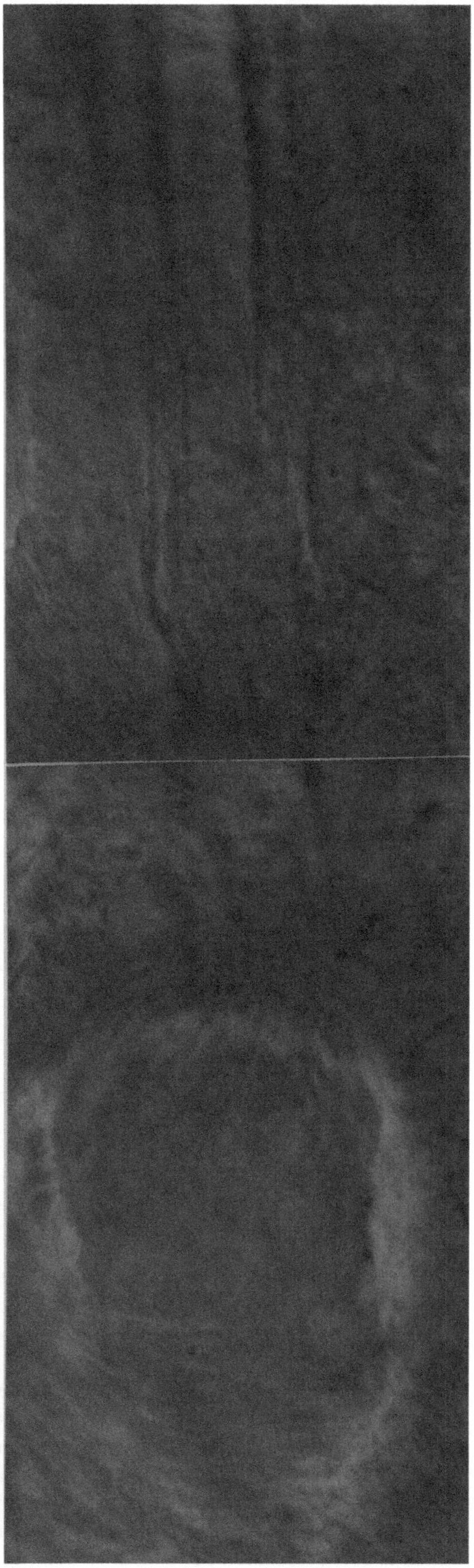

b

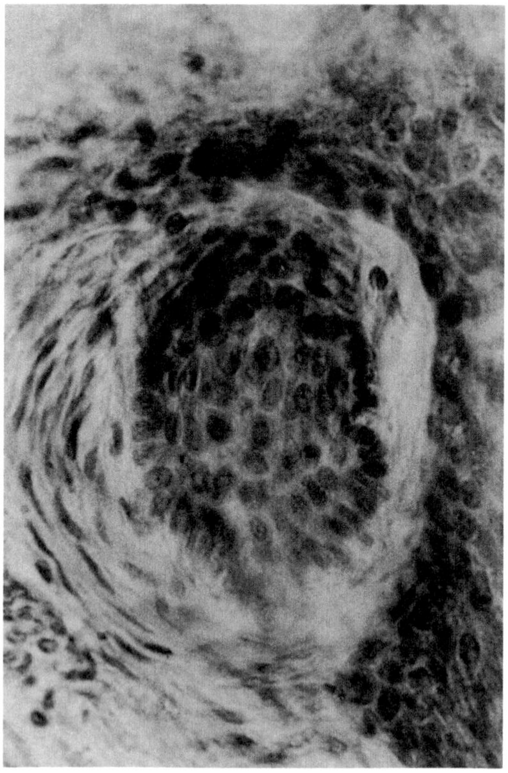

c

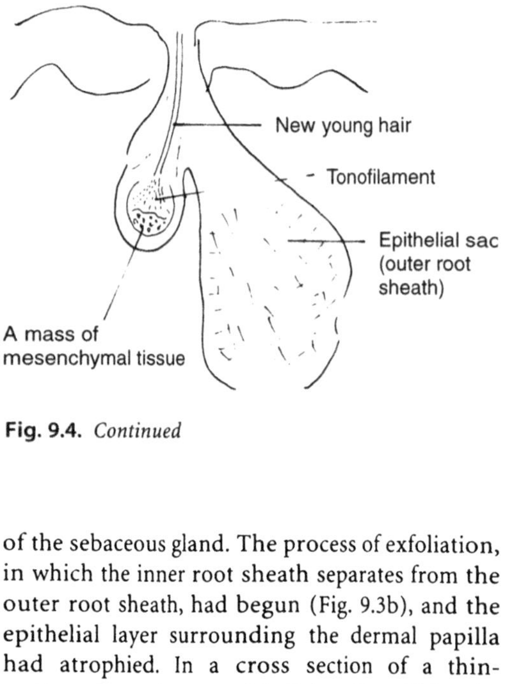

d

Fig. 9.4. *Continued*

of the sebaceous gland. The process of exfoliation, in which the inner root sheath separates from the outer root sheath, had begun (Fig. 9.3b), and the epithelial layer surrounding the dermal papilla had atrophied. In a cross section of a thin-sectioned specimen epithelial cells within the trichilemma, protruding from the outer root sheath, were seen in the upper isthmal portion (Fig. 9.3c,d).

Vigorous mitotic activity had occurred in the trichilemma directly below the duct opening of the sebaceous gland. Melanin granules remaining there had been broken up by this very active cell division process. This process had also begun at the opening of the secretory duct of the sebaceous gland in the upper isthmal region of the follicle. Corrugation was sometimes quite clear within the trichilemma in the isthmal area (Fig. 9.3d).

Six days after the hair plucking, the follicles characteristically showed a cyst-like bulge close to the sebaceous duct (Fig. 9.4a). At higher magnification (Fig. 9.4b), filamentous structures had formed from the bottom of the epithelial sac (cyst-like bulge) in fibrous new young hairs. Masses of mesenchymal cells (the future dermal papilla) had formed at the lower tips of the newly-formed follicle buds (Fig. 9.4c,d).

In specimens observed 8 days after plucking, it was clear that new follicles had developed in the dermis layer below the sebaceous gland (Fig. 9.5a); the lower portion of these follicles was multilobular (Fig. 9.5a,b). The epithelial layer (matrix) surrounding the masses of mesenchymal cells (future dermal papilla) had atrophied (Fig. 9.5b). Keratinized new hairs were clearly visible within the trichilemma, and filamentous structures had developed in the lower regions of these multilobular epithelial sacs. Inner root sheaths had also formed at the same time (Fig. 9.5c).

Cuticle had formed around the cortex of each new hair and had interlocked with the inner root sheath, which adhered to the surrounding trichilemmal epithelium. This interlocking fusion prevented the hair from moving upward; instead, it was forced to elongate downward by mitotic (cell division) activity. Vigorous mitotic activity forced young hairs downward until they reached the final site of the bulb in the subcutaneous tissue, where, as matrices, they enveloped masses of mesenchymal tissue that had become the new dermal papilla. This process, along with the compression exerted by the inner root sheath, caused the initially filamentous structures to become fibrous (Fig. 9.5c,d).

The absence of melanin granules in the hair cortex, the stem-like (not club-like) configuration of the lower part of the hair root (cortex), and the multilobular condition of the lower follicle portion all indicate that this was the anagen (not catagen) stage.

Fifteen days after plucking, newly-formed hair follicles could be seen. The multilobular follicles had generally become simple follicles (Fig. 9.6a). The hair root (cortex) was covered with keratinized inner root sheath. This phase of anagen stage could be confused with catagen stage, since the filamentous structures observed resemble the keratinized rootlets of the club hair phase in catagen stage (Fig. 7.2b). However, these filamentous structures were aggregated only at the tips of the hair roots, and then became fibrous. Melanin granules were not visible in the cortex. At this time, formation of the hair cuticle was clearly visible (Fig. 9.6b).

Cuticle had formed around the cortex of each new hair and had interlocked with the newly-formed inner root sheath by pegging downward due to vigorous mitotic activity.

Three weeks after plucking, the inner root sheath of each follicle had become thick and long. The inner and outer root sheaths in the downward elongating hair follicle had wrapped around masses of mesenchymal tissue at the follicle tip to form the hair bulb and dermal papilla (Fig. 9.7a). The outer root sheath was pressed outward and its lower part was still quite thick, with the hair bulb incompletely formed. Epithelial matrix cells had begun to form at interfaces with the dermal papilla.

The follicle continued to elongate and develop downward until the formation of the hair matrix was complete. The number of melanocytes increased and a few melanin granules were visible in the hair cortex. As soon as the matrix was formed, the inner root sheath and hair cortex began to ascend simultaneously. Changes of configuration were seen in the outer root sheath in this later phase of the bulbous peg development stage.

By the time the new young hair had ascended to the skin surface, melanin granules had increased in number to give it a normal color on outward appearance (Fig. 9.7b,c).

This process of regeneration of axillary hairs after plucking, carefully observed with three-dimensional, thick tissue slide preparations, clearly revealed that regeneration of the new young hair

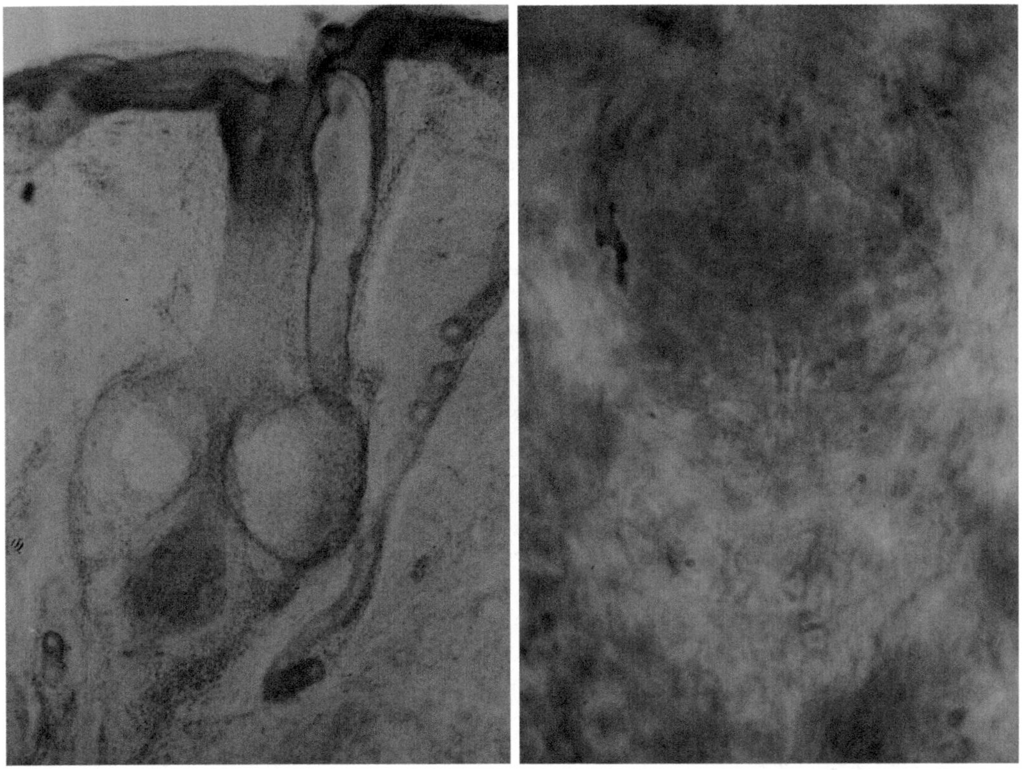

a b

Fig. 9.5. a Eight days after plucking. Keratinized new hair is clearly visible, a multilobular new bud has developed, and a distended apocrine duct is seen. ×75 **b** Higher magnification of **a**; the lower portion of the follicle has not yet become a bulb. The epithelial layer surrounding the future dermal papilla is seen to have atrophied. ×125 **c** Higher magnification of the lower portion of a newly-formed hair follicle. The lower portion of the new bud has become multilobular. Filamentous structures, which have developed in the lower regions of these multilobular epithelial sacs, have changed to tonofibrils, and the upper portion of the lower filament has become the cortex. The inner root sheath has also formed at the same time. ×135 **d** Events 8 days after the plucking of a hair. Filamentous structure is formed from the lower portion. In the Henle layer inside the inner root sheath, the filamentous structure contracts, becoming fibrous. The upper portion of this fibrous structure becomes the cortex. The new young hair is prevented from pegging upward due to interlocking fusion between the hair cuticula and the sheath cuticula, and it thus pegs downward. Pegging takes place as a result of vigorous mitotic activity in the lower portion of the hair follicle. This particular developmental process, explains why the filamentous structure becomes fibrous

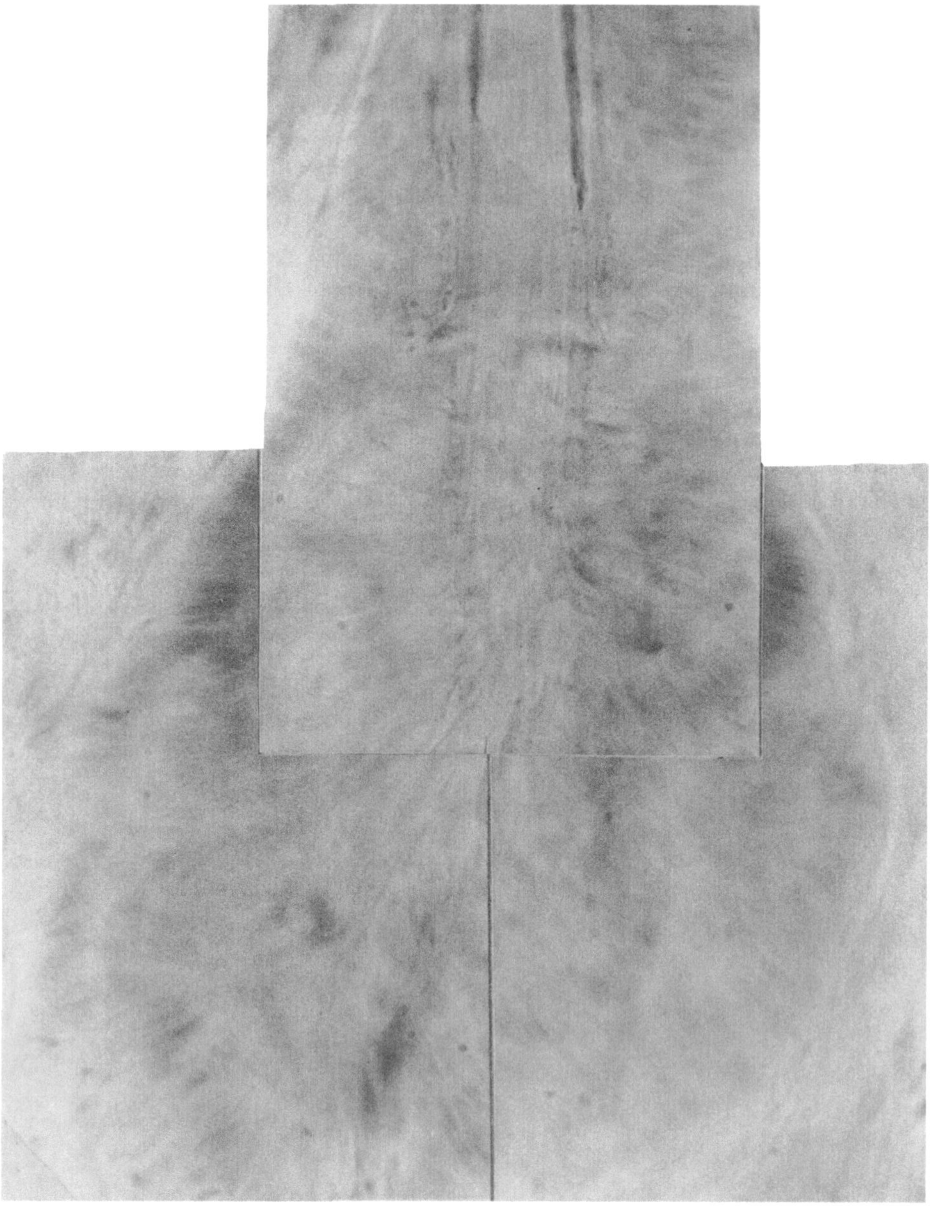

c

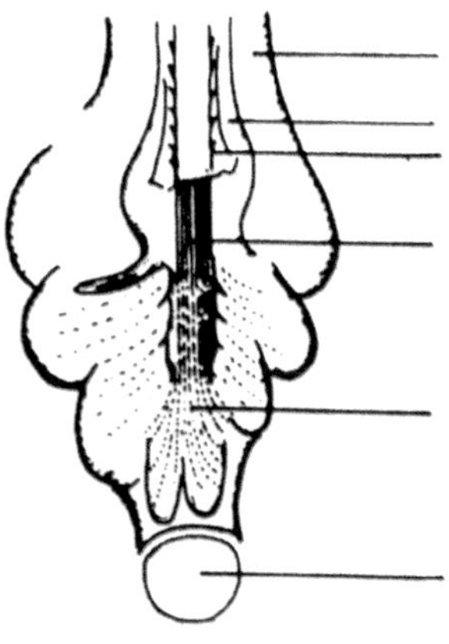

d

Fig. 9.5. *Continued*

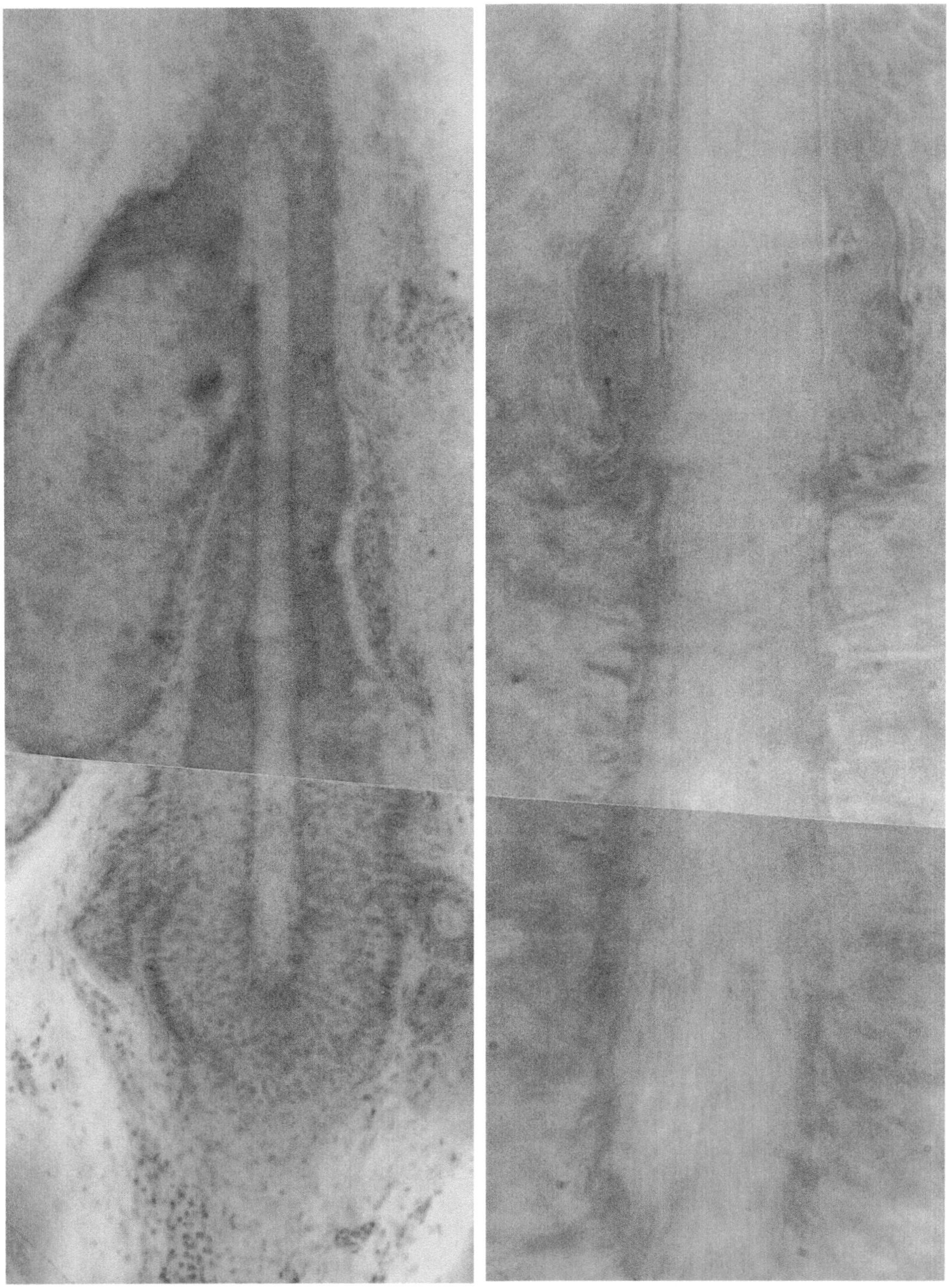

a b

Fig. 9.6. **a** Fifteen days after plucking. Newly-formed hair follicle in anagen stage can be seen descending between the lobes of the sebaceous gland. The multilobular follicle has gradually become simple follicles. This phase of anagen stage could be confused with catagen stage. ×75 **b** Higher magnification of hair roots. Filamentous structures aggregate only at the tips of the hair root and have become fibrous due to the pressure of the inner root sheath. The process of cuticula formation is clearly visible. ×180 **c** Events 15 days after the plucking of a hair (peg stage)

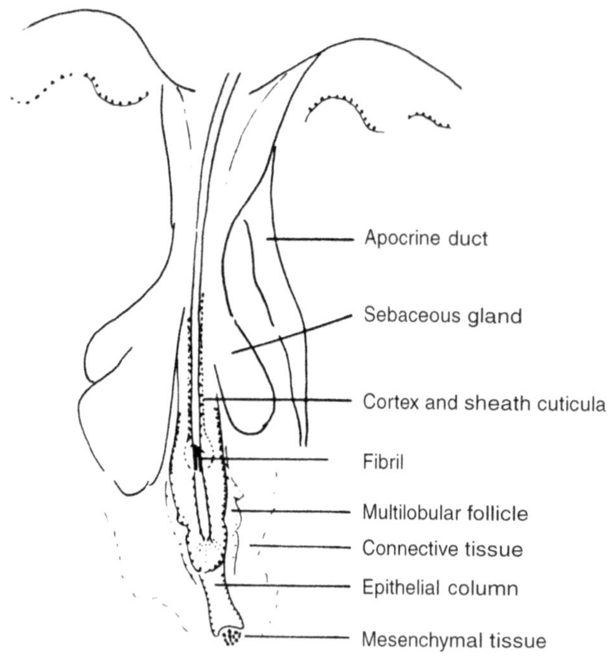

c

Fig. 9.6. *Continued*

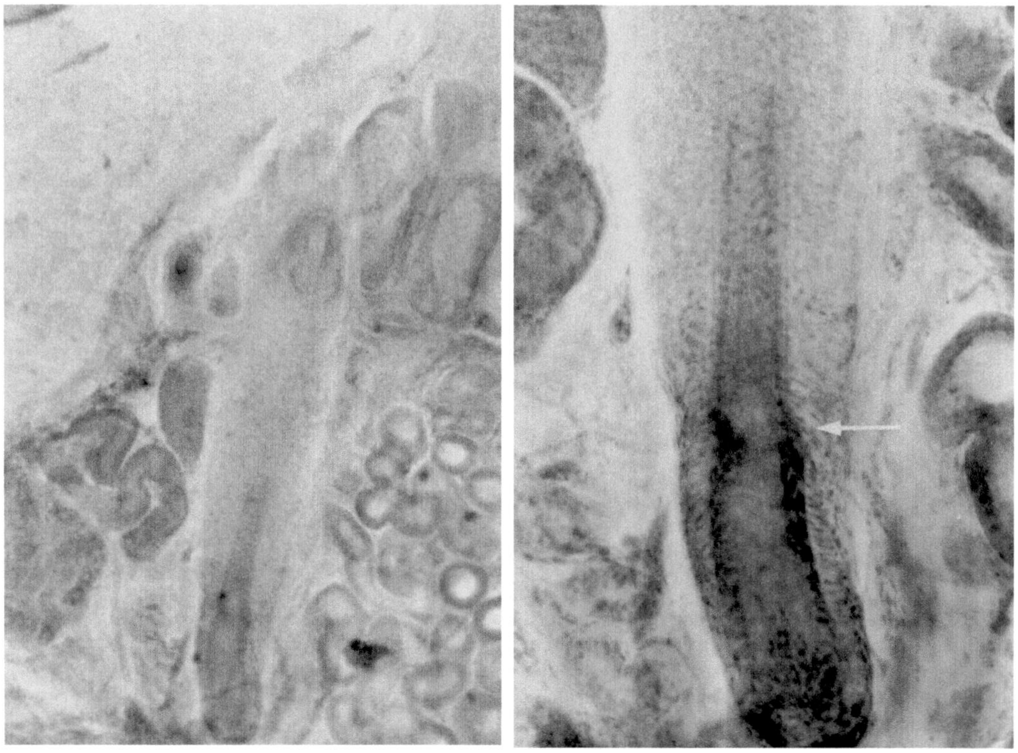

a b

Fig. 9.7. **a** Three weeks after plucking. The inner root sheath has become long, and covers a mass of mesenchymal tissue; this forms the hair bulb and the dermal papilla, but this structure keeps descending until the matrix is completed (late stage in bulbous peg stage). ×75 **b** Higher magnification of the lower portion of **a.** The matrix has begun to form as a bulb: As the cortex and inner root sheath begin to grow upward, bending takes place (*arrow*). ×125 **c** Schematic of **b. d** Hair has stopped pegging with the completion of the matrix. The inner root sheath and hair tissue ascend toward the skin surface. Melanin granules can be seen clearly. ×75 **e** Inside the cortex, dendritic melanocytes and melanin granules can be seen. ×135

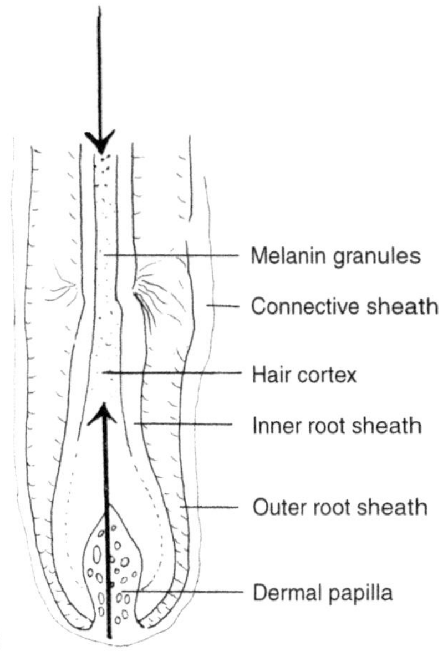

c

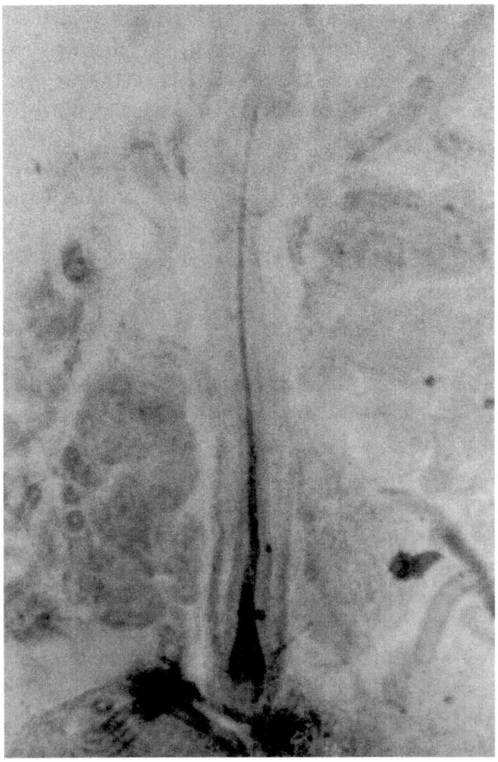
d

Fig. 9.7. *Continued*

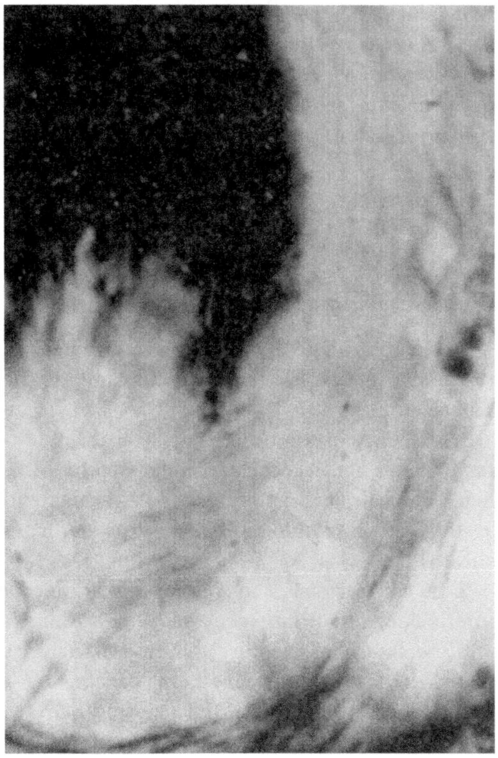
e

begins in the upper isthmal portion of the hair follicle close to the duct opening of the sebaceous gland.

It is interesting to note that it takes around 4 weeks for the new hair follicle to be completely formed. This is the same time it takes for the epidermis to be keratinized from its basal layer.

Plucking does not, of course, permanently remove axillary hairs. New growth may be visible on the skin surface within a very short time after plucking. Rapid regeneration of hairs then begins from the outer root sheath in the isthmal portion of the hair follicle.

Reports from other sources tend to support our findings. As stated above, Lyne (1957) has reported that, in certain marsupials, the hair cycle in the classic sense is the exception. He found that, in these animals in most cases, when a hair had completed its growth, a new hair follicle budded and grew downward from the level of the sebaceous duct. Oliver, in his study of rat whiskers (1966a), found that new dermal papillae and hairs grew to normal size despite removal of the hair bulb. Oliver concluded that hairs can regrow from outer root sheaths. Dry (1926) found that, in the mouse, the first cells of inner root sheaths (hair cones) formed when follicles were very short. Pinkus (1958) reported the same finding in human embryonic follicles. We have found that when vellus hairs change to coarse hairs during puberty, new hair follicles emerge from the isthmal portions of the vellus hairs (Inaba et al. 1980b). In other words, new coarse hairs begin to form in the epithelial sacs (outer root sheaths), emerging from the upper isthmal portions.

9.2 Summary of Our Findings

Our findings may be summarized as follows:

1. Keratinization starts from a certain part of the upper isthmus close to the duct opening of the sebaceous gland.
2. A follicle forms about 6 days after the plucking of a hair, and becomes a multilobular hair follicle. The hair fiber and inner root sheath form at the bottom of the epithelial sac (outer root sheath).
3. A hair peg starts to develop as a result of interlocking fusion between the cuticles of hairs and sheaths that occurs due to the mitotic activity of cells in the lower part of a new hair follicle.
4. About 20 days after the plucking of hair, masses of mesenchymal tissue at the tip of descending pegs are wrapped and covered by inner root sheaths and hair to form hair bulbs. Follicles continue to descend until new matrices are complete. After the matrix is completed, the hair shaft begins to grow upward as a new terminal hair.

These findings have provided us with information of clinical value in that we can set our shaving instrument to assure either regrowth or no regrowth of axillary hair, as the patient prefers. The findings have far more importance, of course, in defining a more accurate model of the human hair cycle.

9.3 Process of Hair Follicle Formation After Subcutaneous Tissue Shaving and Hair Plucking

In the process of hair regeneration, hair germs, formed at the portion of the hair follicle adjacent to the excretory duct opening of the sebaceous glands (upper isthmal portion), continue to grow, going through the hair peg and bulbous peg stages, finally becoming terminal hairs. This finding has been supported by several studies (Inaba et al. 1981a,b; Inaba 1985).

Until quite recently, the formation of the six regions of the inner root sheath and the hair tissue after hair bulb development was not clear. We now know that the six regions can be observed in the hair germ stage and that the germinal cell layer (hair matrix) is formed as it gradually wraps around the dermal papilla. These observations indicate that tissues of different morphologies are not generated from the matrix below Auber's critical line in the hair bulb (Fig. 4.4), as was previously believed (Inaba and Inaba 1990b).

9.3.1 Mechanism of Regeneration of the Hair Follicle from the Upper Isthmal Portion

The conventional theory states that no hair regeneration would occur if the portion above the lower end of the hair follicle had been removed. However, we have confirmed that hair regeneration did occur from the upper isthmal portion of the hair follicle (essential hair cycle, Inaba and Inaba 1990a, 1992a). Yet it was still impossible to elucidate how the hair germ was formed from the upper isthmal portion to induce hair regeneration.

According to Pinkus (1981a), keratinous cysts in the scalp region (thick-walled cutaneous cystwens) have been recognized as having their prototype in the outer sheath (trichilemma) at the level of the follicular isthmus. Thus, trichilemmal cysts are common, and are most frequently encountered on the scalp. In these cysts, fine granules are diffusely distributed in the cytoplasms in the granular layer of the epidermis. In the isthmus, beneath the orifice of the sebaceous glands, keratohyaline granules are usually not noticeable at a glance but, when carefully examined, fine round granules are found grouped in some portions.

Histologically, the epithelium in young cysts consists of large, rather palely stained cells (H&E). When a trichilemmal cyst forms, the large vesicular nucleus fades, and the cell joins the dense central mass of keratin. Keratohyalin usually is absent but may occur in occasional cells. Trichilemmal keratinization represents a trichilemmal cyst.

As in the case of the trichilemmal cyst, a new hair bud is assumed to form from the upper isthmal portion.

9.3.2 Trichilemmal Keratinization

As early as 1895, Maurer had already noted trichilemmal keratinization, and Auber (1952) observed the corrugation in the isthmal portion. Straile's zone of sloughing (Straile 1965) in which the inner root sheath disintegrates is perhaps due to the presence of a keratinolytic enzyme (keratinase).

Fig. 9.8. Longitudinal sections of the upper isthmal portion of the hair follicle. The formation of the corrugation in the isthmal portion can clearly be seen. The inner root sheath has begun to disintegrate from the outer root sheath (*arrow*). *TK*, Trichilemmal keratinization. ×135

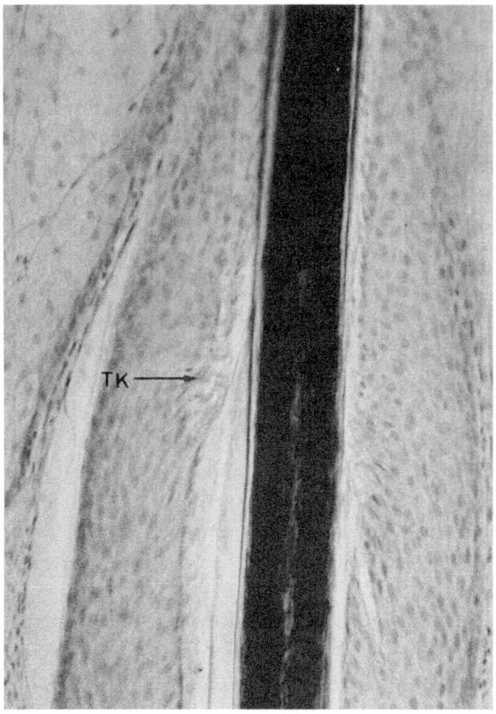

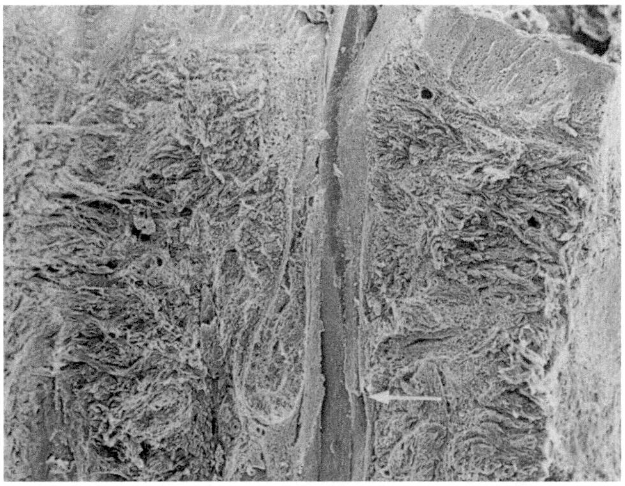
a

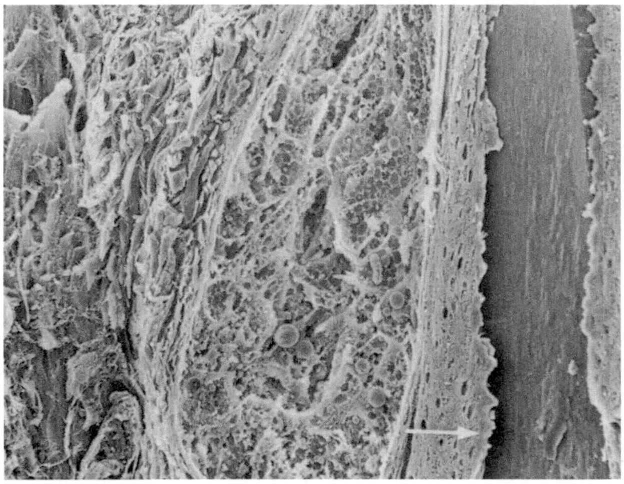
b

Fig. 9.9. a Longitudinal section of portion of an axillary hair at the level where degraded cells of the inner root sheath slough into the follicle lumen (*arrow*). ×75 **b** Higher magnification of **a**. Adjacent cells, which are part of the outer root sheath, undergo cornification and degradation and also slough into the follicle lumen (*arrow*). ×135

Pinkus (1969) reported that the human outer root sheath, which does not keratinize as long as it is covered with the inner sheath, does keratinize in a specific situation in the follicular isthmus of anagen hairs, in which the inner root sheath has disappeared (Figs. 9.8, 9.9a,b). The stratified epithelium progresses to dense keratin through an intermediate stage of voluminous non-nucleated cells, without the formation of visible keratohyalin. It appears justified to conclude that the stratified trichilemmal epithelium with its specific mode of keratinization is the prototype for the wall of the wen, which therefore is neither a sebaceous nor a pilar cyst, and certainly not an epidermoid cyst, but may be termed a trichilemmal cyst. The wall cells seen in steatocystoma multiplex closely resemble these cells, and therefore, steatocystoma multiplex is strongly suggested to be a cyst originating from the outer root sheath of the isthmus.

Pinkus (1969) also stated that the outer sheath cells exposed to the inner root sheath in the cavity of the isthmus were rapidly keratinized as a whole, not through keratohyalin granules, and not through flattening of the cells, and that an intercellular bridge remained between the cells, this being an extremely specific type of keratinization. Pinkus named this "trichilemmal keratinization." However, Hashimoto (1976) found it noteworthy that, on electron microscopic examination, keratohyalin granules were also observed in the isthmus as fine, round granules.

Further, it was ascertained by Hashimoto (1976) that keratohyalin granules were present, though in small numbers, in the portion where the inner root sheath still remained and covered the outer sheath. It was therefore presumed that the outer sheath cells undergo the same keratinization process, morphologically, as the epidermis, although their characteristics differ greatly from those of epidermal keratinocytes. The inner root sheath cells of the outer root sheath in the isthmus, however, have eosinophilic cytoplasm and protrude hemispherically or cylindrically into the follicular cavity, and are morphologically fairly characteristic. Whether this trichilemmal keratinization leads to the formation of a hair bud is still unclear.

As a corollary, some other conclusions may be drawn. It has always been said that, in addition to epidermis-like keratin in the infundibular part, the hair follicle produces six distinct variants of keratin or keratin-like substances. All of these arise in the hair matrix and are found in the medulla, cortex, and cuticle of the hair, and in the cuticle, and in Huxley's and Henle's layers of the inner root sheath. Trichilemmal keratin is a distinct seventh variant arising not in the hair matrix, but in the stratified epithelium of the outer root sheath.

Regeneration After Electrical Epilation of the Hair

10

10.1 Basic Principles of Electrolysis and Electrocoagulation

Physical therapy has been used in the treatment of axillary bromidrosis by axillary hair epilation. The fact that hairs frequently regrow despite the supposedly complete destruction of hair roots has been attributed in many cases to a failure to destroy the hair, or the dermal papilla, or to the presence of short hair roots in the telogen stage. Studies were conducted to examine the supposedly complete epilation by electrocoagulation (Inaba et al. 1979b; McKinstry 1979). These studies showed that permanent epilation was possible only when the upper isthmal portion of the hair follicle and sebaceous gland was destroyed.

In order to confirm this finding, we investigated the destruction of those portions only, inserting the needle obliquely at a 5-mm distance from the hair canal (Fig. 10.1). Histological examination of hair regrowth after epilation by electrocoagulation showed that, if the upper isthmal portion remained intact after the lower portion of the follicle was destroyed, new hair roots began to form in the isthmal region of the follicle. On the other hand, if this isthmal portion was destroyed by electrocoagulation, the lower portion of the hair follicle rapidly changed into a premature telogen stage, finally becoming a terminal hair, despite the fact that the dermal papilla and hair bulb receive their blood supply from below. It has been thought that blood was supplied to hair follicles by candelabra vessels from the lower blood plexus to the dermal papilla and by the cutaneous blood plexus diverging from the dermis layer (transverse vessel branches) or by a vascular system, in a form similar to a basket net, directly surrounding the hair follicles from the musculocutaneous arteries (Durward and Rundall 1958; Montagna and Ellis 1957) (see Chapter 16).

Figure 10.2 shows that only the apocrine glands remain. The sebaceous gland is usually connected to the hair follicle close to the skin surface, while the apocrine gland has a secretory tract connected to the skin pore above the duct opening of the sebaceous gland. If only the isthmal portion is destroyed by electrocoagulation with an obliquely inserted needle 5 mm distant from the hair canal, the associated hair follicle completely vanishes. This finding suggests that the central portion of hair regeneration lies in the upper isthmal portion.

The shock of destruction in the isthmal region may lead to an imbalance in blood supply to the lower portions of the follicle following electrocoagulation. This occurrence suggests that the dermal papilla is affected by the isthmus region in some obscure way related to blood vessels, nerves, or the sebaceous gland. This, in turn, suggests that the destruction of the follicular isthmus and the sebaceous gland by electrocoagulation is critical to permanent epilation of axillary hairs.

Hinkel and Lind (1981), in their exposition of electrolysis, note that the technique has relied on the assumption that destruction of the dermal papilla terminates hair growth, but they have not been able to point to specific research for confirmation. Their explanation of hair regrowth after electrolysis is curiously similar to ours in declaring that an entirely new follicle is regenerated after unsuccessful epilation, and that its source is the outer root sheath of the upper follicle.

Barber and Jackson (1982) cite our hypothesis in their discussion of "Basic Principles of Electrolysis" in *Skin Surgery* as follows: "It appears that the previous theory requiring destruction of the papilla in order to destroy the hair may be inaccurate. These studies suggest that the proximal portion of the hair follicle including the isth-

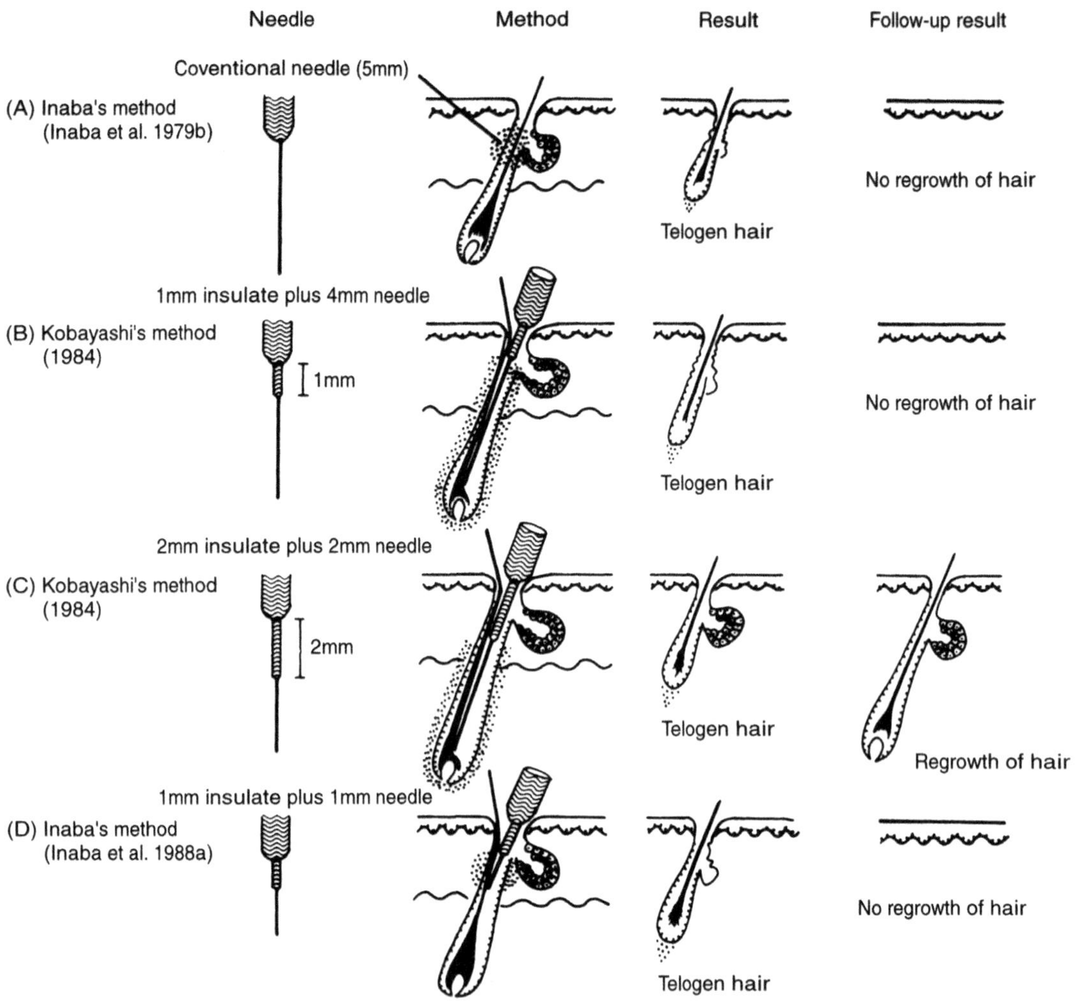

Fig. 10.1. Modifications of electrocoagulation needles used by Kobayashi and Inaba et al. indicate the need to destroy the upper isthmal portion of the hair follicle to achieve permanent epilation. (Reproduced from Inaba et al. 1988b)

mus must be destroyed to stop regeneration of the papilla and subsequent regrowth."

Recently, the authors (Inaba and Inaba 1992a) have indicated that this destruction leads to the destruction of the upper stem cell of the hair follicle, and then epilation becomes permanent.

10.2 Supportive Findings for Basic Principles of Epilation Treatment

An earlier report (Marton 1940) of permanent epilation by coated-needle electrocoagulation states that effective, permanent epilation requires positioning of the needle close to the skin surface. This, however, can cause small scars to form on the skin.

To perform non-scarring epilation, therefore, Kobayashi (1984, 1985) used a coated needle of a new construction (Fig. 10.1B). He found that when the coating was only 1-mm long (K-type needle), the needle destroyed the upper portion of the hair follicle (upper isthmal portion) and that epilation was permanent. However, when the needle was coated to a length of 2 mm, the coating protected the middle portion of the hair follicle and the sebaceous gland, leaving both intact, and subsequent hair regrowth was observed (Fig. 10.1C). This finding also indicated that the upper isthmal portion of the follicle was the essential center of hair regrowth.

In order to confirm the efficacy of this new type of needle, Inaba et al. (1988a) used the 1-mm insulate with a shorter needle; this destroyed the isthmal portion with subsequent permanent epi-

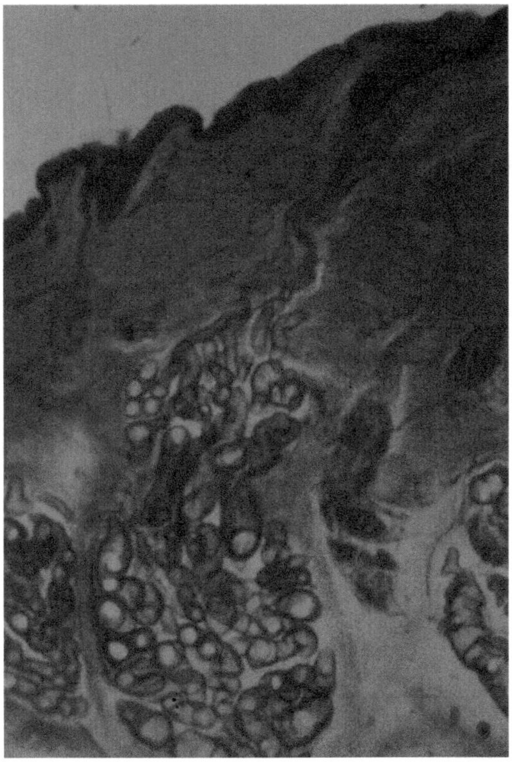

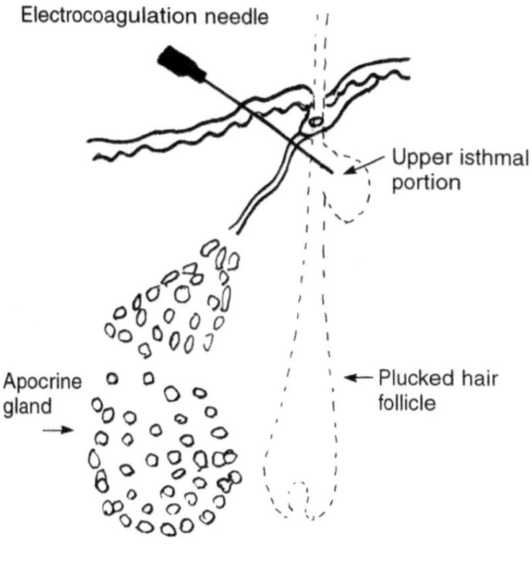

b

Fig. 10.2. **a** Only apocrine glands remain after destruction of the upper isthmal portion of the hair follicle. The associated hair follicle has completely vanished. **b** Diagrammatic view of **a**

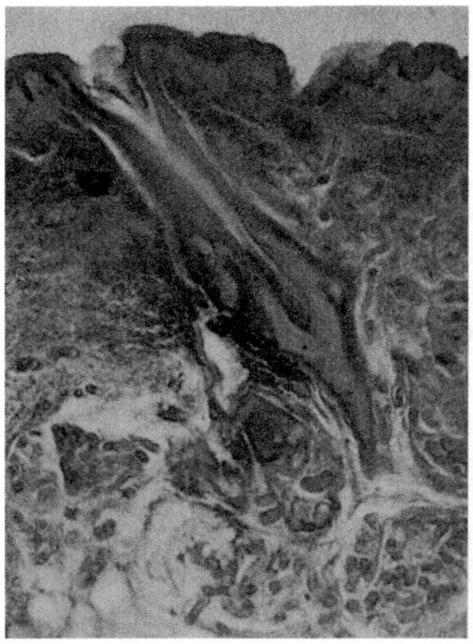

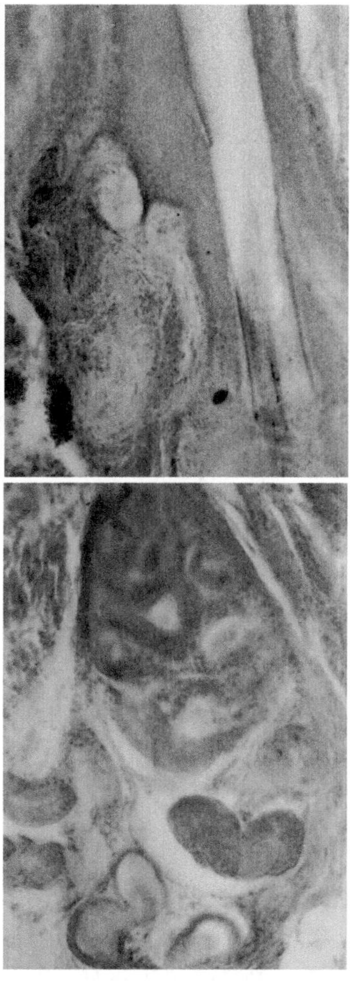

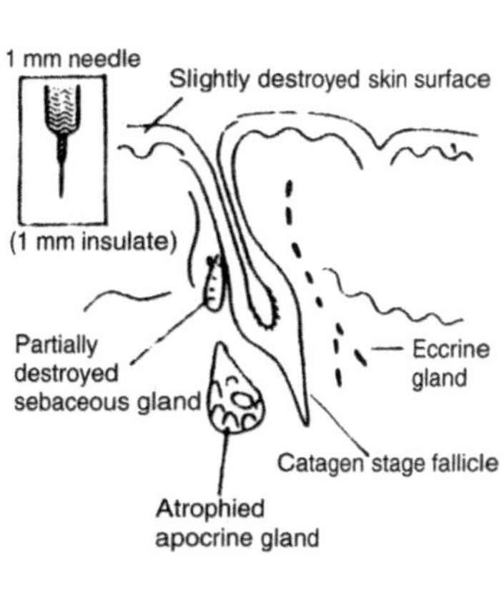

a

Fig. 10.3a,b. Histological review of skin treated with a specially designed needle. **a** Histological findings 10 days after electrocoagulation with 1-mm insulate plus 1-mm needle. Sebaceous glands partially remain after the use of the special needle. On follow-up, axillary hair was shown to have regrown. **b** Histological findings 2 weeks after electrocoagulation with 1-mm insulate plus 1-mm needle. Sebaceous glands have been completely destroyed after the use of the special needle. Axillary hair does not regrow

Fig. 10.3. *Continued*

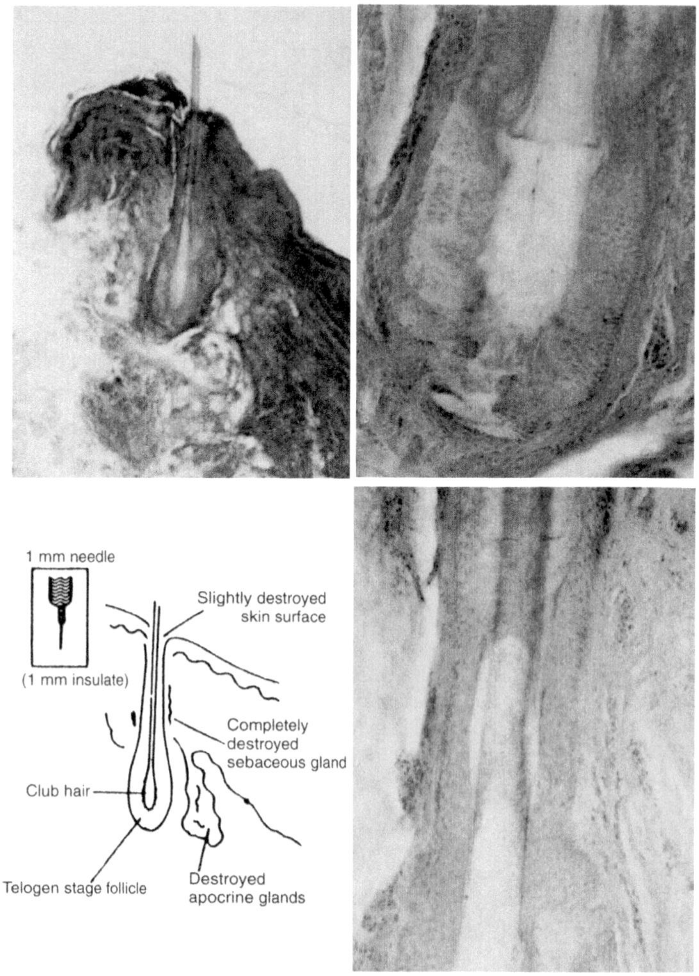

b

lation. As Fig. 10.3 shows, destruction of the isthmal portion and the sebaceous gland by electrolysis using the 1-mm insulated needle is essential for permanent epilation of axillary hair without damaging the skin surface. A histological review of skin treated with this specially developed needle shows that if some of the sebaceous gland cells remain (Fig. 10.3a), hair regeneration was observed, within 2 months after treatment. As shown in Fig. 10.3b, when this needle was used at the upper isthmal portion of the hair follicle the follicle completely vanished and the sebaceous gland was destroyed and lost. No regeneration of hair was observed on follow-up 2 months after the treatment.

This finding indicates that destruction of the upper isthmal portion leads to permanent epilation.

Regeneration of Scalp Hair

11

The authors decided to extend their histologic studies to include scalp hair, as well as axillary and body hair (Inaba et al. 1980a).

Surprisingly, not much is known about scalp hair growth in humans, mostly because the investigation of this phenomenon is tedious and unexciting and has therefore failed to capture the interest of investigators.

According to Montagna and Parakkal (1974), except for individual variations, hair growth patterns in the scalp remain the same from infancy to puberty. From about 16 to 46 years of age, however, hair density and thickness in the scalp decrease progressively in both sexes, most noticeably in the vertex. The number of telogen follicles, which are smallest at puberty, increases with age in both sexes and is greater in the central than in the peripheral areas of the scalp. In both sexes, hair grows faster between the ages of 16 and 46 than in older age. After the age of 50, hair density decreases, in both sexes. In this age group, the individual hairs are thicker and a higher proportion of follicles are in telogen phase (Barman et al. 1965). According to Montagna and Van Scott (1958), for the hairs of the human scalp, the time required for follicles to grow is 147 days.

In our studies of the process of scalp hair regeneration, we (1990b, 1992a) found that, based on the common hair cycle (Fig. 7.1) the process began from the lower tip of the epithelial sac in telogen stage. On the other hand, we also observed regeneration beginning from the upper isthmal portion, based on the essential hair cycle. Previous series of studies on the regeneration of axillary hair had also tended to confirm that the process does, in fact, begin from the upper isthmal portion (Chapters 9 and 10).

11.1 Hair Stages

11.1.1 Hair Germ Stage

Figure 11.1a–c shows that the new hair follicle (hair germ) is regenerated from the common neck of the lobes of a multilobular sebaceous gland.

11.1.2 Hair Peg Stage

In Fig. 11.2 we can see the three lobes of a multilobular sebaceous gland. A new hair follicle is forming from the common neck of these lobes. At higher magnification (Fig. 11.2b), the tip of the new follicle is clearly visible between two of the lobes. In a further enlargement of the tip, we see that the bulb has not yet formed (Fig. 11.2c).

Figure 11.2d,e shows the new young hair clearly forming within the follicle. The hair has a stem-like configuration typical of the anagen stage.

In another case (Fig. 11.3a) the sebaceous gland is shown in multilobular configuration. To its right is a typical catagen stage hair follicle. Remnants of melanin granules are clearly visible in the lower portion of the follicle. To the left of the follicle is a cluster of melanin granules. A high-power view of this specific area of the same serial thick section (Fig. 11.3b) shows the same cluster of melanin granules in the bottom left corner. The authors could see a new young hair forming from the upper isthmal portion of the catagen stage follicle on the left. Within the follicle, the new hair was being formed. There was no visible trace of melanin granules within the hair cortex (Fig. 11.3b,d). Figure 11.3d is a higher magnification of the newly-formed anagen hair, showing the lower portion of the new hair root. It appears to be in a typical anagen stage configuration. A filamentous structure has been formed from the epithelial cells

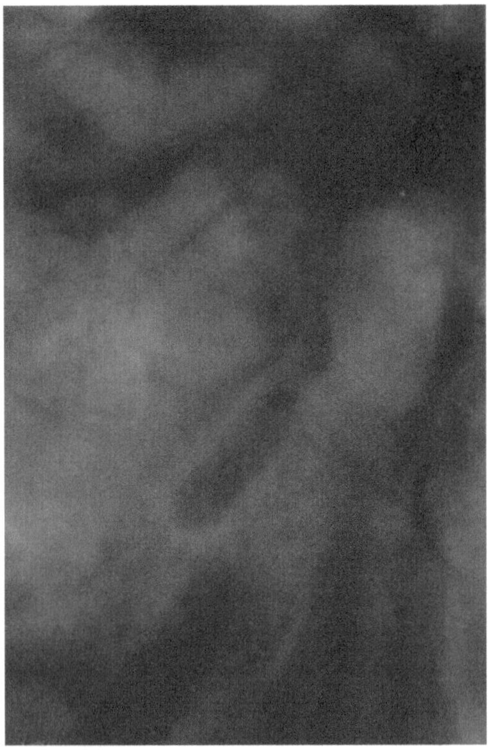

a

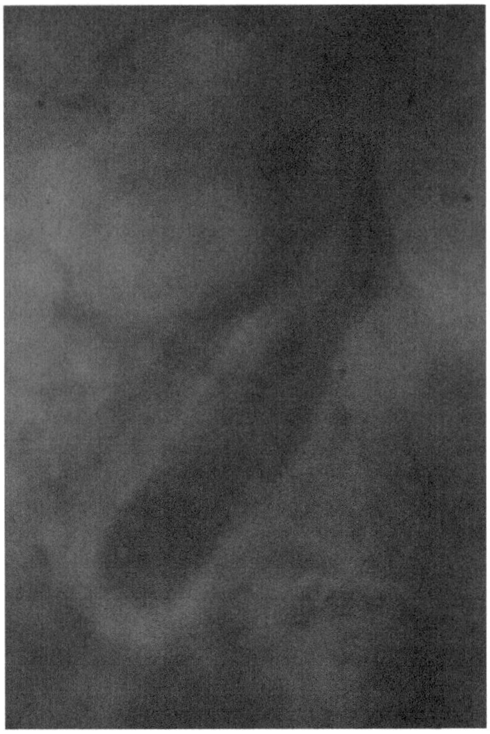

b

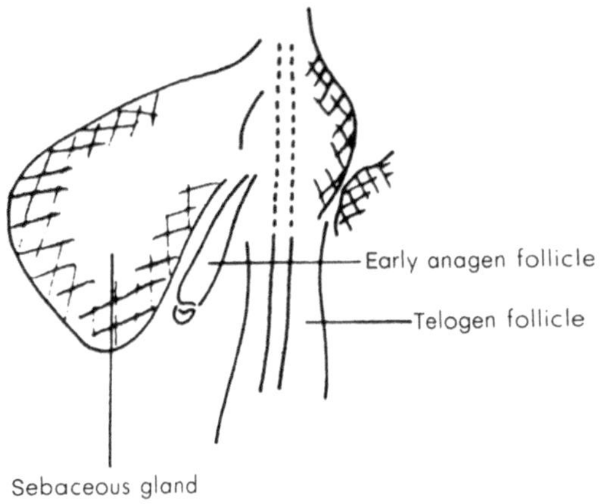

c

Fig. 11.1. **a** A new hair follicle is regenerated from the common neck of the lobes of a multilobular sebaceous gland (hair germ stage). ×135 **b** Higher magnification of **a**. Hair germ and a mass of mesenchymal cells can be seen, but no hair is yet generated. ×400 **c** Schematic representation of **a** and **b**

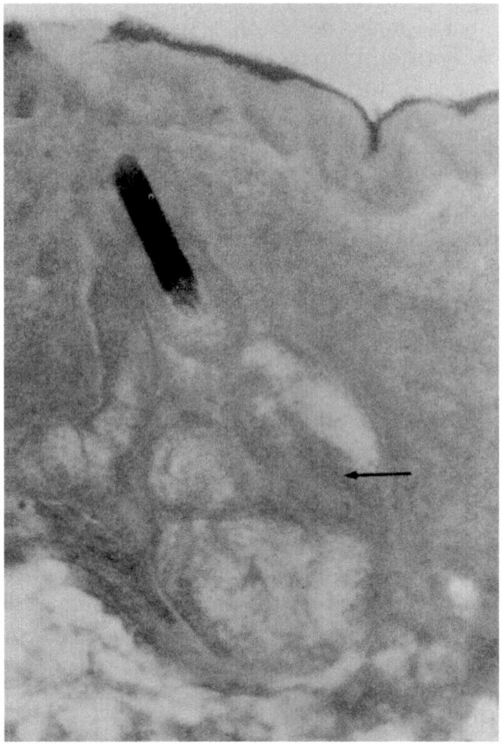

a

Fig. 11.2. **a** Sebaceous gland in multilobular configuration. A new young hair follicle is forming from the common neck of the three discernible lobes. One can see an anagen stage hair root at the upper portion of the multilobular sebaceous gland (*arrow*). ×135 **b** Higher magnification of **a**, showing the new young follicle. ×400 **c** Further magnification of the new young hair follicle (**b**) showing that the bulb has not yet formed. A mass of mesenchymal cells is clearly visible at the follicle tip. **d** Another perspective of high-power view in **b** shows a new young hair root visibly forming within the follicle. It has the stem-like configuration typical of the anagen stage. Also see Fig. 11.3d. ×400 **e** Schematic representation of significant findings in **a**, **b**, **c**, and **d**

b

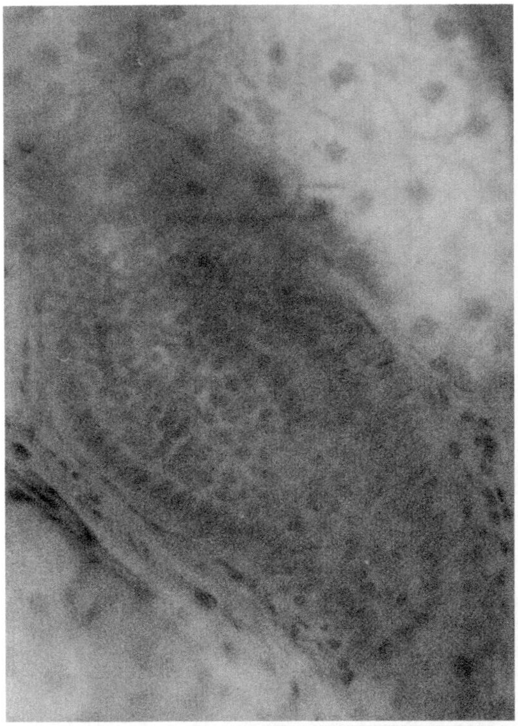

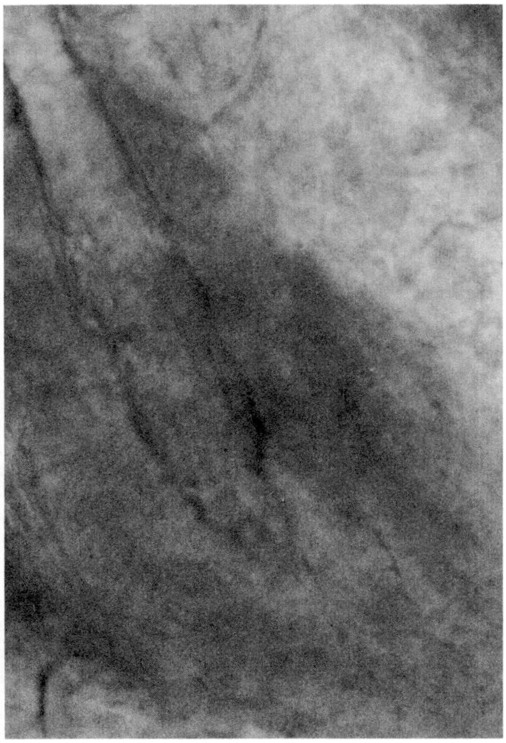

d

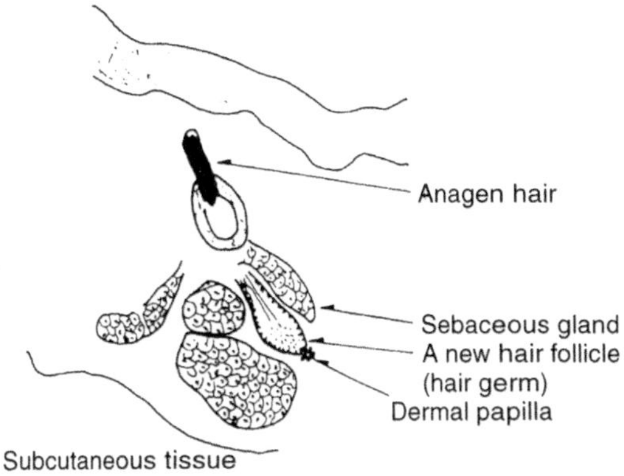

e

c

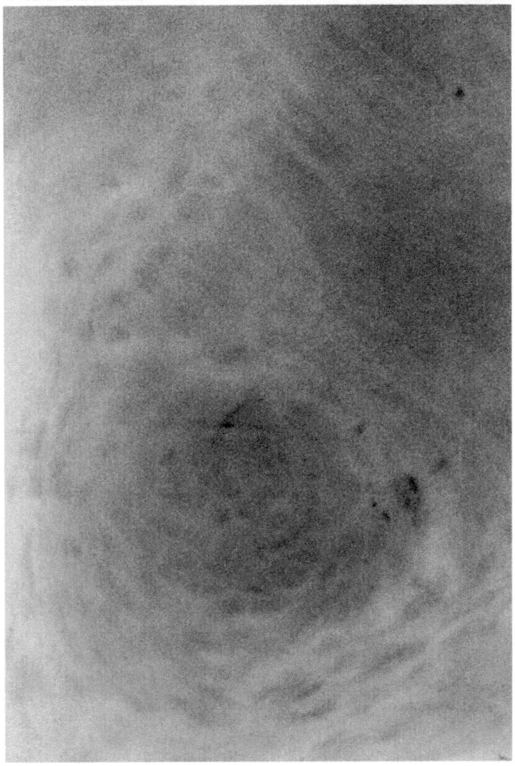

Fig. 11.2. *Continued*

of the lower tip of the epithelial sac. The inner root sheath was apparently formed at the same time. Keratinization of Henle's layer of the inner root sheath takes place; this is followed by formation of the hair fiber, and the upper portion is keratinized to become the hair cortex. Cuticle forms around the cortex and interlocks with the inner root sheath that adheres to the surrounding trichilemmal epithelium. This interlocking fusion of cortex and inner root sheath prevents the newly forming hair from pegging upward. The follicle, instead, pegs downward. The lower tip of the hair

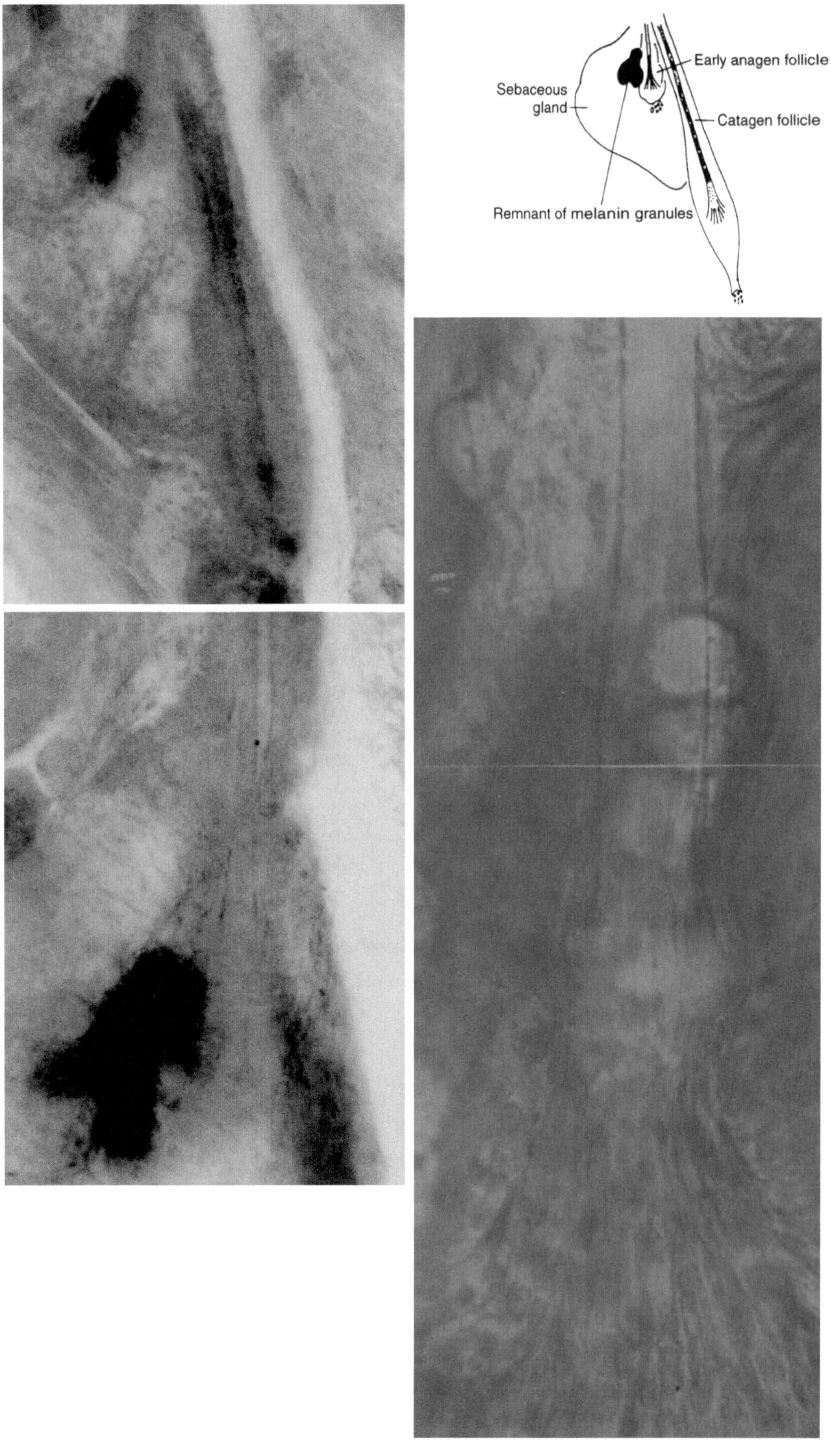
Early anagen follicle
Sebaceous gland
Catagen follicle
Remnant of melanin granules

a

b

c

d

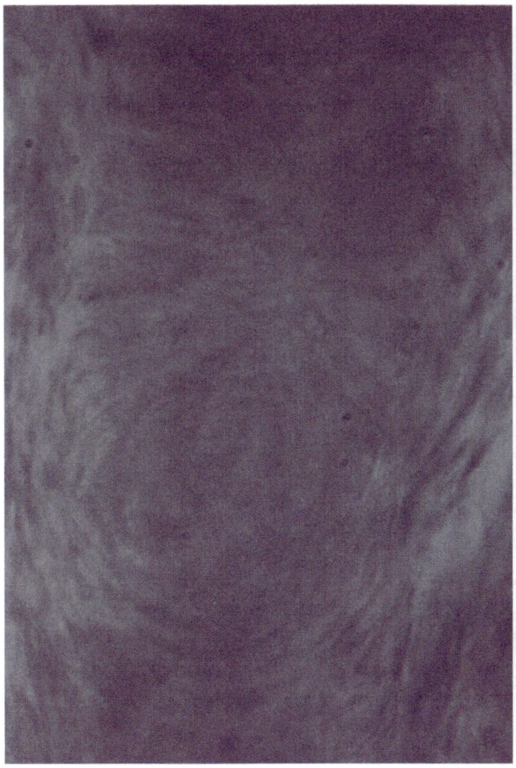

e

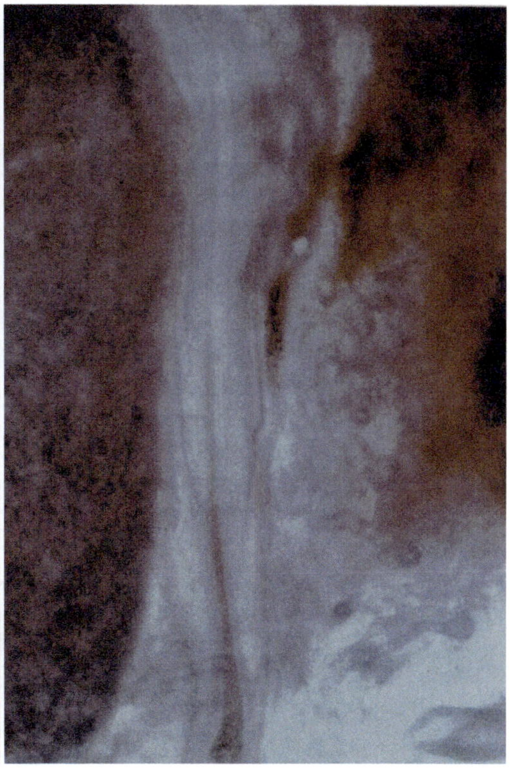

f

Fig. 11.3. **a** The cluster of melanin granules visible at *upper left* beside this catagen stage follicle indicates that an old hair (club hair) has fallen out. ×135 **b** The same cluster of melanin granules appears at the *lower left* in this high-power view of the upper left portion of **a**. A new young hair root (in anagen stage) can be seen between the cluster and the catagen follicle. ×400 **c** Schematic representation of significant findings in a and **b**. **d** High-power view of the lower portion of the new young hair root in a typical stem-like anagen configuration that is clearly dissimilar to the broom-like club hair in the catagen stage. ×600 **e** Aggregation of mesenchymal cells at the tip of the epithelial sac; this aggregation will develop into a new dermal papilla. **f** Late bulbous peg stage. ×135

root, at this stage, has a straight, stem-like configuration, with rootlets projecting from the tip. There is no visible trace of melanin granules in the cortex. Figure 11.3e shows an aggregation of mesenchymal cells at the tip of the epithelial sac; this aggregation will develop into a new dermal papilla.

11.1.3 Bulbous Peg Stage

Both scalp hair and axillary hair exhibit the same growth pattern in these later stages. When the forming hair reaches a level near the permanent site of the dermal papilla, the epithelial cells grow around the mass of mesenchymal tissue, thereby pressing the outer root sheath outward. Consequently, the outer root sheath becomes thin, and at its bottom has only one to two layers. The hair bulb is formed at this stage. The mass of mesenchymal tissue is wrapped by the inner and outer root sheaths and hair tissues and becomes the dermal papilla. When the epithelial matrix cells are fully formed on the surface of the dermal papilla, melanocytes increase and melanin granules are deposited in the hair cortex.

11.1.4 Terminal Stage

The hair follicle stops descending, and the hair begins to ascend toward the skin surface. Hair and inner root sheath grow at the same speed, and the terminal hair grows according to the classical rules of the hair cycle.

11.2 Supporting Findings

The foregoing phenomenon has been observed clinically by Fukuda and Ezaki (1975) in that, they found that hair may grow from split-thickness scalp skin transplanted in reconstructive surgery for microtia.

Clodius and Smahel (1979), in their work with scalp hair split-thickness transplants for reconstructive surgery to correct skin defects in the beard area, have also reported regeneration of hair despite the removal of the lower portions of hair follicles when taking a skin flap from the scalp area.

Fujita et al. (1960) have reported that, with first-degree burns, there is no hair loss, but that with second-degree burns, when the middle portion of the follicle is destroyed, hair growth does not recur, even though the hair matrix remains intact. This finding also indicates that the middle (including the isthmal) portion of the follicle is essential for hair regeneration.

These reports tend to support our own findings that scalp hair can be regenerated from the upper isthmal portion of the hair follicle.

Hair Regeneration in the Mouse After Application of Anti-Cancer Agent, Particularly in Terms of Epithelial-Mesenchymal Interaction

12

12.1 Anti-Cancer Agents and Hair Loss

Most anti-cancer agents currently in use are aimed at suppressing the growth of cancer cells and the accretion of tumors. Since the mechanism of cellular growth is the same in both normal and cancer cells, most of these agents can exert toxic effects on normal cells, especially on bone marrow mucous membrane and epithelial cells, which divide rather rapidly during the S phase. The anti-cancer agents may infiltrate the nucleolus and toxically transform the DNA structure. Sebaceous epithelial cells and hair matrix cells are therefore greatly affected by such agents. The phenomenon of hair loss is an often observed side effect of anti-cancer agents.

Inaba et al. (1991) and Inaba and Inaba (1992a) studied the effects of various anti-cancer agents on the pilosebaceous unit; the effects of methotrexate, 1.3-bis [2-chlorethyl]-1-nitrosourea (BCNU), 5-fluorouracil (5-Fu), daunomycin, cytarabin, and cyclophosphamide on the hair follicle were examined.

It was found that the process of hair regeneration after the follicle had been damaged by the anti-cancer agent could be fully elucidated by the common hair cycle theory (Montagna and Parakkal 1974) alone. We conducted a study of the process of hair regeneration. The epithelial-mesenchymal interaction is an especially important factor in hair growth and, therefore, the regeneration of mesenchymal cells (dermal papilla) was the major subject of our study.

In experiments in which various anti-cancer agents were applied, we used female ICR Swiss mice about 65 days old, in good health, and with hair follicles on the back in telogen stage. Solutions containing various anti-cancer agents were applied twice daily for 7 days.

For the preparation of thick tissue specimens, we used the cellotape method developed by Inaba et al. (1978d) (Chapter 2).

12.2 Regeneration of Hair Follicle After Application of Anti-Cancer Agent

We attempted to study the process of regeneration by applying an anti-cancer agent (methotrexate, etc.) to mouse body skin surface, thus experimentally creating telogen hair follicles (Inaba 1985). It has been thought that the new hair bud (germ) in the regeneration process begins to form from remnants of the dermal papilla or from a secondary hair germ in telogen stage (Fig. 12.1a,b). However, the authors recognize from recent studies (Inaba et al. 1991) that the regeneration of the hair germ does not necessarily occur from a secondary hair germ and the remnants of the dermal papilla, but that can it can be formed from the upper isthmal portion close to the duct opening of the sebaceous glands (Fig. 12.1b).

These findings are explained as follows. As shown in Figs. 12.1a and 12.2a, the lower portion of the single hair indicates that this is a typical club hair in the telogen stage. In the medium portion of the follicle, the sebaceous gland cells and their nuclei can be observed. From between the two lobes of the sebaceous gland, i.e., from the upper isthmal portion, the epithelial cells (hair germ) regenerate as if to wrap around the lower portion of the club hair. No hair germ seems to be seen at the lower end of the telogen follicle (Fig. 12.1b). As already described in Section 1.5.2.3, no mass of mesenchymal cells can be seen at the lower portion of the telogen hair follicle.

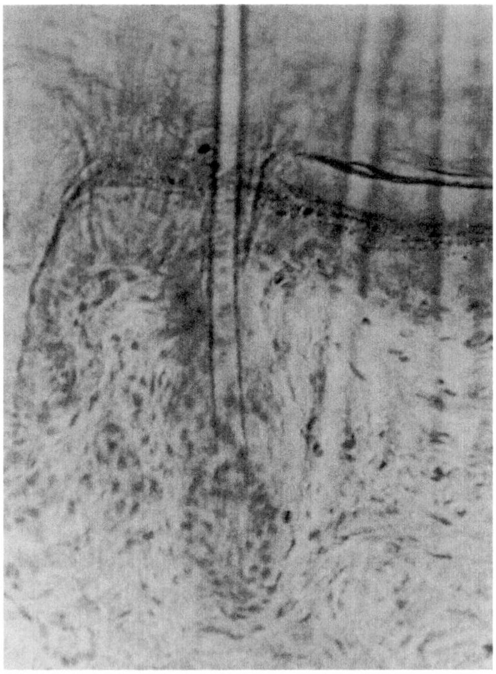

a

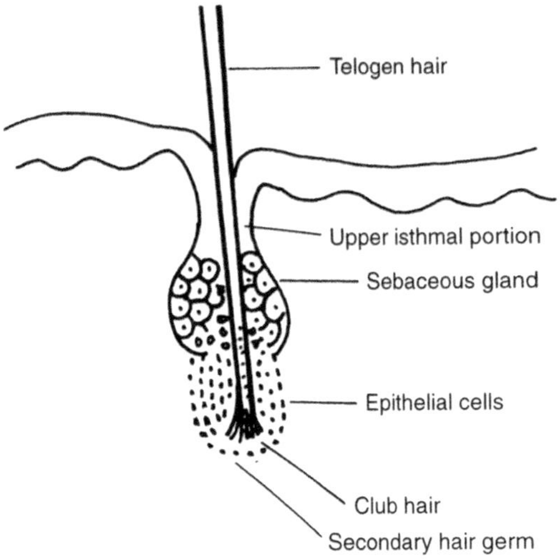

b

Fig. 12.1. **a** Vigorous mitosis can be observed over the club hair surface from the upper isthmal portion of the hair follicle. Mesenchymal cells are not visible, and are formed later. ×250 **b** Diagram of features in **a**

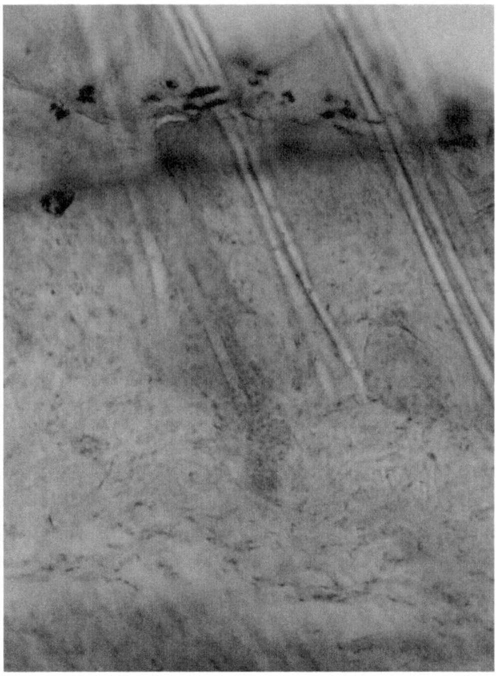

a

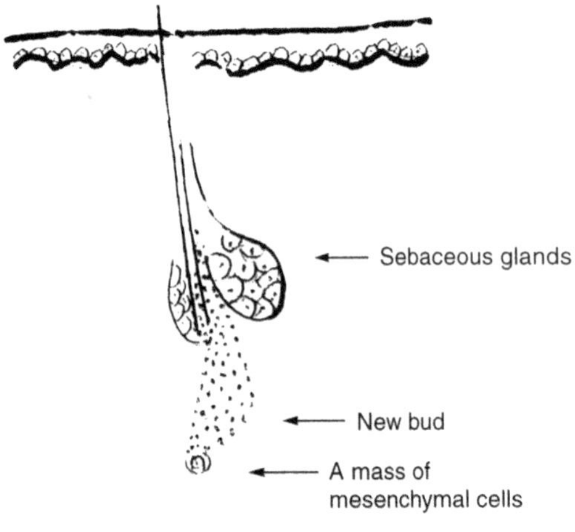

b

Fig. 12.2. **a** A newly-formed epithelial bud regenerates from the upper isthmal portion. A mass of mesenchymal cells may be formed later at the lower tip of the new bud. **b** Diagram of essential features in **a**

In Figure 12.2, a more advanced hair bud also regenerates from the upper isthmal portion. A mass of mesenchymal cells can be seen at the lower tip of the newly-formed epithelial bud. From these mesenchymal cells the future dermal papilla may be formed later. Figure 12.3 shows regeneration of the hair peg stage: a club hair can be seen at the lower end of the telogen hair follicle. The lower hair follicle surrounding the club hair has atrophied and thinned. No presence of a hair germ, as asserted by Montagna, can be seen. The hair germ does not seem to have regenerated from the rem-

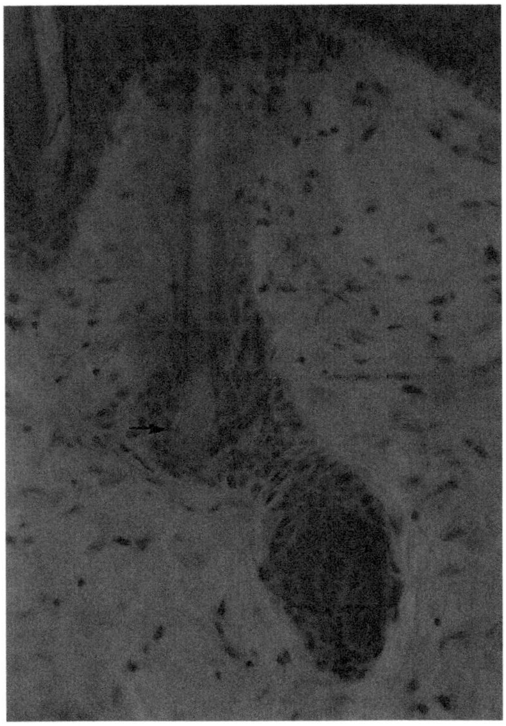

Fig. 12.3. View of hair follicle in hair peg stage. No hair germ can be observed in the lower end of the telogen follicle (*arrow*). At first glance, the new hair germ could appear to regenerate from the bulge area, as suggested by Cotsarelis et al. (1990). However, in the outer region of the bottom of the follicle presumably newly-formed epithelial cells are developing from the upper isthmal portion of the sebaceous gland

nant dermal papilla, which is assumed to be present at the lower end of the telogen hair follicle, but, rather, a hair germ has newly formed outside the lower end of the telogen follicle, and the epithelial cells in the upper new bud seem to develop from the upper isthmal portion. The lower portion of the newly-formed follicle has become bulbous, as if to wrap around the dermal papilla. This is the bulbous peg stage. At a glance, it appears that the new bud seems to be formed from the bulge in which Cotsarelis et al. (1990) suggest follicular stem cells reside in the bulge region. However, it is possible that the upper portion of the hair bud may be formed from the upper isthmal portion (sebaceous isthmus). (See Section 14.1.4.)

Figure 12.4 shows regeneration of the follicle bulbous peg stage. A follicle can be observed to develop and peg down from the upper isthmal portion, clearly demarcated from the telogen follicle, presenting a view of the bulbous peg stage. A gap between the lower portion of the telogen hair follicle and the new young hair follicle can be clearly seen. In other words, the hair matrix wraps around the dermal papilla to form a hair bulb and then pegs downward (late bulbous peg stage).

Regarding the regeneration of the hair follicle, it was thought that cell division occurred in the lower tip of the telogen stage epithelial sac (secondary hair germ) (Section 7.1.2, Fig. 7.3a,b). However, in our studies, we applied anti-cancer agents to the mouse skin surface and observed

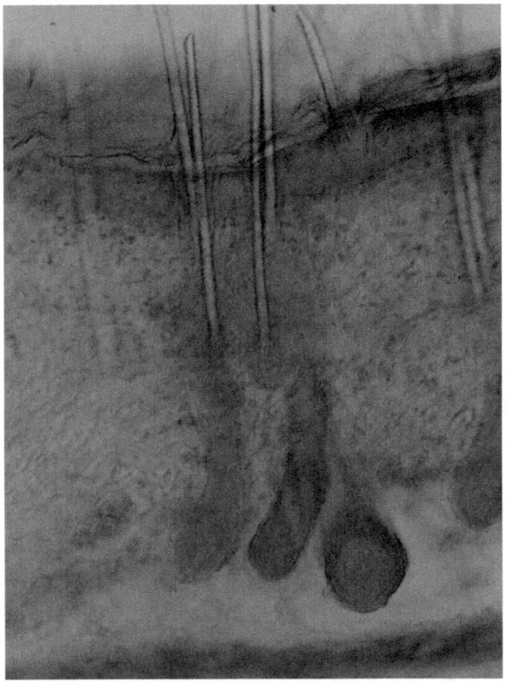

a

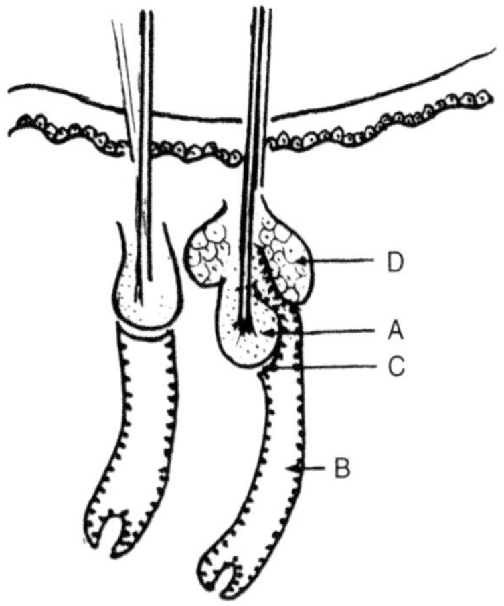

b

Fig. 12.4. **a** View of hair follicle in bulbous hair peg stage. A bulbous hair peg stage follicle developed from the upper isthmal portion can be observed, clearly demarcated from the lower end of the telogen follicle. **b** There is a gap (*C*) between the lower portion of the telogen hair follicle (*A*) and the new young hair follicle (*B*). *D*, Sebaceous gland. **c** This finding is similar to that shown in **a**. **d** High-power view of **c**

c

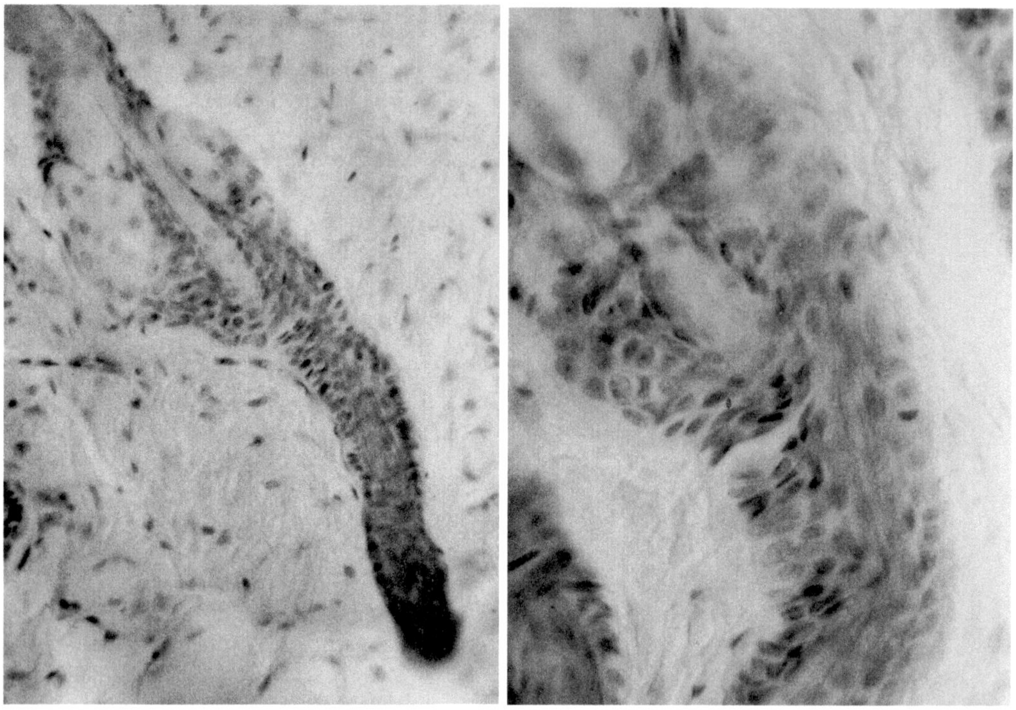

d

Fig. 12.4. *Continued*

regeneration of hair. This regeneration seemed to occur, at first impression, from the tip of the telogen hair follicle. Further, the generation of a mass of mesenchymal cells was later found in the lower tip of the newly-formed epithelial bud and the epithelial cells, connecting with an area adjacent to the secretory opening of the sebaceous gland of the hair follicle (upper isthmal portion) (Fig. 12.2a,b). This finding also indicates that this regeneration is closely related to the sebaceous isthmal portion and the vascularization of the hair follicle (Inaba 1985).

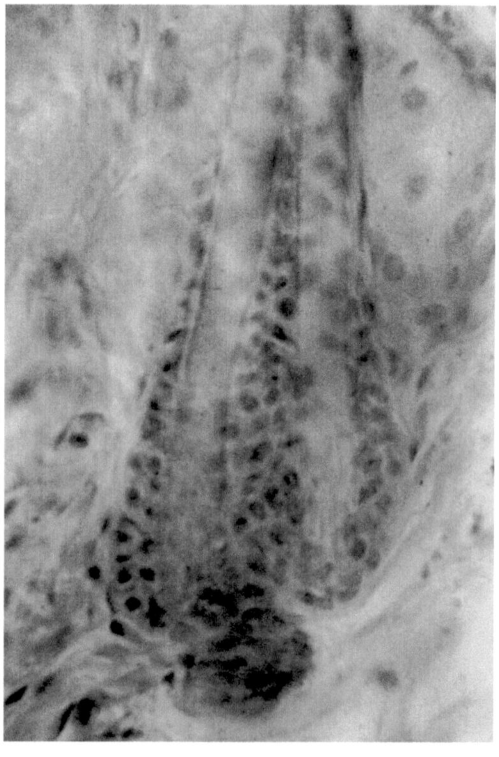

a

Fig. 12.5. **a** Hair regeneration after the formation of bundle telogen hair follicles. Despite the presence of bundle telogen hair, a single mass of mesenchymal cells has formed at the lower tips of the bundle telogen hair follicles above which the epithelial cell layer has already formed from the sebaceous isthmal portion. The mesenchymal cells will develop afterwards below the epithelial bud. **b** Only one mass of mesenchymal cells can be observed at the lower end of the compound hair follicle. This seems to be related to the regeneration of the sebaceous gland cells. **c** Diagram of essential features in **b**

Fig. 12.5. *Continued*

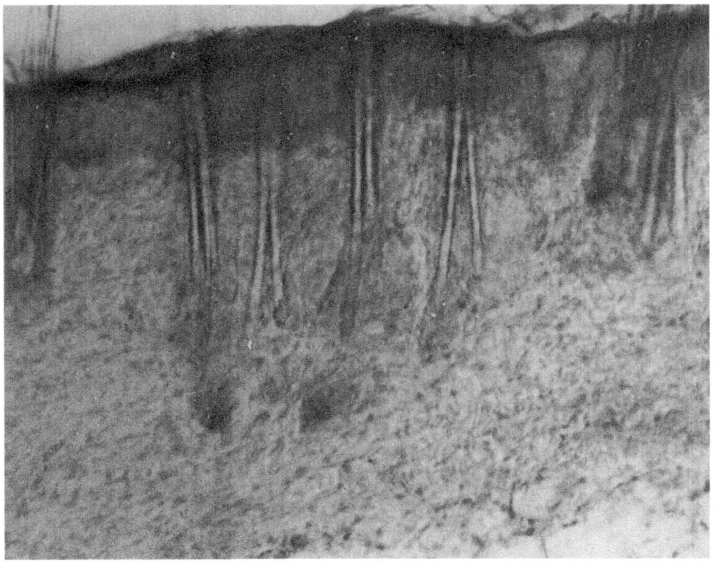

b

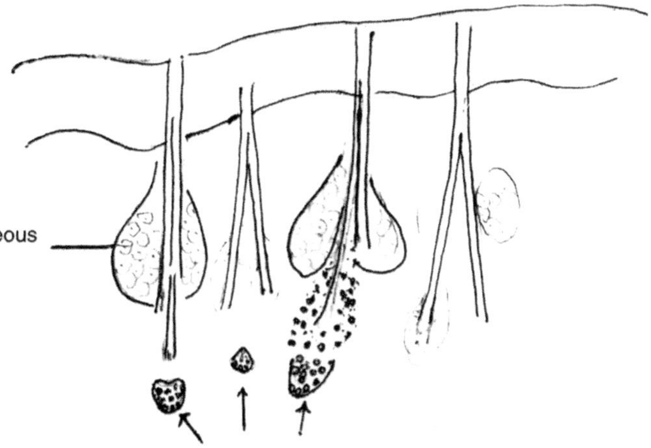

c

12.3 Regeneration from Remaining Bundle Telogen Hair Follicles

The common hair cycle theory states that during the telogen stage, hair regeneration starts from the lower end of the compound hair follicle. Contrary to this, our finding is that a single mass of mesenchymal cells is sometimes newly formed at the lower end of compound hair follicles, above which the epithelial cell layer will migrate from the upper isthmal portion (Fig. 12.5) (see Figs. 1.13 and 12.10). This finding suggests that the generation of the mass of mesenchymal cells does not necessarily start from the remnant of dermal papilla cells or from the secondary hair germ present in the lower portion of the telogen follicles, but that the mesenchymal cells will develop afterwards below the epithelial bud and the recovery of the vascular system surrounding the follicles may precede the above phenomenon.

As shown in Fig. 12.6 the new hair bud does not regenerate from the lower portion of the telogen hair follicle, but regenerates from the upper isthmal portion close to the duct opening of the sebaceous glands. This finding has elucidated the phenomenon of thinning of the hair in males during adulthood. (See Chapter 21)

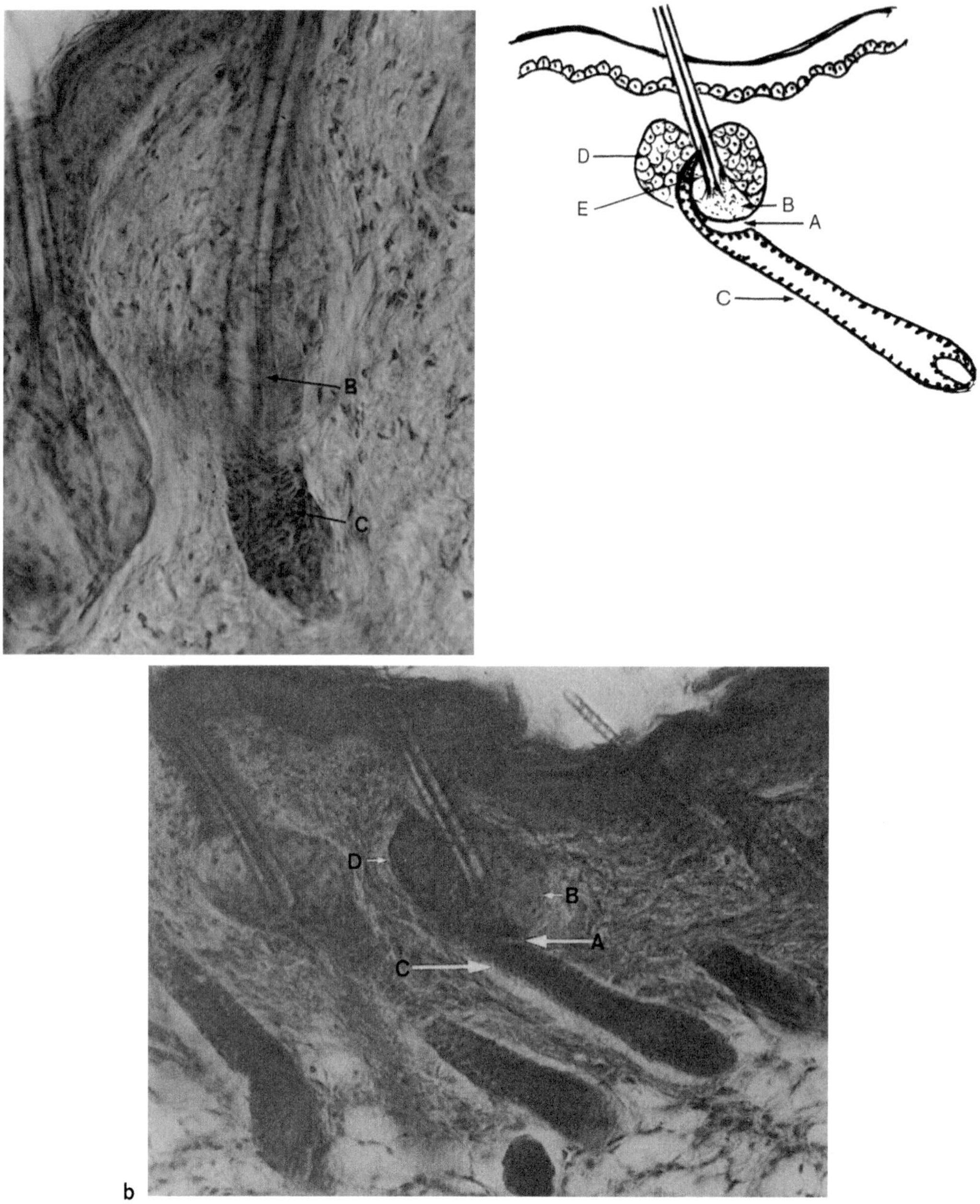

a

c

b

Fig. 12.6. **a** The new hair bud does not regenerate from the lower portion of the telogen hair follicle, but regenerates, instead, from the upper isthmal portion. **b** The formation of new hair: *arrows* indicate (*B*) telogen hair follicle; (*E*) upper isthmal portion; and a gap (*A*) between the lower portion of the telogen hair follicle (*B*) and the new young hair follicle (*C*). **c** The new follicle regenerates from the upper isthmal portion of the telogen hair follicle. There is a gap (*A*) between the lower portion of the telogen follicle (*B*) and the new young follicle (*C*). (*D*), Sebaceous gland

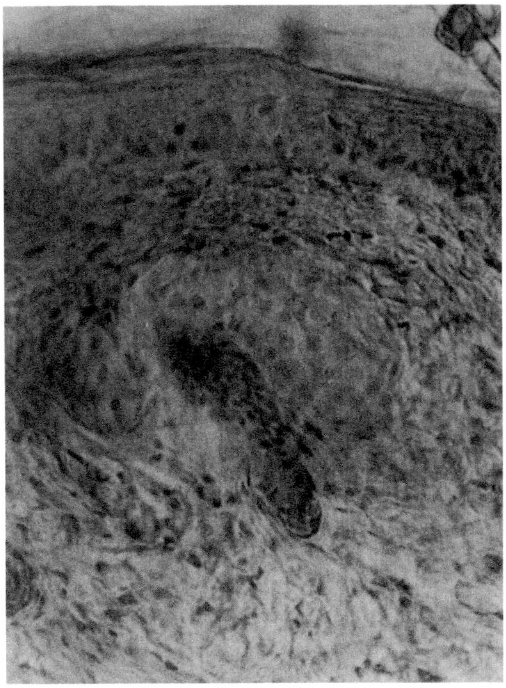

a

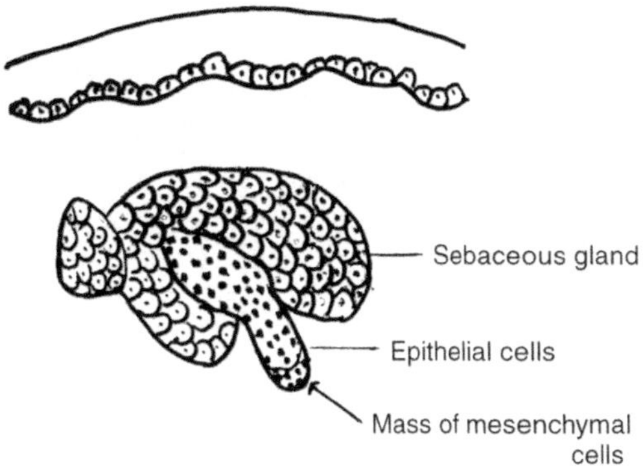

b

Fig. 12.7. a Regeneration of a new hair germ can be observed at the upper isthmal portion after the hair is plucked. **b** Schema of micrograph in **a**

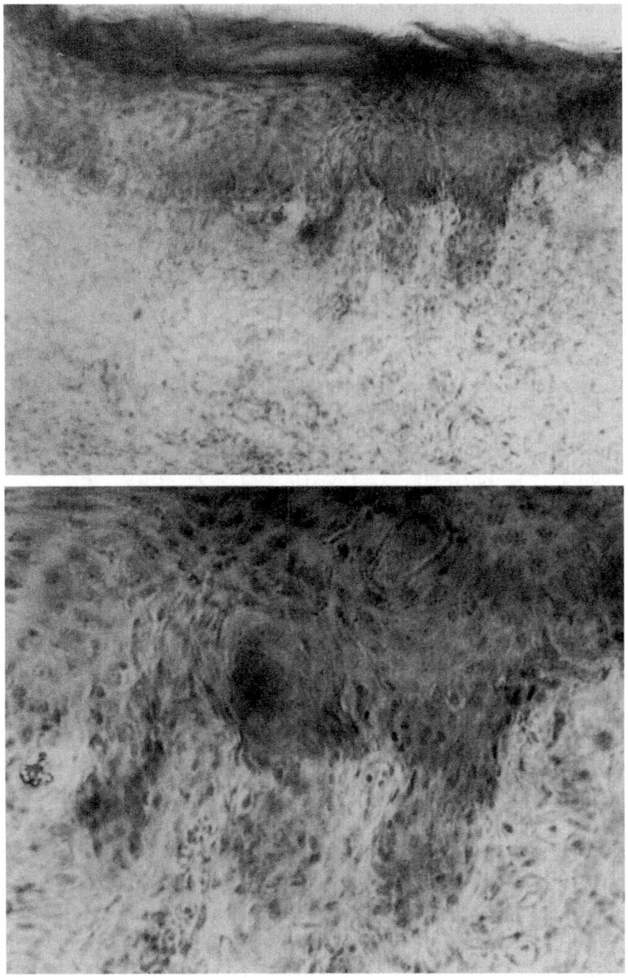

a

b

Fig. 12.8. a When the sebaceous gland and lipocytes have been destroyed and lost, no regeneration of the mass of mesenchymal cells is induced, resulting in permanent epilation. **b** High-power view of **a**. No regeneration of the mass of mesenchymal cells is observed

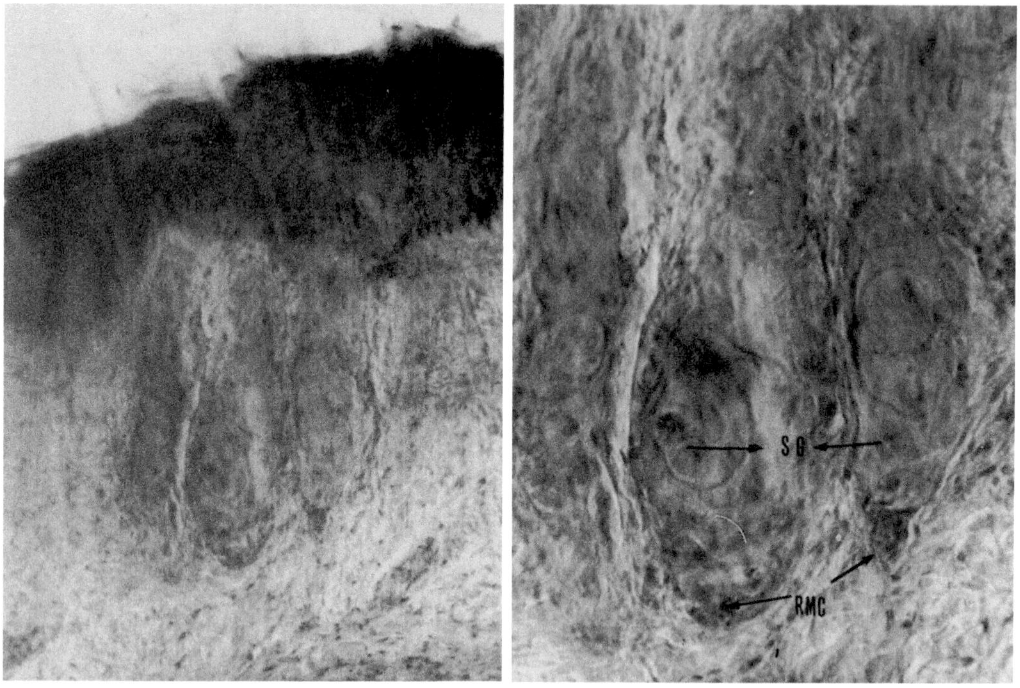

a b

Fig. 12.9. **a** If damage caused by the anti-cancer agent is severe, the sebaceous gland is destroyed; however, even a small remnant of lipocytes is enough to induce the possible generation or regeneration of the mass of mesenchymal cells. **b** Higher magnification of **a**. *SG*, Lipocyte in sebaceous gland; *RMC*, regenerated mesenchymal cells

12.4 Regeneration from the Upper Isthmal Portion After the Plucking of Telogen Hair

If the telogen hairs have been epilated, hair generation is observed to start from the upper isthmal portion close to the duct opening of the sebaceous gland (Fig. 12.7, Fig. 12.10c[i]). The sebaceous gland is slightly damaged and the vascular system below the epidermis (subpapillary blood vessel) is preserved; the epithelial bud then regenerates from the upper isthmal portion.

12.5 Regeneration After Destruction of the Sebaceous Gland

If the sebaceous gland is severely damaged and atrophied due to the application of an anti-cancer agent, this leads either to permanent epilation or to hair regeneration, depending on the degree of damage.

12.5.1 Complete Loss of Sebaceous Gland

As seen in Fig. 12.8a,b, the follicles gradually atrophy from the right to the left and finally disappear. This observation indicates that when the anti-cancer agent severely damages the sebaceous gland, the sebaceous gland in the follicle will be lost. As shown in Fig. 12.8, the lipocytes have been destroyed, so the follicles will gradually atrophy and disappear and the formation of the mass of mesenchymal cells is not observed at the lower end of the follicle.

12.5.2 Incomplete Loss of Sebaceous Gland

Figure 12.9a shows three remaining atrophied hair follicles; the hair has already escaped and disappeared. The higher magnification in Fig. 12.9b reveals a small remnant of lipocytes in the sebaceous lobule; the nuclei are not clearly identified. As seen in this case, only a small remnant of sebaceous lipocyte is capable of inducing the formation of the mass of mesenchymal cells (future dermal pa-

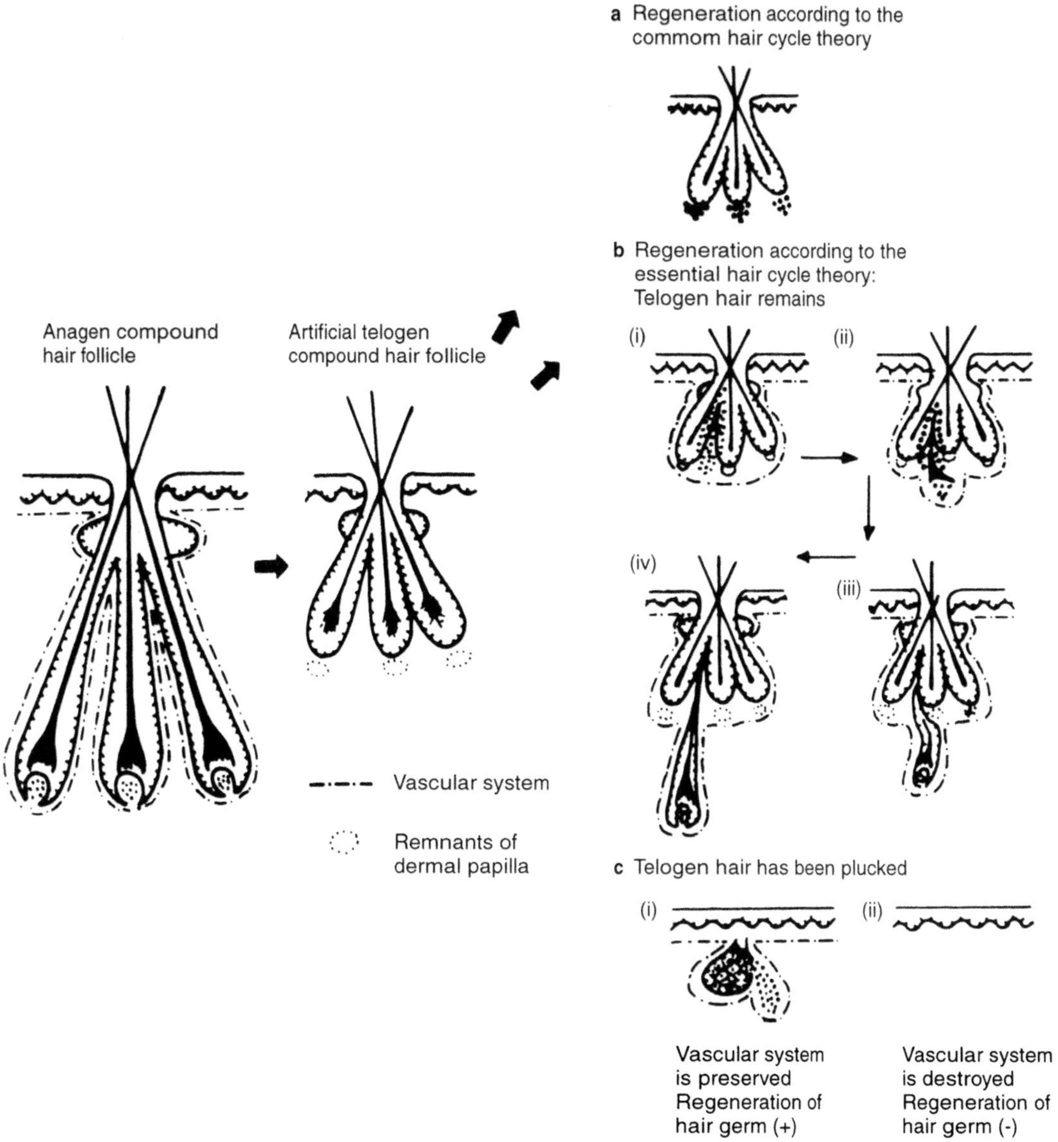

Fig. 12.10a–c. Regeneration and vascular system after application of the anti-cancer agent. The hair germ cannot regenerate from the remnant dermal papilla of each telogen hair follicle. The hair germ is formed from the sebaceous isthmal portion and the mass of mesenchymal cells may be formed later (from Inaba et al. 1990a)

pilla) observed in Fig. 12.9b to be vividly stained at the lower end of the follicle.

12.6 Hair Regeneration in the Mouse

The above findings can be summarized as follows (Fig. 12.10).

The common hair cycle theory states that during the telogen stage, hair regeneration starts from the lower end of the compound hair follicle, where 2–3 hairs are present in a single hair follicle (Fig. 12.10a).

However, we have found that regeneration from remnants of the dermal papilla does not occur by the formation of a hair germ at the lower portion of the bundle (compound) hair follicle in the telogen stage (Fig. 12.10a). Our finding is that a single mass of mesenchymal cells (hair germ) is newly formed at the lower end of compound hair follicles above which the epithelial cell layer has already stemmed from the sebaceous isthmal portion (Fig. 12.10b[i]). This suggests that generation of the mass of mesenchymal cells does not necessarily start from the remnant of dermal papilla cells or secondary hair germ present at the lower portion of bundle telogen follicle, but can be also formed from newly-formed epithelial cells from the sebaceous isthmal portion, and mesenchymal cells will develop completely in a later period (Fig. 12.10b[ii], [iii], [iv]). The recovery of the vascular system surrounding the follicles may precede the above phenomenon.

Hair regrowth depends upon whether the sebaceous gland remains (Fig. 12c).

New Concept of the Hair Cycle (Sebaceous Gland Hypothesis)

13

The cycle of alternating periods of rest and activity passed through by follicles of all types was first described in detail by Dry (1926) in the mouse standard model (Fig. 13.1a). During anagen (the active phase) the dermal papilla is almost enclosed by the cells of the matrix, which divide rapidly. Daughter cells move upward and differentiate to form the concentric layers of the hair itself and of the inner root sheath. A few epithelial cells are destined to become incorporated in the outer root sheath. Eventually, in the relatively short catagen phase, mitosis in the matrix ceases, and the base of the hair is keratinized to form the brush or club end, which then rises until it comes to rest just below the level of one-third of the anagen hair follicle. The follicle then passes into the resting phase (telogen), during which the inner root sheath of the lower portion of the follicle is no longer present and the club hair is retained in the follicle.

In histological sections, the cells of both the hair germ and the dermal papilla appear inert during telogen phase, and Silver and Chase (1970, 1977) have shown that neither DNA nor RNA is synthesized until the last few days before the beginning of a new anagen phase.

13.1 Common Hair Cycle Theory Subject to Revision

According to Uno et al. (1985), a new follicular cycle always starts from the end of telogen phase. Epithelial cell budding opposing condensed mesenchymal cells in the lower portion of a telogen follicle is the first sign of new follicular growth (Figs. 7.3a, 13.2). Cellular proliferation and differentiation inside the budding structure form a follicle in which a new bulb begins to produce a new matrix of hair. Subsequently, an elongation of the newly growing follicle proceeds towards the lower part of the dermis.

According to Pinkus (1981b), when regrowth of hair begins, the new germ closely resembles the fetal hair germ, except that it now forms at the base of the trichilemmal sac. Its axis is at an angle with the axis of the old hair, a useful sign for differentiating a follicle in early anagen phase from telogen.

Cotsarelis et al. (1990) state that, inconsistent with the view that hair follicle stem cells reside in the bulge region, label-retaining cells exist exclusively in the bulge area of the mouse hair follicle.

As noted above, Uno et al. (1985), Pinkus (1981b), and Cotsarelis et al. (1990) stated that regeneration starts not precisely from the lower end of the telogen follicle, but from a slightly lateral region of the lower follicle. This finding has been described in Sections 1.5.2.3 and 9.3.1; i.e., regeneration does not start only from the secondary hair germ at the lower end of the telogen follicle, but that a follicular epithelial layer may be formed from the upper isthmal portion close to the duct opening of the sebaceous gland (sebaceous isthmus) (Fig. 13.1b). Then a mass of mesenchymal cells may be formed later at the slightly lateral region of the telogen follicle. It then pegs downward as it goes through the hair peg and bulbous peg stages to become a terminal hair. We further confirmed that this regenerated follicle is clearly demarcated from the telogen follicle.

13.2 New Concept of the Hair Cycle in Humans

The above findings may suggest that the common hair cycle theory is still incomplete. Our proposi-

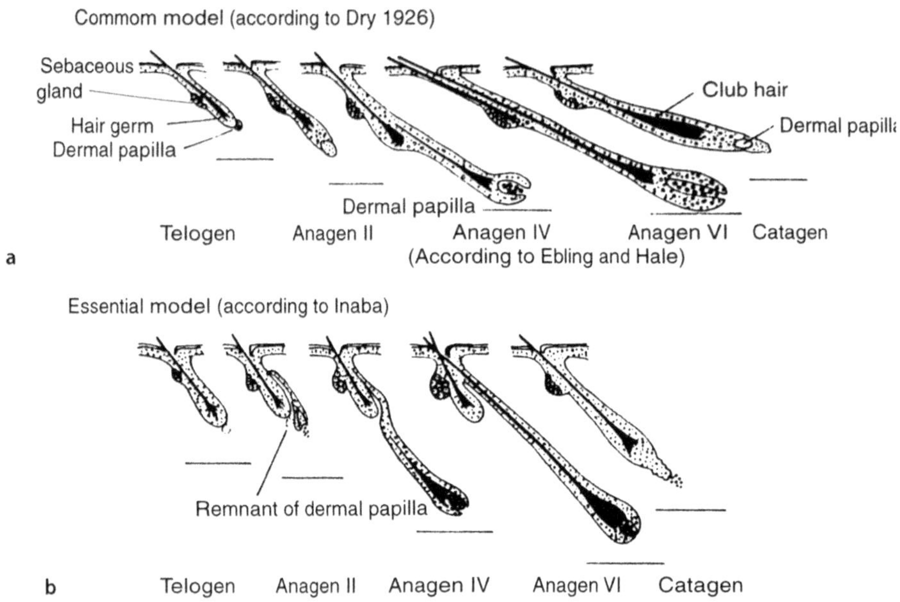

Fig. 13.1a,b. Models of the hair cycle (from Inaba and Inaba 1992a, reproduced with permission from Springer-Verlag)

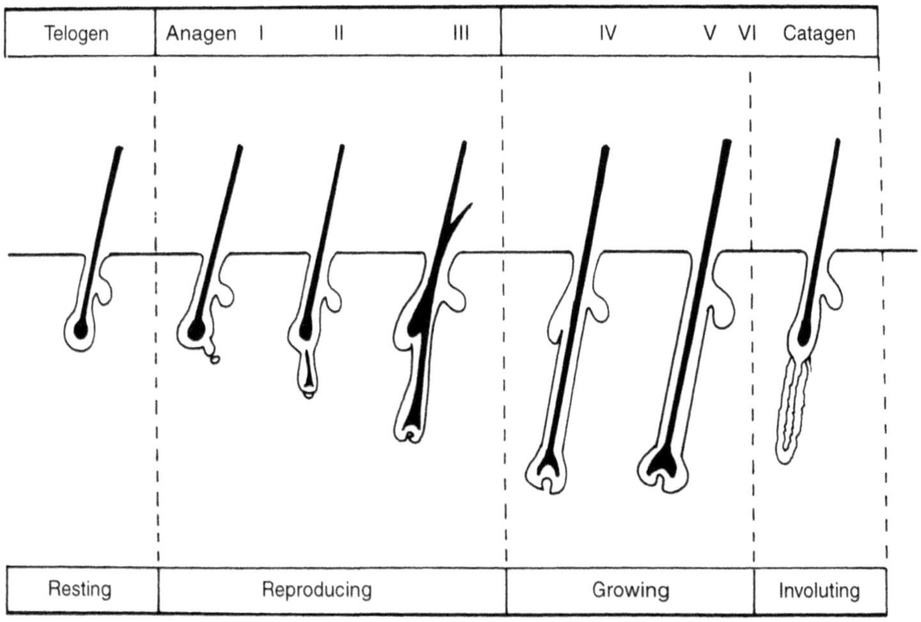

Fig. 13.2. Models of the human hair cycle (from Uno et al. 1985) (reproduced with permission from Raven Press, New York). According to Uno et al. (1985), a new bud cannot regenerate from the lower end of the telogen hair follicle. Its axis is at an angle with the axis of the telogen hair follicle (Anagen I). The hair bud then pegs downward as characteristic of the common hair cycle

tion that the true hair center is sited at the sebaceous isthmus, that is, the upper isthmal portion close to the duct opening of the sebaceous gland, then appears to be more reliable (Inaba 1985). Our suggestion is that the hair cycle should be divided into four stages: anagen, catagen, telogen, and isthmal (Fig. 7.1b) (Inaba 1985).

Formation of the early anagen stage from the lower end of telogen follicles as observed in axillary hair and human scalp hair is compatible with the common hair cycle theory. Yet in our observation of typical telogen hairs, we found that early anagen did not necessarily form from the lower telogen follicles, but that it was also regenerated from the upper isthmal portion of the follicle adjacent to the secretory duct opening of the sebaceous gland. The hair follicle has been theoretically divided into two portions, transient and permanent, at the lower telogen hair follicle point of attachment to the arrector muscle (Montagna and Parakkal 1974) (Fig. 8.4). The common hair cycle theory would seem valid if regeneration were to start from this remnant of dermal papilla cells or from the secondary hair germ that is present at the lower telogen follicle sac. The regeneration from the hair germ depends on the size of the telogen hair because, in some cases, the telogen hair follicle retracts within the lobes of the sebaceous gland instead of extending to the site of attachment of the arrector pili muscle. We found, specifically, that if the telogen hair was plucked, regeneration was observed to start from the upper isthmal portion of the hair follicle adjacent to the secretory duct opening of the sebaceous gland (Inaba and Inaba 1990b, 1992a).

The point of regeneration in our essential hair cycle theory is thus sited at the upper isthmal portion of the telogen hair follicle (essential hair cycle) (Fig. 7.1b).

13.3 Essential Hair Cycle Hypothesis and Supportive Findings

Montagna and Parakkal (1974) separated the hair follicle into two parts: the permanent and transient portions. Pinkus (1969) proposed separating it into three parts: the upper portion (from the epidermis to the duct-opening site of the sebaceous gland), the middle portion (from the duct-opening site of the sebaceous gland to the lower portion of telogen phase), and the lower portion (the same as the transient portion of Montagna and Parakkal) (Fig. 8.4).

The central portion of the hair follicle was believed to lie at the lower portion of the telogen stage follicle. It is now evident that this central portion is, instead, situated precisely at the isthmal portion close to the duct opening of the sebaceous gland. The hair bud can be formed from the upper isthmal portion. Hair regeneration depends on whether both the vascular system of the pilosebaceous unit and the upper isthmal portion of the sebaceous gland are left intact.

Pinkus and Mehregan (1981) cited our hypothesis (Inaba et al. 1979a) in their book (*The Guide to Dermatohistopathology*, 3rd edn): "This general scheme of the hair cycle has recently been challenged by Inaba et al., who found that axillary hair of Japanese is newly formed in the region of the sebaceous duct when dermal papilla and the entire lower part of the hair follicle have been surgically removed."

Other Important Findings in the Hair Follicle

14

14.1 Location of the Central Portion of Hair Regeneration

14.1.1 Replacement of Damaged Skin and Hair Regeneration (Follicular Stem Cell)

Breedis (1954) has reported the formation of many new hair follicles from the epidermis of healing wounds on the backs of rabbits.

Eisen et al. (1955) investigated the process of wound healing, and stated that regeneration of the epidermis began at the point of the sebaceous duct opening in the outer root sheath of the hair follicle, the eccrine duct, and the basal layer in the surrounding epidermis (Fig. 14.1a). In other words, if and when the basal layer is completely destroyed, it can be replaced by new daughter basal cells formed by these primary basal cells. The rate of regeneration of an epidermal site is proportional to the numbers of retained hair follicles: experimental outgrowth from hair follicles can regenerate full-thickness epidermis showing normal differentiation (Lenoir et al. 1988).

Kligman and Strauss (1956) have described the apparent new formation of vellus hair follicles from the reconstituted epidermis of facial skin abrasions.

Montagna and Chase (1956) found that X-irradiation could destroy the hair matrix, but that cells in the outer root sheath could regenerate a complete hair bulb. Based on this finding, Montagna (1962) suggested that the seed, or germinative source, of each generation of hair follicles must reside in the outer root sheath and not in the bulb. Studies of irradiated skin have shown that there is a significant proliferative cell population within the hair follicle that can contribute to epidermal regeneration (Withers 1967; Al-Barwari and Potten 1976). It has also been shown that some outer root sheath cells contribute towards new skin epidermis during wound healing (Sanford et al. 1965). Starico (1960) studied the destruction and regeneration of the sebaceous gland in cases of skin abrasion, and likewise found that regeneration began in the same region.

In vitiligo, when amelanotic melanocytes are activated by such agents as X-rays and trauma, the next growth phase (repigmentation) takes place (Starico 1961; Withers 1967; Al-Barwari and Potten 1976; see Section 4.4).

Amelanotic melanocytes divide, proliferate, and migrate upward along the hair follicle surface to a site close to the epidermis, where they continue to move radially. During this migration, the melanocytes gradually mature in both function and morphology.

Occasional observations of abnormally directed accessory hair roots in skin biopsies have also been noted (H. Pinkus, personal communication, 1977). This finding seems to indicate that such follicles have grown from the upper isthmus of scalp hairs. This upper isthmus area, which lies at the same level where the sebaceous glands originate, seems to be the most common site for the formation of milia and the epithelial collar of mantle hairs in certain mammals.

Furthermore, there is a strong phenotypic correlation between basal cell carcinomas and cells of the hair follicle outer root sheath, as well as some peculiar kinetics observed in the experimental development of skin tumors (Lane et al. 1991).

Stem cells are, by definition, present in all self-renewing tissues, and are thought to play a crucial role in tissue homeostasis and tumorigenesis (Cairns et al. 1976; Lajtha 1979, 1983). Primary stem cells are believed to exist in all organisms, and they are thought to be present in the skin and bone marrow (hematopoietic stem cells; Lajtha

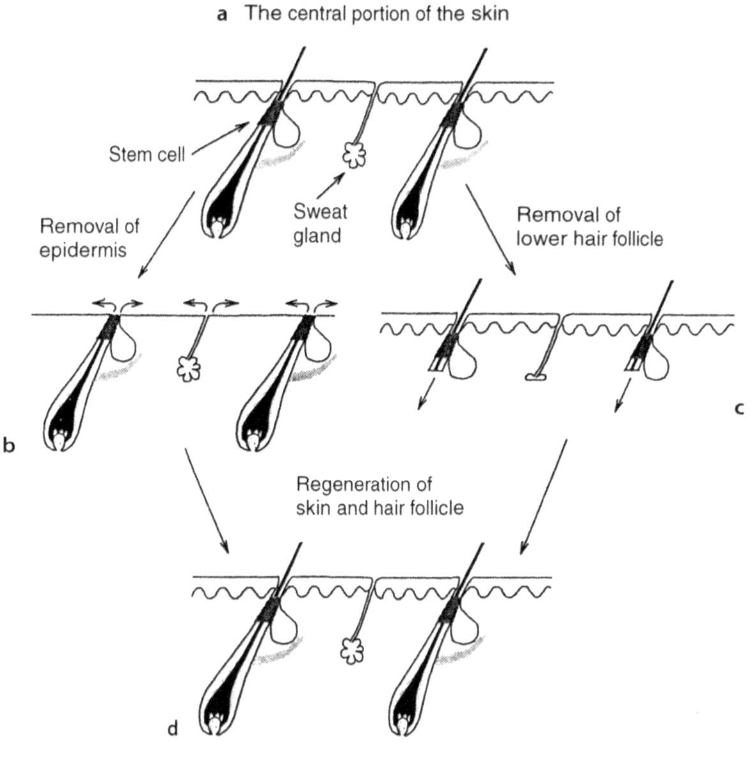

Fig. 14.1a–d. Replacement of damaged skin and hair generation. **a** Normal structure. **b** Wound healing: regeneration of epidermis occurs from the upper isthmal portion, the eccrine duct, and surrounding epidermis. **c** After removal of the lower portion of the hair follicle, regeneration begins from the upper isthmal portion. **d** Hair has fully regenerated

1979), in the intestinal epithelium (Potten et al. 1987; Schmidt et al. 1985), in the filiform papillae on the tongue (Hume and Potten 1980), and in the limbus in the corneal epithelium (Cotsarelis et al. 1989).

14.1.2 Stem Cells of the Skin and the Hair Follicle

Numerous studies have attempted to identify the location of stem cells in the epidermis (Bickenbach and Mackenzie 1984; Cotsarelis et al. 1989). Some aspects of morphological heterogeneity have been interpreted as indicative of stem cells (Klein-Szanto 1977; Lavker and Sun 1981). On the other hand, in hairy skin, there is very little variation in the morphology of interfollicular basal cells, and basal cell heterogeneity is more easily correlated with relative states of differentiation and impending progression into the suprabasal compartment (Schweizer et al. 1984; Roop et al. 1987) than with proliferative capacity (reviewed by Lane et al. 1991).

Keratin analysis can yield information about the state of differentiation of a single keratinocyte. Thus, in the epidermis, the 56.5-/65- to 67-kD keratin markers of skin-type differentiation are made predominantly by suprabasal cells (O'Guin et al. 1986). The few basal cells (<5%–10%) expressing these two keratins are considered to be partially differentiated cells about to leave the basal layer (Schweizer et al. 1984).

The derived keratinocytes are able to generate a full-thickness, normally differentiating epidermis after partial thickness excision. Lenoir et al. (1988) reported that outer root sheath cells of human hair follicles are able to regenerate a fully differentiated epidermis in vitro.

Consistent findings were obtained by Oliver (1966a, 1967a,b) and Ibrahim and Wright (1982), who showed with one-third of the rat vibrissal hair follicle being surgically removed, a new hair bulb could regenerate in response to the implantation of a new dermal papilla. If less than the lower third was removed, the dermal papilla regenerated either from the outer root sheath or from the connective tissue of the dermal sheath surrounding it, and a vibrissa grew. This result strongly suggests that hair follicular stem cells are located in the upper half of the follicle. According to Kobayashi (1987), the skin tissue in the grafts containing the upper one-half or two-thirds of the follicle could be preserved in good condition, but no regeneration of the dermal papilla was recognized, even after long-term observations, and a vibrissa did not grow.

The defining properties of a stem cell, according to Alberts et al. (1989) (Fig. 14.2) are:

1. It is not itself terminally differentiated (that is, it is not at the end of a differentiation pathway).

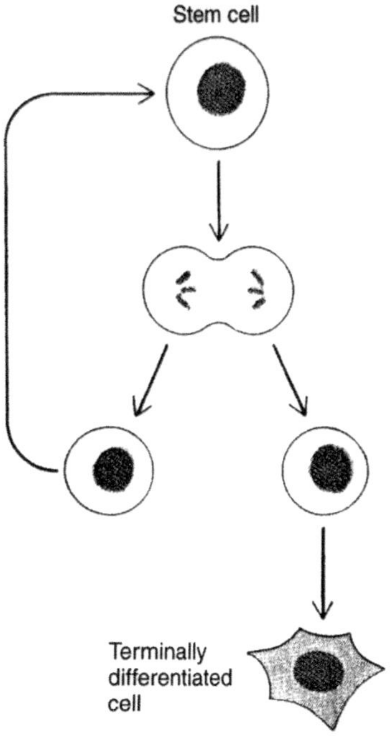

Fig. 14.2. Definition of stem cell. Each daughter produced when a stem cell divides can either remain a stem cell or go on to become terminally differentiated (from Alberts et al. 1989, reproduced with permission from Garland Publishing Inc.)

2. It can divide without limit (or at least for the lifetime of the animal).
3. When it divides, each daughter cell may either remain a stem cell or may begin a course leading irreversibly to terminal differentiation.

According to Cotsarelis et al. (1990), stem cells:

1. Are relatively undifferentiated, both ultrastructurally and biochemically.
2. Have a large proliferative potential and are responsible for the long-term maintenance and regeneration of the tissue.
3. Are normally slow-cycling, presumably to conserve their proliferative potential and to minimize DNA errors that could occur during replication.
4. Can be stimulated to proliferate in response to wounding and to certain growth stimuli. They are often located in close proximity to a population of rapidly proliferating cells corresponding to transient amplifying (TA) cells.
5. Are usually found in a well-protected, highly vascularized and innervated area.

In this respect, most of the structures and cell layers that characterize growing follicles are lacking in telogen follicles, and a morphologically distinct germinative cell population cannot be identified in the lower epithelial sac, while follicular stem cells are thought to reside somewhere for the next generation (for details, see Section 7.2).

14.1.3 Bulge Activation Hypothesis (Cotsarelis et al. 1990)

Recently, Cotsarelis et al. (1990) suggested that follicular stem cells reside in the bulge region; this idea has provided new insights into how the hair cycle may be regulated. During late telogen or early anagen, the normally slow-cycling stem cells of the bulge area are activated by dermal papilla cells (bulge activation hypothesis; Fig. 14.3a).

In human embryonic hair (15–17 weeks), the bulge is a prominent structure, sometimes being even larger than the hair bulb (Stöhr 1904; Pinkus 1958; Unna 1976). However, it is relatively inconspicuous in routine sections of adult follicles (see Section 3.1.3). Madsen (1964) identified outer root sheath bulges in human trunk and neck skin. However, bulges are less conspicuous in the follicles of the scalp. Consequently, the bulge has attracted so little attention in the past that it is rarely mentioned in histology textbooks (Cormack 1987; Stenn 1988). As mentioned above, the realization that hair follicle stem cells may reside in the bulge area provides new insights into how the hair cycle may be regulated (Cotsarelis et al. 1990).

Light and transmission electron microscopic findings (Cotsarelis et al. 1989) indicate that the bulge was not just an outpouching of outer root sheath (ORS) cells. In fact, it is now clear that (at least in the mouse) the bulge area is not only kinetically but also morphologically distinct from other ORS cells. At the light microscopic level, cells within the bulge are generally smaller than surrounding ORS cells, and they have markedly convoluted nuclei. Ultrastructurally, bulge cells have a cytoplasm primarily filled with ribosomes, are devoid of aggregated keratin filaments, and have a surface distinguished by numerous microvilli (Lavker et al. 1993).

Cotsarelis et al. (1990) have incorporated these findings and other known important histologic and kinetic events occurring during different stages of the hair cycle in a schematic model (the "bulge-activation hypothesis"). This hypothesis consists of four important elements: (i) Bulge cells are normally slow-cycling but can be stimulated/activated by the dermal papilla to undergo transient proliferation during early anagen. (ii) During anagen IV, dermal papilla cells undergo transient proliferation and de-condensation, possibly in response to a matrix signal. (iii) Matrix cells, being derived from the bulge (stem) cells, are transient amplifying cells and thus have only a limited proliferative potential. (iv) The upward movement of

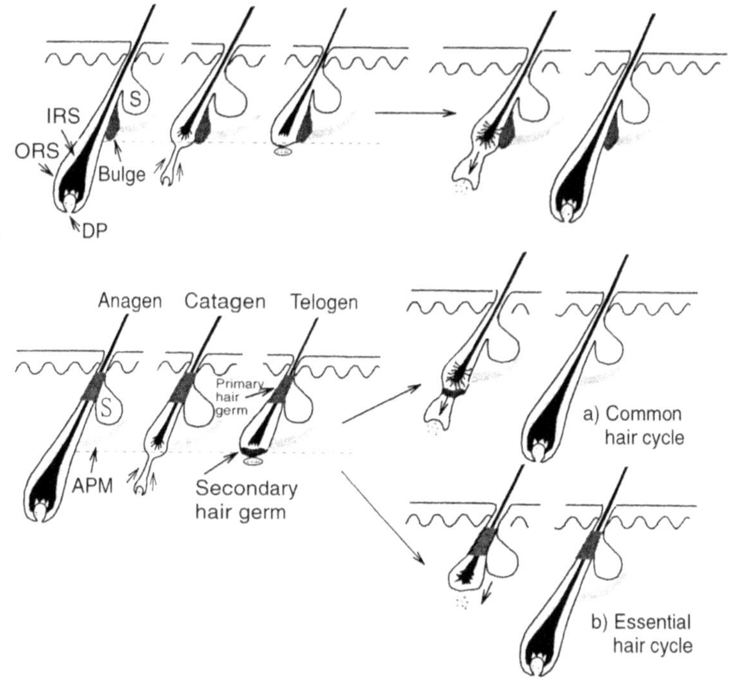

Fig. 14.3. **a** Bulge activation hypothesis (Cotsarelis et al. 1990). **b** Sebaceous gland hypothesis (Inaba 1985; Inaba and Inaba 1994). *ORS*, Outer root sheath; *DP*, dermal papilla; *APM*, arrector pilli muscle; *IRS*; inner root sheath; *S*, sebaceous gland

the dermal papilla (DP) during late catagen is crucial for allowing the subsequent physical interaction or activation of the resting bulge cells by DP cells, and for starting a new cycle of hair growth.

Concerning the activation of bulge stem cells by the dermal papilla during late telogen, Cotsarelis et al. (1990) suggest the following: During late telogen or early anagen, the normally slow-cycling stem cells of the bulge area are activated by dermal papilla cells. The mechanism underlying this activation is not known, but could involve a diffusible dermal papilla, which phenomenon is known to occur during a comparable stage in embryonic hair formation (Robins and Breathnach 1969).

In this respect, Sugiyama and Kukita (1976) researched the ultrastructure of the hair follicles in early and late catagen, with special reference to the alteration of the junctional structure between the dermal papilla and epithelial component. They found that the diffuse dermal papilla could be activated by a derived growth factor and/or by direct cell-cell contact. This activation leads to the proliferation of some cells in the bulge area, which then form a downgrowth (Chase 1954).

As the dermal papilla is pushed away from the bulge by this newly formed epithelial column, the bulge stem cells, presumably, return to their normally quiescent, slow-cycling state in mid-anagen.

According to Lane et al. (1991):

1. Immunohistochemistry with keratin antibodies indicates flexibility of differentiation across the Wulst (bulge) region. The Wulst cells are distinct from outer epidermal keratinocytes, in that the basal cells express keratin 19. Although the Wulst is not as morphologically well defined in the fully developed adult follicle as it is in fetal tissues, it retains its identity into adult follicles by this expression of keratin 19 (Stasiak et al. 1989).
2. The morphology of this region of the hair follicle can be very variable. There is a marked increase in the number of basal keratin 19-positive cells.
3. The regenerative essence of the cycling follicle probably resides much higher up than the hair bulb. Regrowth in anagen begins as a peg of epithelial cells growing down from this Wulst zone, and the keratin 19-positive cells are retained throughout the cycle.
4. The arrector pili muscle is attached to this site of keratin 19-positive cells.
5. The Wulst is a region where cell proliferation occurs, as evidenced by mitotic figures. Asada et al. (1990) also reported that CK19, a marker of undifferentiated stem cells, was found in outermost cells of the outer root sheath at the upper isthmus and in some cells of the lower outer root sheath.

14.1.4 Bulge Activation Hypothesis Reconsidered

According to Montagna and Parakkal (1974), the cells of the outer root sheath in early catagen stage begin to transform into germ cells. In telogen

a

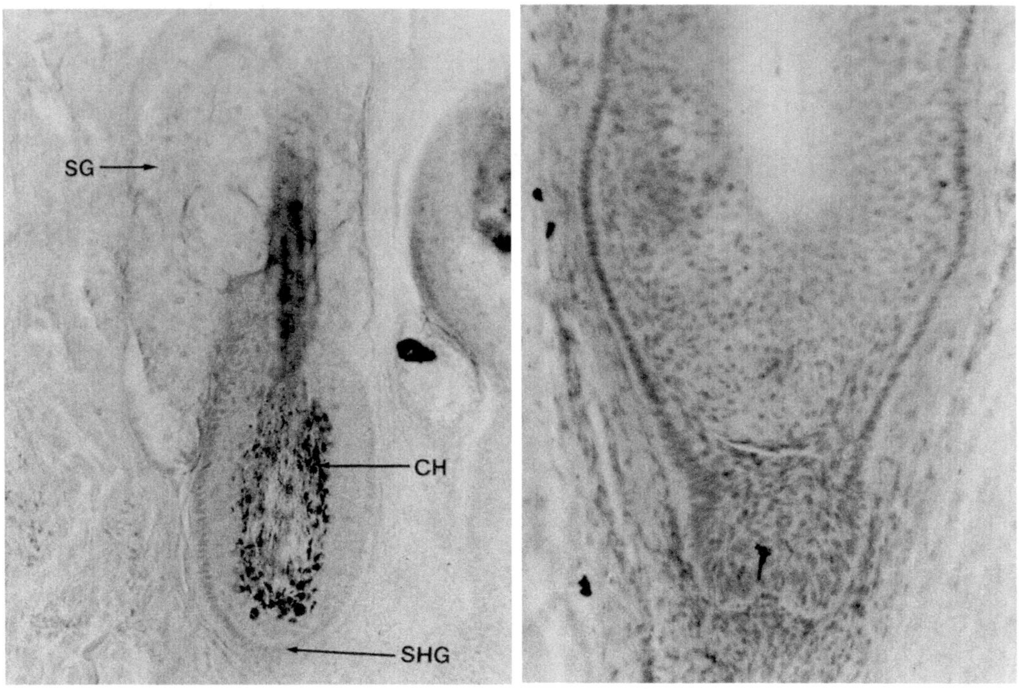

b

Fig. 14.4. a Thick tissue specimen observations. Secondary hair germ (*SHG*) starts to regenerate from the lower tip of the telogen hair follicle, but not from the bulge area. No changes can be seen in the lower follicular epithelial cells. *CH*, Club hair; *SHG*, secondary hair germ; *SG*, sebaceous gland. ×135 **b** Higher magnification of more advanced stage of regeneration of the secondary hair germ. ×400

stage, ultimately two or three layers of germ cells surround the club hair, forming a capsule or germ sac. These seeds for the next generation of hair have been thought to be the important part of the resting follicles. Histologically, the hair germ has been defined as a group of cells located at the base of the telogen follicle in close contact with the dermal papilla (Montagna et al. 1952a; Silver and Chase 1977). We also confirmed the presence of a secondary hair germ at the lower end of the telogen follicle in observation of a thick-tissue specimen (Fig. 14.4a,b). We then recognized that a hair germ was formed from here (in close relation with the lower end of the telogen follicle), but not from the bulge area, finally turning into a terminal hair, after going through hair peg and bulbous peg stages (common hair cycle: Figs. 14.3b, 7.1a). We confirmed that the hair germ was not formed from the bulge area, as has been advocated by Cotsarelis et al. (Fig. 14.3a).

It has recently been reported that, during epidermal regeneration, there was a high incidence of irregularity, suggestive of locally increased cell proliferation (Lane et al. 1991). However, we do not recognize this irregularity in the bulge area, but in the lower portion of the telogen hair follicle. Cotsarelis et al. (1990) claim that the presence of the dermal papilla is a prerequisite for the formation of the hair follicle, and Oliver (1970) and Reynolds and Jahoda (1990) reported that the dermal papilla component of the follicle could induce the formation of hair-producing follicles containing germinative and outer root sheath epidermis.

If germinative cells, including the tip area and bulge area of a telogen phase follicle, are lost (or destroyed) towards the end of each cycle, they are replaced by outer root sheath cells at the initiation of the next regeneration (Reynolds and Jahoda 1991a).

On the other hand, we (Inaba et al. 1979a; Inaba and Inaba 1992a) have reported that after subcutaneous tissue shaving, a new hair germ had begun to generate from the sebaceous isthmus, that is, the upper isthmal portion close to the duct opening of the sebaceous gland (Fig. 8.6). We also recognized new young follicles generated from the duct opening of the sebaceous glands (Fig. 14.5a–d).

Cotsarelis et al. (1990) stated: "Surgical removal of human axillary hair follicles up to a level near the sebaceous gland did not prevent the regeneration of new hair follicles (Inaba et al. 1979a). This again suggests that hair follicle stem cells are located in the upper half of the follicle in an area

Fig. 14.5. **a** Secondary hair germ starts to regenerate from the upper isthmal portion after the telogen hair has been plucked. ×60 **b** Higher magnification of the secondary hair germ follicle. *UIP*, Upper isthmal portion; *SHG*, secondary hair germ. ×135 **c** Secondary hair follicle starts to generate from above the duct opening of the sebaceous gland. ×60 **d** New young hair follicle is already in bulbous peg phase. ×135

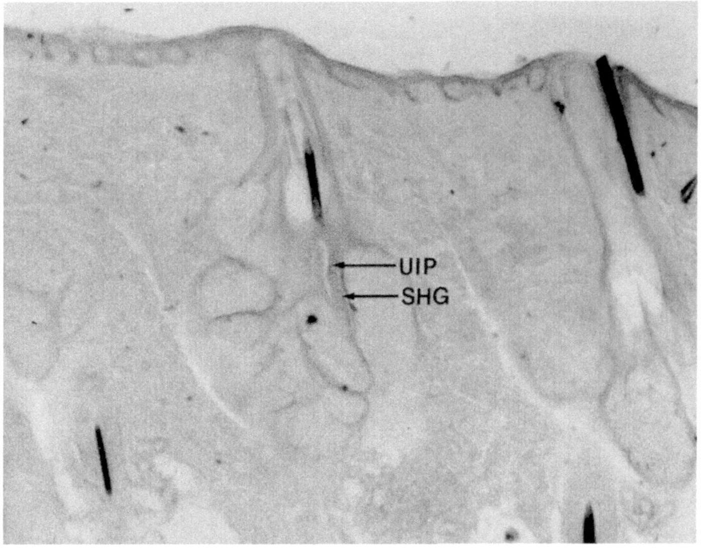

a

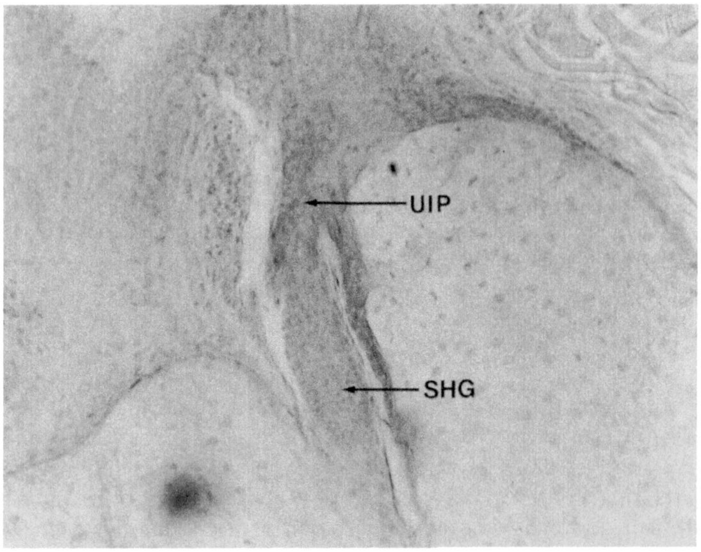

b

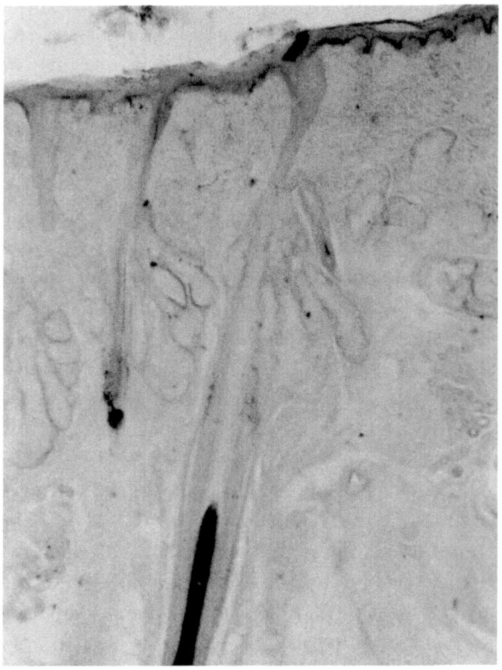

c

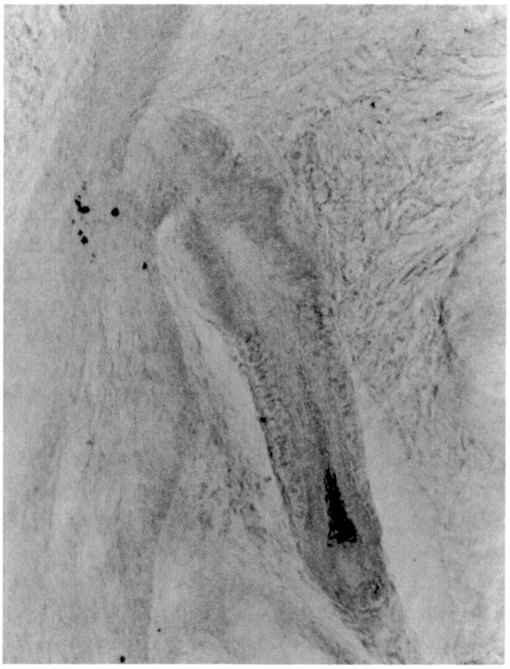

d

immediately below the sebaceous gland opening, i.e., the region of the bulge."

As the bulges usually lie immediately below the sebaceous gland in the mouse, they may have misunderstood the site of regeneration. In murine skin, follicular neogenesis does not occur until after birth (Chase 1954). During this (postnatal) follicle formation, the bulge does not become a recognizable entity until 7–9 days after birth. However, once formed, it is easily recognizable during all stages of the hair cycle, and is present throughout the life of the mouse (Lavker et al. 1992).

As described above (Section 1.5.2), the mesenchymal cells are not necessarily required for the generation and regeneration of the hair follicle; the new hair germ (epithelial tissue) generates from crowding of nuclei in the epidermis (Fig. 1.9) or from the sebaceous isthmus, that is, the upper isthmal portion close to the duct opening of the sebaceous gland, as proposed by the authors in their sebaceous gland hypothesis (see Chapter 13, and Figs. 1.12 and 1.13a,b). Mesenchymal cells will develop completely at a later period. Subsequent development of initiated follicles occurs under the influence of mesenchymal cells (dermal papilla) associated with each of the growing follicles.

As mentioned above, we have been suggesting that the stem cell, which plays a vital role in hair regeneration, resides not only in the lower end of a telogen follicle but in the upper isthmal portion close to the secretory duct opening of the sebaceous gland. In connection with this finding, Morohashi (1968) noted that keratotic epithelium was observed in this area and suggested that cohesive hyperkeratinization occurred under the influence of a male hormone.

In the replacement of vellus hair by coarse hair (Section 6.4.2, Figs. 6.5a, 6.6a–c, and 14.6 [I]) and in the development of bundle hair (Section 6.4.4; Fig. 14.6II), we suggested that the stem cells at the outer root sheath close to the duct opening of the sebaceous gland (sebaceous isthmus) could be activated by stimulation from hyperkeratinization due to hormonal influence (Fig. 14.6).

We attempted to study the process of regeneration by applying an anti-cancer agent (methotrexate, etc.) to mouse body skin surface, thus experimentally creating telogen hair follicles. The new hair bud (germ) in the regeneration process had been thought to begin to form from remnants of the dermal papilla or from a secondary hair germ in telogen stage (Fig. 12.10a).

However, we (Inaba 1985) recognize from recent studies that the regeneration of the hair germ does not necessarily occur from the remnants of the dermal papilla, but that the hair germ can be formed from the newly-formed epithelial cells developing from the sebaceous isthmus (upper stem cells) and later from mesenchymal cells (Fig. 12.1a,b, Fig. 12.10b).

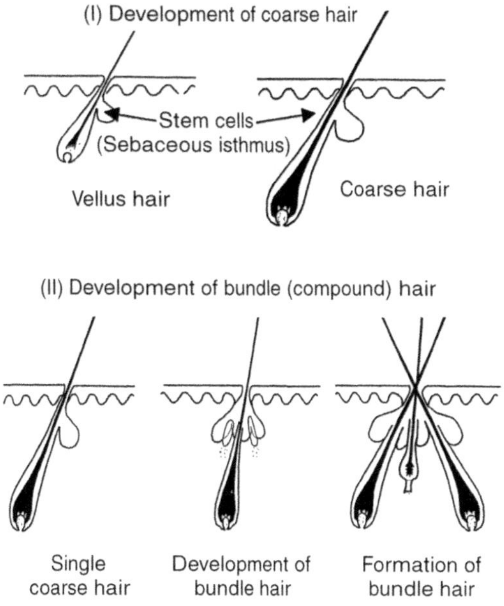

Fig. 14.6. In replacement of vellus hair by coarse hair (*I*) and in the development of bundle hair (*II*), the stem cells at the outer root sheath close to the duct opening of the sebaceous gland (*sebaceous isthmus*) may be activated by stimulation from hyperkeratinization due to hormonal influence

At a glance, the new hair germ could be thought to regenerate from the bulge area, as suggested by Cotsarelis et al. (1990) (Figs. 12.3, 12.6a), but this finding also indicates that this regeneration is closely related with the upper isthmal portion (upper stem cells) (Fig. 12.10b) and vascularization of the hair follicle (Inaba 1985).

The common hair cycle theory states that, during the telogen stage, hair regeneration starts individually from the lower end of the compound hair follicle where two to three hairs are present in a single hair follicle (Section 12.2, Fig. 12.10a).

However, we have found that regeneration from remnants of the dermal papilla does not occur by the formation of a hair germ at the lower portion of bundle (compound) hair in the telogen stage (Figs. 12.5, 12.10b, Section 12.3).

Our finding is that a single mass of mesenchymal cells (hair germ) is sometimes newly formed at the lower end of compound hair follicles above which the epithelial cell layer has already formed from the sebaceous isthmal portion (Fig. 12.10b). This finding suggests that the generation of the mass of mesenchymal cells does not necessarily start from the remnant of dermal papilla cells or from the secondary hair germ present in the lower portion of bundle telogen follicles, but that the hair germ can also be formed from newly-formed epithelial cells derived from the sebaceous isthmal portion, while mesenchymal cells will develop completely in a later period. Recovery of the vascular system surrounding the follicles may precede the above phenomenon.

Based on our extensive research, we cannot support the bulge activation hypothesis (Inaba and Inaba 1994a). Holecek and Ackerman (1993), who cited the "bulge activation hypothesis: is it valid?", reported as follows: "Before it can be validated, serious challenges to it, some from experimental work performed decades ago, must be answered. The most telling argument against the bulge-activation hypothesis comes from the experiments of Oliver, who showed that a whisker in the absence of that part of a follicle that houses the bulge, and of Inaba and collaborators, who demonstrated in humans that follicles could regenerate in the absence of a bulge."

Our research indicates that the stem cells lie at the lower portion of telogen follicles (secondary stem cells) and the sebaceous isthmus (primary stem cells).

Thus the hair cycle must be categorized into two types, that is, the common hair cycle and the essential hair cycle.

14.2 Mechanism of the Descending Hair Follicle

Although the hair follicle is an extension of the germinal layer of the epidermis, the mechanism by which the structure of the outer root sheath descends downward in its initial formation stages, can be elucidated as follows.

Earlier reports (Chase 1954) of this process sug-

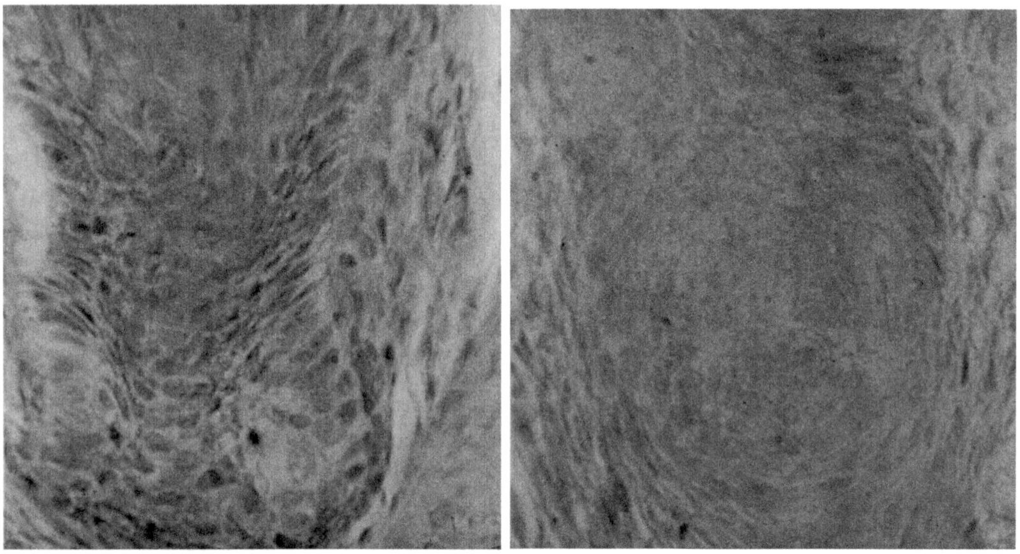

a c

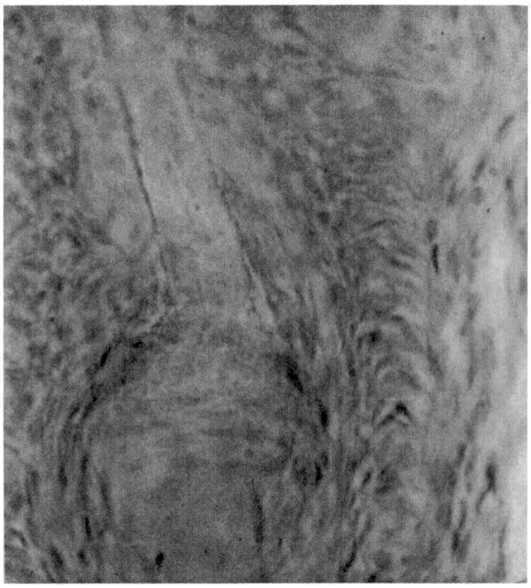

b

Fig. 14.7. **a** The lower portion of hair follicle. New young hair germ can be formed from the lower portion of the outer root sheath (germinal layer). ×400 **b** New hair germ is formed. Upper portion is keratinized to form a new young hair. ×400 **c** Mesenchymal cells can be seen in the lower portion of the hair germ. ×400 gested that the follicle was elongated downward into the dermis by vigorous mitotic activity in the lower epithelial sac, which activity pulled the growth process downward via a leading tip consisting of a mass of mesenchymal cells.

Moretti (1965) and Sato (1976) report much the same findings: Sato remarks that "before movement of the hair occurs, the inner root sheath has begun its upward climb. This upward force exerts pressure on the hair, which nevertheless grows downward ... The mechanism of pegging is unclear."

Montagna and Parakkal (1974) and Serri and Cerimele (1990) have described this phenomenon as follows: When and as cuticle cells arise from the matrix, they move upward from the bulb and increase in volume. They become firmly attached to the cortex on the axial face rather than laterally to the cuticle cells of the inner root sheath. Since the sheath cuticula appears to grow at the same rate as the hair, its cells are likely to increase in volume at a rate faster than the cells of the hair cuticula. This sheath cuticula may then exert pressure inhibiting ascent of the hair. The oblique penetration of the hair germs into the dermis seems to be directed by the cluster of mesenchymal cells which accumulate beneath it.

The discrepancies between the in vivo findings and the transition of anagen to catagen in vivo indicate that factors in the outer root sheath other than epidermal growth factor (EGF) must be important in vivo. Reynolds and Jahoda (1991b) have speculated that, in anagen hair follicles, the outer root sheath cells may undergo downward migration towards the hair follicle matrix and Moore et al. (1991) have suggested that, as EGF receptors are located in the outer root sheath of hair follicles, EGF may be responsible for generating the cell lineages that populate the matrix. However, thus far, little experimental evidence has been provided to support these ideas. Experimental findings presented by Philpott et al. (1992) indicate that ORS cells can, under certain conditions, undergo downward migration within the hair follicle. Tezuka et al. (1991) reported that cells in the outer middle group positively labeled with bromodeoxyuridine (BrdU) and stained immunohis-

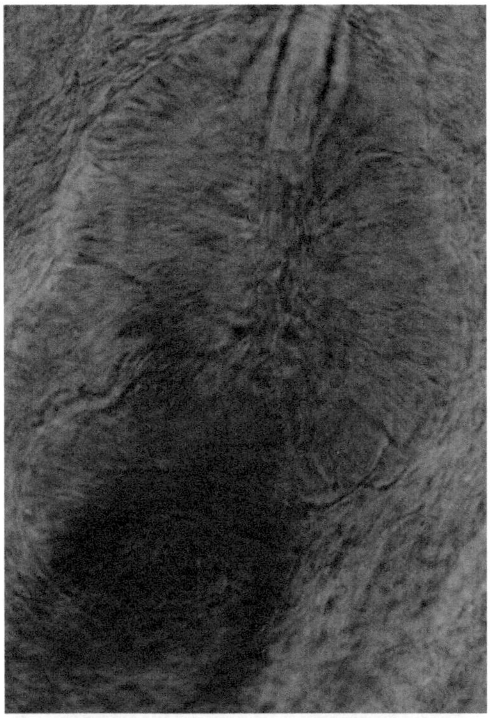

a

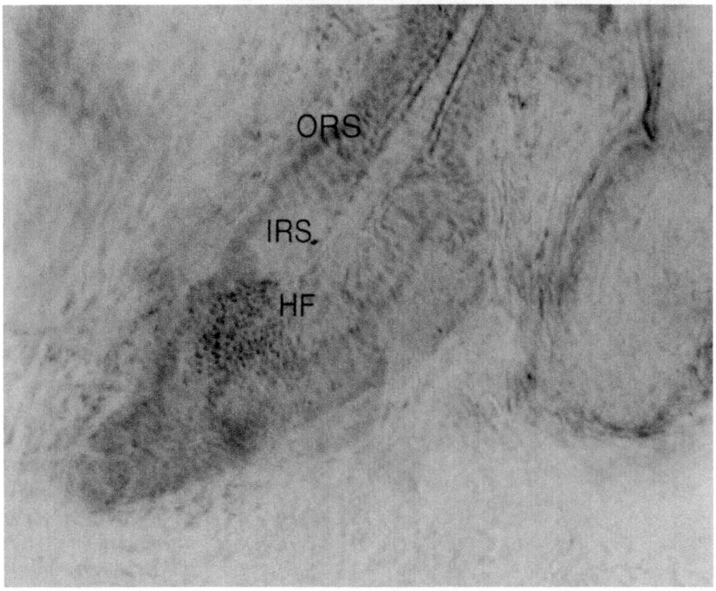

b

Fig. 14.8. **a** New hair germ can be seen descending downward from the outer root sheath. New young hair can already be formed from the aggregating filamentous structure. ×400 **b** Outer root sheath descends downward, to form a hair germ stage follicle (see Fig. 9.5d). *ORS*, Outer root sheath; *IRS*, inner root sheath; *HF*, hair fiber. ×135 tochemically with anti-BrdU monoclonal antibody may be important for the elongation of the hair apparatus and for the production of outer root sheath cells. These findings have not been clarified in regard to the mechanisms responsible for the development of the descending hair follicle. In regard to these mechanisms we considered the following features:

(a) Mechanism of Elongation Downward in Initial Stage. New hair germ descends downward from the outer root sheath (germinal layer). Filamentous structures aggregate from the newly-formed germinal layer and then become fibrils by suppressing the inner root sheath. The upper portion of the fibril becomes a new keratinized hair. In the initial stage, the follicle is elongated downward into the dermis by vigorous mitotic activity in the lower epithelial sac (Fig. 9.5d). Then the outer root sheath descends downward to become a hair follicle (hair peg stage) (Fig. 8.9, Fig. 8.12). Observing this process in more detail, we suggest that the outer root sheath is elongated by the newly-formed epithelial sac.

As shown in Fig. 14.7a, the lower portion of the outer root sheath begins to separate. This finding

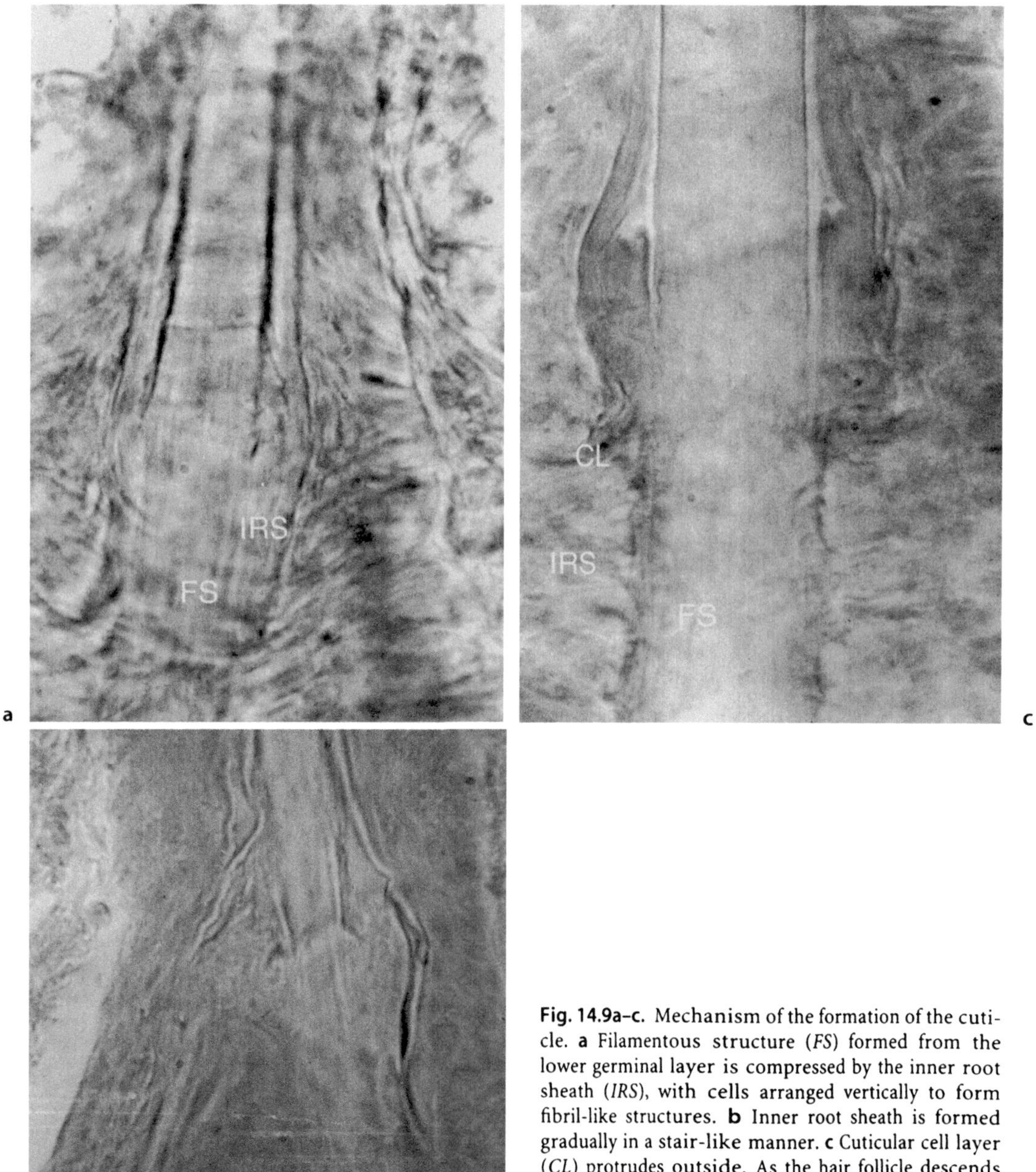

Fig. 14.9a–c. Mechanism of the formation of the cuticle. **a** Filamentous structure (*FS*) formed from the lower germinal layer is compressed by the inner root sheath (*IRS*), with cells arranged vertically to form fibril-like structures. **b** Inner root sheath is formed gradually in a stair-like manner. **c** Cuticular cell layer (*CL*) protrudes outside. As the hair follicle descends downward, the sheath cuticula cell layer becomes flattened and exhibits interlocking fusion with the hair cuticula. ×400

shows that the new epithelial germ can be formed inside the elongated outer root sheath (Fig. 14.7b). New young hair can already be seen at the upper portion of the epithelial sac.

(b) Elongation Downward in Hair Peg Stage. The outer root sheath has also been reported to have a new mechanism of downward elongating hair regeneration. The filamentous structure from which the hair is formed is compressed firmly by keratinization of Henle's layer in the inner root sheath; this filamentous structure is thus arranged in vertical fibrils, with the upper part keratinized to form the cortex of the hair root (Fig. 14.8a,b).

(c) Mechanism of the Formation of the Cuticle. The outer root sheath descends downward to form a hair germ stage follicle (Fig. 14.8b, Fig. 8.12a, Hair germ stage). The inner root sheath is newly-formed in a stair-like manner (Fig. 14.9a,b). The sheath cuticle cells protrude outside. Then, as the hair follicle descends downward, the sheath cuticula becomes flattened and exhibits interlocking fusion with the hair cuticula (Fig. 14.9c).

Observing this process in more detail, we find that the hair cuticula, which is the outermost layer of the hair root, shows interlocking fusion with the interfacing sheath cuticula (Fig. 1.6). This interlocking fusion prevents the newly forming hair from growing upward. The follicle is forced to elongate downward until it has reached the level of the future hair bulb. This downward growth is caused by the vigorous mitotic activity of the hair germ cells in the lower portion of the epithelial sac (Fig. 14.10a). As the hair follicle stops descending and the hair bulb is completely formed, the hair and inner root sheath grow at the same speed upward toward the skin surface, with the prior obstacle of interlocking fusion between hair cuticula and sheath cuticula no longer preventing upward growth (Fig. 14.10b).

14.3 How Is the Hair Matrix Formed?

When the germinal cell layer of the epidermis is differentiated to change and grow into columnar shape, the epithelial cells of the follicle become restricted to the germinal layer that surrounds the mass of mesenchymal tissue (Fig. 8.12c). The outer root sheath is pressed outward by the descending inner root sheath. Consequently, the outer root sheath is thinned, so much so that, at its bottom, it has only one or two cell layers. The hair bulb is formed mostly by the inner and outer root sheaths, including the dermal papilla, and becomes complete (Fig. 14.10b). Hair growth is the result of the intense proliferative activity of hair matrix cells surrounding the dermal papilla within the hair bulb.

A group of germinative cells at the base of the follicle end bulb region has long been considered to be an epidermal stem cell population with a pluripotential nature, since, during each period of active hair fiber growth, they give rise to a number of distinct cell lines as they differentiate, including hair medulla, cortex, cuticles, and Huxley's and Henle's layers (Fig. 14.11a,b) (Bullough and Laurence 1958; Montagna and Van Scott 1958; Epstein and Maibach 1969; Montagna and Parakkal 1974; Chapman 1986; Powell et al. 1989).

From the aspect of formation of the hair bulb, Birbeck and Mercer (1957) studied the hair matrix in detail by electron microscopy. They found, as shown in Fig. 14.12a, the germinal layer wrapped around the dermal papilla below Auber's borderline (the critical level). In this figure mitotic activity is visible in section D (the divided region) and keratinization has begun in the undifferentiated matrix (section U) above section D. This activity results in differentiation of the inner root sheath and the hair at each level.

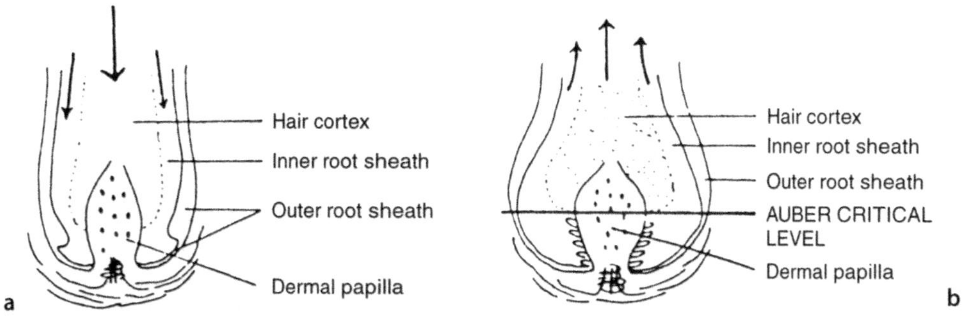

Fig. 14.10. Formation of the hair matrix. **a** Early events in the replacement of vellus hairs by coarse hairs. Descending hair follicle wrapped around a mass of mesenchymal cells. The inner root sheath elongates downward to form the hair bulb. **b** Later events in the full formation of the hair bulb with appearance of pigmentation by melanocytes. (Inaba 1981, 1985)

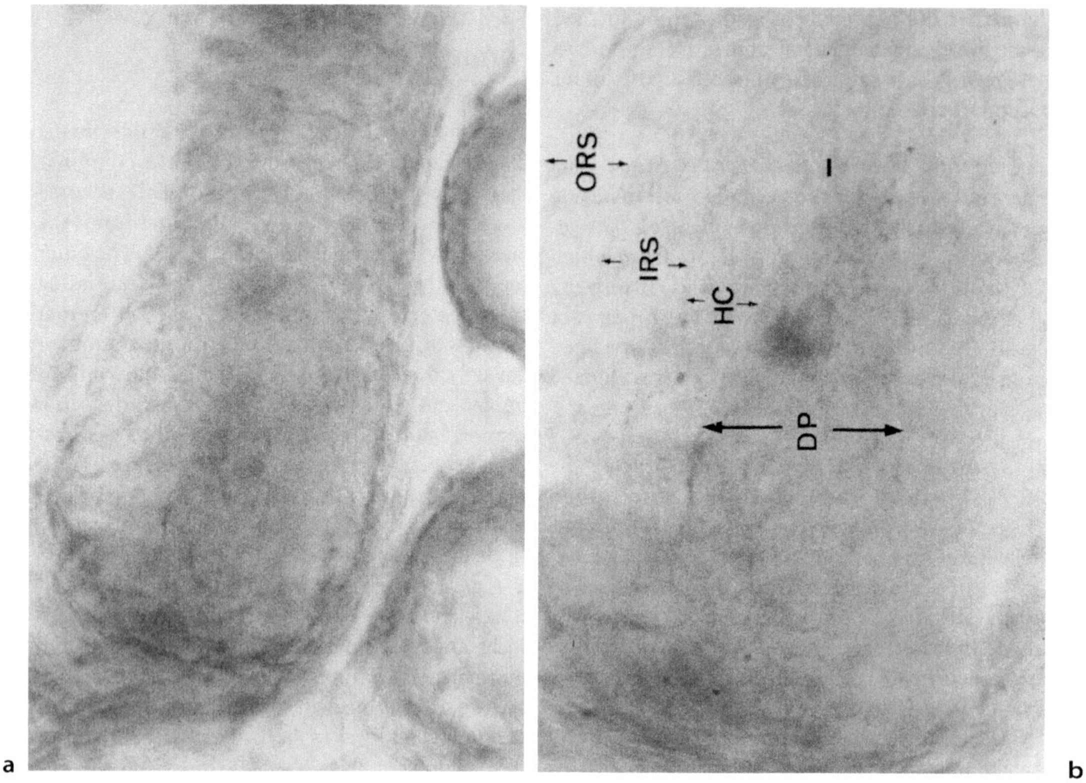

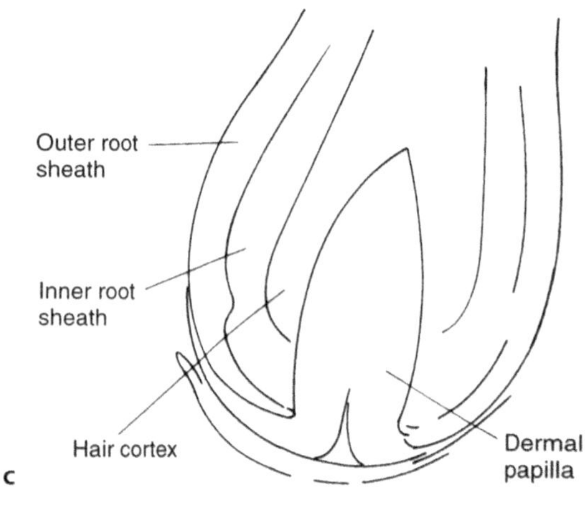

Fig. 14.11a–c. **a** Bulbous peg stage. Descending hair follicle wrapped around a mass of mesenchymal cells. ×135 **b** High-power view of portion of **a** showing the four distinct layers of outer root sheath (*ORS*), inner root sheath (*IRS*), hair cortex (*HC*), and dermal papilla (*DP*). ×400 **c** Schematic representation of significant findings

According to Kinebuchi (1972), all the keratinized cells below Auber's borderline can be said to constitute an immature keratinized region (section IK in Fig. 14.12c), because they are morphologically identical, but it cannot be presumed from morphological observations alone which cells will form which structures, as observed in section UK (undifferentiated region) (Fig. 14.12c).

Earlier autoradiographic studies of anagen hairs have demonstrated most of the DNA synthesizing cells to be matrix cells surrounding the upper and, in particular, the lower, segment of the dermal hair papilla. The DNA-labelling indices of hair matrix cells were determined to be about 28%, most of the cells being located below the Auber's level (Sherad and Marks 1977; Van Scott et al. 1963).

A DNA flow-cytometric study (DNA-FCM analysis) carried out by Kiesewetter et al. (1989) clearly demonstrated that the application of both microsurgical dissection of anagen hairs and DNA-FCM analysis was suitable for the investigation of cell proliferation in different anagen hair compartments Kiesewetter et al. (1990). As expected, the highest S-phase (14%) and proliferation index (PI) (PI, S + G2 + M) percentages were found in the lowermost segment of the hair bulb, decreasing to 7.6% S-phase cells at Auber's level and 5.9% S-phase cells at the follicle isthmus.

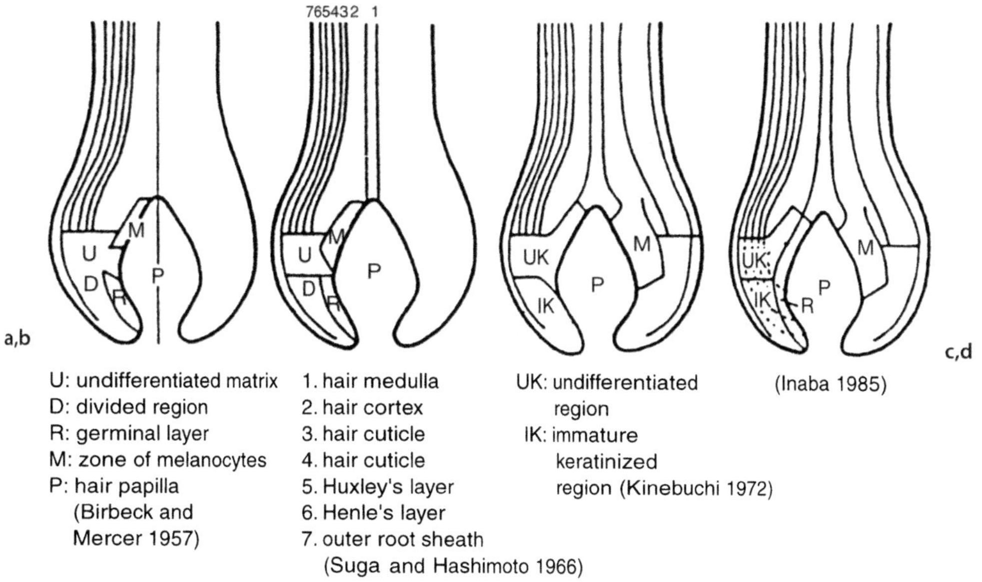

Fig. 14.12a–d. Various schematics of the hair matrix

These results confirm earlier autoradiographic studies (Van Scott et al. 1963).

Our observations suggest that the inner root sheath and the keratinized fiber (the hair) are formed independently from the epithelial cells (germinal layer) in the hair germ (Fig. 8.12). The germinal layer is restricted to the lower portion of the follicle in the hair peg stage; the hair cone (inner root sheath) and hair fiber are evidently formed from this germinal layer, and then continue to peg downward until formation of the hair bulb is complete (Fig. 14.10a,b).

It is also evident that the germinal layer surrounding the dermal papilla may be divided into six distinct regions: Henle's layer, Huxley's layer, sheath cuticula, hair cuticula, hair cortex and hair medulla (Figs. 8.12, 14.11a,b).

Further evidence supporting our own findings includes the observations of Epstein and Maibach (1969) in studies conducted with tritiated thymidine showing some mitotic activity in the epithelial cells surrounding dermal papilla.

14.4 Comparison of Epidermal and Follicular Cells

The processes that take place within the epidermis and the hair follicle may be, in order of occurrence, almost the same. The germinal layers of the outer root sheath of the follicle and epidermis are both continuous.

Skin and hair follicle germinative cells could be similar. Skin basal epidermal cell first extraction fluid (FEF) extracts contained a protein similar to that in the hair follicle, but in lower amounts (Moll et al. 1982, 1984).

Beneath the germinal layer, we find the papillary dermis in the dermis and the dermal papilla in the bulb. The keratohyalin granules which appear in the keratinization of epidermis are similar to the trichohyalin granules found in the inner root sheath.

Based on the authors' own findings, the development of the follicle occurs thus: the germinal layer becomes localized in the lower portion of the follicle above the mass of mesenchymal cells (future dermal papilla), and then generates the hair cone (future inner root sheath) and new young hair, even if the follicle is very small, in a manner quite similar to that of epidermal keratinization (Fig. 8.12).

As the differentiating cells stream upward from the bulb of an actively growing hair follicle, histochemical research has shown that the first cytoplasmic inclusions to develop are the trichohyalin granules in the cells of the inner root sheath and of the medulla, when it is present (Rogers 1983), including citruline—an arginine—rich precursor protein. However, the granules found in the inner root sheath show many differences from those in the medulla. Trichohyalin granules in the inner root sheath are replaced by long filaments. This occurrence led to the view that the granules were precursors of the filaments (Rogers and Roth 1967). Granules in the medulla cells are markedly different; the apparent filamentous transformation does not take place, with the granules aggregating into larger conglomerations as the cell dies.

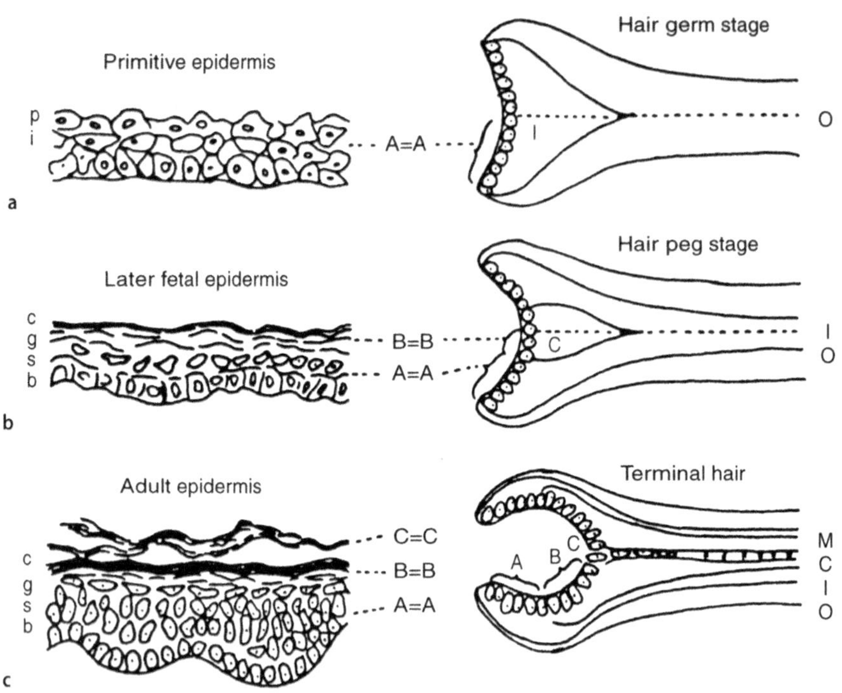

Fig. 14.13a–c. Comparison of epidermis and follicular cells. The processes that take place within the epidermis and the hair follicle may be almost the same. *p*, Periderm; *i*, intermediate layer; *c*, cornified layer; *g*, granular layer; *s*, spinous layer; *b*, basal layer; *O*, outer root sheath; *I*, inner root sheath; *C*, cortex; *M*, medulla

Ultrastructurally, the medulla appears amorphous after its partial cornification superior to the level of the insertion of the hair erector muscle. The loosely aggregated cells of the hair medulla contain melanosomes, empty vacuoles, citrulline-rich granules, and immature filaments embedded in an electron dense material.

The development of the hair cone (Fig. 14.13a) in the hair germ stage resembles the development of the primitive epidermis. The primitive epidermis, which consists of two layers, (periderm, intermediate layer), is called the periderm. Beneath the periderm, basal keratinocytes constitute the only layer of the epidermis as such. In the 2nd fetal month, the progeny of basal cells form the first intermediate layer. Once the granular layer is established in the 6th month, the intermediate cells become known as spinous cells (Holbrook 1983). The first cornified layer is seen at the end of the second trimester. At first it consists of only a few cell layers, but it increases in thickness during the third trimester (fetal epidermis) and, at birth, is approximately as thick as the adult cornified layer.

Considered in comparison to the development of the epidermis, the hair cone may be said to correspond to the state of the primitive epidermis. The new young hair inside the hair cone may be said to correspond to the cornification that takes place in the epidermis (Fig. 14.13b). The differentiation of cells at the tip of the dermal papilla gives rise to a few columns of cells, consisting of vacuolar structures of various sizes and of tonofibrils in irregular arrangement to the level of the attachment of the hair erector muscle (Moretti 1965) (Fig. 14.13c). However, this type of medulla is not characteristic of all human hairs. In fact, the me-

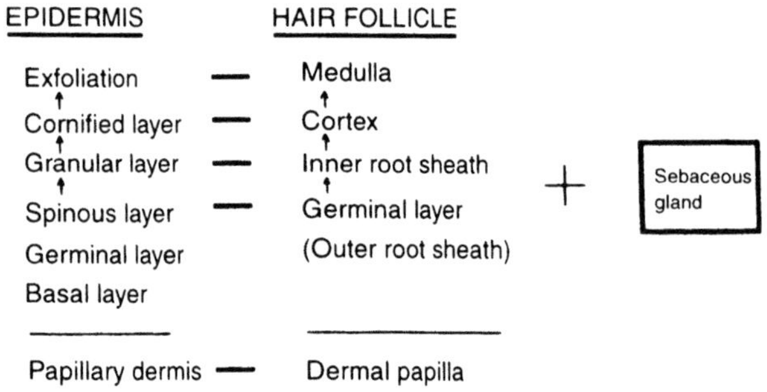

Fig. 14.14. Comparison of keratinization of epidermis and hair follicle. Keratinization in the epidermis and hair follicle is quite similar. The sebaceous gland, present only in conjunction with the follicle, seems requisite to the process of keratinization which produces a new hair. Differences in the keratinization process between the hair and the epidermis seem to depend on whether the sebaceous gland is present

dulla is not visible in fetal and vellus hair and becomes more marked with age. This finding can be explained in terms of the keratinization process being quite similar to the corneal exfoliation occurring in the epidermis. Although human hairs are differentiated and keratinized as already described, the authors suggest that the difference in the keratinization process between the hair and the epidermis seems to depend on whether the sebaceous gland is present and functioning normally (Fig. 14.14). It is increasingly clear, in light of histological findings, that the sebaceous gland is closely involved in the process of follicular keratinization.

14.5 Why the Growth (Anagen) Stage and Regressive (Catagen) Stage Are Confused

Hair follicles in the early anagen and telogen stages can seem quite similar, although close observation does, of course, reveal very significant differences.

In the past, however, many investigators of the outer root sheath have mistaken one of these stages for the other, causing confusion as to exactly what does occur in each of these stages. Much of this confusion has been due to the universal reliance on thin tissue preparations which do not reveal differences between the two stages in sufficient detail to clearly distinguish one from the other.

In thick tissue preparations these differences are immediately evident. First of all, in the anagen follicle, mitotic activity is vigorous in the surrounding dermal layer; moreover, the follicle has a distinctive multilobular form similar to that of a bell pepper (Figs. 14.15a, 14.16).

A fiber-like structure is formed when the filamentous structure formed from the lower germinal layer is compressed by keratinization of Henle's layer within the formed inner root sheath, with cells arranged vertically in palisade shape to form fiber-like structures which appear strikingly "stem-like" (Figs. 14.15b, 14.17A). The upper portion of the fiber-like structure has already become cortex. At first glance, the picture is similar to the telogen stage because it suggests the keratinized rootlets seen in the hair club in telogen (Fig. 14.17B). The cortex of the hair root shows no melanin granules at all in this stage. A mass of mesenchymal tissue (future dermal papilla) is seen at the lower pole but it is not wrapped in hair bulb manner (Fig. 14.17A).

a

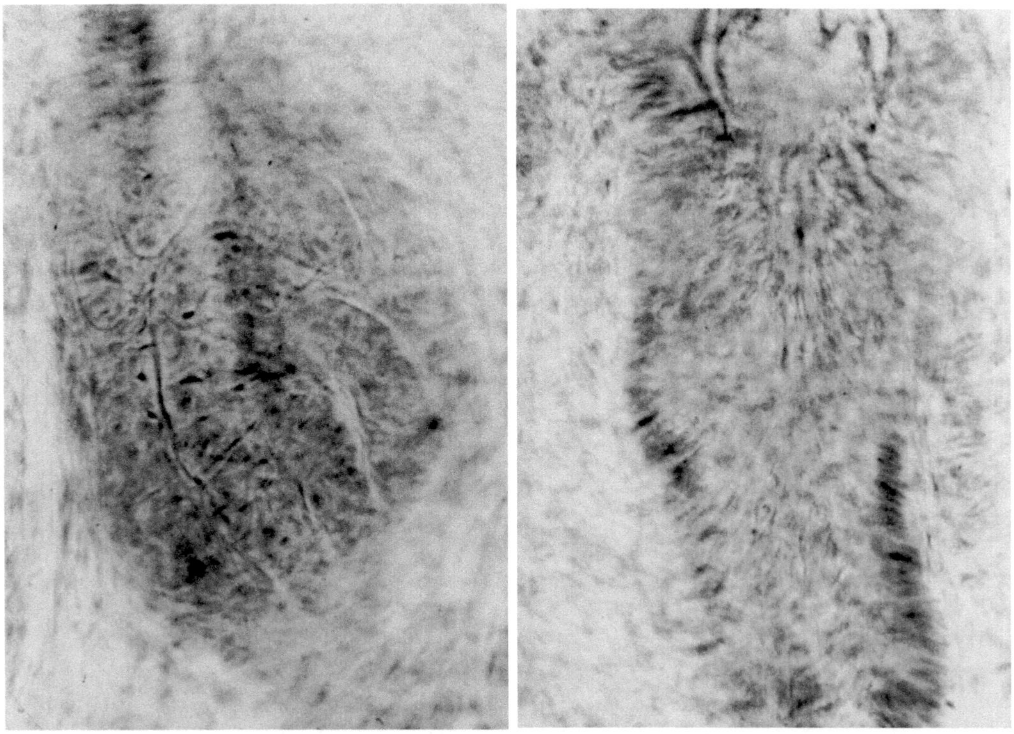

b

Fig. 14.15. a Early anagen hair follicle shows multilobular configuration. Cross section is starfish-like. ×400 **b** Filamentous structures formed from the lower germinal layer are aggregated to form the fiber. This configuration is not club hair, but is stem-like. ×400

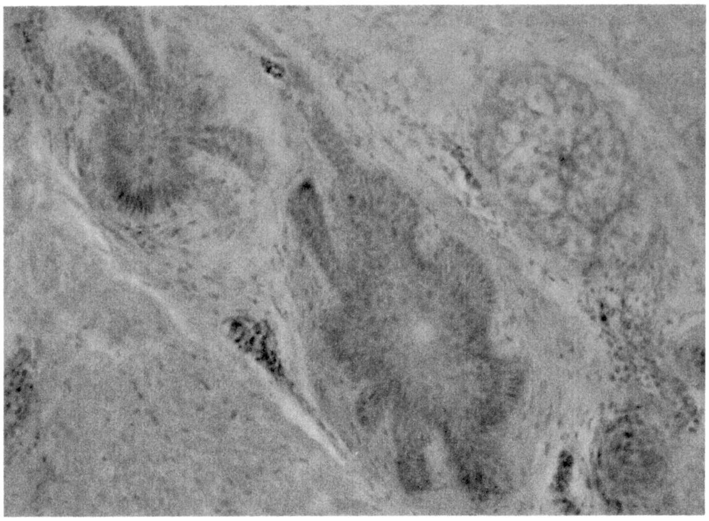

Fig. 14.16. The lower portion of early anagen hair follicle is like a starfish in cross section. ×135

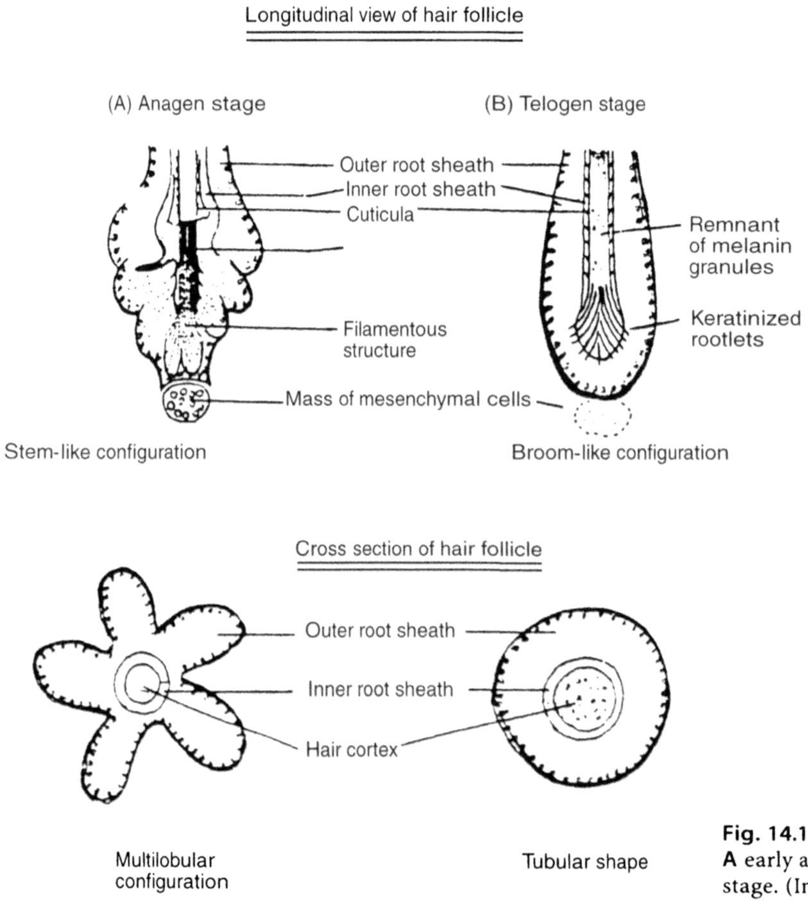

Fig. 14.17A,B. Comparison of **A** early anagen and **B** telogen stage. (Inaba, 1985)

In contrast, the follicle in catagen stage lacks the multilobular starfish-like configuration and instead has a simple tubular shape, the lower part of which is notched because of atrophy (Fig. 14.17). When the lower portion of the follicle collapses, its epithelial sector becomes like an attenuated cord, while the mesodermal sector (glassy membrane) is wrinkled in thick folds. The hair itself is foreshortened and the bottom of the hair root, progressively surrounded by keratinous rootlets (keratinizing trichilemma) (Pinkus 1969), is called a club hair. This hair root, at its bottom, takes on a brush-like or broom-like shape. Melanin granules are still clearly visible in the cortex of the hair root, so that the root preserves some vestige of pigmentation.

Finally, in the telogen stage, the follicle becomes about one-half to one-third the length of the anagen follicle. The dermal papilla, which is reduced to a ball of cells located immediately below the capsule of the telogen follicle, becomes atrophied. Because this distinction between early anagen and telogen stages has not been clearly observed in the past, the false conclusion was drawn that the hair could be formed only from the matrix in the hair bulb.

Inaba and Inaba (1990b), as noted earlier, have suggested that follicular stem cells are sited at the outer root sheath of the duct opening of the sebaceous gland (sebaceous isthmus). If the subcutaneous tissue is removed only up to, and not including the sebaceous gland, axillary hair regenerates because the upper isthmal portion and the secretory duct opening of the sebaceous gland of the follicle are left intact. In contrast, if the upper isthmal portion of the hair follicle and the sebaceous gland are removed, no regeneration occurs (see Section 8.1). We therefore asserted that the hair cycle should be classified into four stages rather than the conventional three: anagen, catagen, telogen, and isthmal (essential hair cycle) (Fig. 7.1) (Section 13.2). At the same time, we confirmed that regeneration also occurred from the hair germ at the lower end of the telogen follicle (secondary hair germ) or from the remnant of the dermal papilla; thus, there are two patterns of hair cycles, common and essential (Inaba and Inaba 1990b, 1992a).

To sum up, the assertion made by Oliver (1966a) that the center of regeneration is sited at the lower third of the follicle simply cannot be subsumed under the same concept of the common hair cycle proposed by Dry (1926) and Montagna (1962). Moreover, neither Dry nor Montagna suggested that the hair center was located at the upper isthmal portion close to the secretory duct opening of the sebaceous gland (sebaceous isthmal portion) as asserted by Inaba et al. (1979a).

14.5.1 Mammalian Vibrissal Hair

We feel that it is rather odd that recent studies on hair have been influenced by such studies as Oliver's on vibrissa (1966–1990), since vibrissa have characteristics different from those of body hair. Was the rat vibrissa chosen as the subject of study because it is thicker than the body hair? It seems that a great many papers have been read on rat vibrissa and that it has become a dominant influence at present. It is questionable whether this special sensory organ, namely, vibrissa, can be utilized in an experiment to observe hair generation and regeneration. At any rate, it is unquestionable that the mesenchymal cells play a very important part in hair formation. However, it remains to be seen whether, in this mesenchymal-epithelial interrelation in hair formation, the mesenchymal cells congregate, as induced by the hair germ, or whether the hair germ is differentiated from the mesenchymal cells by some still unknown function (Kobayashi 1987).

The outer root sheath has been reported to show the development of mesenchymal cells (Section 1.5.2). The mesenchymal cells are not necessarily needed in the generation and regeneration of the hair follicle, but a new hair germ (epithelial tissue) generates from the crowding of nuclei in the epidermis and a new bud regenerates from the upper isthmal portion close to the duct opening of the sebaceous gland (sebaceous isthmus), as proposed by the authors in their sebaceous gland hypothesis, calling the theory set forth by Montagna (1962) and Oliver (1970) into question.

14.5.2 Structure of Vibrissal Hair

Mammalian vibrissae serve as a tactile sense organ. On the upper lip, the major vibrissal follicles are arranged in a constant pattern of dorsoventrally and anteroposteriorly aligned rows; a vertical row of four large follicles alternates with five horizontal rows, in which the follicles vary in number. In rows 1 and 2 on the upper lip, there are always four large follicles, and there are five in row 3. There are always at least six and eight follicles, graded in size, in rows 4 and 5, respectively. A variable number of vibrissal follicles is interspersed among those of the pelage at the anterior end of rows 4 and 5 (Danforth 1925; Davidson and Hardy 1952).

However, the vibrissal follicle is different from the pelage (body) hair follicle (Fig. 14.18a–e). The epithelial follicle of the vibrissa is surrounded by connective tissue connected to the dermal papilla and also by the huge upper and lower blood sinus located inside the connective tissue. Further, another feature distinguishing the vibrissal follicle from the pelage hair follicle is that the vibrissal follicle is again enveloped by an outermost thick sheath of connective tissue and receives abundant trigeminal neurofibers, ending at the pacinian corpuscle. A thick connective tissue capsule surrounds these hairs, enclosing a blood sinus around the hair follicle. The upper part of the blood sinus is called the ring sinus (ring Wulst) and there are no internal partitions in this part of the sinus. The

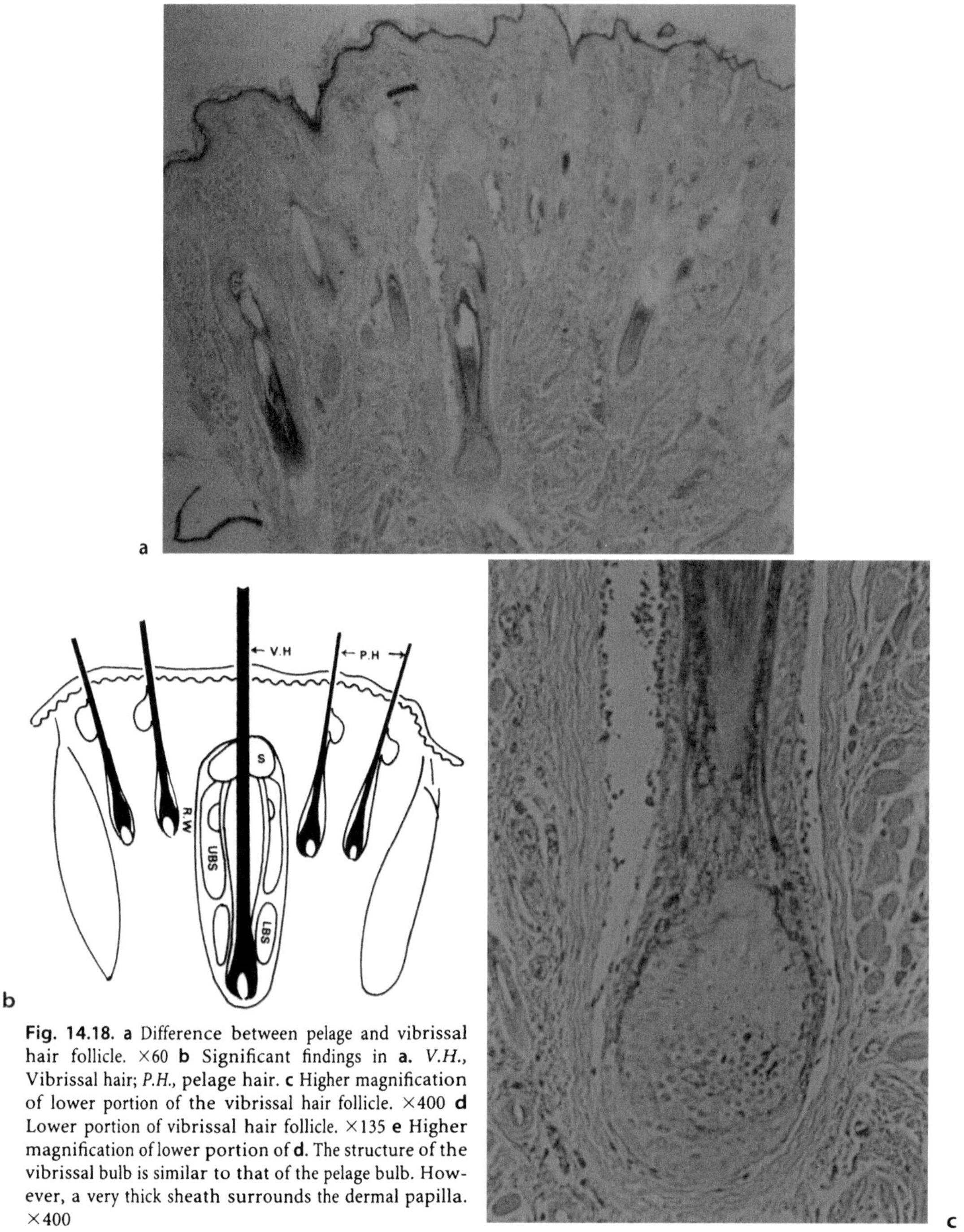

Fig. 14.18. **a** Difference between pelage and vibrissal hair follicle. ×60 **b** Significant findings in **a.** *V.H.*, Vibrissal hair; *P.H.*, pelage hair. **c** Higher magnification of lower portion of the vibrissal hair follicle. ×400 **d** Lower portion of vibrissal hair follicle. ×135 **e** Higher magnification of lower portion of **d.** The structure of the vibrissal bulb is similar to that of the pelage bulb. However, a very thick sheath surrounds the dermal papilla. ×400

lower part of the blood sinus is divided into chambers and is called the cavernous sinus (Halata 1990).

14.5.3 Differences Between Mammalian Vibrissal Hair and Pelage (Body) Hair

Pelage hair follicles are long and thin, and of rather uniform diameter. The vibrissal follicles which produce longer and thicker hair are themselves larger and stouter, and, due to two thickenings of the outer root sheath, have an hourglass shape. The outer root sheath consists of a single outer layer of basal cells, together with three or four more layers of epidermal cells. At the level of the sebaceous gland, the vibrissa is anchored by the most distal cell of the inner root sheath. The dermal sheath of connective tissue surrounding

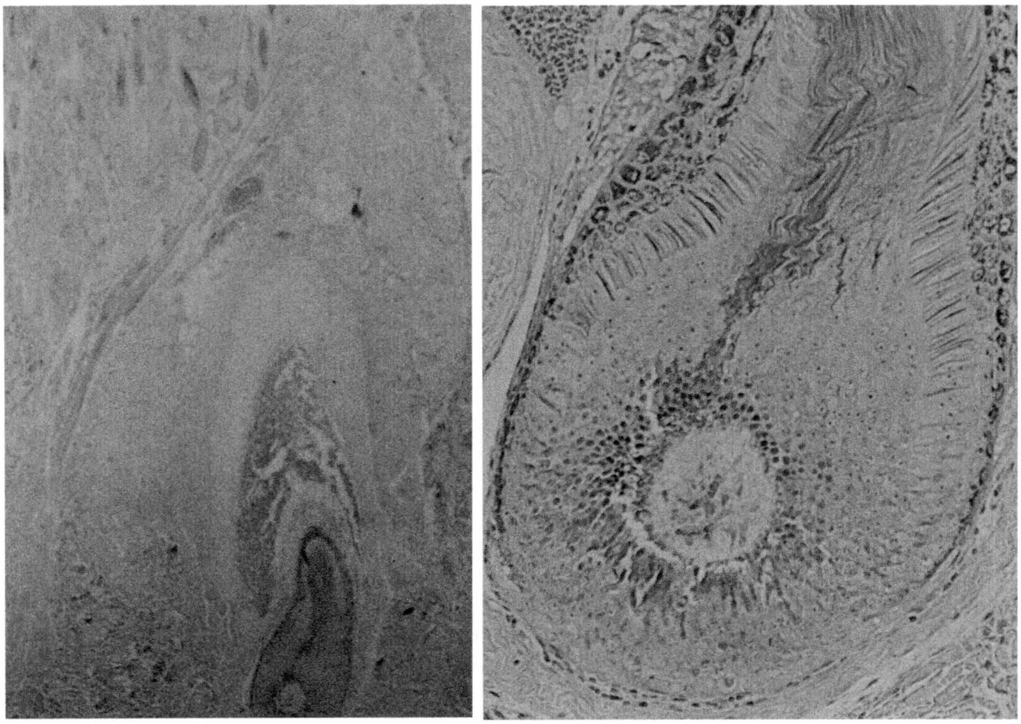

Fig. 14.18. *Continued*

the pelage hair follicle is insignificant, but a very thick sheath surrounds the vibrissal follicle (Fig. 14.18d,e). Within this sheath lie the blood sinuses, which are characteristic of all tactile hair follicles, but are absent from pelage hair follicles. The cavity of the more superficial upper or ring sinus contains the Ringwult, which is attached to the dermal sheath adjacent to the follicle wall, forms a collar surrounding the follicle, and is penetrated by nerve branches and blood capillaries (reviewed from Davidson and Hardy 1952).

According to Yohro (1985, 1988), the vibrissa around the mouth is a sensory organ, receiving approximately 100 neurofibers and containing several sensory nerve ends. The neurofiber leading to the vibrissa is a dendrite which elongates from the nerve cell in the trigeminal ganglion toward the periphery. Another dendrite extends to the center from the same nerve cell and ends at the trigeminus sensory nucleus in the medulla. This dendrite further ascends to the thalamus and then to the fourth layer of the cortex in the brain, around the end of which the neurofibrillae gather to form a cortical barrel (Woolsey and Van der Loos 1970; Weller 1972; Johnson 1977).

The configuration of this barrel corresponds exactly with that of the vibrissa around the mouth. Morphological and functional relationships between sinus hairs and cortical barrels have been documented in mice (Woolsey and Van der Loos 1970; Killackey et al. 1976) and in rats (Killackey et al. 1976). The barrel structure is formed after birth; it is lost if the vibrissal hair is destroyed within 3 days after birth. However, it is not lost if the hair is destroyed on or after the 5th day after birth. If excessive vibrissal hair is generated, formation of barrel structure will correspond to it. A clear correspondence has been established between the arrangement of sinus hairs and that of barrels (Yamakado and Yohro 1979).

Vibrissae are found only in mammals. They are usually sited at the place where the dermal branch of the trigeminal nerve first reaches the skin. As stated above, the hair follicle structure is different from that of pelage (body) hairs. Multiple neurofibrillae are distributed over the hair root. The vibrissa differs from common hair in that it has a large blood sinus in the hair root. These hairs communicate their motion directly to nerves and indirectly through pressure on blood-filled sacs (blood sinus) around the follicles (Fig. 14.19).

Embryologically, the vibrissa is generated as a result of the interrelational action between the epithelial cells and the neuroblast, which forms the mesenchyma of the vibrissa (neural crest-related mesenchyme). In contrast, pelage hair is formed as a result of the interrelational action between the mesenchyma of the mesoblast and the epithelial cells (Fig. 14.20). It is presumed that the

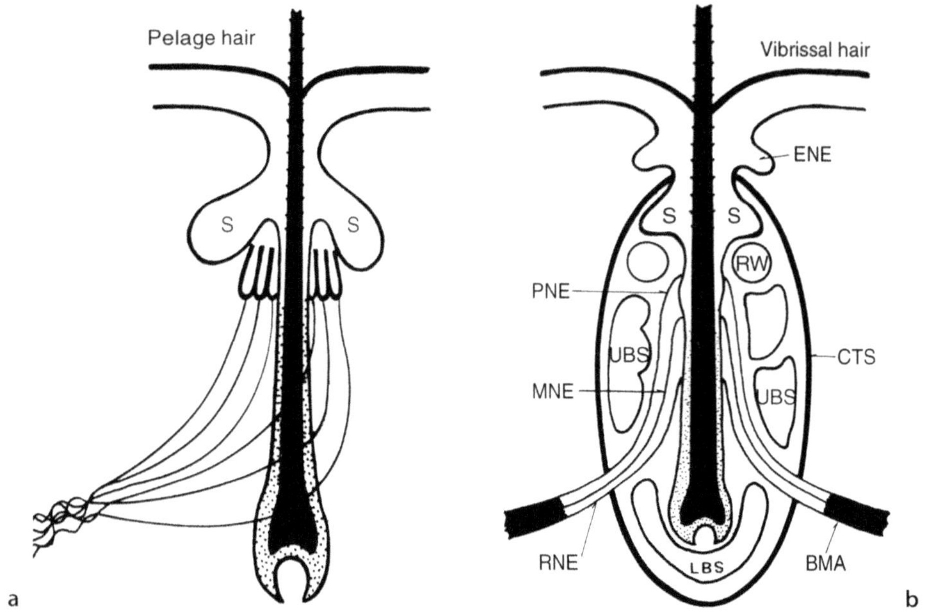

Fig. 14.19a,b. Difference between pelage and vibrissal hair follicles. **a** Guard or pelage hair (Montagna and Parakkal 1974) showing the arrangement of nerve end-organs around the hair follicle. The upper parts of these nerves often branch into plump packed terminals like the tines of a fork (Montagna and Giacometti 1969). **b** Sinus hair (Halata 1990). A thick connective tissue capsule surrounds the hair, enclosing a blood sinus around the hair follicle. The upper part of the blood sinus is called the ring sinus. The lower part of the blood sinus is divided into small chambers and is called the cavernous sinus. *BMA*, Bundle of myelinated axons; *CTS*, connective tissue sheath; *ENE*, epithelial nerve endings; *LBS*, lower blood sinus; *MNE*, merkel nerve endings; *PNE*, perifollicular nerve endings; *RNE*, Ruffini nerve endings; *RW*, ring wulst (sinus); *S*, sebaceous gland; *UBS*, upper blood sinus

Vibrissa	Pelage Hairs
↑	↑
Epithelium	Epithelium
↑ ↓	↑ ↓
Neural Crest-related Mesenchyme	Mesoblast-related Mesenchyme
↑	↑
Lateral-line Organic System	Scale

Fig. 14.20. Generation of vibrissal and pelage hairs (from Yohro 1969, 1988, with permission)

mesenchyma induces the formation of epithelium (Pisansarakit and Moore 1986; Yohro 1988). This hypothesis is illustrated in Fig. 14.20 (Yohro 1988).

As can be seen from the above description, there is a fundamental difference between vibrissal and pelage (body) hairs both from the anatomical and functional standpoints. A number of reports have addressed the mesenchymal-epithelial interaction in vibrissal hair; however, it still remains to be seen whether vibrissal hair can be placed in the same category as pelage hairs such as the scalp hair.

Hormones Classified According to Secretory Organ of Origin

15

Hormones are classified according to the secretory organ of origin:

a. Gonadal (steroid) (sex hormones and adrenal cortical hormones)
   Male
   Female
   Adrenocortical
b. Adrenal cortical (steroid)
c. Non-steroid
d. Adrenomedullary
e. Thyroid
f. Pituitary
g. Others

The male and female hormones, adrenocortical hormone, and thyroid hormone have a direct relationship with the hair follicle and the sebaceous gland.

15.1 Male Hormones

Testosterone is an androgen, and is considered the principal testicular hormone produced in human males. It is a steroid hormone produced by the interstitial Leydig cells, and it is also normally produced by the adrenal cortex in both men and women. It can be prepared synthetically by conversion of other steroids, most notably cholesterol.

In women, the adrenal and ovarian steroids, 4-androstenedione and dehydroepiandrosterone, are the most abundant circulating proandrogens. A prohormone is a 19-carbon steroid that arrives at the target tissue and is converted to the active hormone.

Testosterone is necessary for the normal development of the wolffian duct system and its derivatives, namely the epididymis, vas deferens, and seminal vesicles.

Testosterone enhances the growth of the tissues it affects, and also acts to stimulate blood flow. As a stimulant and promoter of the development of secondary sexual characteristics, it is essential for normal sexual development, function, and behavior, including the growth of the phallus and scrotum and penile erection. It plays a major role in the normal growth and development of the male accessory sex organs, and is responsible for deepening the male voice between puberty and adulthood, male muscular development, the appearance of beard and pubic hair, and adult male fat distribution. Testosterone also affects many other metabolic activities.

15.1.1 Hormonal Control of the Skin

Figure 15.1 shows the major possible androgenic steroid pathways in the skin. The gonadotropins facilitate the synthesis of certain enzymes in the human body which catalyze various steps of steroidal biosynthesis.

Testosterone can be formed in the testes, ovaries, and adrenal cortex. In women, testosterone is produced in the adrenal glands and ovaries. Normal males have testosterone levels ten times higher than those found in normal women (Montagna and Parakkal 1974).

Human skin is an important site for the biotransformation and metabolism of androgens. Androgenic steroids can be metabolized in the skin, as shown in Fig. 15.1.

Testosterone (T) secreted by the testis is the principal androgen circulating in the plasma in men, whereas in women, the adrenal and ovarian steroids, 4-androstenedione and dehydroepiandrosterone (DHEA or DHA), are the most abundant circulating proandrogens. Proandrogens have the potential to enzymatically convert pri-

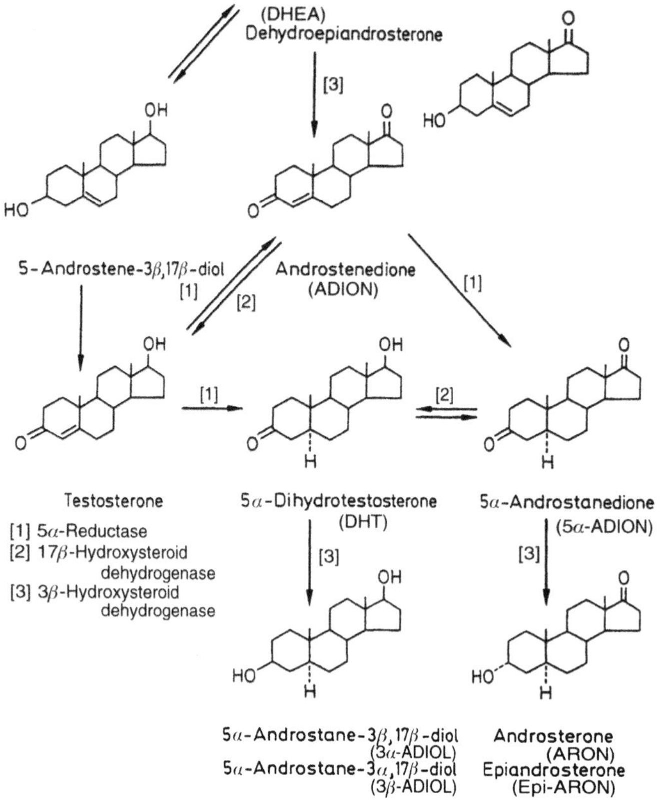

Fig. 15.1. Possible pathways for androgen metabolism in the skin (modified from Ebling 1990)

mary adrenal androgen DHEA to dehydroepiandrosterone, then to T, and then to 5α-dihydrotestosterone (DHT). We agree with the published report of Ebling and Hale (1983) that pretestosterone androgens contribute significantly to total androgenization in women, especially in the second and third decades of life when dehydroepiandrosterone and its sulfate are at their highest lifetime levels.

Androstenedione (ADION), androsterone (ARON), and epiandrosterone (Epi-ARON) are formed from testosterone (Wotiz 1956). Many researchers have studied the pathways of androgenic steroids. Cameron et al. (1966) have shown that testosterone and androstenedione are formed from DHEA in human cutaneous tissue. Gallegos and Berliner (1967) also showed that androstenedione, testosterone, and DHEA sulfate were all formed from DHEA incubated with human male skin in vitro.

In a series of studies by Hsia et al. (1965), human skin was shown to possess Δ4-5α-steroid reductase activity for testosterone and Δ4-andostenedione. Further studies in rat skin showed that 17β-hydroxysteroid dehydrogenase activity was also present in cutaneous microsomes (Davis et al. 1972). Eppenburger and Hsia (1972) were able to show the presence of binding protein in skin cytosol for testosterone, dihydrotestosterone, estradiol-17β, and progesterone.

Wilson and Walker (1969) showed that there were differences in 5α-reductase in various body areas. Regional differences in 5α-reductase activity in the skin may play a role in the expression of secondary sex characteristics. In the syndrome of testicular feminization, there is a deficiency of 5α-reductase activity in the skin (Mauvais-Jarvis et al. 1970). A deficiency in 5α-reductase, which results in diminished formation of DHT in the genital tissue of the embryo, can lead to male pseudohermaphroditism (Walsh et al. 1974; Peterson et al. 1977). There is evidence for an androgen receptor in the cytosol of human skin (Bonne et al. 1977) (see Section 15.1.9 of this chapter). Stewart et al. (1977) investigated the in vitro metabolism of testosterone by the scalp and back skin of human subjects. A major metabolite identified from both sites was 5α-androstane-3-β,17β-diol.

Hay and Hodgins (1978) studied the distribution of androgen-metabolizing enzymes in human skin. They found 17β-, 3β-, and 3-α hydroxysteroid dehydrogenase; 3-β-hydroxysteroid dehydrogenase Δ4-5 isomerase; and 3α- and 3β-ketoreductases in human skin; the 3α- and 3β- ketoreductases converted 5α-DHT into 3α-

and 3β-diols, respectively. Farthing et al. (1982) found that facial hair growth was correlated with plasma DHT but not with plasma testosterone concentration.

Puerto and Mallol (1990) reported that when 17β-hydroxysteroid oxoreductase was measured using either testosterone or DHT as substrate, levels of androstenedione formed from T were higher in hairy skin than in areas of alopecia. Levels of androstenedeione formed from DHT were also higher in areas not showing alopecia.

According to Itami et al. (1991a), human plucked hair follicles, containing predominantly follicular epithelial cells, can metabolize testosterone to DHT, which is biologically the most potent androgen (Fazekas and Lanthier 1971; Takayasu and Adachi 1972a; Schweikert and Wilson 1974a). DHT, however, is not necessarily a major metabolite of testosterone in the hair follicle. Besides, the activity of 5α-reductase in plucked hair follicles does not appear to correlate with androgen-mediated hair growth (Takayasu and Adachi 1972a; Schweikert and Wilson 1974a). Dermal papilla cells, which are a mesenchymal component of the hair bulb, are considered to play a fundamental role in the induction of epithelial differentiation (Oliver 1967b; Jahoda et al. 1984).

15.1.2 Hormonal Control of Sebaceous Gland Function

Androgens are the major stimulators of the sebaceous glands and are probably responsible for the development and enlargement of the glands that occurs at puberty.

Hamilton (1951a) was the first to report a definite relationship between sebaceous gland development and androgen activity in humans. He observed that skin oiliness and acne appeared in male castrates who had been treated with testosterone, and concluded that androgen was the principal factor behind the sebaceous gland activity responsible for those particular skin conditions.

The effects of androgen have also been reported in animal studies. For example, testosterone increased the size of the sebaceous glands in immature female rats (Ebling 1948) and methyl testosterone stimulated sebum secretion in prepubertal male rats, and the sebaceous glands became markedly enlarged (Strauss and Kligman 1961). These findings have been reconfirmed by many subsequent researchers.

Human sebaceous glands appear to be responsive to androgens other than testosterone. Human castrates secrete only half the amount of sebum compared to that in normal males, but they produce much more than prepubertal male children (Pochi et al. 1962). It appears that sebaceous gland activity in castrates is dependent on adrenal rather than on testicular androgens, which they lack.

This feature of sebaceous gland activity may also occur in women, since it has been reported that both ovarian androgen activity and sebum secretion in post-menopausal females decrease markedly after the age of 50 (Pochi et al. 1962; Pochi and Strauss 1974) (Fig. 6.3).

Topical application of testosterone under carefully controlled clinical conditions can promote enlargement of sebaceous glands at the application site (Strauss et al. 1962). Both DHEA and ADION have been found to stimulate sebum secretion in estrogen-suppressed test subjects, even though androsterone was shown to be ineffective (Pochi et al. 1963).

Several androgens may also be active in maintaining sebaceous gland activity, as observed in animal experiments conducted by Ebling et al. (1971). DHEA is closely related to the secretion of sebum (De Peretti and Forest 1976).

According to Caballero et al. (1990) and Puerto and Mallol (1990), there is a specific binding protein for 3β-androstanediol (βD10L) in the sebaceous glands of the alopecia-seborrhoeic scalp. It is possible that βD10L, but not DHT, could be the specific active metabolite of testosterone in the sebaceous gland and that androgen-transforming enzymes are involved in the etiopathogenesis of male pattern baldness.

It has been shown that testosterone and 5α-DHT significantly stimulated the proliferation of human facial sebocytes in a dose-dependent manner; 5α-DHT exhibited the strongest effect. The proliferation of non-facial sebocytes, in contrast, was inhibited by testosterone, whereas 5α-DHT enhanced their growth. However, the stimulatory effect of 5α-DHT was more prominent on facial than on non-facial sebocytes. The effects of testosterone and 5α-DHT on the proliferation of cultured human sebocytes may depend on the localization of the sebaceous glands in different skin regions (Akamatsu et al. 1992).

15.1.3 Androgen Response to Pilosebaceous Unit

15.1.3.1 Mechanism of Response to Androgen Stimulation

The same androgenic stimulus enhances growth and differentiation to terminal hair in certain target areas such as the axilla, mons pubis, and beard, and causes regression from terminal to vellus hair in the frontal, temporal, and crown regions of the scalp in genetically susceptible individuals. To explain such phenomena, the target end-organ, i.e., the pilosebaceous unit, needs to be studied.

Testosterone is considered the most active androgen. However, a number of research studies have indicated that DHT, a testosterone metabolite, rather than testosterone itself, may be the active androgen agent in various target tissues.

DHT is considered to be the major effector hormone in certain androgen-responsive tissues, particularly in the pilosebaceous unit of skin (Hay and Hodgins 1974; Sansone-Bazzano et al. 1972; Kuttenn et al. 1977).

Of the various testosterone metabolites, 5α-DHT is the most potent; it is about four times more active than testosterone (Dorfman and Dorfman 1962). In another study, Bruchovsky and Wilson (1968) found that the predominant androgen in the prostate gland was not testosterone, but dihydrotestosterone, which is formed in the prostate.

Anderson and Fulton (1973), as well as others, have shown that receptors in cells will specifically retain dihydrotestosterone but not testosterone. Adachi and Kano (1970) have found that the binding of dihydrotestosterone to specific receptor proteins is a critical factor in mediating the effects of androgens. These findings suggest that the stimulating action of androgen is due to its activation of specific RNA and protein synthesis.

Lucky (1988) and Schweikert and Wilson (1974a) studied the metabolism of labeled testosterone and androstenedione in individual hair roots from balding and hairy scalp areas and, in general, found higher levels of 5α-DHT-reduced metabolites and 17-ketosteroid metabolites in balding men. It has been reported (Gomez and Hsia 1968; Hay and Hodgins 1973) that, in the hair follicles of patients with androgenetic alopecia, the activation of both 5α-reductase and 17β-hydroxysteroid dehydrogenase (HSD) is high. However, it was not made clear whether these changes were primary or secondary to the balding process. These studies have examined androgen metabolism in skin homogenates, but only a little work has been done in studying isolated hair follicles or sebocytes, comparing androgen metabolism in different anatomic locations or physiologic states.

Sawaya et al. (1988a) have shown that the enzyme 3β-hydroxysteroid dehydrogenase (3β-HSD), which converts DHEA to Δ^4-androstenedione (Ad), as well as converting androstenedione to testosterone (T), has greater activity in balding than in hairy scalp samples. They added the precursor androgen [^{3}H]DHEA to isolated sebocytes and measured the amounts of the more potent androgenic metabolites, [^{3}H]androgen (A) and [^{3}H]T, which were then produced. Lucky (1988) found that this dichotomy of activity was mirrored in the specific 3β-HSD activity of the cytosolic fraction of sebocyte homogenates. Oddly, although the microsomal fraction possessed the highest specific activity of 3β-HSD, there was no difference between hairy and balding scalp. In previous studies comparing acne-prone and acne-free skin (Hay and Hodgins 1974), it was never firmly established whether increased androgen metabolic activity was simply due to the presence of a greater number of sebocytes or whether the sebocytes had higher specific activity.

Sawaya et al. (1988b) have also emphasized that sebocytes are perfectly capable of metabolizing the so-called "weak" androgen, DHEA, to much more potent metabolites such as T. DHEA itself is a product primarily of the adrenal gland and its effect has often been disregarded clinically because it is intrinsically such a weak androgen. The finding that the skin can convert DHEA to T has been documented before (Hay and Hodgins 1978; Milne 1969; Sansone-Bazzano and Reisner 1974). However, these studies confirming the capacity of human scalp skin to metabolize DHEA to other potent metabolites and showing differences between balding and hairy skin should make us more aware of the potential role that elevated or even high-normal range amounts of circulating DHEA may play in balding.

It is well established that there are androgen receptors in sebocytes (Adachi 1974; Lucky et al. 1985); however, it has been much more difficult to firmly localize such receptors and/or enzymatic systems in the hair follicle.

There are virtually no data localizing androgen receptors or enzyme systems to specific cell types within the hair follicle (Lucky 1988).

15.1.3.2 Mechanism of Testosterone Conversion to Dihydrotestosterone (DHT) (Fig. 15.2)

In a study by Price (1975), it was found that free testosterone, or androstenedione, entered a peripheral target cell and was reduced to dihydrotestosterone by 5α-reductase. Reduced nicotinamide adenine dinucleotide phosphate (NADPH) was also present as an essential cofactor.

Hsia et al. (1965) have shown that human skin exhibits 5α-reductase activity for testosterone and DHEA. This enzymatic activity was localized in the 100 000 ×g pellet (microsomal fraction).

This reductive activity seems to occur on the nuclear membrane. The newly-produced DHT is then bound to a specific high-affinity receptor pro-

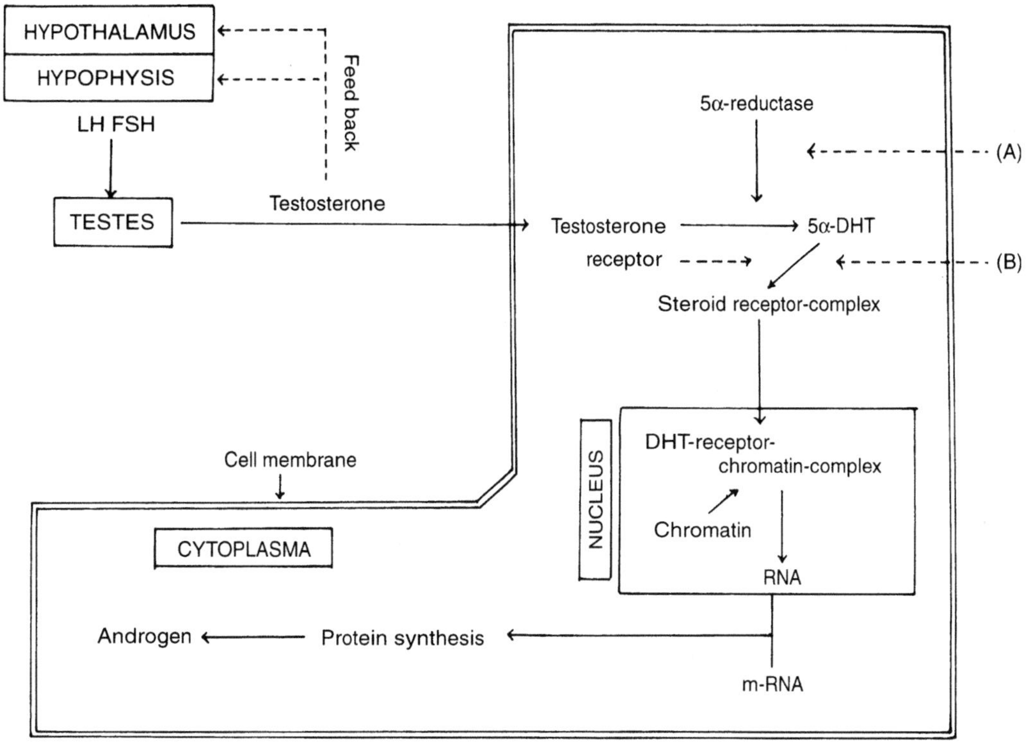

Fig. 15.2. Mechanism of androgen action. (*A*), Point of inhibition by antiandrogens which inhibit 5α-reductase; (*B*), point of inhibition by antiandrogens which block receptors. *LH*, Luteinizing hormone; *FSH*, follicle-stimulating hormone; *DHT*, dihydrotestosterone

tein that carries DHT into the cell nucleus. There it is bound to chromatin and stimulates the transcription or translation of stored genetic information (Fig. 15.2).

In normal men and women, 5α-DHT can be further metabolized by certain target cells. In the liver, this can occur by conversion of 5α-DHT from androstanediol, which is excreted in the urine.

It is quite possible, on the basis of studies made thus far, that the androgen-dependent conditions of acne vulgaris, male pattern baldness, and idiopathic hirsutism may all result from increased 5α-reductase activity in the androgen target cells of the skin, leading to a local increase in the rate of 5α-DHT formation. The bald scalp has a greater capacity than the non-bald scalp to convert testosterone to 5α-DHT in vitro (Bingham and Shaw 1973).

Takayasu and Adachi (1972a) reported that 5α-reductase activity was greater in anagen than in telogen follicles. However, according to Schweikert and Wilson (1974a) and Takayasu et al. (1980), no difference in 5α-reductase activity was observed between the frontal region which was likely to become bald, and the occipital region which was not. Also, no high level of activation was observed in the beard, chest, or pubic hair follicles, all of which are related to sexual maturity. In other words, there was no significant correlation between male hormone levels and 5α-reductase activity in hair growth, i.e., this activity was not male hormone-dependent. Also, 5α-reductase activity in beard, chest, and pubic hair follicles was considerably lower than this activity in male hormone-dependent tissues, such as the sebaceous gland or the apocrine gland.

Dissection studies of freeze-dried skin specimens have shown that 5α-reductase activity is concentrated mostly in the sebaceous and apocrine sweat glands, while 5α-reductase activity in the hair follicle was significantly lower. Identified metabolites were DHT, 5α-androstane-3β, 17β-diol, and 5α-androstanedione (Takayasu et al. 1980).

As mentioned above, testosterone is a male hormone that is likely to be metabolized to Δ^4-androstenedione, which is less affected by DHT than 17β-HSD. This indicates that the epithelial cells of the hair follicle are not a target tissue in terms of male hormone metabolism (Takayasu et al. 1980).

Since 5α-reduction is irreversible and oxidation at carbon 17 is favored, androstenedione (ADION) was found to be the principal intracellular androgen in human hair roots.

However, Hay and Hodgins (1978) stressed the significance of the 17-oxysteroids (DHEA, androsterone, etc.) as androgenic compounds and have questioned the importance of DHT, which has secondary significance in sexual development.

Caballero et al. (1990) demonstrated the absence of a specific DHT receptor in scalp biopsies of bald subjects.

15.1.4 Levels of Steroid Metabolic Enzymes Related to Male Pattern Baldness

According to Sawaya (1991), the enzymes in the steroid metabolic pathway are Δ-5,3β-hydroxysteroid dehydrogenase (3β-HSD), 17β-hydroxysteroid dehydrogenase (17β-HSD), and 5α-reductase (5α-R); these convert weak androgens such as DHEA and androstenedione (AD) to T and DHT, whereas aromatase (A enzyme) converts T to estrogens, namely estradiol. 3α-Hydroxysteroid dehydrogenase (3α-HSD) converts DHT to a less active androgenic metabolite that is less potent than DHT, called 3α-androstanediol (AL). AL also has an affinity for the androgen receptor protein (ARP) and can stimulate androgen actions similar to those seen with T. The conversion of androgens by these enzymes is dependent on the oxidized-reduced pyridine cofactors in the outer root sheath, i.e., nicotinamide-adenine dinucleotide (NAD), reduced NAD (NADH), and NADPH.

The A enzyme (cytochrome P-450 aromatase enzyme) converts androgens such as androstenedione and testosterone to estrone and estradiol (Ryan 1982; Sawaya et al. 1990). Sawaya et al. (1990) suggested that females with androgenetic alopecia (AGA) had more than twofold the levels of 5α-reductase in the frontal hair follicle than in the occipital hair follicle. However, less than half the amount of the enzyme found in females with AGA was found in men with AGA. In men with AGA, levels of 5α-reductase in the frontal hair follicle are almost twofold those in the occipital hair follicle, with minimal A enzyme. Females may have sparing of the frontal hairline due to increased A enzyme, limiting the formation of 5α-reduced substrates that may bind to the androgen receptor protein to initiate androgenic cellular events. The elevated 5α-reductase and low A enzyme levels seen in men with AGA may be due to the formation of reduced products which decrease the amount of available substrate for A enzyme utilization.

15.1.5 Is Dihydrotestosterone Only a Stimulator?

It seems rather paradoxical that in most cases of stimulated growth, androgen acts to stimulate such growth, but in the cases of androgenic alopecia, androgen acts to suppress the growth process. This results in the progressive shrinkage of predisposed hair follicles. It is not clear why androgen should have these disparate polar effects on hair follicles in specific instances of hirsutism and male pattern baldness.

Adachi et al. (1970) reported circumstantial evidence that human scalp hair follicles have the capability to produce 5α-DHT in vitro. They also reported that 5α-DHT (but not T) markedly inhibited adrenal cyclase activity in the normal terminal hair follicle.

This inhibitory effect tends to decrease the intracellular concentration of cyclic adenosine monophosphate (c-AMP) (Butcher et al. 1968). In turn, this decrease has varied effects on the various pathways of energy metabolism. One of these effects is a decrease in the glycolytic rate, which is mediated by phosphofructokinase inhibition. It is quite likely that this decrease could result in inhibition of the normal rate of hair growth by limiting the energy supply.

The low c-AMP level found in affected hair follicles may cause a fall in efficacious protein (enzyme) synthesis by inhibiting the release of protein from polysomes, and so forth.

Adachi et al. (1970) and Adachi (1973) proposed that the main action of DHT in hair follicles may be as a rate-limiting factor for the adenylcyclase system.

15.1.6 Testosterone Metabolism in the Pilosebaceous Apparatus, Especially the Difference Between the Upper Portion and the Lower Portion of the Isolated Hair Follicle

To study the testosterone metabolism in the pilosebaceous apparatus, Choi et al. (1990a) used a single hair collected from the occipital area in an experiment. In this experiment, we divided the single hair into two fractions, the hair-bulb portion, and the isthmal portion, with the sebaceous gland. The metabolism of testosterone was determined in two fractions of isolated hair follicle. The samples were incubated with ^{3}[H]testosterone and an NADPH-generating system. The testosterone metabolites were separated by thin-layer chromatography on silica gel, and counted in a Packard 300c liquid scintillation spectrometer.

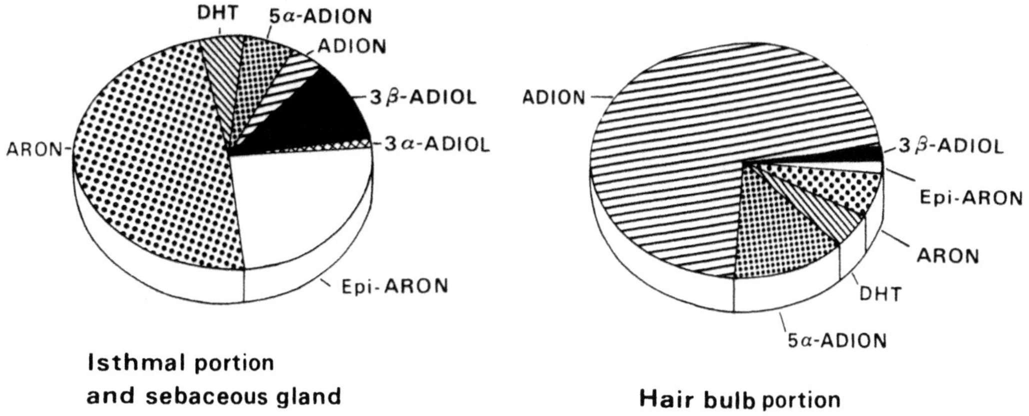

Fig. 15.3. Testosterone metabolism

As shown in Fig. 15.3, ADION, formed by the enzyme 17β-hydroxysteroid dehydrogenase from testosterone, was the major metabolite in the hair bulb portion, followed by 5α-ADION (5α-androstenedione), ARON (androsterone), and DHT. ARON is the metabolite of 5α-ADION. Epi-ARON and 3,β-ADIOL were observed in much smaller amounts. In the sample of the isthmal portion and sebaceous gland, the predominant metabolites were ARON, Epi-ARON ADION, 5α-ADION, and 3β-ADIOL. There was no difference between the two samples regarding the amount of DHT.

Schweikert and Wilson (1974a) found that isolated hair roots produced mainly ADION. This ADION is biologically inactive in the hair follicle (Bruchovsky and Wilson 1968). Stewart et al. (1977) found 5α-androstane-3β-17β-diol (3β-ADIOL) to be the major metabolite when they incubated skin from the back or scalp with [^{3}H]testosterone.

In our experiment (Choi et al. 1990a), a far greater amount of ARON and 3β-ADIOL was observed in the sample of the isthmal portion and the sebaceous gland than in that of the hair bulb. This was probably due to the presence of the sebaceous gland, in which 5α-reductase is produced in large amounts, resulting in the rapid formation of DHT and the greater amount of ARON and 3β-ADIOL conversion.

15.1.7 Effects of Azelaic Acid on 5α-Reductase

Azelaic acid is a naturally occurring, straight-chained saturated dicarboxylic acid (1.7-heptane-dicarboxylic acid). It is a competitive inhibitor of

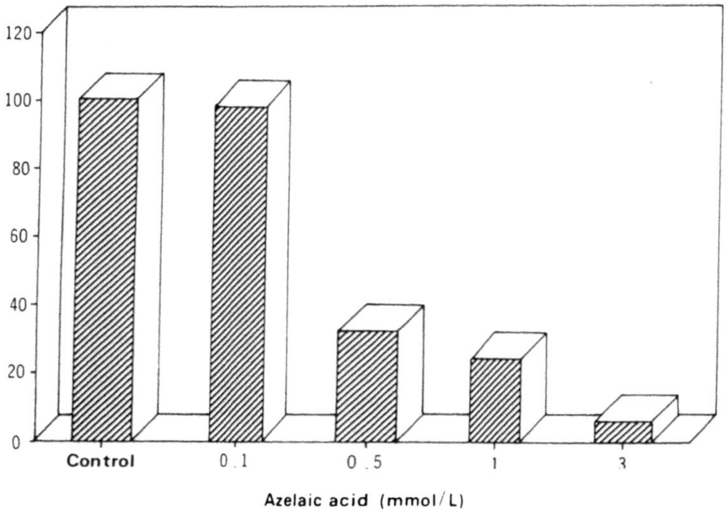

Fig. 15.4. Effect of azelaic acid on 5α-reductase activity

tyrosinase in vitro (Nazzaro-Porro and Passi 1978). While treating cases of chloasma with topical application of a 15% azelaic acid cream, Nazzaro-Porro et al. (1983) observed that acne lesions within the areas being treated showed significant improvement. They also examined the effect of azelaic acid on 5α-reductase activity in sebaceous glands, and found that azelaic acid was a potent inhibitor of 5α-reductase (Fig. 15.4). Dicarboxylic acids containing 8–13 carbon atoms under β-oxidation have been shown to be potent inhibitors of oxydoreductases. It has been proposed that azelaic acid could competitively occupy the NADPH-binding site of 5α-reductase, thus resulting in inhibition of the enzyme (Breathnach et al. 1984). Topical application of azelaic acid has been reported to have beneficial effects on acne vulgaris (Nazzaro-Porro et al. 1983). As mentioned above, 5α-reductase activity in the sebaceous gland may possibly be inhibited by the application of azelaic acid in future treatment of male pattern baldness.

15.1.8 Androgen Receptors in Human Skin and in the Pilosebaceous Unit

Classic endocrinology focused on the isolation and characterization of hormones and on the control of their synthesis, secretion, and catabolism. More recently, attention has turned to the way in which hormones affect target tissues, especially those tissues that control the response to the hormones that essentially bathe all organs. It is now believed that hormones act by combining with specific protein receptors either within cells or on their surfaces, and that this interaction changes the workings of the whole cell thereby causing hormonally induced cellular alterations (reviewed in Epstein 1983).

Androgens cause beard growth, the development of male pattern baldness, enlargement of the sebaceous glands, and increased sebum production. It is also known that androgens are metabolized in the skin. Dehydroepiandrosterone is converted to T, and T is rapidly converted to the biologically active androgen—DHT—by 5α-reductase (Wilson and Walker 1969). The action of T and DHT is mediated by an androgen-receptor protein, the presence of which has been demonstrated in skin cytosol (Bonne et al. 1977; Michel 1979; Mowszowicz et al. 1982) and in skin fibroblasts derived from various anatomic sites in both male and female subjects (Marrs and Voorhees 1971; Jensen et al. 1976; Aiman and Griffin 1982; Kaufman et al. 1982).

In skin cytosol, as well as the androgen-binding receptor, another binding protein, testosterone-estradiol binding globulin (TeBG), has also been found (Powell et al. 1971; Mowszowicz et al. 1981); TeBG binds to androgens with an affinity similar to that of the androgen-binding receptor, and a higher capacity.

Sex hormone binding-globulin (SHBG) is thought to reduce the tissue availabity of hormones such as testosterone. SHBG binding is required for steroid hormones to bind their tissue receptors. SHBG values were found to be significantly lower in Japanese men than in American white and black populations (Siiteri and Simberg 1986).

Both T and DHT bind to the androgen receptor, DHT showing higher affinity for the receptor than T. Other sex hormones, such as estrogen and progesterone, also bind to androgen receptors, although with much lower affinity than is the case with T and DHT (reviewed from Ponec 1987).

Hair growth and sebum production are known to be androgen regulated. The androgen dependency of sebaceous glands has been studied in model systems of the hamster flank organ (Giegel et al. 1971; Takayasu and Adachi 1972b; Takayasu 1978) and the rat preputial gland (Sherins and Bardin 1971).

Androgen receptors have been detected by ligand-binding assays in cultured skin fibroblasts (Griffin et al. 1976; Herfert et al. 1980) and skin cytosol (Mowszowicz et al. 1981; Razel et al. 1985). Although skin fibroblast cultures have proven to be excellent models for the study of androgen receptor concentration and function both in normal skin and in various androgen-dependent disorders, no direct evidence of androgen receptors in other types of skin, e.g., testicular feminization (Brown and Migeon 1981), has been published.

However, it has become possible to isolate cells from rodent and human papillae and to grow them in culture (Jahoda and Oliver 1981; Messenger et al. 1986), providing an opportunity to examine hair growth regulation in great detail. Katsuoka et al. (1986) have suggested that androgen receptors are present in papilla cells and that DHT in culture media enhances both DNA and protein synthesis. The dermal papilla cells contain androgen receptors, and thus may represent a promising target for androgen-mediated hair growth regulation (Arai et al. 1990).

Katsuoka (1991) also reported that androgen receptors were present in cultured papilla cells (PCs) and that these PCs had keratinocyte-chemotactic factors. The elucidation of human androgen receptor structure (Chang et al. 1988; Trapman et al. 1988) and the concomitant development of specific anti-androgen receptor antibodies (Lubahn et al. 1988; Trapman et al. 1988; Liang et al. 1993; Diani and Mills 1994) have made it possible to develop immunohistochemical methods for the localization of androgen receptors in target tissues. Blauer et al. (1991) reported the histochemical localization of these receptors in the nuclei of prostatic cells, and in their dermatological investigation, found that in nongenital skin, androgen receptors were also expressed in the nuclei of basal cells and glandular cells of sebaceous glands, in the outer root sheath of the hair follicle, and in eccrine sweat glands. The method they used was based on a polyclonal anti-androgen receptor antibody directed against the human androgen receptor (Lubahn et al. 1988; Trapman et al. 1988; Chang et al. 1989).

It is well established that there are androgen receptors in sebocytes (Adachi 1974; Lucky et al. 1985); however, it has been much more difficult to firmly localize such receptors and/or enzymatic systems in the hair follicle. There are virtually no findings localizing androgen receptors or enzyme systems to specific cell types within the hair follicle (Lucky 1988).

Sawaya et al. (1988a,b) observed that, in male pattern baldness, androgen receptors were increased in the sebaceous glands of the frontal region.

Randall et al. (1993) reported that specific saturable androgen receptors were present in all human papilla cells examined, with higher levels being noted in cells from androgen-dependent follicles, for instance, in the beard, than in control nonbalding scalp cells.

15.1.9 Deficiencies of Body Hair

According to Ebling and Hale (1983a), absence or sparsity of sexual hair occurs in forms of pseudohermaphroditism in genetic males in which either the androgen receptor or the enzyme 5α-reductase is lacking or deficient. 5α-Reductase is essential for male differentiation in embryogenesis and for some, though not all, responses to androgen in the adult. Three conditions in which there are defects in androgen receptor or 5α-reductase have been defined:

(1) Complete Testicular Feminization. In this disorder, there is a complete absence of androgen receptors (Keenan et al. 1974; Griffin and Wilson 1977). In consequence, the phenotype is feminine at birth and remains so. Pubic hair is completely absent in the adult, even though the plasma testosterone is two to four times the normal level. 5α-Reductase is lacking in areas of skin such as the pubic region, where it is androgen dependent (Mauvais-Jarvis et al. 1976), but is present in regions where it is independent of androgens, e.g., the perineum.

(2) Type I Incomplete Pseudohermaphroditism (F1MP, Type I). This condition, which is inherited through a recessive gene on the X chromosome, involves a partial deficiency of the androgen receptor (Griffin and Wilson 1977; Andersson et al. 1989). The phenotype is variable, and virilization is incomplete. There is some pubic and other body hair. The activity of 5α-reductase is normal in the perineal region but reduced in the pubic region.

(3) Type II Incomplete Pseudohermaphroditism. (F1MP, Type II). This condition, which is transmitted through an autosomal recessive gene, involves a deficiency in 5α-reductase (Walsh et al. 1974; Moore and Wilson 1976; Peterson et al. 1977; Kuttenn et al. 1979; Andersson et al. 1989). The subjects are generally feminine at birth, but partial virilization occurs at puberty. Although the plasma testosterone in the adult is normal or even slightly elevated, the sexual hair remains sparse and the prostate does not develop at all.

It appears that muscle development and the breaking of the voice are dependent on testosterone, without any requirement for 5α-reductase. On the other hand, the growth of facial hair, in common with development of the prostate, is dependent on 5α-dihydrotestosterone. Since subjects with 5α-reductase deficiency do not suffer from seborrhea or acne, it seems likely that enhanced sebaceous activity in the acne-prone areas similarly requires 5α-reductase, although if this were the case, it would not establish that sebaceous activity in general is dependent on 5α-reduction (reviewed from Ebling and Hale 1983a).

According to Itami (1993) 5α-reductase activity has a narrow optimum pH in close proximity to pH 5.5, and it decreases between pH 6 and 9.0. This can be observed only in pubic fibroblast cells (Type II 5α-reductase).

Contrary to this, in the male hormone-independent dermal papilla cells in the occipital area, no sharp highs and lows of 5α-reductase activity are observed (Type I 5α-reductase). Also, in both sexes, the level of 5α-reductase in the dermal papilla cells of axillary hairs that grow after adolescence is almost equal to that in the occipital area. In testicular feminization, no male hormone receptor is present, and therefore no androgenization phenomena, as shown in Table 15.1, can be observed. In F1MP II, androgenization of various degrees is recognized. Conspicuous phenomena of masculization, such as the growth of beard or chest hair and the male pattern type of hair loss, is not observed in either of these deficiencies, which finding indicates that both the male hormone receptor and type II 5α-reductase

Table 15.1. Characteristics of skin in patients with androgen deficiencies

	Testicular feminization (receptor deficiency)	FIMP, type I (partial receptor deficiency)	FIMP, type II (5α-reductase deficiency)
Axillary hair Pubic hair	–	+	+
Acne vulgaris	–	–	±
Androgenetic alopecia	–	–	–
Beard Chest hair	–	–	–

FIMP, Familial incomplete pseudohermaphroditism. (From Itami 1993, with permission)

are indispensable for the growth of axillary and pubic hairs (reviewed from Itami 1993).

15.2 Estrogens

The estrogens have a number of important effects on uterine development and on the cyclic endometrial changes associated with ovulation. Estrogens are also said to be responsible for secondary female sex characteristics. They are bound and retained in their target organs by combining with a specific macromolecule, the estrogen receptor.

High concentrations of estrogen-binding protein have been observed in the uterus, vagina, and mammary glands. The receptor is in the cytosol fraction of target cells.

In human males, the testes produce both testosterone and estradiol, but the actual amount of estradiol produced is only about 1/13 the amount of testosterone.

Androstenedione is converted directly to estrone; alternatively it may form testosterone which, in turn, is converted to estradiol. It has been found that low concentrations of 17β-estradiol were ineffective, while higher doses (180 μm) of 17-estradiol were effective in increasing the rate of growth of all skin cell types, especially of papilla cells compared with dermal fibroblasts (Kiesewetter 1992).

Estrogens definitely suppress human sebum secretion (Strauss et al. 1962; Strauss and Pochi 1963). The question remains whether the effect is physiological or pharmacological, and whether estrogens play any role in the normal control of sebum secretion.

Extensive studies have been directed at the effect of estrogen on various skin tissue components. Estrogens have been found to suppress sebaceous gland activity and hair growth (Bullough and Laurence 1960; Ebling 1973; Stumpf et al. 1974). They can interact with cytoplasmic protein target tissues and translocate into the nucleus. There they bind to acceptor sites in the chromatin to induce gene expression and set off a sequence of events leading to altered cell function (Eppenburger and Hsia 1972; Ebling 1973; Jensen and De Sombre 1972; Stumpf et al. 1974).

Jarret (1955) seems to have found the first clear indication that estrogen administration can reduce sebum secretion in both men and women. It has been shown that large, unphysiological amounts of estrogens inhibit sebaceous gland secretion in both humans and animals (Strauss and Pochi 1963; Ebling 1973; Pochi and Strauss 1974).

Contrary to the evidence in animals, estrogen in humans does not inhibit androgenic stimulation at the sebaceous gland itself, but rather reduces circulating levels of androgens. Whereas androgens stimulate both mitosis and lipogenesis, estrogen primarily inhibits lipogenesis. Ebling (1974) also demonstrated that antiandrogens not only inhibit lipogenesis but also markedly reduce cell mitoses. Ebling and Skinner (1967) have reported that topically applied estradiol inhibits sebaceous gland activity in intact male rats.

The topical application of estrogens has been less effective than systemic administration in inhibiting sebum secretion. Ethinylestradiol topically applied to the forehead reduced sebum secretion in normal males. However, the concentration required to obtain that effect in a hydrophilic ointment was 1% or more, enough to produce feminization due to systemic absorption. Topical estrogens are ineffective unless applied in doses high enough to achieve pharmacological systemic levels. They then work through a systemic mechanism, increasing androgen-binding globulin and reducing gonadotropins and total testosterone production. They do not work through direct local action on the hair follicle.

Furthermore, their action does not occur at the peripheral level (Strauss et al. 1962). Strauss and Pochi (1963) have suggested that the systemic action could arise from the suppression of gonadotropin and the reduction of endogenous androgen levels.

It is now possible to detect the presence of extremely small quantities of estrogen receptor, by using a radioisotope (Hasselquist et al. 1980; Press and Green 1984). Various authors (Mowszowicz et al. 1982; Hasselquist et al. 1980; Punnonen et al. 1980) have reported the presence of estrogen receptors in the cytosol of whole skin; however, the estrogen receptor levels were very low. The highest levels were found in the face, and the lowest in the breast and thigh (Mowszowicz et al. 1982). The receptors showed high affinity and high specificity for estrogen and diethylstilbestrol. No correlation was observed between estrogen-receptor levels in the skin and serum estradiol or progesterone levels during the normal menstrual cycle, suggesting that the cellular estrogen receptor level is not regulated by plasma levels of estrogen and progesterone (Punnonen et al. 1980).

15.3 Progesterone

Progesterone, which is produced and secreted by the corpus luteum, a small yellow body that develops in the ruptured ovarian follicle, can also be prepared synthetically. It is responsible for the changes that occur in the uterine endometrium in the latter half of the menstrual cycle. Its effects on the vaginal epithelium and on cervical mucous secretions are quite the opposite of those of estrogen.

Physiological doses of progesterone do not seem to have any effect on human sebaceous secretion, although, under some conditions, large doses may produce an observable response. The reported effects of certain synthetic progesterones on the sebaceous gland may be attributed to androgenic activity (Strauss and Kligman 1961).

Ebling (1948) was unable to confirm any increase in sebum secretion unless extremely high doses of progesterone (10 mg/day) were used. Even then, the increase in gland size was small, and there was no change in sebum secretion.

The cutaneous metabolites of progesterone have been shown to be 5α-derivatives. These findings are similar to those obtained with testosterone and suggest that cutaneous microsomal 5α-reductase can metabolize both testosterone and progesterone (Sulzberger and Witten 1952).

Progesterone receptors have been found in cytosol fractions of whole skin, and variations in their level with anatomical site have been observed. For instance, the highest progesterone level has been found in the cytosol of skin from the breast, followed by that from the retroauricular area, with the lowest level being found in the pubic skin (Mowszowicz et al. 1982).

Our study (Inaba et al. 1988b) showed that the distribution of receptors for progesterone was the same as that for estrogen receptors.

15.4 Distribution of Estrogen and Progesterone Receptors in Scalp Tissue

The authors (1988b) and Chung (1994, personal communication) investigated the distribution of estrogen and progesterone receptors in relation to scalp region, age, and sex as one means of observing receptor distribution.

15.4.1 Method of Measurement

Approximately 1 g of dermal tissue was obtained from biopsy dermal tissue specimens taken from the frontal, temporal, parietal, and occipital scalp regions of patients who had undergone operations for traumatic injuries to the head.

In order to observe the distribution of estrogen and progesterone according to the patients' age and sex, five males and five females in their twenties, thirties, forties, fifties, and sixties were selected.

Reagents used in the investigation were [2.4.6.7.-3H(N)]-estradiol [3H(E); 99 ci/mmol]; [17a-methyl-3H]-promegestone (3H-R5020; 86.9 ci/mmol); diethylstilbestrol (DES); cortisol; dihydrotestosterone (DHT), Norit A charcoal (activated powder), Dextran T-70, ethylene diaminetetraacetic acid (EDTA), dithiothreitol (DTT), and bovine serum albumin.

All procedures were conducted at temperatures between 0°C and 4°C. The materials used were stored at a temperature of −70°C prior to measurement. After fatty tissue was removed from the scalp specimen, the specimen was cut into pieces measuring approximately 1 mm; these pieces were then placed in a buffer (buffer A). The formula for buffer A was 10 m*M* Tris-HCl, 1.5 m*M* EDTA in H_2. The buffer solution contained 10 m*M* Tris-HC1. 1.5 m*M* EDTA pH 7.4. DTT was dissolved in this solution to a final concentration of 1 m*M* per 1.6 ml of solution, and this was then refined for 5 s with an Ultra-turrax homogenizer (Polytron PT10ST "OD" S Knematica, Lucerne, Switzerland). This process was repeated three times at 45-s intervals.

This fine tissue solution of 1000 × g was centrifuged lightly and the supernatant solution of 60 000 × g removed was centrifuged for 60 min with an ultra-high-speed centrifugal separator (Beckman L8-70, Palo Alto, CA, USA). The supernatant solution produced is lipid-free Cytosol. The solution was then adjusted with buffer A to a concentration of 2–3 mg/ml of protein suitable for receptor measurement.

15.4.2 Measurement of Estrogen Receptors

For measurement of estrogen receptors, three types of solutions were prepared: 50 μl 8 n*M* ^{3}H-Estradiol (8 n*M* $^3H[E_2]$) was added to 200 μl Cytosol solution for a total binding. One hundred times the amount of $^3H[E_2]$ concentration of diethylstilbestrol (DES) was added to the above-mentioned solution for a nonspecific binding. Lastly, 50 μl of $^3H[E_2]$ and 200 μl buffer solution were mixed for a total counting. (However, no Cytosol was contained in the total count.) These solutions were reacted for 16–18 h at a temperature of 4°C. When the reaction was completed, 400 μl of DCC (Dextran-coated charcoal) (0.5 g Norit A charcoal, 50 mg Dextran T-70 in buffer A) was added to the total binding and nonspecific binding. The solutions were then left for 30 min at a temperature of 4°C so that the isolated hormone could be adsorbed to the charcoal.

The isolated hormone thus adsorbed to charcoal was then centrifuged and its supernatant of 500 μl was mixed with 10 ml of scintillation cocktail, a mixture of PPO (2,5-diphenyloxazole) 5.5 gm, dimethyl-POPOP (1,4-bis [5-phenyl-2-oxazolyl]-benzene; 2,2-p-phenylene-bis 5-phenyloxazole) 0.5 g, and Triton X-100 300 ml with toluene 667 ml. The radioactivity in the solution was measured with a liquid scintillation counter (Packard, CA, USA).

The density of the estrogen receptor was calculated by dividing the specific binding, i.e., the total binding minus the nonspecific by the total count (Total binding − nonspecific binding/Total counting = Density of estrogen receptor).

The unit used to express the receptor density was the amount of protein, which was femtomoles per milligram of Cytosol protein (fmol/mg Cytosol). When the amount of estrogen exceeded 5 fmol/mg Cytosol protein, it was expressed as estrogen receptor positive (Lowry et al. 1951).

15.4.3 Measurement of Progesterone Receptors

Fifty microliters of 16 n*M* [^{3}H]R5020 was added to 200 μl of Cytosol solution (the same solution used in the estrogen receptor) for a total binding to prepare the Cytosol solution. Fifty microliters of solution containing 26.7% 16 n*M* [^{3}H]R5020, 1.34 *M* Cortisol, 133 n*M* DHT, and 534 n*M* R5020 was added to buffer A solution for a nonspecific binding. Then 200 μl of buffer A solution was added to 50 μl of 16 n*M* [^{3}H]R5020 for a total count. The solution was treated as had been done for the estrogen receptor to determine progesterone receptor positive and negative.

15.4.4 Results

The distribution of estrogen and progesterone receptors in five men and five women according to age and scalp region is shown in Table 15.2. In the case of a 15-year-old female, the estrogen receptor (ER) level in the frontal region was 1.30 fmol/mg protein and the progesterone receptor (PR) level was 1.42 fmol/mg protein; temporal parietal ER was 0.58 and PR was 0.15 fmol/mg, while the occipital region ER was 0.20 and PR was 0.10 fmol/mg.

There was no significant difference in the measured amounts of ER and PR in the 29-, 44-, 55-, and 66-year-old women and in the 15-year-old girl. In the case of a 21-year-old man, the amounts were: ER 0.54 and PR 0.36 fmol/mg protein in the

Table 15.2. Distributions of estrogen receptors (*ER*) and progesterone receptors (*PR*) in human scalp

Case no.	Age (years)	Sex	Site of biopsy: Frontal	Temporal parietal	Occipital
			ER and PR (fmol/mg protein)		
1	15	♀	1.30 (1.42)	0.58 (0.15)	0.20 (0.10)
2	29	♀	0.79 (0.62)	0.32 (0.21)	0.20 (0.00)
3	44	♀	1.24 (0.72)	9.24 (0.11)	0.00 (0.00)
4	55	♀	0.16 (0.12)	0.42 (0.20)	0.45 (0.20)
5	66	♀	0.22 (0.10)	0.78 (0.25)	0.62 (0.32)
6	21	♂	0.54 (0.36)	1.20 (1.76)	1.26 (0.36)
7	33	♂	0.82 (0.78)	0.72 (0.21)	0.85 (0.23)
8	46	♂	0.10 (0.00)	0.22 (0.10)	0.12 (0.45)
9	58	♂	0.75 (0.25)	0.72 (0.22)	0.70 (0.22)
10	62	♂	1.22 (0.20)	0.71 (0.48)	0.78 (0.32)

Numbers in parentheses indicate distribution of PR.

frontal region, ER 1.20 and PR 1.76 fmol/mg in the temporal and parietal regions, and ER 1.26 fmol/mg PR 0.36 fmol/mg in the occipital region. Again, there was no significant difference in the amounts in terms of age differences and dermal tissue. As a result of our study, we found that extremely small numbers of estrogen- and progesterone-positive cells were distributed in scalp tissue.

Studies of the distribution of estrogen and progesterone in human dermal tissue rarely have been conducted in the past. Because the skin is formed by hard protein, chemical analysis was extremely difficult in terms of its contact or interaction with exterior elements, the differences in regions, and, especially, its fibrous nature.

During the extraction of the particular type of protein, steroid hormone receptor, dealt with in this study, the protein is degraded by the heat produced during the process of tissue destruction, making it difficult to confirm its existence.

Since the late 1970s, however, it has become possible to produce steroid hormones by radioisotope marking, and a technique has been developed to extract tissues and cells at comparatively low temperature. That development has played a very important role in the progress of studies in this particular field.

Hasselquist et al. (1980) observed the distribution of estrogen in human dermal tissue. They reported that higher quantities of estrogen were present in facial skin than in the breast area or the limbs, although the total amount was very small. They thus suggested that the facial region was more affected by sex hormone than other regions. Studies on the effects of sex hormone on the generation and growth of scalp hair have shown remarkable progress. As scalp hair generation, i.e., the relation between MPB and male hormone, began to attract attention, the antagonizing female hormone (estrogen) was used for the purpose of preventing hair loss.

However, recent chemical analysis has revealed that the hormone bound with the steroid receptor in cell substance is transmitted into the nucleus, and affects the nucleic acid, causing the enzyme system to change.

Therefore, to fulfill the purpose of formulating a local remedy for the prevention of hair loss by applying female hormone on the skin surface in order to antagonize the male hormone, further biochemical analysis and study are deemed necessary.

In our study described in this chapter, we found extremely small quantities of estrogen and progesterone in the scalp, regardless of age and sex, and no regional difference was observed.

Further studies will compare differences between regions where coarse hair persists and regions where no coarse hair is observed, along with further research on the male hormone receptor.

For observation of the distribution of estrogen and progesterone receptors in human scalp tissue, we biopsied dermal tissue from each scalp region in five males and five females of different ages, extracted estrogen and progesterone receptors in the protoplasm, and then measured them by the radioisotope method.

Comparatively small amounts of these receptors were found in the scalp irrespective of age.

15.5 Adrenal Steroid Hormones

The adrenal gland is a triangular body that is adjacent to and covers the superior surface of each kidney. The cortex secretes a group of hormones (collectively called adrenal cortical hormone) which can vary in both quantity and quality. The adrenal cortex plays a central role in the development of the hair pattern, particularly in women. All of these adrenal cortical hormones are synthesized from cholesterol; they are grouped according to their chemical structure and biological activity. The glucocorticoids (cortisol, corticosterone), for instance, act principally on carbohydrate metabolism, while the mineral corticoids (aldosterone, dehydroepiandrostenedione), the androgens (17-ketosteroids), the estrogens (estradiol), and the progestines (progesterone) are all of importance to the physiology of reproduction.

An adrenalectomy can result in a decrease in sebum secretion. On the other hand, DHEA and Δ^4-androstenedione, both of which are chiefly adrenal androgens, can act to increase sebaceous gland activity (Pochi and Strauss 1974).

Moreover, suprarenal hyperandrogenemia has been documented by elevated levels of dehydroepiandrosterone sulfate (DHEAS) in a small group of patients. Only limited information regarding hyperandrogenemia in male pattern baldness can be derived from the hitherto known data (Pitts 1987).

Prednisone, which has no detectable effect in normal men, can act to decrease sebum production in castrated men and, to an even greater degree, can do so in women (Pochi and Strauss 1967). In estrogen-treated, sebum-suppressed subjects, neither prednisone nor hydrocortisone, unlike testosterone, can overcome this inhibition, indicating that prednisone and hydrocortisone lack an androgen-like effect (Pochi et al. 1963). Also, hydrocortisone does not have significant effects on the sebaceous glands of children (Strauss and Kligman 1959). Replacement therapy with hydrocortisone in Addison's disease resulted in an increase in sebaceous gland secretion, suggesting that glucocorticoid functions in a permissive capacity for the action of androgen. This decrease is probably due to inhibition of adrenal androgens, because no direct effect of glucocorticosteroids has been discovered (Pochi et al. 1963).

15.6 Thyroid Hormone

Thyroid hormone activity stimulates follicular activity. Administration of thyroxine speeds up molting and inhibition of the thyroid slows it down (Ebling and Johnson 1964). Of great practical importance are hair symptoms connected with functional thyroid disorders (Church 1965; Saito et al. 1976; Sterry et al. 1980). Since the thyroid hormone influences the metabolism of almost all cells and determines the metabolic transformation of protein, carbohydrates, fats, and minerals, it is not surprising that metabolically active cell groups such as the hair matrix are affected by both a lack and an oversupply of this hormone. Thyroidectomy in rats and mice slightly reduces the growth rate of hair and retards anagen stage in resting hair follicles (Houssay et al. 1965). Freinkel and Freinkel (1972) studied the relative proportions of telogen to anagen hair in the scalps of hypothyroid subjects with hair loss and found that thyroid hormone deficiency was associated with an increase in the percentage of telogen hairs in all instances. After 8 weeks of treatment with thyroid hormone, the counts were restored to normal. Thyroidectomy in sheep reduces wool growth by 25%–45% but has no effect on the shaft diameter of wool fibers (Rougeot 1965; Thody and Shuster 1975). In the rat, thyroid hormone stimulates the sebaceous gland, whereas ablation of the thyroid decreases sebaceous glandular function (Ebling 1974; Shuster and Thody 1974). In contrast to stimulation of sebum production, thyoxine decreased the mitotic activity of the sebaceous glands in castrated rats receiving testosterone (Ebling 1974).

Thyroid hormones influence the hair growth and the duration of the hair cycle. DNA flow cytometry data (Kiesewetter 1992) revealed statistically significant differences between the peaks of S-phase and proliferation index (PI) values in hyperthyroidism: [S: 10.3%, PI (S + G2 + M): 18.3%] and hypothyroidism (S: 7.5%, PI: 13.9%). A correlation between peak T3 plasma levels and S-phase values was obvious. These results are in agreement with previous autoradiographic studies which demonstrated an increase of the epidermal mitotic rate in hyperthyroidism (Holt and Marks 1977).

15.7 Anterior Pituitary Gonadotropins

The anterior pituitary gland consists of six or seven different types of secretory cells that can function independently in producing their characteristic hormones. These hormones are thyroid-stimulating hormones (TSH), adrenocorticotropic hormone (ACTH), luteinizing hormone (LH), follicle-stimulating hormone (FSH), melanocyte-stimulating hormone (MSH), prolactin (PL), and growth hormone (GH).

Considerable interest has been directed toward the interaction between neuropharmacologic agents and releasing factors. Several neuropharmacologic agents have been found to alter anterior pituitary secretion by acting on the elaboration of hypothalamic releasing factors. The neurons that secrete the releasing factors seem to be located in the ventral hypothalamus (Goth 1978), and various neurotransmitters have a role in regulating their activity.

It has been suggested that 5α-reductase activity is dependent on the pituitary (Ebling et al. 1971). This view was based on the observation that DHT, but not testosterone, was effective in stimulating sebum secretion in hypophysectomized rats.

Sebaceous gland activity is reported to decrease in patients with decreased pituitary activity, such as gonadotropin deficiency (Pochi and Strauss 1974, 1977). In patients with acromegaly, sebum secretion is increased (Burton et al. 1972; Pochi and Strauss 1977).

Shuster and Thody (1974) suggested that pituitary factors were quite likely the ultimate controlling factors of sebaceous gland function, but that androgenic hormones were the agents that act directly on sebaceous glands. In men, the testes are the source of these androgenic hormones. In women, sebaceous gland secretion is probably stimulated by both adrenal and ovarian androgens.

The decrease in sebaceous gland activity after menopause is apparently related to a decrease in ovarian androgens. The pituitary can exert indirect effects on sebaceous activity, since it influences other endocrine organs, such as the gonads and thyroid, whose secretions in turn affect the sebaceous glands. The action of ACTH is mediated, in part, via the adrenals, so a direct action on the sebaceous glands is a possibility (Thody and Shuster 1971).

Growth hormone (GH) increases sebum secretion in hypophysectomized rats, and this appears to be related to its somatotropic action (Nikkari and Valavaara 1969; Silman et al. 1976). Melanocyte-stimulating hormone (MSH) is an important sebotropic hormone in the rat. Removal of the pars intermedia, the source of MSH, decreases sebum secretion, and this is restored after administration of α-MSH (Thody and Shuster 1975; Shuster et al. 1973).

Neuronal and Other Factors That Influence the Hair Follicle 16

The cutaneous innervation includes unmyelinated efferent sympathetic nerves that supply arterioles, eccrine glands, apocrine glands, and hair erector muscles, and mostly myelinated somatic sensory nerves that supply specialized end-organs (e.g., Meissner corpuscles and Pacini corpuscles), Merkel cells, hair follicles, and free dermal nerve endings (Jakubovic and Ackerman 1985).

Perifollicular nerve endings were observed early, either by silver impregnation methods (Szymonowicz 1909; Straile 1960; Seto 1963; Mann 1968), or by histochemical techniques (Seto 1963; Winkelmann 1968; Montagna and Parakkal 1974).

According to Montagna and Giacometti (1969), regardless of size, every follicle is surrounded by nerve fibers from the base of the bulb to its junction with the epidermis (Fig. 14.19a). Some nerves lie parallel to the follicle; other finer ones form a sock-like net around it. At the level of the bulge of large follicles and the bulb of small, vellus follicles, a "basket" of blunt parallel nerve fibers forms a collar or stockade; the upper parts of these nerves often branch into plump, packed terminals like the tines of a fork.

These light microscopic studies have revealed that human hairs, particularly vellus hairs, are richly endowed with networks of nerves. It was also found that the greatest concentration of the nerve network encircles the follicle at the level of the sebaceous gland (Hashimoto et al. 1990).

In our interpretation of the review by Hashimoto et al. (1990), the disadvantage of silver impregnation methods is that they may stain miscellaneous fibers other than nerve fibers. Although the histochemical method which stains acetylcholine is specific for nerves, the final reaction product tends to diffuse out, so it is often difficult to delineate delicate nerve fibers. With either method it is difficult or even impossible to determine the topographical relationship of the nerve endings to the follicular epithelium since this epithelium is not stained by these methods; even when counterstained, the follicle is only poorly visualized.

A more recent development in histochemistry is immunohistochemistry; very specific monoclonal antibodies against neurofilament and myelin basic protein have become available (Aso et al. 1985). Using either monoclonal antibody to neurofilament or myelin basic protein, the fine details of perifollicular innervation and nerve endings can be specifically demonstrated.

Although the staining is precise and specificity is absolute, these nerve endings still do not seem to touch the follicular epithelium (reviewed from Hashimoto et al. 1990).

In an electron microscopic investigation, Yamamoto (1966) reported that, in mouse skin, there was a palisade-like arrangement of terminal sensory fibers attached to the follicle at the level of the sebaceous gland. Subsequently, Orfanos (1967), Orfanos and Ruska (1968), Hashimoto (1973), and Ishibashi and Tsuru (1976) described a similar end-organ in the human skin (reviewed from Hashimoto et al. 1990).

The permanent structure of a hair follicle is considered to be that part from the secondary hair germ sited at the lower portion of the telogen follicle and the sebaceous isthmus; this part of the follicle is little affected by the hair cycle that modifies the lower follicle. The perifollicular nerve endings are attached to the permanent part of the follicle.

However, as the authors note, the stem cell may reside in the sebaceous isthmus (see Section 14.1.2). Thus, dysfunction of the nerve ending may affect the sebaceous isthmus and sebaceous gland.

Since follicles grow without nerves, the innervation of the follicle must be sensory. The abundance of nerves clearly indicates that they are the most important elements of the sensory mechanism (Winkelmann 1959).

The nerves of the skin, on the other hand, have both somatic sensory and sympathetic autonomic fibers that are distributed together (Stenn and Bhawan 1990).

The function of the blood vessels and sweat glands within the skin may be governed by bundles of mixed sensory and autonomic nerve fibers. Since the hair follicle has the same basic structure as the skin, it is possible that the so-called sensory nerve plexus attached to the follicle also includes autonomic nerve fibers, and is not merely a sensory nerve plexus. If this is so, then atrophy of the sebaceous gland, induced by stress that affects the autonomic nerve fibers in the terminal nerve plexus, could lead to the destruction of the upper stem cells in the sebaceous isthmus and to the secondary inhibition of matrix function, with alopecia areata as the eventual end result (see Section 22.1.1).

In the past, it has been suggested that regulatory factors from the sebaceous gland (duct) act on the dermal papilla (the matrix), and that there is a relationship between regulatory factors in the hair follicle and the neuroendocrinological system, e.g., the activity of the thymus and hypophysis, or lymph circulation (Imura 1982; Chung, personal communication 1994). Such regulatory factors are not well defined and remain as objectives for intensive study and clarification.

The pituitary gland plays a central role in the hormonal regulation of a wide variety of processes, and thus it has been one of the most extensively studied of all endrocrine glands. Pituitary function is under the control of the hypothalamus. The interaction of the pituitary and hypothalamus is an excellent example of the interaction between the nervous and endrocrine systems (Phoades and Pflanzer 1989).

However, as described in Chapter 5, we reported a microcirculatory system originating from the subpapillary blood plexus below the epidermis and surrounding the follicular appendix; we noted that this vascular system was of prime importance, with the principal blood supply coming from the subpapillary blood to form the microcirculation around the pilocebaceous unit. From this finding, it can be surmised that enzyme and hormone activity takes place continuously in the sebaceous gland.

Dysfunction of the sebaceous gland induced by nervous stress influences the dermal papilla. Both alopecia androgenetica and alopecia areata may be induced by this mechanism.

Androgenetic Alopecia

17

17.1 Definition of Androgenetic Alopecia

The term "androgenetic" was coined by Ludwig (1962), who combined the words "androgen" and "genetic". In youth, the scalp is covered by thick pigmented terminal hair. Normally, all human beings become progressively balder. The course of androgenetic alopecia (A.a) is progressive in the middle decades of life; the transition into senile involution alopecia follows later in life. A major distinction between long-term normal balding and the condition known as is that the more advanced and obvious signs of pattern baldness appear at an earlier age.

This characteristic in humans appears to be heritable. Increased levels of androgen in adolescent males are thought to be a factor that triggers the development of baldness: prepubertal castration or a deficiency of steroid 5α-reductase counteracts this hereditary phenomenon (Burton and Marshall 1979a).

Androgenetic alopecia usually manifests itself in both sexes. In the male, this may lead to complete baldness (male pattern baldness, calvities hippocratica), but extensive diffuse alopecia of the male pattern may also occur in women. This androgenetic alopecia has previously been referred to in many terms, such as "seborrheic alopecia," "premature alopecia," "common baldness," and "diffuse alopecia of the female".

The physiology of both types of baldness, i.e., A.a and alopecia areata, is the same. During the balding process, not only does the telogen resting stage of the hair follicle cycle become progressively longer, but the follicles themselves gradually shrink in size. The change occurs over several successive generations of hair cycles. At each cycle, the size of the follicle at anagen becomes smaller. With each diminution, the hair generated by the follicle becomes shorter, thinner, and less pigmented. This process continues until the size of the follicle has reached that of the vellus state, in which the hair produced is a minute, colorless filament, almost invisible to the eye.

Although hair follicles in the bald scalp appear atrophic, their number does not change. The scattered follicles that regress through normal aging produce imperceptible vellus hairs that are interspersed with the long, thick pigmented hair covering the scalp.

Thus, the phenomenon of androgenetic baldness is generally considered to be an effect primarily of diminution in size of hair follicles and not of disease. On the other hand, alopecia areata involves pathological changes in hair follicles.

Androgenetic alopecia usually manifests itself in both sexes at an early age and progresses slowly. However, the pattern established is different. Male pattern baldness typically manifests itself as an M-shaped outline on a receding hairline. Concurrently, a balding patch appears on the crown and increases in size, eventually meeting the receding hairline. In its final stage, the entire scalp is exposed, except for a ring of hair circling its lower sides and rear. Female pattern baldness, on the other hand, is more limited, rarely reaching the extent of its male counterpart. Known as diffuse hair loss in women, it can be characterized by a general rarefication of hair throughout the scalp and depilation in the crown. In women, however, A.a follows a moderate course and rarely leads to the development of lanugo hair and to true baldness.

The terms "common baldness" and "male pattern baldness" do not actually correspond to the clinical picture and course of androgenetic alopecia in females.

17.2 Occurrence and Frequency

Androgenetic alopecia is the most frequent form of hair loss in humans. Its appearance is, in fact, a sign of sexual maturity, since A.a does not occur in children, in men with testicular insufficiency, before menarche, or in early castrates. In certain animal species (stump-tailed macaque, *Macaca speciosa*), it appears regularly as a sign of normal sexual development in puberty. The onset of synthesizing androgen hormones is evidently responsible for this, as was first emphasized by Hamilton (1942); however, increased responsiveness and availability of receptors located in the hair follicles, e.g., in the frontal and the central parietal area, is a necessary prerequisite for the development of androgen-dependent alopecia, whereas occipital hair is generally preserved. Since every sexually mature male has a sufficient amount of androgen, androgenetic alopecia develops only when there is a genetic predisposition. In the female, minimal amounts of circulating androgen alone evidently do not suffice to induce telogen effluvium; here, both the degree of genetic predisposition, i.e., the presence and responsiveness of receptors, and the levels of circulating androgen play a role. Precise results are not available from statistical studies of the incidence of androgenetic alopecia in different population groups. In early reports, a receding hairline past the temples was found in about 62.5% of all middle-aged men; in the age group up to 30 years, there was predilection for the male sex (men 47%, women 19%; Hamilton 1951a), whereas this difference was no longer demonstrated in older age groups (men 80%, women 75%; Beek 1950). It appears that the incidence is higher by 25% in whites compared to blacks (Setty 1970). Men of other races more rarely become bald. For example, baldness occurs in only 15% of Chinese males (Hamilton 1951a; Salamon 1966). In women, common baldness usually begins later in life than in men. The pattern of thinning is much more diffuse, involving, primarily, the frontocentral scalp and sparing the peripheral margins (Ludwig 1977). Parietotemporal recession usually is not prominent, and severe thinning is infrequent. Androgenetic alopecia in women, which may lead to a bald pate, occurs in patients with idiopathic hirsutism or pathologic disorders related to increased androgen stimulation and therefore should alert the physician to check for an endocrine disorder.

In a group of 564 normal women, frontal and frontoparietal recession was found in 13% of those who were premenopausal and in 37% of those who were postmenopausal, a total of 50% overall (Venning and Dawber 1988); in his study of the types of androgenetic alopecia occurring in women, Ludwig (1977) found more diffuse vertical recession. Orfanos (1990) estimated that about two-thirds of all men and one-third of all women in the German population display clinically visible androgenetic alopecia. However, in the dermatologist's office, the ratio of men to women is almost 1:1, evidently because women more readily consult a physician for hair loss than men do.

Sperling and Winton (1990), in their study of the transverse anatomy of androgen alopecia, reported that up to 30% of telogen hairs were found in females.

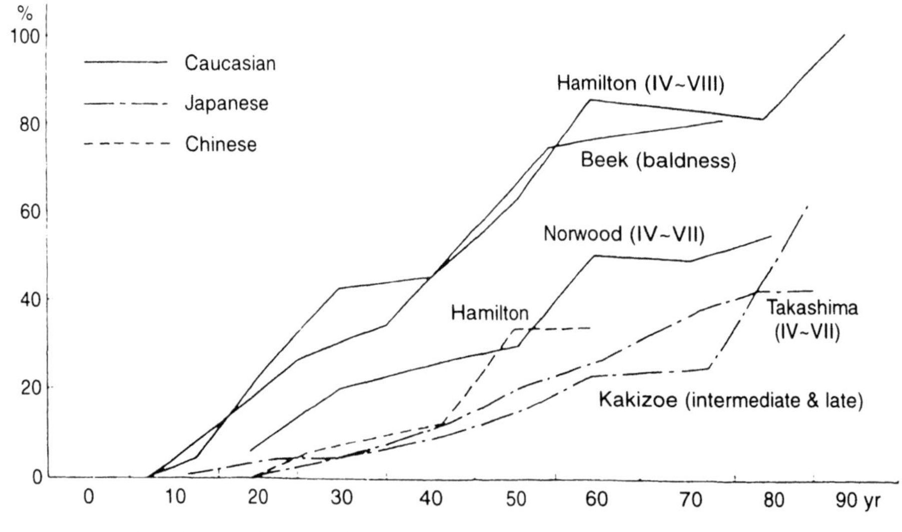

Fig. 17.1. Age-specific incidence of advanced baldness in Caucasians, Japanese, and Chinese (from Takashima et al. 1981, with permission)

Following Norwood (1975), Takashima et al. (1981) collated findings for advanced baldness, Hamilton (1951a) types IV and over (see Section 1.6.1), together with findings in Beek's (1950) and Kakizoe's (1969) studies. In Fig. 17.1, all curves show a similar tendency, advanced baldness increasing with aging. Baldness is a function of aging. As shown in Fig. 17.1, the incidence of advanced baldness in Caucasians, in the study of Norwood (1975), was almost 20% lower in every decade, except for the forties to fifties, than the incidence in Chinese in Hamilton's study (1951a). Earlier balding in Caucasian than in Chinese and Japanese men is easily discernible (reviewed from Takashima et al. 1981).

17.3 Incidence of Baldness in Japanese

Hamilton (1951a) carried out extensive studies on the patterns of development of scalp hair in men and women from the prenatal period through the tenth decade. He divided the balding patterns into eight types, with three subdivisions, and then compared the incidence of baldness in Caucasians and Chinese.

Ogata (1953) in Japan suggested that baldness should be classified into six types, as shown in Fig. 17.2. Norwood (1975) revised Hamilton's classification to ensure the result of hair transplant surgery, dividing the patterns into seven (Fig. 17.3), with a type A variant (Fig. 17.4).

Takashima et al. (1981) analyzed the scalp hair types of 1726 Japanese males, aged 15–96 years, who were in- and outpatients of seven hospitals. Patients with any hair disease were excluded from the study. To avoid discordance in judging the patterns, a few hundred patients were also jointly studied and special attention was paid to the classification of type III, the minimal degree of apparent baldness. Takashima adopted the standards of Norwood (1975) for classification. The overall age- and type-specific incidence of baldness in Japanese men, according to Takashima et al. (1981), is summarized in Fig. 17.5 and Table 17.1. type II-vertex was seen in 6.5% of the cases; the rate was not negligible. When type II-vertex through VII is taken to indicate baldness, the incidence in all ages was calculated to be 31.7%. Soon after commencing the work, however, he noted a peculiar type of

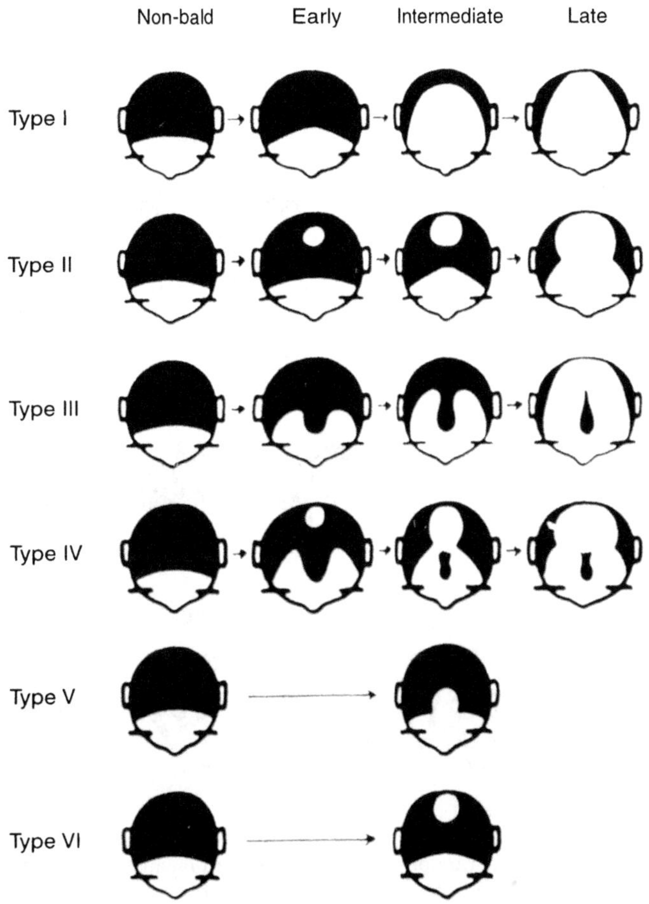

Fig. 17.2. Ogata's (1953) classification of balding patterns (with permission of Kobundo)

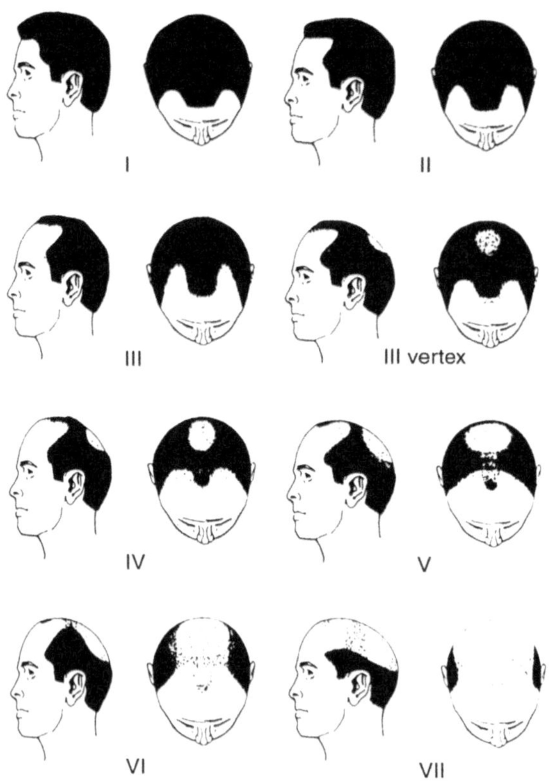

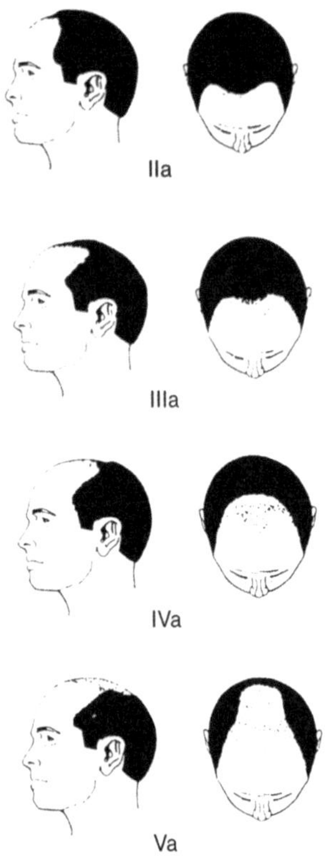

17.3 17.4

Fig. 17.3. Norwood-Hamilton classification of male pattern baldness (from Norwood 1975, with permission)

Fig. 17.4. Standards for classification of type A variant male pattern baldness (from Norwood 1975, with permission)

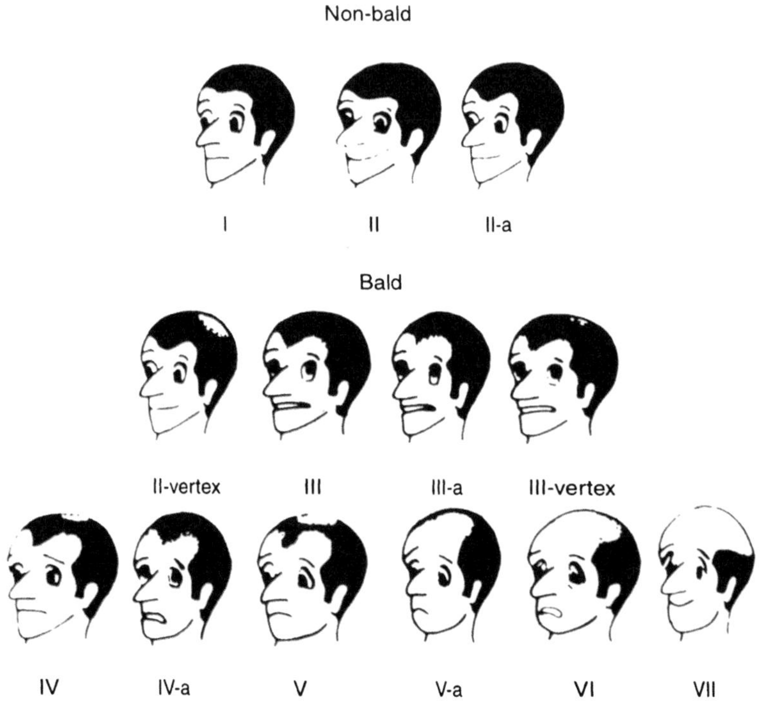

Fig. 17.5. Distribution of male balding pattern in Japan. (According to Takashima, based on Norwood's classification; with permission from Takashima et al. 1981)

Table 17.1. Overall type- and age-specific incidence of baldness in Japanese men. (From Takashima et al. 1981, with permission)

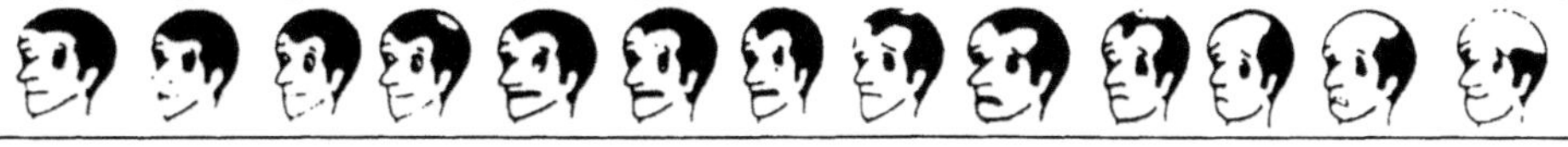

Age (years)	I	II	IIa	IIv	III	IIIa	IIIv	IV	IVa	V	Va	VI	VII	Total
15–19	90[a] 58.4	63 40.9			1 0.7									154
20–29	93 48.5	82 42.8	6 3.1	2 1.0	7 3.6		1 0.5	1 0.5						192
30–39	85 37.7	100 44.2	13 5.9	8 3.5	9 4.1	4 1.7		2 0.8		4 1.7	1 0.4			226
40–49	103 27.8	127 34.2	21 5.7	33 8.9	26 7.0	10 2.7	14 3.8	6 1.6	3 0.8	10 2.7	12 3.2	5 1.3	1 0.3	371
50–59	79 19.9	118 29.7	25 6.3	37 9.3	32 8.1	9 2.3	21 5.3	19 4.8	6 1.5	15 3.8	16 4.0	17 4.3	3 0.7	397
60–69	30 14.1	55 26.0	19 9.0	15 7.1	17 8.0	11 5.2	11 5.2	4 1.9	6 2.8	8 3.8	16 7.5	13 6.1	7 3.3	212
70–79	17 12.1	26 18.7	12 8.6	15 10.7	10 7.1	7 5.0	3 2.1	6 4.3	7 5.0	5 3.6	16 11.4	11 7.8	5 3.6	140
80–	3 8.8	10 29.3	1 3.0	3 8.8	1 3.0	1 3.0			1 3.0	4 11.8	3 8.8	6 17.5	1 3.0	34
Total	500 29.0	581 33.7	97 5.6	113 6.5	103 6.0	42 2.4	50 2.9	38 2.2	23 1.3	46 2.7	64 3.7	52 3.0	17 1.0	1,726 31.7[b]

[a] Upper line: number of subjects; lower line, percentage.
[b] Percentage of types II-vertex through VII for 1726 subjects.

baldness in which an early baldness patch appeared on the occiput while frontotemporal angles were well preserved in the type II or even I category. This type was not listed in either Hamilton's or Norwood's classification; however, in Ogata's study it was called type II-early and VI-intermediate. Takashima named it type II-vertex. This type is probably Japanese-specific.

17.4 Hair Density in the Scalp

The adult scalp (20–30 years) has an average of 615 hair follicles per square centimeter. In the newborn we counted 1135 follicles/cm^2 (cited by Giacometti 1964).

There is a gradual reduction in the density of hair follicles with advancing age. The difference between the 20- to 30-year age group and other groups from 30 to 90 years is statistically significant. The reduction in the number of hair follicles from ages 30 to 40 is considerable. About 40% of the follicles are lost in male pattern baldness. A comparative study of the mean number of follicles in the hairy scalp and in the bald scalp shows, as expected, a significant difference in number.

17.5 Factors Affecting the Hair Cycle

The hair cycle is affected by various endogenous and exogenous factors. In a newborn, much of the hair goes through the anagen stage into the telogen stage several days after birth, and there is significant hair loss in several weeks. The hair cycle is influenced by hormones (Crovato et al. 1975). In human females, hair in the telogen stage decreases during the second to third trimester of pregnancy, and increases after delivery (Munro and Darley 1979). Scalp hair grows faster than hairs on other parts of the body, but the anagen stage is shorter in the summer than in the winter (Saito et al. 1976). As an abnormal process, there is an increase in telogen hair and hair loss following disease in which there is fever and after systemic disease, and this also occurs due to stress in psychiatric disorders (Kligman 1961).

17.6 Various Signs of Scalp Hair Loss

17.6.1 Recognition of Hair Loss with Brushing

Hair is normally lost and regenerated regularly. According to Orentreich (1969), in young adults regardless of sex, 90% of scalp hairs are growing and 10% are in the resting stage; about 100 club hairs would be shed per day. The problem occurs when the loss rate rises considerably higher. Exogenous hair damage through excessive shampooing or manipulation occurs frequently in androgenetic alopecia and may alter the clinical picture. Excessive force used in brushing the hair can pull out more hairs than might fall out naturally. To find the difference between a hair that has fallen out naturally and one that has been prematurely pulled out by excessive brushing, a simple test may be used. Place the hair on a flat glass slide and then stand the glass vertically. A hair (telogen hair) that immediately falls off the slide is naturally lost, as the root sheath is loose or absent. One that sticks to the glass has been pulled out prematurely. The pulled-out hair (anagen hair) still has intact connective tissue covered by the root sheath, and thus retains an adhesive quality (Fig. 17.6a,b). Roots of anagen hair are either of uniform diameter or are broadened at the base, are usually wrapped firmly by the root sheath, and may be angulated. In telogen hair, the lower tips are clublike and invariably straight, and the sheaths are loose or absent.

17.6.2 Receding of Scalp Hair Border

A second sign of incipient baldness is a receding hairline. Baldness has various patterns, but, in general, most of the patterns include a receding hairline. The borders recede increasingly toward the parietal region, making the size of the forehead appear to expand.

17.6.3 Excessive Dandruff and Seborrhea

An abnormal increase in dandruff and seborrhoea is another danger signal. Dandruff is formed as a lipid mixture secreted from the sebaceous gland

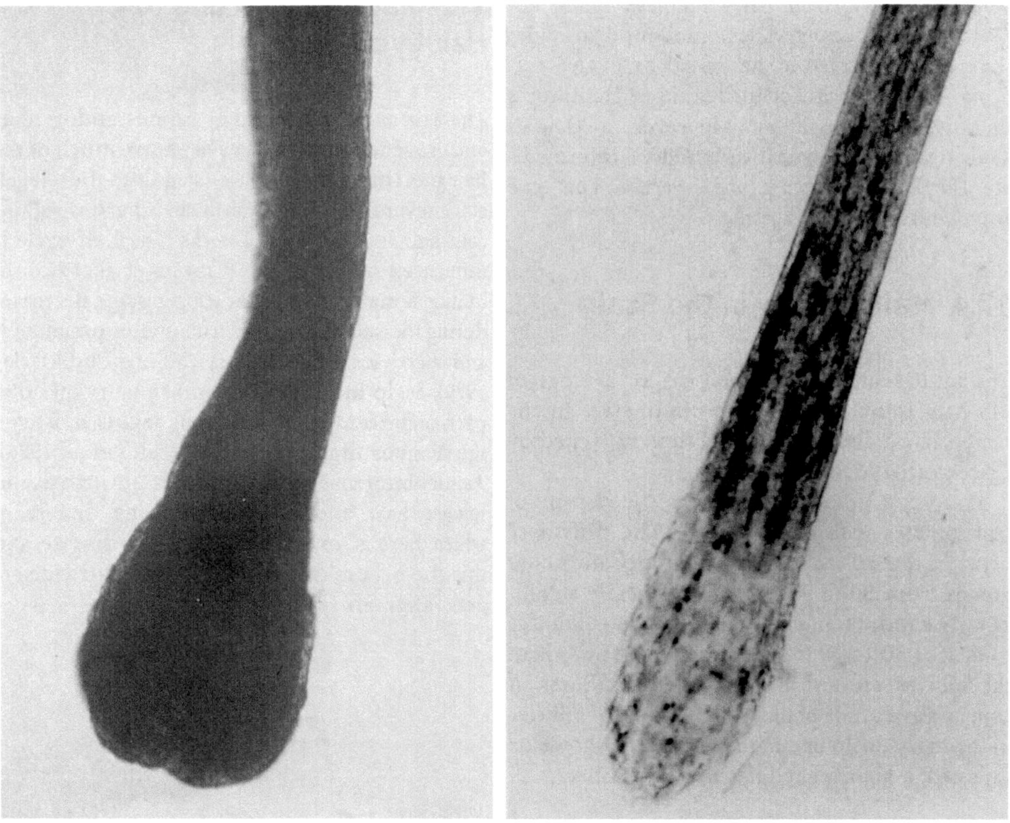

a b

Fig. 17.6. a Anagen hair (pulled-out hair). Hair roots in anagen are either of equal diameter throughout or broadened at the base, are usually firmly encased by the root sheath, and may be angulated. **b** Telogen hair. The lower tips of telogen hairs are clublike, are invariably straight, and the sheaths are loose or absent (seborrhea oleasa). It appears on the scalp skin surface in the corneal layer exfoliated by the lateral epidermis. Dandruff may be either the fatty (seborrheic) type or the dry type. We are concerned with the fatty type, which is caused by hormone activity and hypernutrition.

Androgen or excessive ingestion of fatty acids contributes to enlarging the sebaceous gland and enhancing the sebaceous secretion that forms a fatty membrane (sebum) on the surface of scalp skin; the amount of fatty dandruff is then increased abnormally and is accompanied by itching. When this condition persists for some time, and the dandruff comes to an abrupt halt, excessive loss of hair begins, an indication of growing bald. However, there is no evidence in either humans or experimental animals that any components of sebum are directly derived from ingested fats (Strauss et al. 1991). Prolonged starvation of human subjects (Pochi et al. 1970) decreased the rate of sebum synthesis by about 40% (see Section 23.2 for details).

Seborrhea was found to be present in about three-fourths of all patients with androgenetic alopecia, both males and females (Wüstner and Orfanos 1974). However, there is no direct relationship between androgenic alopecia and seborrhea of the scalp (Ebling and Rook 1972).

17.6.4 Thinning and Solitary (Single) Hairs in Parietal and Temporal Regions of Scalp

A definite danger signal is that hairs in the parietal and frontovertical region have become thinner than those in the temporal region of the scalp. As a result, many secondary vellus hairs are interspread with normal hairs. Such alteration in hair diameter may serve as a marker for androgenetic hair loss.

The loss of hair occurs episodically every few years in some individuals and once or twice per year in almost all subjects. Phases of increased hair loss are followed by periods of relative stability. In youth, the density of scalp hair increases due to the generation of bundle (compound) hairs from one hair canal. However, with aging bundle hairs turn into solitary (single) hairs and the scalp becomes visible.

According to Orfanos (1990), the decrease in hair diameter may be especially pronounced in women. Meiers and Grobbel (1974) postulated that such alterations in hair diameter appear early and may serve as a marker for genetic predisposition to androgenetic hair loss. These measurements obviously express the incipient transformation of thick terminal hair into intermediate and vellus hair types, which arise in miniature follicles. Recent findings on hair density, hair diameter, and hair growth rate in androgenetic alopecia in the male have recently been reported by Runne and Martin (1986).

Jackson et al. (1972) found two equal frequency peaks of decrease in hair diameter at 0.04 and 0.08 mm in female baldness whereas there was one, at 0.08 mm, in a control series.

The authors (Inaba and Inaba 1992a) have elucidated the mechanism underlying the process by which bundle hairs turn into solitary (single) hairs (see Sections 12.3 and 21.4).

17.6.5 Thickening of Body Hairs

Another sign that baldness has begun is a thickening of chest and beard hairs (Fig. 17.7). The generation of axillary or pubic hairs, which is without gender distinction in puberty, depends on stimulation provided by the male hormone (androgen) secreted from the adrenal cortex. The chest or beard hair characteristic of male body hair, on the other hand, is generated as a result of stimulation by another male hormone (testosterone) secreted from the testes. The rate of beard growth is correlated with the amount of 5α-DHT in the plasma, but not with the level of testosterone (Farthing et al. 1982).

The question arises whether male baldness is associated with any other proposed indices of masculinity and whether any hormonal abnormalities are involved.

Men tend to have thicker axillary and pubic hair than women, due to the metabolic effect of testosterone. Some men have thick chest hair and others have little or none. This characteristic depends on the quality and quantity of male hormone production and secretion.

In considering variations between individuals, the extent of the peripheral response may be even more important than the level of circulating androgens. Thus, the rate of thigh hair growth showed no significant correlation with plasma testosterone (T), sex hormone binding globulin (SHBG), or free testosterone, as reflected by T/SHBG, but was correlated with both 5α-dihydrotestosterone and androstenedione (Ebling et al. 1984). One interpretation of these findings is that the capacity of the hair follicles to metabolize testosterone is more important than the amount of free testosterone available.

According to Salamon (1968), thickening of chest hair, which is indicative of increased testosterone secretion, can be a danger signal in respect to the preservation of scalp hairs. On the other hand, much evidence refutes the idea that

a

b

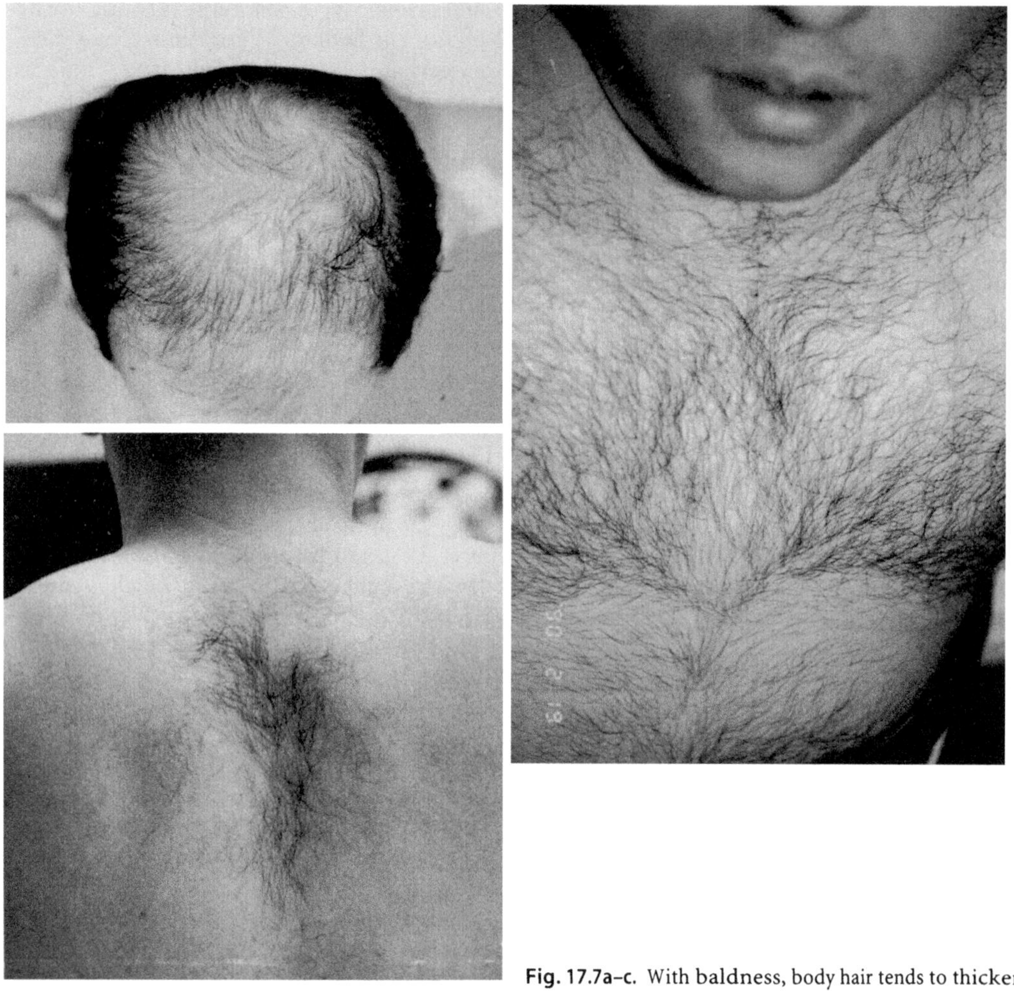

c

Fig. 17.7a–c. With baldness, body hair tends to thicken

baldness is associated with other proposed indices of masculinity such as density of body hair, skin and muscle thickness, and rate of sebum secretion (Burton and Marshall 1979a).

Lookingbill et al. (1991) have reported that increased serum levels of 5α-reduced androgen metabolites in Caucasian vs. Chinese subjects provide circumstantial evidence for a radical difference in 5α-reductase activity and suggest a mechanism for the increased body hair observed in Caucasian men. Increased levels of precursor androgens may also play a role in this phenomenon.

Etiologic Factors in Male Pattern Baldness

18

Many etiologic factors may be involved in the causative mechanisms of baldness. Each of these important factors will be discussed.

18.1 Seborrhea and Dandruff

The epidermis (surface skin) has characteristic metabolic activity. The germinal cells that are responsible for vigorous, cyclic mitotic (cell division) activity in the basal layer of the epidermis push away the cytoplasm that is split off as spinous and granular cells. These cells soon keratinize to form the lateral-corneal layer of the scalp. The corneal portion of the layer, separating away from the lateral portion, then becomes dandruff.

Sebum secretion from the sebaceous gland is mixed with the dandruff; seborrhea is the result of that mixture. Dandruff and sebum produce the condition of seborrhea by clogging the dermal papilla, which then atrophies, and unsaturated fatty acids in seborrheal deposits can accelerate hair loss. However, Bloom et al. (1955) found no abnormalities in the content of squalene or of free or esterified fatty acid in subjects with early male pattern baldness.

Some researchers have suggested that the condition of seborrhea, associated with growing bald, is related to excessive male hormone secretion. Male hormone secretion may be the primary cause of baldness, with seborrhea as a secondary cause. In any case, seborrhea has frequently been considered a progenitor of baldness.

Individuals with androgenetic alopecia did indeed reveal significant elevation of sebum excretion rates in the scalp, particularly during the acute phase of androgenetic hair loss (Thiele 1975). Many authors have observed the association of sebum with baldness and believe that microorganisms are involved in both these phenomena (Sabourand 1929).

In some earlier studies no quantitative differences were found in the amounts of skin surface lipids between patients with androgenetic alopecia and normal individuals (Maibach et al. 1968). A number of investigators, e.g., Kuchinska (1973), have suggested that the auto-oxidation of hair lipids gives rise to substances that exert depilatory or hair loss activity, but the evidence that such substances play any part in ordinary hair loss is unconvincing (Fukuzumi 1986). There is no conclusive evidence that the excessive production of sebum itself affects the basic mechanisms of hair loss.

18.2 Dietary Factors

A number of reports have been published regarding the relationship between baldness and nutrition (Bradfield et al. 1967; Bradfield 1971; Crounse et al. 1970; Gummer 1985). Most of these studies conclude that excessive intake of certain nutrients can cause an increase in blood cholesterol and deterioration of blood flow in the peripheral capillary vessels. The capillary vessels that circulate blood to the dermal papilla of the hair root thus exhibit this deterioration of blood flow and the hair follicle is subsequently deprived of sufficient nutrition.

However, these conclusions fail to explain why women, who ingest the same kinds of nutrients as men, do not grow bald. If cholesterol plays an active role in the onset of baldness, why don't women grow bald as early or as frequently as men? Hypernutrition may be a causative factor in baldness, but the causal process must be considered apart from the cholesterol intake.

In Japan, three men who were wrongly imprisoned for capital crimes, when found innocent and released after 30 years, still had healthy heads of black hair. Another prisoner, 90 years old, had a good growth of white hair after serving a prison term of 35 years. The regular eating habits and prison diet of less than 2000 calories daily seemed to be beneficial to the hair. These dietary factors are described in detail in Chapter 23.

18.3 Genetic Predisposition Theory

The mantle of hair which covers the entire surface of the body is one of the characteristics of mammals. Human beings, unique among the mammals, have mostly vellus hair as body hair, although the hairs of the head, the eyebrows, the nostrils, etc., retain much of their original mammalian form.

Hair type is determined by genetic inheritance. Straight hair indicates inheritance of a recessive gene, which does not express itself and is incapable of suppressing dominant genes. Frizzy or curly hair indicates inheritance of a dominant gene.

Male pattern baldness is a condition which appears only when androgen activity is present. Eunuchs, even those who have a family history of baldness, do not lose their hair unless treated with testosterone (Hamilton 1942). Hamilton also confirmed that there was no difference in the amount of urinary excretion of 17-ketosteroids (17-KS) between bald and nonbald individuals. These findings indicate that the genetic predisposition to baldness is determined by the susceptibility of the hair follicle cells themselves to testosterone and not by excessive blood levels. There is much evidence that baldness can be inherited as an autosomal dominant trait (Harris 1946).

According to Osborn (1916), a sex-linked pair of factors is responsible for the manifestation of androgenetic alopecia. She believed that balding men would be either heterozygotes (Bb) or homozygotes (BB), whereas females would be homozygotes (bb) only.

Smith and Wells (1964) speculated that the expressivity of the gene could be partly determined by the androgen level: the BB genotype may lead to the clinical manifestation of alopecia even at low androgen levels in women, whereas the Bb genotype requires higher amounts of androgen, e.g., as found in males or in the androgenital syndrome in females. The bb genotype remains subclinical in both sexes. Other evidence supports the theory of multifactorial or conditioned inheritance (Salamon 1968). More recently, arguments have been presented in favor of polygenic inheritance of the trait, in contrast to the mendelian BB-Bb model (Kuester and Happle 1984).

Orentreich (1959) discovered the tendency of hair follicles to be donor dominant in transplantation. He introduced punch skin grafts from nonbald occipital or temporal areas to the bald frontal area as a therapeutic measure. The transplanted skin pieces retained coarse terminal hairs long enough for satisfactory surgical results to be achieved.

If male pattern baldness is exclusively hereditary, why has the rate of male baldness in Japan increased considerably since the end of World War II? Although genetic inheritance may be one factor in the tendency toward baldness, it does not seem to be a critical factor. The great variety and quantity of sex hormone stimuli in different men are also inherited.

18.4 Aging

In a young frontal scalp, the proportion of anagen (growth phase) follicles increases with age (Barman et al. 1969). An aging, balding frontal scalp has a greater percentage of telogen follicles: the 5α-reductase activity here can be relatively low: the proportion of weak metabolites such as androstenedione will be relatively high. The course of androgenetic alopecia is progressive in the middle decades of life. The density of scalp hair decreases by more than 50% in individuals older than 60 years of age.

Aging is said to produce a diffuse type of hair loss that is superimposed on the male pattern loss. However, this type of loss is difficult to distinguish from the normal progression of male pattern alopecia. Another parameter showing rapid fluctuation during the balding process in humans is the telogen ratio. The ratio is reported to be 60% in the infant frontal area several weeks after birth; it then decreases to 20% in the adult (Barman et al. 1967), and doubles in the fifth decade (Barman et al. 1965).

18.5 Insufficient Blood Circulation

It is often said that "a tight cap thins one's hair." How can a tight cap influence the condition of the hair? Is blood circulation inhibited by the pressure of a tight cap on the blood vessels?

One amusing notion springing from this simplistic supposition is that the hair follicles in the parietal region suffer from malnutrition due to insufficient blood circulation. Another is that baldness begins in men with an oval-shaped head because it is more difficult to elevate the blood flow to the crown of an oval head.

Another notion is that there are many bald intellectuals, because their brain size is supposedly larger than normal. According to this notion, the larger brain presses against and stretches the cranial bone. The scalp covering the cranial bone is stretched out to the extent that the blood vessels are pinched and blood flow is diminished.

Wadel (1933), in reporting findings of decreased motility of the scalp, was convinced that this decrease was due to androgenetic alopecia patients having a scalp that was both frontally and sagittally too short, and thus the scalp had to be stretched like a too-small cap to cover the relatively overlarge skull.

There have, however, been reports (e.g., Tarnow 1971) that wearing a cap can cause insufficient blood flow due to pressure, thus accelerating hair loss. Therefore, it is plausible that a tight cap, habitually worn, could influence hair loss to some extent.

A bald scalp shows reduced circulation compared to a hairy scalp. This is the result of the reduced metabolic needs of a bald scalp, whose hair follicles are much smaller. If it were the cause rather than the result, one would expect transplants from hair-bearing areas of the scalp to bald areas to atrophy rapidly (Unger 1979). However, hair autografts maintain their integrity and characteristics after transplantation to a new site (Orentreich 1969).

18.6 Scalp Tension

This idea is similar to the blood circulation supposition, except that a tight cap puts external pressure on the scalp while scalp tension pressure is exerted internally. Carefully examined, the scalp shows surface tension, with the skin tight against the bone. Since the scalp skin adheres so tightly to the cranial bone, the presumption is that blood circulation must be suppressed, causing insufficient nutrition and inducing atrophy of the hair follicles.

As shown in the review of Takashima (1990), Schein's hypothesis (1903), that tension of the galea aponeurotica brought about by the chronologically disproportional development of skull and scalp skin causes narrowing of the blood vessels, followed by damage to the scalp hairs, is still alive in dermatology to some extent. One researcher (Young 1947) who sought to give credence to this tension supposition carried out experiments with monkeys. He reported that loss hair occurred when the monkey's scalp was cut off in a long circle and then sutured back again as tightly as possible.

Kessler (1963) introduced "frontalotomy" as a surgical measure to reduce the scalp tension. However, Ponten (1963) reported no objective improvement after frontal galeotomy. If Schein's hypothesis (1903) is correct, one cannot explain how females rapidly develop androgenetic alopecia when they suffer from endocrine disturbances such as arrhenoblastoma, and why adult castrates become bald after testosterone injections (Richter 1963).

One investigator (Engstrand 1965) believes that baldness is caused by pressure on the capillaries of the scalp as a result of the thickening of the tendinous membrane (the aponeurosis of the occipitofrontalis). As men age, this membrane gradually thickens and loses elasticity.

On the other hand, Toshitani (1989) reported a simple treatment of male pattern alopecia: relaxing scalp tension with a scalp tension relaxation (STR) instrument.

18.7 Nervous Stress

The occasional occurrence of alopecia areata (patchy bald spots in the scalp) due to nervous stress has been demonstrated, but is not reasonable to conclude that stress is a major cause of this common type of premature baldness (see Section 22.1).

The annals of war, hate, and strife record many instances of sudden hair loss ensuing after some especially fearful event (Obermayer 1955; Kligman 1961).

Japanese war fugitives, living in constant tension in jungle hideaways for 30 to 40 years after the end of World War II, were subject to extreme psychological stress. The survivors who came home to Japan still had full heads of healthy hair. Thus it is not invariably true that high stress levels over long periods are a major contributory factor in premature baldness. Diet may have played a contributory role in preventing baldness in these men.

18.8 Hair Conditioners

The cuticle of the hair consists of a series of overlapping ring-like cells surrounding the cortex. As mentioned earlier, these cells have a scale-like appearance. When the hair is in good "condition," the series of cells is closed tight to the hair shaft, and is shiny and relatively smooth; the appearance is like a shiny new pine cone. As the hair weathers, or is physically or chemically damaged, it begins to look cracked on the edges and dull, appearing like a pine cone that has dried and opened.

Because conditioners, for the main part, act on the surface or cuticular portion of the fiber, our interest will be mostly focused on this portion of the hair.

Hair pomades and waxes containing vegetable oil as the major ingredient, or petroleum-based conditioners, when used in excess, may cause baldness. Some of these conditioners contain strong surfactant agents, and may have a harmful effect on the dermal papilla, permeating downward through the scalp.

Excessive use of hair conditioners may increase the fatty membrane (sebum) on the surface of scalp skin. Consequent inhibition of sebaceous gland activity results in enlargement of the sebaceous gland.

18.9 Hormonal Factors

18.9.1 Hormone Imbalance

A definite cause-effect relationship between androgenetic alopecia and testicular hormones was suggested by Hamilton (1942), based on gross anatomical observations of the scalp hair pattern of eunuchs and castrates subjected to testosterone injections. The following findings support his conclusion:

a. A male who is castrated before puberty does not grow bald, and males castrated at the ages of 14–19 years exhibit the same effects. However, those who are castrated later in life, at ages 20–40, occasionally grow bald to some degree.

b. The administration of androgen to castrated males whose normal relatives tend to be bald causes progressive symptoms of baldness when androgen treatment is continued. This continues until the androgen administration is stopped.

The above evidence strongly suggests that baldness may be attributable to excessive male hormone secretion. However, other facts cannot be explained by these findings alone. For example, there are many cases in which the parietal region of the scalp becomes bald but the temporal region does not. There are other cases in which the parietal region of the scalp tends to become bald, but beard or chest hairs become conspicuously thicker.

There is no fully acceptable explanation of why androgen activity should cause baldness to occur on the scalp while stimulating thicker hair growth on other parts of the body.

However, in a review by Takashima (1990), Hamilton (1942) confirmed that there was no difference in the amount of urinary excretion of 17-ketosteroid (17-KS) between bald and nonbald individuals. Kakizoe (1969) compared the amounts of urinary excretion of 17-KS with those of estrogens in subjects with and without androgenetic alopecia and found that bald males excreted more 17-KS than estrogens, while hairy males excreted more estrogens than 17-KS. These results suggest that a predominance of androgens may exist in bald individuals.

In contrast, Philipou and Kirk (1981) measured the sexual and adrenocortical steroids in plasma and urine in 15 subjects, and found no difference in the level of circulating androgens between bald and nonbald men, whereas there was a positive correlation both between the urinary excretion of dehydroepiandrosterone (DHA), and androgen precursor, and between the urinary excretion of tetrahydrocortisone and the presence of androgenetic alopecia; mild hyperadrenal activity was revealed in many subjects with androgenetic alopecia.

18.9.2 Other Studies of Hormone Activity and Androgenetic Alopecia

The pathogenetic processes involved in androgenetic alopecia are not yet fully clarified. Basically however, according to the present state of knowledge, two factors are required for the development of androgenetic alopecia: (a) minimal amounts of androgen-like compounds, mostly hormones circulating in the peripheral blood, and (b) the capacity of the pilosebaceous apparatus in the periphery to respond with increased sensitivity to the amount of circulating androgens (Orfanos 1990).

Following this pathogenetic concept, androgenetic alopecia is not an endocrine disorder. Of course, the metabolism of testosterone in the periphery is of major importance (Price 1975), but the levels of the circulating hormones remain within normal limits in the majority of cases; De Villez and Dunn (1986) found total testosterone, DHEA, and androstenediol to be normal in androgenetic alopecia. In contrast, testosterone glucosiduronate was increased in females who exhibited diffuse hair loss (Tamm et al. 1980), and circulating sex hormone binding globulin (SHBG) was found to be reduced in young women with diffuse hair loss (Miller et al. 1982; Georgala et al. 1986) and in bald males (Cipriani et al. 1983). The ratio of total androgens to the transfer proteins to which they bind has been proposed as a major parameter (Gilliland et al. 1981) for assessing peripheral androgenism (reviewed from Orfanos 1990).

In skin, the presence of two important enzymes that catalyze C_{19} steroids, 17β-hydrosteroid dehydrogenase and 5α-reductase, has been confirmed (Hay and Hodgins 1978). Of the various metabolites of sexual steroids, compounds with a hydroxyl group in the 17β-position and hydrogen in the 5α-position have more potent hormonal action than those with a 17-oxystructure and an unsaturated form in the basic A (aromatic) ring. Therefore, 5α-reductase makes steroids more potent while 17β-dehydrogenase makes them less potent. One of the 5α-reduced metabolites of testosterone, dihydrotestosterone (DHT), has been shown to be one of the most potent androgen compounds (Dorfman and Dorfman 1962) (reviewed from Takashima 1990).

When testosterone penetrates hair follicle cells, it is converted to a pair of metabolites: DHT, the most potent, and androstenedione (ADION), which is biologically inactive in the follicle (Bruchovsky and Wilson 1968).

In studies of human scalp not predisposed to androgenetic alopecia, incubation of hair follicles with testosterone showed that ADION was the major metabolic agent in both the anagen (growing) and telogen (resting) follicles (Adachi et al. 1970).

Schweikert and Wilson (1974a) studied the metabolism of labeled testosterone and androstenedione in individual hair roots from balding and hairy scalp areas and, in general, found that levels of 5α-reduced metabolites and 17-ketosteroid metabolites were higher in balding men. However, it was not clear whether these changes were primary or secondary to the balding process.

In a later study, Schweikert and Wilson (1981) investigated the relation between androgens and hair growth, assessing the metabolism of $[^3H]$-testosterone and $[^3H]$androstenedione in isolated human hair roots, using a micromethod. Using this method, it was demonstrated that both anagen and telogen hair roots originating from ten different body sites contained two major enzymatic systems, namely, 5α-reductase and 17β-hydrosteroid dehydrogenase (17β-HSD). No significant relationship was found, with either testosterone or androstenedione as a substrate, between the androgen-mediated growth of hair and the capacity to form 5α metabolites. There was a significantly greater 5α-reductase activity in anagen hairs from the frontal scalp of balding men than in corresponding hairs from the frontal scalp of nonbalding men or women, regardless of whether the hairs were incubated with tesetosterone or androstenedione.

Other studies have revealed that DHT can be formed from ADION, which appears to be a prehormone contained in the hair follicle. Dihydrotestosterone formation has been found to be more active in anagen rather than telogen follicles. Adachi and Kano (1970) have indicated that DHT is the active form that testosterone takes in the hair follicles. They showed that the activity of glucose-6-phosphate-dehydrogenase (G6PDH; a major enzyme in energy production), which is stimulated by cyclic adenosine monophosphate (cAMP), increases considerably during the anagen phase of hair growth. There is a correlation between the degree of progress of alopecia and the level of G6PDH activity in the follicle.

18.9.3 Theories of the Etiological Mechanism of Androgenetic Alopecia

18.9.3.1 Inhibition of Adenyl Cyclase Activity

Adachi (1973) also reported that DHT, but not testosterone, inhibited adenyl cyclase activity in the follicle matrix. The supposition was that male pattern baldness was controlled at the cellular level by 3′,5′-adenosine monophosphate, mediated via adenyl cyclase activity. Adachi and Kano (1970) thus hypothesized that baldness may result from a fall in cAMP levels producing a marked decrease in the activity of the protein kinase system, upon which the consecutive steps of glycolysis and protein synthesis depend. This modification in cellular metabolism may provoke a shortening of the anagen phase with an acceleration in the pilary cycle, exhausting the total number of cycles for which the hair is programmed within a few years.

In young, balding stump-tailed macaques, Takashima and Montagna (1974) found that DHT formation was greater in the hair follicles sited on the frontal scalp than in those in the occipital region; experiments with long-term injections of testosterone induced rapid transformation of terminal hairs to vellus hairs in the frontal scalp.

In humans, Bingham and Shaw (1973) found that in balding areas the affinity of the cytosol receptor for testosterone was greater and the 5α-reductase activity higher; thus, it is possible that bald scalp skin may metabolize greater amounts of androgens into 5α-DHT than nonbalding areas.

18.9.3.2 Defect in the Function of Dehydroepiandrosterone (DHEA)-17β-Hydroxysteroid Oxydoreductase (Fazekas and Sandor 1972, 1973)

Fazekas and Sandor (1972, 1973) observed two apparent characteristics in bald scalp hair follicles when DHEA was used as substrate; in their 1972 study, they reported that dehydroepiandrosterone had a strong inhibitory effect on the activity of 17β-hydroxysteroid oxydoreductase (17β-HO) in the hair follicle. The conversion of dehydroepiandrosterone into 5-androstenediol represents an inactivation step when the enzyme inhibitor becomes deactivated. Consequently, a defect in the function of the deactivating enzyme (17β-HO) would result in a higher intracellular concentration of dehydroepiandrosterone and an inhibition of G6PDH (a key enzyme for both glycolysis and nucleic acid synthesis). This phenomenon, in turn, would slow down the growth of hair and the hair cycle.

In a recent study, Puerto and Mallol (1990) reported similar findings; they studied 3–2, β-hydroxysteroid oxoreductase (3-α, β-Ho), using [^{3}H]DHT as a precursor, and measured the corresponding formed 3-α and 3-β androstanediols (α- and β-DIOL). The β-DIOL was the predominant metabolite, and total 3-α, β-HO activity was higher in the skin of areas showing alopecia than in non-alopecia areas.

18.9.3.3 Increased 17β-Hydrosteroid-Dehydrogenase (17β-HSD) Activity

Schweikert and Wilson (1974b) found that in the frontal hair follicles, the activity of 5α-reductase, as well as that of 17β-hydrosteroid-dehydrogenase (17β-HSD), was vigorous and the 5α-DHT produced was immediately converted to 5α-ADION, with the consequent loss of the male hormone effects. In general, the formation of 5α-reduced metabolites and 17-ketosteroid metabolites was greater in all sites of the scalp in bald men than in hair follicles obtained from corresponding sites in women and non-balding men. The activity of 17β-HSD was significantly higher in the bald frontal area of the bald men.

18.9.3.4 Other Factors

Also, Takashima et al. (1970) and Takashima and Montagna (1974) reported that, when the hair follicle was cultured with DHEA as the substrate, 5α-androstene-3β, 17β-diol was produced in the temporal region, while in the frontal region, the production of 17β-HSD was insufficient and DHEA remained in its original form. Takashima believed that DHEA may have accumulated in balding hair follicles. Since the addition of DHEA to G6PDH in the hair follicle decreases the activity of this enzyme, it can be concluded that a defect in energy metabolism will induce vellus transformation.

Here again, DHT need not necessarily behave as in other target tissues; the hypothesis does not stand against the finding that coarse terminal hairs retain a high rate of DHT transformation from testosterone, and there is no evidence to prove DHT to be a major androgen in the hair follicles of balding scalp skin.

Nikkari and Valavaara (1970) showed that 3β-androstenediol was a more powerful stimulator of sebum secretion in hypophysectomized female rats than DHT. It is possible that 3β-hydroxysteroid oxoreductase (3β-HO), which transforms DHT into 3β-androstanediol (3β-DIOL), could be involved in the localized metabolic disturbances of androgenic hormones in some tissues.

Sebaceous Gland Hypothesis of Androgenetic Alopecia (Inaba 1985; Inaba and Inaba 1992a) 19

If the basic concepts of treatment of male pattern baldness prove to be incorrect, the causative mechanism will not be revealed and effective treatment will not be developed for this condition.

19.1 Review of Hormonal Mechanisms in Hair Regeneration

Hamilton (1942) was the first to report that male hormones play a very important role in hair regeneration. Testosterone originally shows weak hormonal action, but, when it is converted to 5α-DHT (dihydrotestosterone) by 5α-reductase, this compound shows strong hormonal effects (Fig. 15.1).

Testosterone produced in the testes is carried to the hair matrix by plasma circulation and promotes hair formation when it is converted to DHT (Dorfman and Dorfman 1962; Anderson and Fulton 1973) (Fig. 19.1a). It still remains to be seen why DHT inhibits hair growth in the parietal region of the scalp while, on the other hand, it promotes the growth of beard and chest and axillary hair. Adachi and Kano (1970) found that DHT inhibited adenyl cyclase activity and that cell proliferation was inhibited as a result. The apparently contradictory phenomenon of 5α-DHT both promoting the growth of beard and chest and axillary hair and, at the same time, inhibiting the growth of hair in the parietal region has yet to be completely elucidated, and it has generally been accepted that hormonal imbalance plays a vital part in this phenomenon. We (Inaba et al. 1988b) conducted studies on the differences in male and female hormone receptor distribution in various regions of the scalp and at various ages but we found no differences in distribution (Section 15.4). According to Schweikert and Wilson (1974a), more 5α-reductase is present in the hair follicles in bald regions than in those in other regions. Although there have been several such reports, the causative mechanism of male pattern baldness has not yet been clearly elucidated.

19.2 Development of the Sebaceous Gland Hypothesis

The authors developed a radical surgical technique they called the subcutaneous tissue shaving method for the treatment of bromidrosis and hyperhidrosis (Inaba 1976; Inaba et al. 1978a,b). This treatment method has been explained in some detail in Chapter 8, but it is important to note that it is a method by which the sweat glands and hair roots are removed beneath the axillary skin. After the subcutaneous tissue is removed by a shaving technique, the surface skin is then grafted and preserved in place. It was found that when the sebaceous gland appended to the hair follicle was left intact, the hair would grow again, but if the sebaceous gland was removed, the hair would not regrow.

The central portion of the hair follicle was thought to lie at the lower portion of the telogen stage follicle. Clinical and histologic observation led to experimentation and the new hypothesis (sebaceous gland hypothesis) that the central generative site of the hair follicle also lies close to the duct opening of the sebaceous gland, especially in the sebaceous isthmus, in the upper isthmal portion of the hair follicle.

The new young hair is already formed at the lower portion of the germinal layer prior to the formation of a new hair bulb.

Pinkus and Mehregan (1981) cited our sebaceous gland hypothesis (Inaba et al. 1979a) in their book *The Guide to Dermatohistopathology*, 3rd edition: "This general scheme of the hair cycle has recently been challenged by Inaba et al. who found that axillary hair of Japanese is newly formed in the region of the sebaceous duct when dermal papilla and the entire lower part of the hair follicle have been surgically removed." (Inaba et al. 1981b, 1990b; Inaba and Inaba 1992a).

19.3 Mechanism of the Development of Androgenetic Alopecia

Can this sebaceous gland hypothesis shed any light on the onset of baldness? Generally speaking, baldness seems contingent on male hormone activity, but to simply say "the cause of baldness is hormone imbalance" falls short of the mark. In brief, the common explanation for the effect of male hormone activity is as follows. As shown in Fig. 19.1, the male hormone testosterone is produced in the testes, and it is then circulated to the dermal papilla in the hair bulb. Testosterone affects the hair matrix cells and interacts with the enzyme 5α-reductase in the cells. Testosterone is thereby converted into an even more powerful hormone, 5α-dihydrotestosterone (5α-DHT).

This particular hormone is said to accelerate cell division activity by anabolism and to encourage the formation of hair. In men, the phenomenon of body hair (such as the beard) appearing during puberty is a good example of the effect.

According to the hormone imbalance supposition, the parietal region of the scalp is controlled by the female hormone, which normally prevents women from experiencing baldness, whereas excessive production of male hormone, when conveyed to the hair follicle, inhibits the generation of new hairs by producing a hormone imbalance.

The testosterone is conveyed both to the hair bulb and to the sebaceous gland. Any explanation of baldness which excludes this fact can be very misleading.

Within the sebaceous gland, 5α-reductase converts testosterone to 5α-DHT. The blood vessels that surround the hair follicle (see Section 5.3) convey this 5α-DHT to the hair matrix, where, in excessive amounts, it acts to inhibit matrix activity by inhibiting the activity of adenyl cyclase.

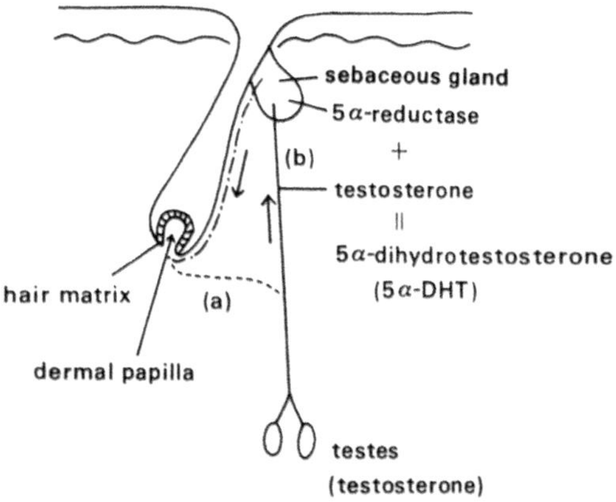

Fig. 19.1. Circulation of testosterone. Testosterone is converted to DHT mainly by 5α-reductase in the sebaceous gland, then binds to the receptors in the sebaceous gland cells, and acts on the nucleus to promote proliferation and enlargement of cells. This DHT acts secondarily on the dermal papilla and the matrix. (Reproduced with permission from Inaba 1985; Inaba and Inaba 1990b)

19.4 Hair Follicles and Sebaceous Glands Relative to 5α-DHT Production

Again, the larger the sebaceous gland becomes, the smaller the hair follicle (Montagna and Parakkal 1974). An abnormally enlarged sebaceous gland produces excess 5α-DHT and this inhibits the hair matrix. The result is that mature terminal hairs become downy (vellus) hairs. The authors believe that this is the principal causative mechanism of male pattern baldness (Inaba 1982a, 1985).

In the healthy hair follicle, the appended sebaceous gland is not large, so that the volume of 5α-reductase within it is normal. The action of this enzyme on testosterone does not cause the formation of large amounts of 5α-DHT. Rather, the formation of 5α-DHT in proper quantities enhances hair growth (Fig. 19.2a).

If, however, the sebaceous gland is enlarged for some reason, such as genetic inheritance, dietary habits, hormone influence, etc., the quantity of 5α-reductase will also increase and more 5α-DHT will be produced. Just as excessive use of fertilizer will stunt rather than enhance the growth of plants, too much 5α-DHT can act to inhibit hair growth. The authors have found that the effect of excessive 5α-DHT on the hair matrix is an inhibition of cell division and gradual atrophy of the hair follicle (Fig. 19.2b). This triggers the onset of baldness. We have said that an atrophied hair follicle is the cause of baldness, but this is not quite the same as loss of the hair root. In fact, the root remains but the hair grows thin and short, as a vellus hair (Fig. 19.2c).

Likewise, baldness does not imply that the sebaceous gland disappears. The hair can regenerate as long as the sebaceous gland exists, as we have already noted in touching on our treatment procedure for the relief of bromidrosis. Our own

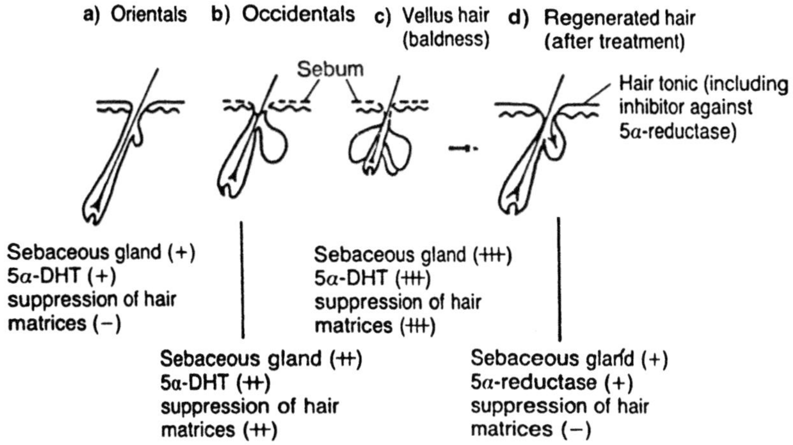

Fig. 19.2a–d. Hair follicles and sebaceous glands relative to 5α-DHT production. Orientals have follicles with quite small sebaceous glands and have a relatively low incidence of premature male pattern baldness (*MPB*). Occidentals, who typically consume much greater volumes of animal fats, have comparatively large sebaceous glands and a relatively high incidence of premature MPB. The vellus hair follicle typical of MPB has a supra-enlarged multilobular sebaceous gland, whereas the follicle of the terminal hair regenerated after treatment has a sebaceous gland of quite modest size. Levels of 5α-DHT production tend to be directly proportional to sebaceous gland size. (Reproduced with permission from Inaba 1985; Inaba and Inaba 1990b)

conviction that baldness can be prevented and cured comes from this particular discovery.

Actual treatment techniques for the relief of baldness will be described in later chapters (Chapter 28). In brief, however, the key factor seems to be the inhibition of excessive 5α-reductase activity in the sebaceous gland, and this provides the chief lead for the development of truly effective remedies.

Common premature baldness is subject to effective remedy. This type of baldness is, of course, quite different from the so-called scar-tissue (alopecia cicatrisata) type which will be described elsewhere (see Section 22.2). We find, in the common type of premature baldness, vellus-like hairs growing where the so-called bald spots appear. This finding points to excess production of 5α-DHT and consequent inactivation of the hair follicle. Accordingly, the hair could, theoretically, be regenerated by inhibiting the secretion of 5α-reductase from the sebaceous gland (Fig. 19.2d).

Once again, premature baldness (MPB) is not a phenomenon in which the hair root and sebaceous gland have died. The hair follicle becomes less active and atrophies, but does not disappear. In this condition, the regeneration of terminal hair, with proper remedial treatment, is not impossible.

19.5 Sebaceous Gland Hypothesis for Male Pattern Baldness; Supportive Findings

The process by which male pattern baldness develops can be explained by the sebaceous gland hypothesis, which proposes that the true hair center is located in the duct opening of the sebaceous gland (sebaceous isthmal portion) (see Section 14.1.4). Testosterone is first converted to DHT mainly by 5α-reductase in the sebaceous gland. It then binds to sebaceous gland cell receptors and acts on the nucleus to promote cell proliferation and enlargement. It may also act secondarily on the dermal papilla and the hair matrix through the vascular system in the connective tissue sheath surrounding the hair follicle (see Chapter 5). In brief, the condition of the sebaceous gland affects the hair root (Fig. 19.2) (Inaba 1985).

Takayasu et al. (1980), in effect, substantiated this finding by reporting that 5α-reductase was detected in greater amounts in sebaceous and apocrine glands than in the hair matrix. More recently, Sawaya et al. (1988a) found that sebaceous glands in the bald areas of male pattern alopecia had greater 3β-HSD (Δ^5-3β-hydroxysteroid dehydrogenase) activity in converting dehydroepiandrosterone (DHA) to Δ^4-androstenedione (Ad), as well as in converting androstanedione to testosterone, than those in hairy scalp areas. In a later study, Sawaya et al. (1988b) found greater androgen-binding capacity in the bald areas of male pattern alopecia than in hairy scalp areas. These findings, taken together, provide a biochemical explanation for the disease mechanism of androgenic alopecia.

As Lucky (1988) points out, the Sawaya findings represent another step forward in deciphering metabolic differences between "balding" and "hairy" scalp skin. The enzyme 3β-HSD, in converting DHA to Ad and androstenedione to testosterone (T), shows more activity in balding than in hairy scalp samples. By adding the precursor androgen [^{3}H]DHA to isolated sebocytes, Sawaya et al. (1988b) measured the amounts produced by the more potent androgenic metabolites, [^{5}H]androstenediol and [^{3}H]T. Moreover, they demonstrated this dichotomous activity, i.e., androgens stimulate the sebocyte stimulation, for the growth of secondary sexual hair and paradoxically for the regression of hair growth in the balding scalp. This was reflected in the specific 3β-HSD activity of the cytosolic fraction of sebocyte homogenates. Sawaya's studies (1988a,b) also illustrate the phenomenon of sebocytes metabolizing the "weak" androgen DHA to far more potent metabolites, such as T. The differences shown between balding and hairy skin indicate a potential role of excessive DHA in promoting baldness (reviewed from Lucky 1988).

Puerto and Mallol (1990) demonstrated that cytosol from the scalp skin of subjects affected by MPB did not bear a specific DHT receptor. They suggest that there is a specific binding protein for 3β-androstanediol (βDIOL) in the sebaceous gland of the alopecic-seborrheic scalp. The possibility is that βDIOL, but not DHT, could be the specific active metabolite of testosterone in the sebaceous gland and the substrate of androgen-transforming enzymes in the causative mechanisms of MPB.

With the development of the radical treatment for bromidrosis, we were able to elucidate a completely new concept of the generation and regeneration of hair, which, we presume, will contribute a great deal to the field of dermatology. The causative mechanisms of male pattern baldness have been found to be related to hereditary factors, hormones, and nutritional factors, and these findings have established a basic concept for the development of completely new hair tonics (Section 28.8.2). It should be noted that the above findings have consequently led to the worldwide approval of various patents related to hair-growing agents.

Histological Findings in Androgenetic Alopecia

20

20.1 Histological Findings

The balding process does not lead to a reduction of the number of hair follicles but to a reduction in their size (Van Scott and Ekel 1958). This phenomenon was first designated "vellus transformation" by Uno et al. (1969).

Apparent similarities between the histological changes in male pattern baldness and those in the skin of the aged have led some investigators to conclude that baldness is an exaggeration of the aging process (Singh and McKenzie 1961). The development of baldness is associated with shortening of the anagen phase of the hair cycle and, consequently, with an increase in the proportion of telogen hairs, which may be detected in trichograms of the frontovertical region before evident baldness is present (Rassner et al. 1963).

Recently, Sperling and Winton (1990) reported that transverse frozen sectioning with toluidine blue staining appeared to be a rapid and reliable tool for studying androgen alopecia.

20.1.1 Early Stages of Androgenetic Alopecia

Clinically visible reduction of the hair density and no significant histological changes are seen in this stage. The epidermis and dermal structures remain unaltered. The occurrence of inflammation in androgenetic alopecia has not been generally reported or emphasized (Lattanand and Johnson 1975). However, Kligman (1988) did report a significant degree of inflammation in patients with androgenic alopecia. Abell (1988) also noted an inflammatory reaction in 75% of balding patients, focal fibrosis in 25%, and destruction of follicular structures in 5%.

On some occasions, moderate infiltrates of mononuclear cells, together with a few mast and plasma cells, can be found around the hair follicle, and in some cases also around some dermal vessels (Allegra 1968; Orfanos 1990). The sebaceous gland and sweat glands appear normal in the early stage.

Sperling and Winton (1990) reported a mild to moderate inflammatory infiltrate at the level of the isthmus and infundibulum; they did not detect obvious inflammation in the lower portion of deeply seated follicles. The inflammation they detected can also be seen in scalp biopsies from normal patients and in those with seborrheic dermatitis. However, in our histological research we did not detect this inflammation (Fig. 20.1a,b).

20.1.2 Advanced Stages of Alopecia

The absence of normal anagen hair follicles and the frequent occurrence of miniaturized hair follicles together with others in telogen stage can be seen (Figs. 20.2a–b, 20.3a–c). A prominent enlargement of sebaceous glands was a constant feature in the middle stage (Allegra 1968) (Fig. 20.1a). Hori et al. (1972) found a decrease in the thickness of the epidermis, dermis, and subcutaneous tissue in advanced MPB, the extent ranging from 24% less than normal skin (Giacometti 1964; Salamon et al. 1975). Lattanand and Johnson (1975) found that the decrease in thickening of the corium was probably related to loss of constituents of the normal hair follicles, as well as to loss of connective tissue itself, and they observed significant gland enlargement in 76% of the specimens examined (Fig. 20.4a). Atrophy of sebaceous glands was not observed. However, Rampini et al. (1968) have stated that they were decreased in size. According to Orfanos (1990), one finds sebaceous glands with

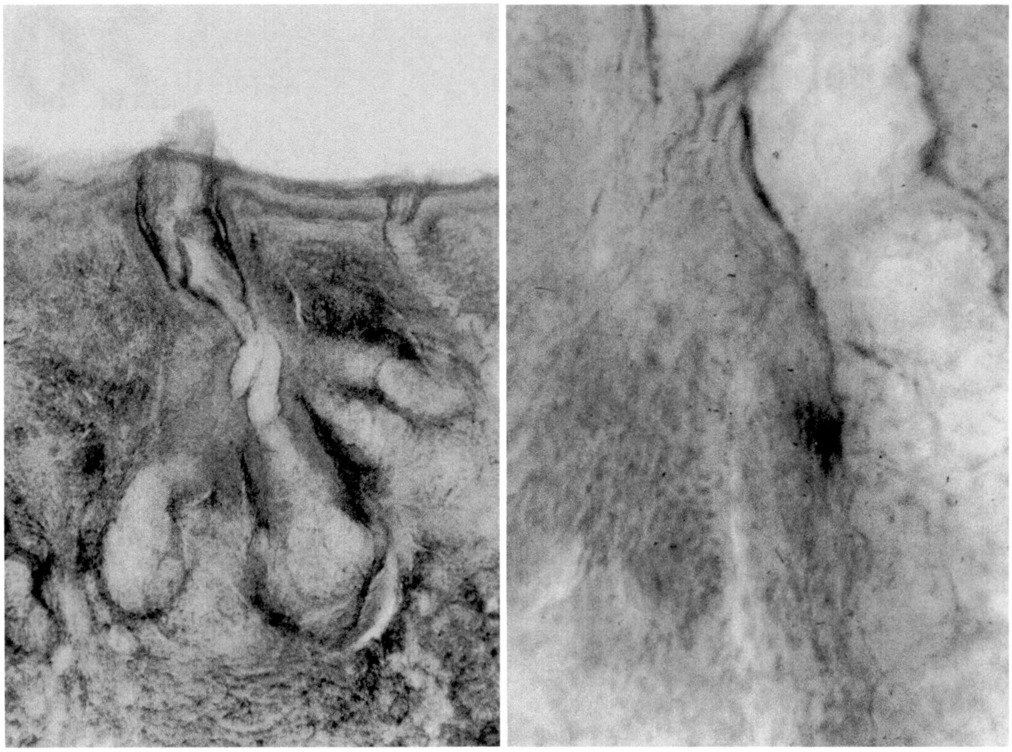
a b

Fig. 20.1. **a** Regenerating stage in the balding scalp hair follicle (hair germ stage). Sebaceous glands become multilobular. Hair germ can be seen to regenerate from the duct opening of two hypertrophic sebaceous glands. Scalp hair has already fallen out. ×135 **b** High-power view of **a**. Hair bud can be seen in hair germ stage. No inflammation can be seen in surrounding new hair germ. ×440

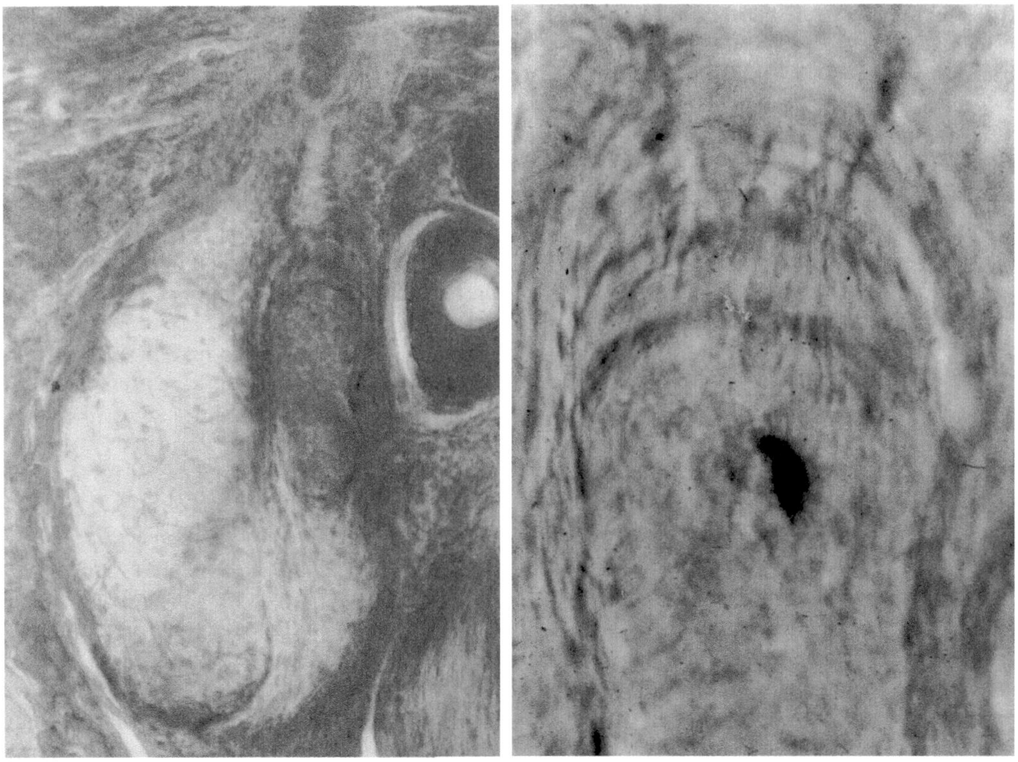
a b

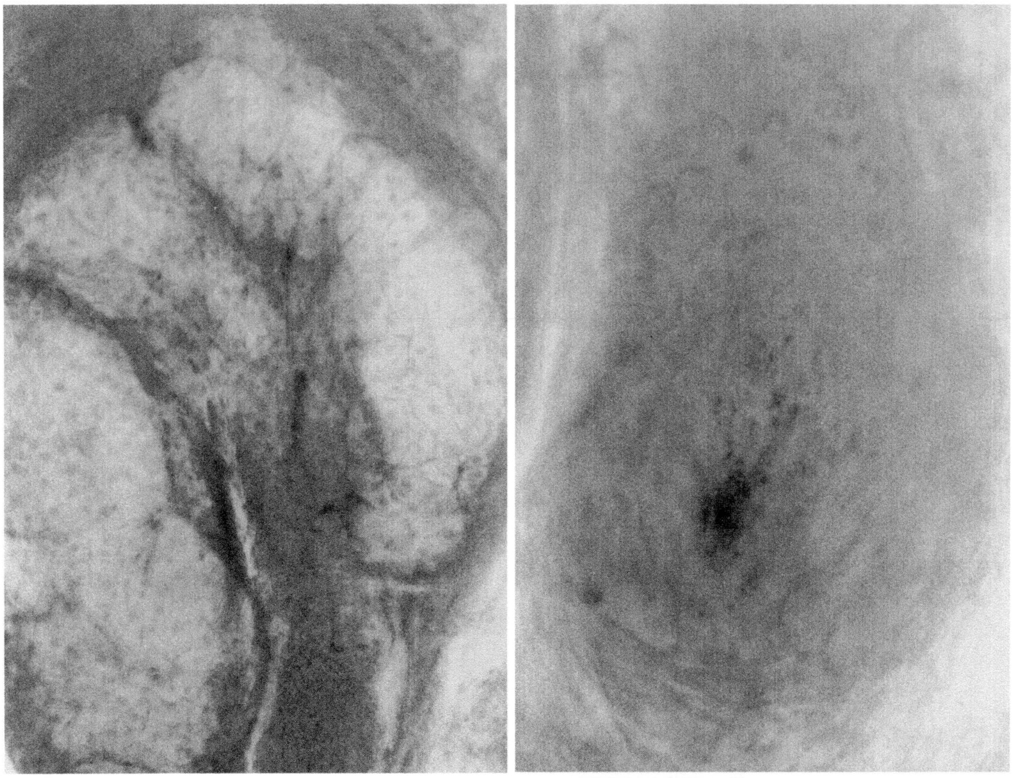

a b

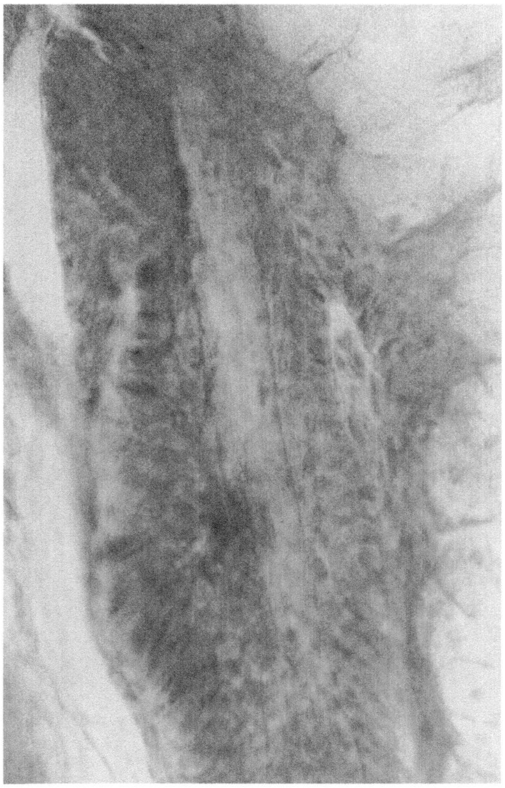

c

Fig. 20.3a–c. Regenerating state (bulbous peg stage). **a** Despite the small regenerating scalp hair follicle, this hair follicle is already in the bulbous peg stage. ×400 **b** *Lower portion* of the hair follicle shows bulbous configuration. Few dendritic melanocytes can be seen. ×800 **c** Vellus hair can be seen in the *upper portion* of the follicle. ×800

Fig. 20.2. **a** Regeneration state in balding scalp hair (hair peg stage). Minor hair buds can be regenerated from the duct opening of the sebaceous glands. Vellus hair can be seen in the upper portion of this hair follicle. ×400 **b** High-power view of **a**. Filamentous structure is formed from the surrounding germinal layer. ×800

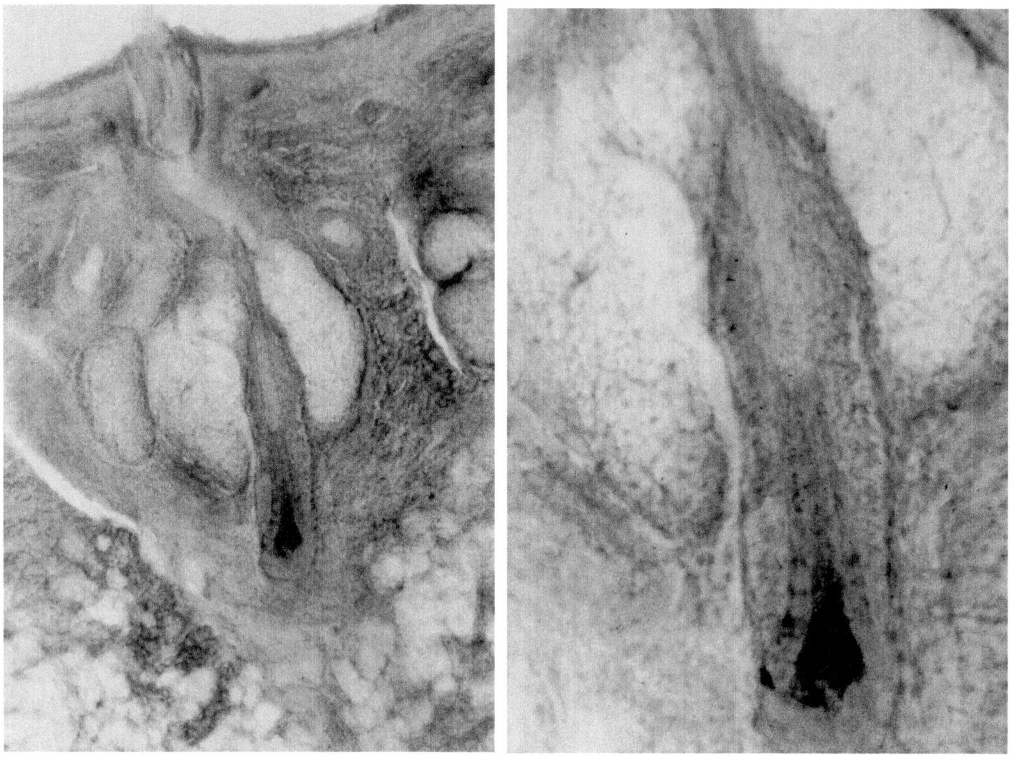

a b

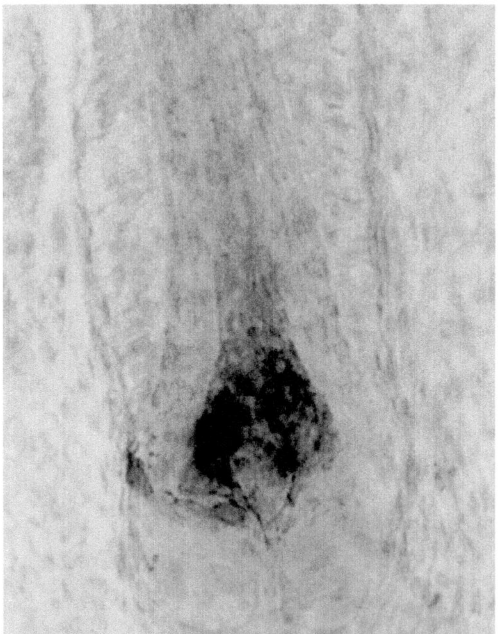

c

Fig. 20.4a–c. Regenerating state (terminal hair stage). **a** Regenerating hair follicle is already in terminal stage. Tiny hair is formed. The decrease in thickening of the carium can be seen. ×400 **b** High-power view of **a**. This miniature follicle shows the terminal phase. Regenerating hair is tiny. ×800 **c** High-power view of the *lower portion* of the newly-formed hair follicle. Dendritic melanocytes are formed from the matrix. ×800 an increased number of lobules in the later stages of androgenetic alopecia.

20.1.3 Transformed Vellus, Miniature Follicle

Transformed vellus follicles are shorter and thinner than those of normal anagen or telogen hairs; Areas of completely developed MPB usually contain only vellus hairs. Connective tissue streamers were present beneath every vellus follicle (Lattanand and Johnson 1975).

Transformed vellus hair follicles differ from true vellus follicles; the former retain an arrector pilarum muscle with or without direct contact to the hair sheath (Uno et al. 1968). Parts of the perifollicular connective tissue network are lost; only the arrector muscles and the enlarged sebaceous glands are then left behind in the middle dermis.

Vascularization of the vellus hair follicles shows only one or two capillaries associated with the hair bulb. The plexus around the sheath becomes obscure (Ellis 1958; Allegra 1968).

According to Orfanos (1990), the histological findings do not support the hypothesis that reduced blood supply may be of pathological significance in MPB. Vascular profiles are present in advanced stages without significant alterations or other signs of disturbed blood circulation. Also, the eccrine glands are never involved.

20.2 Histochemical Findings

Tissue-bound acid mucopolysaccharides were found to be slightly increased in androgenetic alopecia and eventually decreased in long-standing MPM (Crovato et al. 1968).

According to Lattanand and Johnson (1975), some specimens showed an increase in hyaluronic acid in the ground substance of the corium; occasionally this change was prominent.

The blood supply to the follicles, determined by the alkaline phosphatase method, appears to be normal in early MPB and reactive vessels remain in the streamers. Vascular insufficiency does not appear to have a causal role in MPB, but the decreased blood supply of vellus follicles is probably due to the needs of the small hair follicles.

The nerve plexus often remained intact after the follicle had changed to the vellus type and had completely withdrawn, or the nerves made up a part of the streamers. Giacometti and Montagna (1968) found that some perifollicular nerves became independent after miniaturization of the follicle and formed separate nerve endings in the dermis.

Enzyme studies have not shown any significant abnormalities in metabolism in MPB, except for increased enzyme activity, such as that of β-glucuronidase, associated with the degenerative or regressive follicular changes of catagen. Enzymatic activity is quite well represented in the hair follicles, even in baldness: this indicates that enzymatic defects should not be considered important factors in the genesis of MPB and, therefore, that the transformation of terminal to vellus hairs is not a sequence of degenerative changes but merely an irreversible transformation of the hair follicle (Allegra 1968).

There was absence or a decreased number of dopa-positive melanocytes in the bulb of the vellus follicles (Allegra 1968; Uno et al. 1968) (reviewed in Lattanand and Johnson 1975).

Causal Mechanism of Progressive Androgenetic Alopecia

21

Inaba and Inaba (1990a) indicate that the close relationship which exists between the hair follicles and sebaceous glands has special relevance to the incidence of androgenetic alopecia.

21.1 Fetal Period (Fig. 21.1)

The human forehead is first covered by lanugo hair, which is similar to vellus hair but much longer, growing from the forehead and over the scalp in equal distribution during the early fetal period. In the 5th month of gestation, the scalp hair becomes longer than the forehead hair and is in anagen phase (Pecoraro et al. 1964). This can occur under the influence of the maternal progesterone-dominant blood during the terminal stage of pregnancy. However, the borderline between the scalp and forehead hair is still not clear. The lanugo hairs appear to be synchronized in anagen in fetal life at 5 months, but this occurs before terminal hairs appear in all three phases of hair growth (Barman et al. 1967). Between the 10th and 8th week before birth, the hair in the frontal and parietal regions in most cases will be found in catagen or telogen phase and provides the first hair-shedding event for the individual.

In this area, a new growth cycle appears about 5 to 6 weeks before term, so that, at birth, the scalp follicles are in all three phases of the growth cycle (Barman et al. 1964). In the occipital region, however, the follicles remain in anagen until term, when they too change to telogen.

The sebaceous gland is quite well developed by the 3rd or 4th month of fetal body hair growth. With maternal androgen stimulation received through placental infusion, the gland begins to develop in the embryonic stage.

Sebum, the product of the sebaceous gland, makes a significant contribution to the vernix caseosa.

21.2 Neonatal Period

During the first 3 months after birth dihydrotestosterone (DHT) formation in the forehead rises, and then progressively falls, until in the adult, DHT formation is as low as in the foreskin.

The lanugo hair comes to its peak in the 32nd week of the fetal period, after which the hair is gradually transformed to telogen hair and remains as such until about the 15th postnatal week. It is then replaced by coarse hair in the scalp (Lynfield 1960). The hairline between the frontal and parietal area is clearly discernible. The telogen ratio is reported to be 60% in the infant frontal area several weeks after birth and then it decreases to 20% in the adult (Barman et al. 1967).

In the scalp of a neonate, the hairs in the parietal and frontal areas are thinner than those in other areas. Therefore, they acquire an appearance similar to male pattern baldness (infant male pattern baldness) (Fig. 21.2a). Agache et al. (1980) have observed a male pattern alopecia up to Hamilton's type IV occurring in both sexes a few weeks after birth, and spontaneously subsiding by the 3rd or 4th month. This phenomenon of the first hair shedding occurs within 1 year postnatally, irrespective of sex.

From the 18th week of postnatal life, the hair, individually or in groups, manifests a modification of the duration of the cyclic changes, which results in a mixed distribution (mosaicism) of the different phases of the cycle over the entire scalp (Barman et al. 1967).

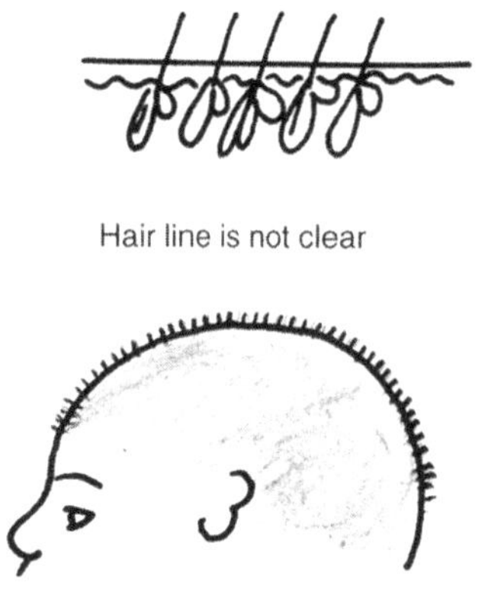

Fig. 21.1. Fetal period. The human forehead in the fetal period is covered by lanugo hair. The borderline between the forehead and the scalp is not clear. (Permission from Inaba and Inaba 1994a)

Emanuel (1936) was the first to demonstrate that the sebum level in newborn babies can be nearly as high as that in adults. The levels then gradually decline, remaining at a very low baseline level until puberty. The skin surface lipid composition in the newborn is similar to that of an adult; cholesterol levels are low and the levels of wax esters and squalene are high (reviewed from Ramastry et al. 1970).

Plasma levels of dehydroepiandrosterone (DHEA) seem to be a plausible sebum stimulus, since they are elevated at birth (by 10–15 times the levels of other androgens) in both sexes equally and they gradually decrease during the first 3 months of life (De Peretti and Forest 1976).

Although there is a wide individual range, sebum levels in the 1st week of life are very high and are of the same magnitude as those in adults. Females display a different pattern of sebum excretion from males. On the 1st day of life, levels in females are lower than in males, but a large increase takes place between the 3rd and 6th day, followed by a fall, bringing the level below that of the males. At 6 months, the levels are low in both sexes (Agache et al. 1980).

21.3 Childhood Period

During childhood, the mosaic pattern becomes consolidated. During the years before puberty an average of 94% of follicles are in anagen stage and 6% in telogen stage, but there are regional variations. In the frontal region, 10% of follicles are in telogen stage, and in the occipital only 3% are in telogen stage (Pecoraro et al. 1964).

The enlarged sebaceous glands characteristic of the fetus begin to gradually shrink in size in the forehead; this can be detected by an increase in the percentage of cholesterol and a decrease in the percentage of wax esters and squalene (Pochi et al. 1977). At the same time, lanugo hairs vanish during infancy and childhood, and become vellus hairs.

21.3.1 Process Underlying the Increase in Scalp Hair

In the scalp crown region during childhood we observe the growth of coarse scalp hairs (Fig. 21.2b). The diameter of scalp hairs tends to increase with the advance of age. It seems to require

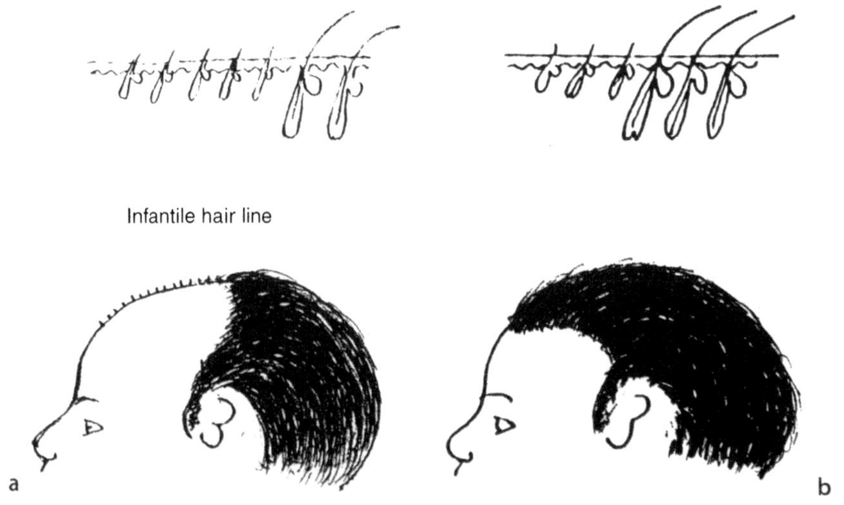

Fig. 21.2a,b. Childhood period, vellus hair. **a** In the scalp of the neonate, the hairs in the parietal and frontal areas are thinner than those in other areas (infant male pattern baldness). **b** The increase in frontal hair density depends on an increase in the diameter of individual hairs. The hairline is clearly discernible

several years before the complete forehead borderline is established. It is evident that androgen acts not only on the hair bulb (matrix) but that it also causes the enlargement of the sebaceous gland. Its secondary effect on the matrix prompts the growth of coarse terminal hairs to replace existing vellus hairs (Inaba et al. 1981d). The hair borderline above the forehead then becomes perfectly distinct. Between the ages of 1 and 2 years, most infants acquire a complete borderline called "the infantile hairline."

21.3.2 Formation of Solitary Coarse Hairs in the Scalp

The appearance of the lanugo hair in infancy and in childhood (infant male pattern baldness) is similar to that of androgenetic alopecia. This lanugo hair is shed, and the coarse hair then appears to be formed from the upper isthmal portion of the follicle. This process may be similar to the formation of solitary coarse hair in the axillary region (see Section 6.4.2).

With the onset of puberty, the sebaceous glands in the axillae are once again remarkably enlarged and take on a multilobular shape similar to that of a bell pepper. The vellus hair dies. Formation of a new hair bud and a new coarse hair begins from the sebaceous isthmus, that is, the upper isthmal portion of the follicle adjacent to the opening of the sebaceous duct (Inaba et al. 1981d). The new hair pegs downward until the formation of a new hair bulb (matrix) is completed. It then grows toward the epidermal surface as a coarse terminal hair (Fig. 21.3a, Fig. 6.6a–d). The same phenomenon may occur in the scalp hairs. This replacement of scalp hair occurs in a hereditary fashion (Fig. 21.3a).

21.3.3 Formation of Bundle Hairs (Groups of Coarse Hairs) (Fig. 21.3b) (Fig. 6.8)

The sebaceous gland has hypertrophied and developed two or three distinct lobes. A new primary central coarse hair follicle descends from the neck of the gland (the sebaceous isthmus of the original follicle). Two or three secondary follicles may later be formed from the same region (similar to the process in axillary hairs) (see Section 6.4).

The new hairs that emerge from the sebaceous isthmus of multilobular sebaceous glands first develop in groups of two or more hairs that emerge from a common ostium. The emergence of these hairs, in close association with the sebaceous gland, is more evidence that new hairs can be formed from the sebaceous isthmus of the hair follicle, requiring no bulb in the initial period of growth. The increase in hair density is accompanied by an increase in the diameter of individual hairs and by the formation of bundle hairs (Fig. 21.3b).

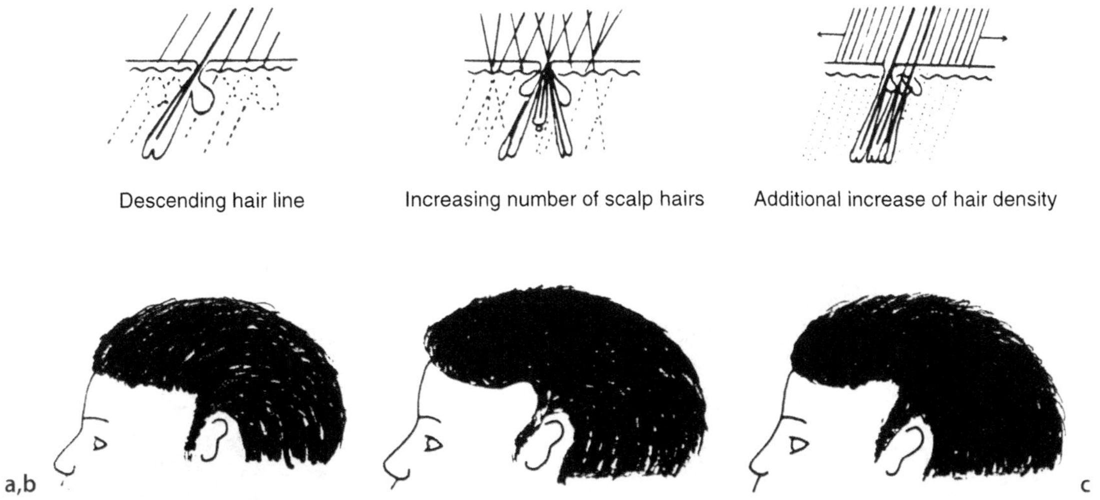

Fig. 21.3a–c. Adolescent period. **a** Formation of single coarse hair. When the sebaceous gland becomes hypertrophied the vellus hair is shed and a single coarse hair then develops. **b** Formation of bundle hair. When the sebaceous gland becomes multilobular, with two or three lobes, bundle hair develops from the duct opening of the sebaceous gland. **c** Formation of independent hairs. Hair bundles pull apart and form a separate ostium, and hair groupings are formed

21.3.4 Formation of Independent Hairs (Stage of Separated Follicle) (Fig. 21.3)

The generally accepted opinion is that lanugo hair grows densely during the fetal period, with new primary or secondary hair follicles formed among the first follicles. Hair grouping, the trio arrangement, becomes gradually inconspicuous as aging advances (Ellis 1958; Salamon et al. 1975). There are no marked changes in the other adnexal organs. True neogenesis of hair does not occur at any time throughout human life after the 7th month of fetal life.

According to Inaba et al. (1982), the secondary follicles develop on either side of the preexisting follicles and usually form groups of three as the skin surface expands.

If this is so, what mechanism underlies the remarkable increase in the density of terminal hairs during and after the childhood years?

If no other follicles are formed, the final number of mature terminal hairs, thus spread far apart, would seem quite sparse as the scalp continues to expand until the adult stage. However, the growth is actually quite dense until late childhood.

Inaba et al. (1981d) (see Chapter 6) have reported that, in childhood, vellus hairs of the axillary regions are formed as individual units equidistant from one another. After puberty begins, coarse hairs emerge in bundles.

In time, some of these hair bundles pull apart and form a separate ostium, with each hair then becoming independent, while other bundle hairs continue to remain in groups of two or more growing from a common ostium. The overall result is the replacement of vellus hairs by coarse hairs in greater abundance and a variation in the growth pattern (Fig. 6.14).

21.4 Adult Period (Fig. 21.4)

No generation of new hairs is observed, in contrast to the process in adolescence. However, with the emergence of bundle hairs (compound bundle hairs), scalp tension, and the separation of bundles, the hair density in the scalp increases. Some of the independent hairs are again grouped to form bundle hairs, increasing the density of scalp hair, which appears thick and glossy, making it the symbol of youth (Fig. 21.4).

The thickness of the scalp hair shaft is at a peak between the ages of 22 and 27 years and declines steadily thereafter. According to Montagna and Parakkal (1974), from about 16 to 46 years of age, hair density and thickness in the scalp decrease progressively in both sexes, most noticeably in the vertex.

21.5 Balding Period (Solitary Coarse Hairs) (Fig. 21.5)

In alopecia areata, hairs fall out in clear circles, while in male pattern baldness, the scalp skin sur-

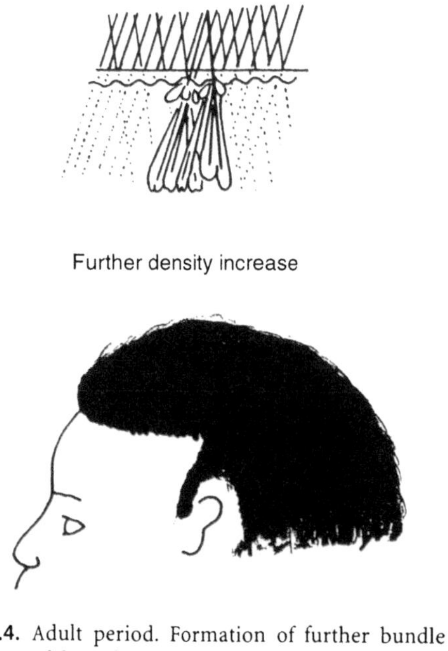

Fig. 21.4. Adult period. Formation of further bundle hair. Some of the independent hairs in the hair grouping again form bundle hairs. Scalp hairs increase during this period

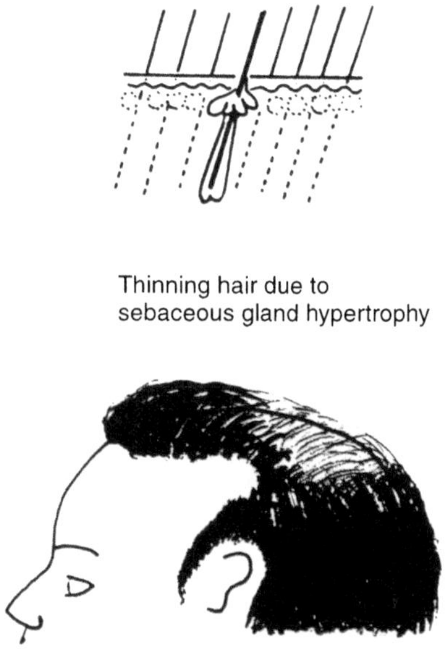

Fig. 21.5. Balding period. Formation of solitary coarse hair. When the sebaceous glands become hypertrophied, only solitary coarse hairs develop.

face gradually becomes more and more visible as the compound hairs become solitary coarse hairs. This is the omen of male pattern baldness (Fig. 21.5).

A definite danger signal is that hairs in the parietal temporal regions have become thinner than those in the lateral region of the scalp. Thinning hairs are a definite sign that the process of baldness has begun.

Increased responsiveness and availability of receptors in the hair follicles, e.g., in the frontal and the central parietal area, is a necessary prerequisite for the development of androgen-dependent alopecia, whereas occipital hair is generally preserved (Orfanos 1990).

21.5.1 Mechanism of Solitary Coarse Hair Formation

According to Giacometti (1964), coarse hairs will become softened and compound (bundle) hairs will become solitary hairs. In normal healthy individuals, the number of hairs per unit area will be reduced by about 38% between the ages of 30 and 80 years.

In order to find why compound hairs become solitary coarse hair, the authors (Inaba and Inaba 1990b) attempted to study the process of regeneration by applying an anti-cancer agent (methotrexate) over the skin surface of a mouse, thus experimentally creating solitary hair follicles (Fig. 12.10) (see Section 12.3).

According to the conventional hair cycle theory, regeneration starts individually from the lower end of each compound hair follicle (two to three hairs are present in a single ostium). Contrary to this expectation, Inaba and Inaba (1990b, 1992a) found a single mass of mesenchymal cells to be newly formed at the lower end of the compound hair follicle, and the epithelial cell layer (hair bud) migrated from the sebaceous isthmus by the recovery of the vascular system surrounding the compound hair follicle and the remaining sebaceous glands. Generation of the mass of mesenchymal cells (future dermal papilla) does not necessarily start from the remnant dermal papilla cells or secondary hair germ located at the lower end of telogen follicles. This finding is supported by the regeneration from a remaining single hair follicle shown after the follicle was damaged by an anti-cancer agent (see Section 12.3, Fig. 12.10). Therefore, no secondary hair germ is seen at the lower end of the telogen follicle, but it may possibly be formed by newly-formed epithelial cells derived from the upper isthmal portion, in particular, the sebaceous isthmus, and mesenchymal cells may be formed later (Section 12.2).

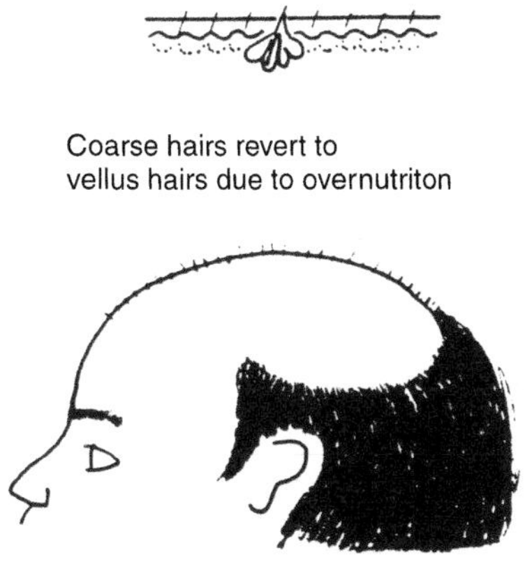

Fig. 21.6. Complete baldness. The sebaceous gland becomes more and more enlarged. Large amounts of dihydrotestosterone (*DHT*) produced in the sebaceous gland act to inhibit hair growth, and coarse hairs revert to vellus hair

When the sebaceous glands become enlarged, or at the onset of disorders in their function in the scalp hair cycle, only solitary coarse hairs regenerate, due to inhibition of secondary or third hair follicle formation by large amounts of DHT produced in the sebaceous gland (see Chapter 7). No compound hair follicles are formed in scalps with a predisposition to MPB. The hair density decreases, making the skin surface visible. On the other hand, when the sebaceous glands are smaller, and become functional, two to three coarse hairs may regrow to the former state.

21.6 Complete Baldness

(Fig. 21.6)

If the sebaceous glands become more and more enlarged, or at the onset of disorders in their function, large amounts of DHT produced in the sebaceous glands can be conveyed to the hair bulb through the system of blood vessels in the connective tissue that surrounds both the glands and the follicles. This is the circulatory connection between the sebaceous glands and the dermal papilla (bulb matrix). It is quite evident that most of the testosterone conveyed directly from the testes goes into the sebaceous glands, where the 5α-reductase enzyme converts it into DHT, which acts to inhibit hair growth by restricting adenyl cyclase activity to such a degree that the follicle regresses from terminal to vellus hair conditions (Adachi 1973) (see Section 19.2; Inaba and Inaba 1990b, 1992a).

Differential Diagnosis (Types of Baldness Other than Male Pattern Baldness)

22

22.1 Alopecia Areata

The differential diagnosis of androgenetic alopecia will sometimes not be easy to establish, particularly because centroparietal thinning based on telogen effluvium is not specific.

Alopecia areata is a "round spot" type of baldness (alopecia areata with single patch). Alopecia areata may begin with and simulate diffuse hair loss, whereby circumscribed lesions will appear only after a few weeks or months. Its site is almost always the occipital region of the scalp. If all the hair on the scalp is lost, the condition is called alopecia totalis. If, in addition, there is complete or virtually complete loss of body hair, then the disorder is designated alopecia universalis. Alopecia aphiasis, in which large bald patches with clear borderlines appear along the hairline of the occipital to temporal regions, in particular, is often observed in infants. Sometimes only the thick terminal hairs are lost, so that, with a hand lens and cross-lighting, vellus hairs can be seen.

In alopecia areata, the hair follicles do not undergo normal cyclic changes but remain at approximately the anagen IV stage of growth. In a fresh lesion of alopecia areata, there is often a unique hair shaft. Hair follicles may become like an exclamation mark in appearance or be precipitated into catagen and telogen stages (Van Scott and Ekel 1958).

Frequency of recurrence is high in alopecia areata with multiple patches, alopecia totalis, alopecia universalis, and alopecia aphiasis and low in alopecia areata with a single patch. The rate of recurrence is about 40%, and this occurs within a few months to 5 years after a temporary cure (Sato 1981). It is not accompanied by much soreness or itching, and may go unnoticed until brought to the individual's attention by a barber or by other people.

Another characteristic of alopecia areata is its clear borderline. Inside this border, hairs come out easily when pulled. If left alone, the condition may return to normal with a new growth of terminal hairs. However, occasionally, the bald spot spreads rapidly over the entire head. In rare cases, the overlapping of androgenic alopecia with alopecia areata may occasionally occur, and differential diagnosis may give rise to considerable difficulties.

This type of baldness can occur quite early in life; for example, during adolescence or in the prime of life, when mental and physical activity is vigorous. It occurs in Japanese teenagers when they are involved in the extremely stressful competition for high marks in school examinations. This lends some credence to the supposition that baldness can be caused by psychosomatic stress.

22.1.1 Possible Etiologic Mechanism of Alopecia Areata

The etiology of alopecia areata has not yet been clarified, although immunological factors are now considered as causative mechanisms (Sato 1981; Gollnick and Orfanos 1990). This is because complications may be observed in patients with thyroid disease, diabetes, or various endocrine diseases. In addition, it has also been reported that alopecia areata may be due to the destruction of hair matrix cells brought on by an autoimmune mechanism in which lymphocytes heavily infiltrate the periphery of the hair bulb (Fig. 22.1) (Ebling and Cunliffe 1986; Gollnick and Orfanos 1990). However, at present, the production of autoantibodies has not been proven (Calver et al. 1992; Klaber and Munro 1978; Schenk 1980).

Alopecia areata, the most common form of pathological hair loss, still poses a number of a 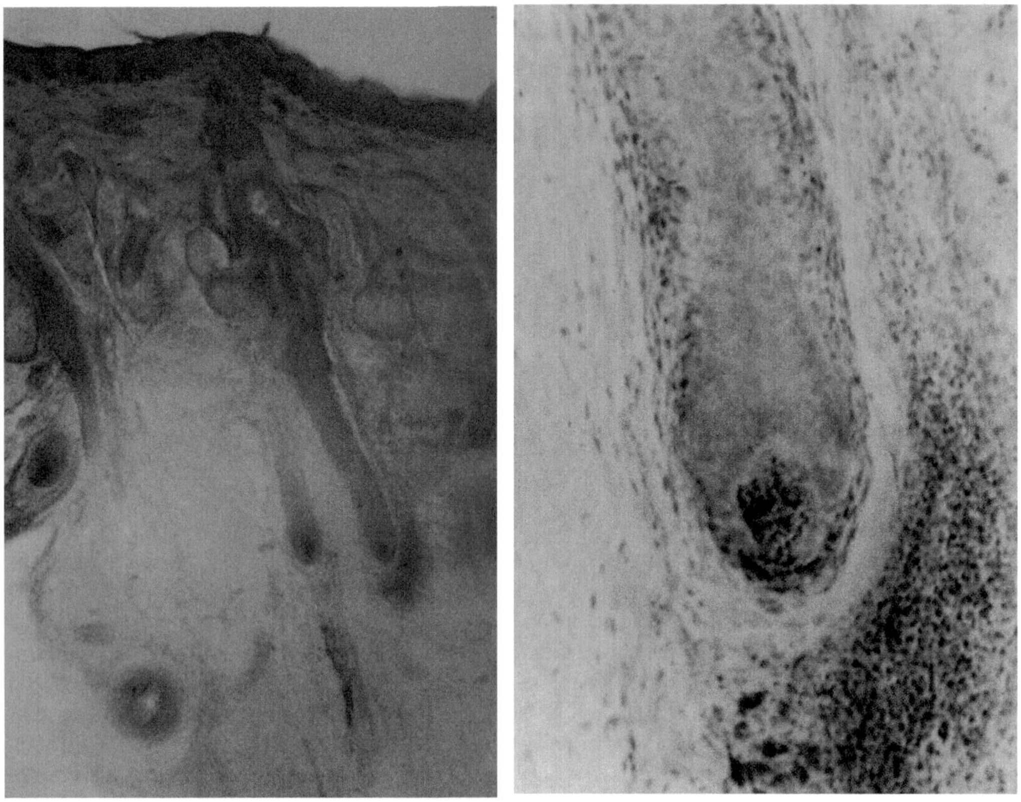 b

Fig. 22.1. **a** Onset of alopecia areata. Lymphocyte infiltration can be seen below the hair bulb. ×135 **b** High-power view of **a**. ×400

problems. Immunofluorescent studies have been negative for the deposition of immunoglobulin in the hair follicles of alopecia areata (Igarashi et al. 1980).

In 1977, Rook hypothesized that alopecia areata may be a heterogenous syndrome, in the light of the different findings of various authors regarding family background, the presence of other disease, age of onset, and response to therapy. The presence of autoimmune (Mitchell and Krull 1984; Editorial 1984) disease has also been implicated, and there may be an association with atopy (Lutz et al. 1988). Undoubtedly, heredity also plays an important role in alopecia areata (Ebling and Cunliffe 1986).

A high rate of HLA antigen B12 was reported by Kianto et al. (1977) to be characteristic of this condition. However, Kuntz et al. (1977) and Gollnick and Orfanos (1990) reported no definite association of alopecia areata with a particular HLA antigen.

Recently, Imai et al. (1994) investigated the populations of activated (HLA-DR+CD_3+) cells and natural killer (CD57-CD16+) cells in the peripheral blood of patients with various types of alopecia areata. They indicate that both HLA cells in the peripheral blood of patients with alopecia areata may be correlated with the disease activity of alopecia areata.

In terms of the relationship of primary factor T cells to cellular immunity, Brown et al. (1980) reported a decrease in the T-cell count in the peripheral circulatory system in blood samples taken from alopecia areata patients. Gianetti et al. (1978) reported a significant decrease in the number of circulating T cells in patients with alopecia areata, while B cells and Null cells did not significantly differ in numbers from those found in controls.

Inaba (1985) reported that the number of T cells remained the same in alopecia areata patients, not decreasing in comparison to the normal population, except in quite severe cases of alopecia totalis and universalis, when a slight decrease was noted (Tables 22.1 and 22.2).

Van Baar et al. (1994) reported cytokeratin expression in alopecia areata hair follicles. They compared the expression of cytokeratins in normal hair follicles to that of alopecia areata using immunohistology with monoclonal antibodies. A number of cytokeratins were specifically ex-

Table 22.1. Distribution of lymphocyte populations in peripheral blood of patients with alopecia areata (A.a.)

Clinical form of alopecia areata	No. of cases	T cell	B cell	Monocyte	Double marker cell (D cell)	Null cell
A.a. with single patch	5	79.4 ± 7.2	7.8 ± 2.7	1.9 ± 0.71	1.1 ± 1.5	9.8 ± 6.4
A.a. with multiple patches	13	75.9 ± 13.3	13.5 ± 9.4	2.42 ± 1.6	0.65 ± 0.69	7.5 ± 6.7
A. totalis	11	66.3 ± 11.3	18.4 ± 11.7	2.68 ± 2.7	1.18 ± 1.3	11.4 ± 7.3
A. universalis	15	68.6 ± 11.6	15.9 ± 7.2	3.06 ± 1.7	1.2 ± 1.7	11.3 ± 8.1
Total	44	71.4 ± 12.3	14.9 ± 9.2	2.64 ± 1.9	1.02 ± 1.1	10 ± 7.3
Normal population		58–74.2	13.1-23.5	2.4–8.3	1.0–3.0	3.4–13.9

Table 22.2. Distribution of three different lymphocyte populations in peripheral blood of normal subjects

Subject No.	T cell (%)	B cell (%)	Monocyte (%)	Null cell (%)
1	80.0	6.5	3.5	10.0
2	85.5	9.5	1.0	2.5
3	70.0	12.5	0.5	16.5
4	82.0	8.5	3.0	6.0
5	75.0	5.5	2.0	16.5
6	68.5	14.5	2.0	14.5
Mean	76.83	9.50	2.00	11.00
± SD	6.21	3.16	1.04	5.34

pressed in defined anatomical parts of the follicle; however, no gross qualitative or quantitative differences were found between normal and diseased scalps. Interestingly, the expression of cytokeratin 16, which is modulated by conditions that affect the rate of keratinocyte proliferation, was found to be unchanged in the outer root sheath of alopecia areata follicles. This is in contrast with earlier observation of a decrease in the expression of the proliferation-associated Ki-67 nuclear antigen.

Anderson (1950) reported that 23% of his patients with alopecia areata had a shock or another acute anxiety experience in their personal history and that an additional 22% suffered from mental disturbances; the notion that mental stress causes degeneration of the connective tissues surrounding the blood vessels that feed the hair papilla (Greenberg 1955) is no longer commonly believed (Muller and Winkelmann 1963).

Masters (1984) mentioned a dramatic increase in the number of alopecia areata patients during the last weeks before the Allied invasion of Normandy in the summer of 1944 during World War II.

There are various other suppositions about the mechanisms and processes involved in this factor of psychosomatic stress (Invernizzi et al. 1987). One explanation points to autonomic nervous system imbalance. The autonomic nervous system controls the activity of the blood vessels and physical motion. It can be negatively affected by excessive psychosomatic tension, causing nervous system instability.

This instability can trigger off continuous spasms in the capillaries surrounding the dermal papilla at the hair root and can aggravate blood circulation in the vicinity of the papilla, with the result that the hair root area becomes undernourished.

In alopecia areata, metabolic activity is inhibited mainly in the connective tissue (Pierard and de la Brassinne 1975) whereas, in the hair bulbs, the synthesis of DNA and RNA is not changed. The same process is also observed within the large undifferentiated compartment of the sebaceous glands.

In a series of papers, Inaba and Inaba (1990b, 1992a) have reported a hypothesis that the true center of hair generation is not only located in the hair root, but also in the upper isthmal portion of the hair follicle close to the duct opening of the sebaceous gland (sebaceous isthmus). It was noted that nerve plexuses, which could innervate hair follicles, were found in the upper isthmal portion, close to the secretory duct opening of the sebaceous gland, and that these plexuses contained both sensory and autonomic nerves. A further suggestion has been made that nervous stress induces atrophy of the sebaceous gland, resulting in its dysfunction and leading to the onset of alopecia areata (see Chapter 16).

A few important reports have noted sebaceous gland activity in alopecia areata. Although the sebaceous glands in this condition have usually been considered as normal in size, in contrast to the usual enlargement in male pattern baldness (MPB), a general reduction in the volume of sebaceous glands has been reported to occur during hair loss caused by alopecia areata (Moretti et al. 1963). Okochi (1968) has studied sebum secretion and perspiration at the lesion sites of skin disease. He found that sebum was secreted in small amounts immediately after the onset of hair loss, when vellus hair was not visible, and reported that the secretion of sebum was normalized at the growth stage when vellus hairs emerged.

Brown et al. (1982) examined the gonadal status in ten alopecia areata patients and found unilateral testicular atrophy in two and bilateral testicular atrophy in one, showing dysfunction with oligospermia to aspermia. This testicular atrophy may induce atrophy of the sebaceous gland.

In prolonged alopecia areata, the secretory activity of the sebaceous glands declines with the duration of the disease (Schweikert 1967).

Inaba (1985) has found that sebum secretion generally tends to decrease in patients with alopecia areata. Enhancement of sebum secretion with androgen agents stimulates hair regrowth in affected regions.

On observing the nerve plexus on the hair follicle in detail, it can be seen that the nerve end has the shape of a fork at the point where the duct opening of the sebaceous gland comes into contact with the hair follicle's upper isthmal portion (Ishibashi and Tsuru 1976). It is precisely from this upper isthmal portion that hairs deprived of a lower hair root can begin to regenerate. The fact that the nerve end is located here is very suggestive of the causative mechanisms of alopecia areata (see Section 14.1.2, Stem Cells). Up to now this nerve plexus has been considered only a sensory nerve. However, if it also has autonomic characteristics, it would be subject to dysfunction. If so, we would have an important clue concerning trophopathy of the hair follicle and the sebaceous gland.

The marked contrast of alopecia areata to premature baldness may be due to the sebaceous gland beginning to atrophy due to nervous stress. This explanation agrees with the finding reported by Okochi (1968) that enzyme is excreted from the sebaceous gland in small amounts in the early period of hair loss. In stable, stress-free conditions, trophopathy may also come to a halt and the lipid condition in the scalp would gradually normalize in association with activation of the sebaceous gland. This coincides with the finding that sebaceous gland excretion is enhanced at the stage of vellus hair growth.

Inaba and Inaba (1990b, 1992a) do not attribute alopecia areata to autoimmunity, but postulate that the disease is caused by injury of the upper hair stem cells resulting from stress-induced atrophy of the sebaceous isthmus close to the duct opening of the sebaceous gland (see Section 14.1.2, Stem Cells).

Goldsmith (1991) states that an intrinsic abnormality in a follicle component, for example, in follicular keratinocytes or melanocytes, is responsible for triggering the immune reaction, which then causes internal damage to the hair follicle sufficient to prevent hair fiber production.

22.1.2 Various Treatments for Alopecia Areata

As described above, the lack of understanding of the basic mechanism underlying the inhibition of hair growth in alopecia areata is reflected by the absence of a consistently effective therapy (Perret and Happle 1990). The most promising approach is topical immunotherapy, and corticosteroids still seem to have, at least under certain circumstances, a limited place in the treatment of this condition. Cyclosporin has serious side effects. Other therapeutic agents, such as topically applied minoxidil, have gained much attention (see below). To date, many treatments for alopecia areata have been examined, treatment with a contact allergen, in particular, psoralen (oral) with long-wavelength ultraviolet light (PUVA) therapy, being regarded as the most efficaceous. The first report on the treatment of alopecia areata with 8-methoxypsoralen and sunlight was made by Rollier and Warcewski (1974). However, the effectiveness of PUVA therapy is controversial (Weissmann et al. 1978; Lassus et al. 1980; Amer and El-Garf 1983). The therapeutic value of topical minoxidil in alopecia areata has been investigated in recent years, with variable results (Toda 1989). There have been reports of a decrease in the perifollicular infiltrates of mononuclear leukocytes, particularly T lymphocytes, which decrease characterizes this condition in patients responding to minoxidil (Fenton and Wilkinson 1983). However, Khoury et al. (1992) reported that, interestingly, no significant differences in the extent or composition of the perifollicular infiltrates were detected at week 12 between patients receiving minoxidil (5%) and placebo, or between the week-12 and week-24 biopsies of those patients who first received placebo and then minoxidil. These findings indicate that, in alopecia areata, the reduction in perifollicular T-cell infiltration associated with cosmetically acceptable hair regrowth is not attributable to an effect of topical minoxidil.

The authors believe that, by improving the blood flow of the subpapillary blood plexus by irritating the scalp skin, as is done in the PUVA therapy, the microcirculation to the hair follicle is improved and the stem cells in the sebaceous isthmus are stimulated to induce hair regeneration (see Section 5.2; Fig. 22.2a–c).

However, immunological factors may operate in the heterogenous syndrome or surrounding hair follicle as a result of the remaining degenerated hair.

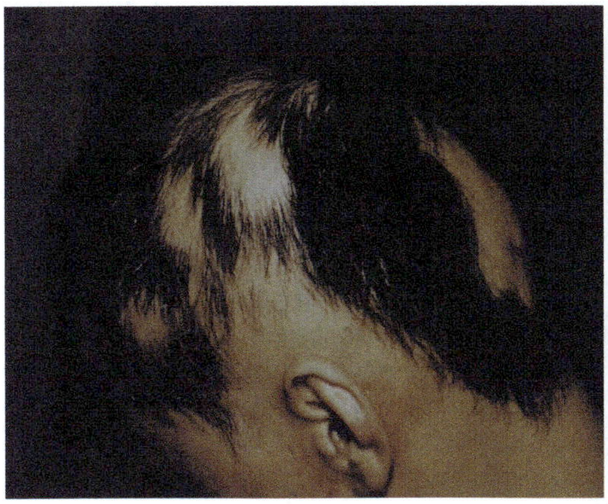
a
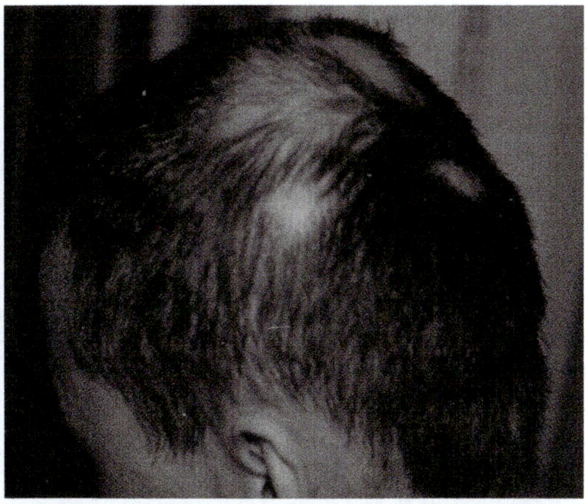
b
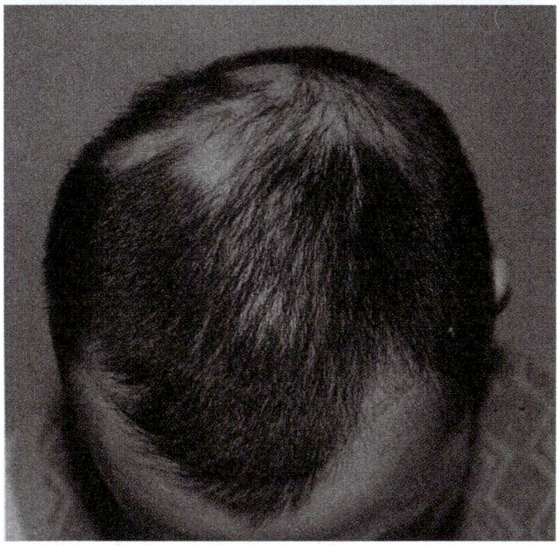
c

Fig. 22.2. **a** Alopecia areata with multiple patches. **b** After 1-year treatment, patches have become smaller. **c** Frontal view of Fig. 22.1b. The area has been almost cured except for the parietal region

22.2 Alopecia Cicatrisata

Premature baldness and alopecia areata do not include loss of the hair root in addition to enlargement or atrophy of the sebaceous gland and the hair follicle; on close observation, vellus hair growth can be found in the bald area in these conditions.

Alopecia cicatrisata (baldness due to scarring) in contrast, is baldness in which the skin is cicatrized due to accident (e.g., in traffic accidents) or other trauma such as burns, radiotoxicity, or infectious tumor disease. The hair root and follicle are completely lost. Even vellus hair is extinguished, and it is impossible to expect hair regeneration. In order to conceal the scar, hair transplantation in this area has been attempted. This has always been unsuccessful; however, in scalp surgery, the authors have developed a new suture method in order not to leave linear scars in the excision scar tissue (see Chapter 32).

22.3 Alopecia Gradus Induced by Hairstyling

The chignon style was once popular in France. This style was also popular among women of the Japanese upper classes in the late nineteenth century, along with the rapid westernization of Japan in that era. The shape of the chignon was similar to that of the more traditional Japanese hair bun, but the fact that the style was popular in France was attractive to these upper-class women.

However, chignon styling over a long period caused a gradual thinning of the hair and even baldness in the frontal, temporal, and parietal regions. This type of baldness became well known as chignon alopecia.

The ponytail hairstyle, more recently popular among young women, also has the hair pulled backward tightly in the same areas. Baldness does not, of course, occur in 1 or 2 days, but after a period of years.

Continued hair dressing can, likewise, cause red, bean-sized bald spots to appear. This type of baldness is called alopecia gradus. What is pertinent here is that the flow of blood and lymph surrounding the hair follicle is inhibited, and both the hair follicle and papilla can develop aplastic atrophy.

Krstic et al. (1981) reported that prolonged and intensive hair traction was followed by a perifollicular inflammatory process, damaging the hair papilla, which later became atrophic. If this happens, it is possible that hair will be lost in a manner similar to that in alopecia cicatrisata.

22.4 Baldness Due to Syphilis

Baldness is caused not only by scalp disease or local injury, but also by other types of disease. Syphilis is representative. Baldness caused by syphilis differs from the premature baldness which starts at the frontal region. Syphilitic baldness characteristically occurs at random spots in the occipital and temporal regions of the scalp. Baldness occurs in the secondary stage of syphilis. If this condition is discovered, the disease itself must be treated immediately.

Loss of hair due to drugs or secondary syphilis may also be accompanied by elevated numbers of telogen hairs, but dystrophic hair roots (about 10%) will be seen in the trichogram under these conditions, requiring serological tests to exclude suspected syphilis (Orfanos 1990).

22.5 Other Contributory Diseases in Baldness

Baldness can also appear in patients with Hansen's disease. In myxedema (hypothyroidism), caused by dysfunction of the thyroid gland (which gland excretes a hormone that governs metabolism), the scalp metabolism may be affected, with baldness beginning much the same way it does in male pattern baldness.

Distinct alterations of the hair cycle occurring in relation to pregnancy provide evidence for the effects of circulating estrogen. Given the increased estrogen levels during the second half of pregnancy, there is marked lengthening of the anagen phase, which shortens abruptly when the levels fall to normal values postpartum. A large number of growing hairs then pass into the telogen phase and cause telogen effluvium after 6–8 weeks. "Postpartum alopecia" is thus a physiological model for temporary androgenetic alopecia.

Diseases in which high fevers are manifested, as well as other types of disease, when at a serious stage, can cause occasional transient baldness. Copious bleeding can also cause baldness. These types of baldness occur as a result of physical exhaustion. In most cases, hair growth returns to normal with recovery of health.

In women with a pronounced male pattern baldness, thorough endocrinological investigations are indispensable to exclude androgenic alopecia caused by androgen-producing tumor or other endocrine abnormalities in which there are elevated levels of androgens of gonadal or adrenal origin (Orfanos 1990).

Thyroid disease (mostly hypothyroidism), hepatopathies, syphilis, drugs, and exogenous trauma may simulate the clinical picture of female pattern androgenetic alopecia. In such cases, withdrawal of all drugs with resting androgen-like properties, e.g., progestogens in contraceptives, other hormones, and appetite depressants, as well as laboratory work-up, are required (Orfanos 1990).

In conclusion, the differential diagnosis of androgenetic alopecia will sometimes not be easy to establish, particularly because centroparietal thinning based on telogen effluvium is not specific.

Relationship of Diet to Androgenetic Alopecia

23

23.1 Malnutrition and Androgenetic Alopecia

It has been thought that diet plays a minor role in androgenetic alopecia. It is conceivable that consumption of androgen-containing foods could exacerbate male pattern baldness in some women, but it is unlikely that men would experience any deleterious effects, because of high levels of endogenous androgens. Although proteins, carbohydrates, vitamins, and minerals are essential for normal hair growth, their absence may not produce male pattern baldness, but a rather characteristic diffuse hair loss.

The effect of protein-calorie malnutrition on hair growth has been studied in adults. Male subjects aged 24–29 years were fed equicaloric (2800) diets with or without adequate protein (Bradfield et al. 1967; Calloway and Margen 1966). In subjects deprived of protein, severe atrophy of up to 50% of the anagen hair bulbs occurred (Kaufman 1976; Spencer and Callen 1987).

Marasmus is the result of an extremely low caloric diet in children. In this condition, amino acids are utilized from skeletal muscles and other less essential tissues to maintain essential body functions. Clinically, the marasmic child is emaciated and shows extreme muscle wasting and atrophy of most organs, although histological changes are minimal. Hair changes are less severe than those seen in kwashiorkor. The most consistent finding is an overall shift to the telogen phase (up to 50% of anagen follicles); the remaining bulbs often show various degrees of atrophy of bulb diameter. The hair is dry and lusterless, and there is a reduction in shaft diameter. Changes in hair color do not always occur (Gummer 1985).

Nine adults on "crash" diets experienced profuse hair loss 2–5 months after starting a vigorous weight reduction program resulting in a weight loss of 11.7–24.75kg (Goette and Odom 1976). Telogen counts of 20%–50% were observed; the normal scalp telogen count is about 10%. Regrowth of hair occurred within several months. Of these patients, three had experienced hair loss closely following a successful weight reduction program on several occasions.

On the other hand, the almost normal hair of yogis, such as Buddha, who meditated for 6 months, eating only one bean a day, contradicts these findings. Patients suffering from nutritional edema due to starvation lost hardly any hair (Bhattacharya et al. 1977). Today, many yogis and householders in India fast for 1–3 months with no food and only sips of water in preparation for spiritual pursuits, without noticeable hair loss or gross changes.

Hair changes in starvation are minimal; however, the hair may be dry and lusterless (Davidson et al. 1975) or it may be thin, grow slowly, and fall out prematurely, and, occasionally, it may become gray (McLaren 1971).

Bradfield (1971) found that anagen roots displayed a rapid reduction in diameter, leading to atrophy within about 11 days after protein deprivation; this was reversed after protein supplement. However, Johnson et al. (1976) reported significant differences only between the hair of well-nourished and severely malnourished children, whereas the hair of patients with kwashiorkor did not show marked differences in hair morphology.

23.2 Relationship of Animal Fat Intake to Androgenetic Alopecia

A definite contributory cause of male pattern baldness is the excess consumption of animal fat. A

Table 23.1. Comparative thickness of individual hair. (Steggerda 1940)

Caucasians (Europe, North America)	Thin
Afghans and Aryans	Thin
Asians (Japan, Asian mainland)	Thick
Latins, Africans	Average

diet high in animal lipids can contribute to baldness by causing enlargement of the sebaceous gland.

Hair thickness in different ethnic groups (Table 23.1) appears to be related to diet. Miyamoto (1981) classified traditional diets around the world into six main cultural zones (Table 23.2). The whole grain diet culture shown in the table includes Japan to the Korean peninsula, the northern Indochinese peninsula, China, and the eastern sector of the Indian subcontinent. The staple foodstuffs in this area consist mainly of rice plants or other whole grain cereals, with little intake of dairy products. The inhabitants are traditionally agricultural. Until recent times, they did not engage in hunting and did not consume animal fats or proteins as a daily food source. Meat (or fish) was eaten only at dinner on special feast days. The zone of ground or powdered grain culture shown in the table extended westward from much of the Indian subcontinent and the Middle East to Europe, and these populations also engaged in animal husbandry from ancient times. They traditionally ate bread made from ground flour as a food staple, with livestock meat as a side dish, and consumed a large quantity of dairy products. Accordingly, their diet was high in animal lipids and protein.

It appears that Caucasians and the Afghan/Aryan peoples, who had characteristic thin, soft hair (Table 23.1), subsisted on a diet of ground or powdered foods and a significant quantity of animal fats or protein. Asian peoples had thick, stiff, tufty hairs and subsisted mostly on whole-grain foodstuffs, without much consumption of animal fats or protein.

We can surmise that thin individual hairs, accompanied by enlarged sebaceous glands, is one indicator of incipient baldness, and is closely linked to traditional diets. Thin hairs are most characteristic of people who consume animal flesh and dairy products. A reduction in fat intake has been reported to reduce circulating testosterone concentrations in humans (Hill and Wynder 1979).

The saturated fatty acid contained in animal fats seems to induce enlargement of the sebaceous gland and to precipitate the onset of baldness. In that context, the high incidence of baldness observed in European and North American men is somewhat understandable.

Table 23.2. Six main dietary zones (until the fifteenth century)

Dietary culture zone	Area	Staple food	Dry products	Side dishes
Whole-grain culture	Eastern Asia	Rice, Italian millet, millet, dry land rice, beans	Almost none	Scant
Potato-meal culture	Islands in southern Asia	Dry land rice, taro, banana, cassava	Almost none	Pork
Cassava culture	Upper Amazon river	Cassava, banana, Indian corn	None	Monkey, crocodile, insects
Powdered gruel cake culture	Africa, south of Sahara desert	Milk, dairy products, cereals	Butter, cheese, cream	Camel, goat, sheep
Ground or powdered grain culture	Indian subcontinent, Middle East, Europe	Bread	Butter, cheese, cream,	Camel, goat, sheep
Carnivorous culture	Arctic circle	Fish, animal meats	Scant	Seal, caribou

Classifies traditional diets around the world into six main cultural zones. (Modified from Miyamoto 1981, with permission from Shibata Shoten)

23.3 Japanese Diet

According to Abe (1983), the average energy intake required per day for a Japanese is 2000 kcal. The total individual intake of protein in the Japanese population between 1911 and 1915 was 50 g, which was far from ideal both from the qualitative and quantitative standpoints. In 1981, the average protein intake was approximately 80 g. The percentage of protein in the essential nutritive elements was 15%, more than half of which was animal protein (Table 23.3).

Fat intake between 1911 and 1915 was 13 g (5.6% of the essential nutritive elements) compared to the 1981 figure of 55 g (23.4% of the essential nutritive elements), most of which was animal fat. Table 23.3 shows the changes in the percentage components of energy intake in terms of essential nutritive elements, indicating that the percentage of carbohydrates has gradually decreased, while those of protein and fat have increased. In the case of Americans, the ratio of carbohydrates is still smaller and that of fat much greater.

Figure 23.1 shows the changes in essential food intake starting from 1967, indicating the decrease in rice intake and the increase in the intake of meat, eggs, milk, and dairy products. In the present era of economic growth, the dietary pattern is showing a decrease in the intake of carbohydrate foods (cereals, potatoes) and an increase in the intake of animal products, i.e., a shift from vegetable to animal foods. The typical Japanese diet of rice, soy bean soup, and pickles is gradually changing to the western diet (Fig. 23.1).

The recommended energy intake should not exceed the amount necessary for maintaining average weight (height: cm—100) × 0.9 kg. For adults, carbohydrates (cereals, sugar) should total about 60% of all energy intake, and fat 20%–25%. The ideal amount of fat per day would thus be 40–50 g, and the ratio of animal to vegetable fat would be 1:2. Protein is essential for building the body, and a fixed amount must be taken each day. Animal protein intake in Japan was once very low, and the Japanese were advised to consume more. Dietary habits have improved since then, and the

Table 23.3. Changes in energy intake of essential nutritive elements in the Japanese population compared with USA

Year	Protein	Fat	Glucide (%)
1911	9.5	5.6	84.9
1955	12.7	7.5	79.8
1965	13.1	14.8	72.1
1975	14.6	21.4	64.0
1981	15.0	23.4	61.6
USA 1977	12	42	46

Modified from Abe (1983), with permission from Mainichi Life

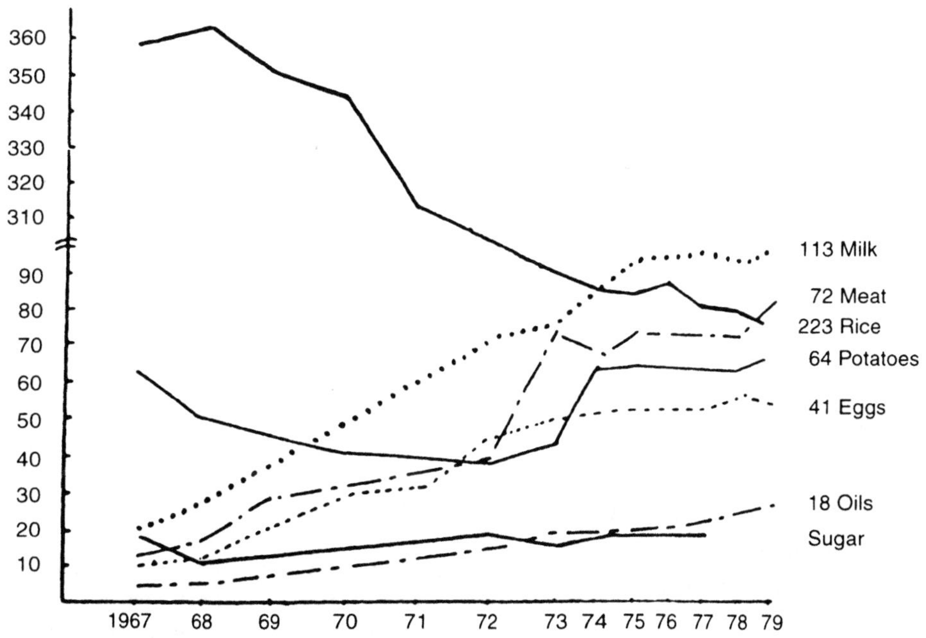

Fig. 23.1. Changes in intake of various foodstuffs per capita (Japan national average; survey by Ministry of Health and Welfare). The graph shows the decrease in rice intake and the increase in the intake of meat, eggs, milk, and dairy products. (Modified from Abe 1983, with permission from Mainichi Life)

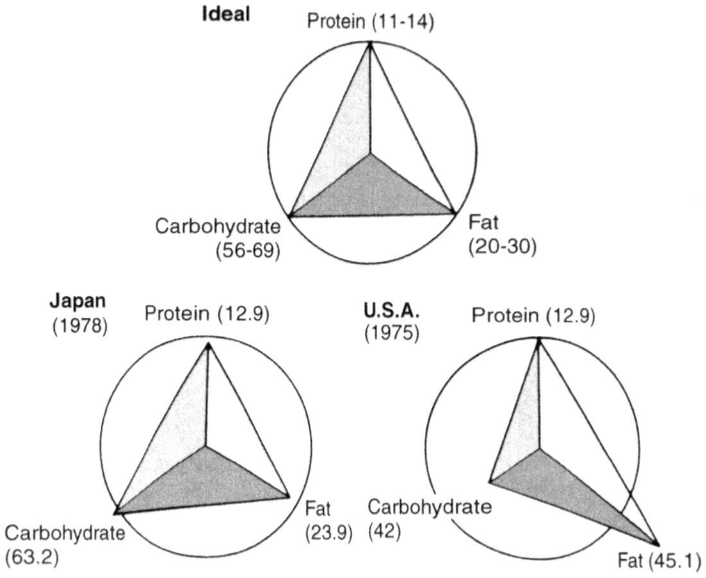

Fig. 23.2. Comparison of caloric intake (%). Comparison of typical caloric intake in the diet in Japan and the United States shows less than optimum intake of carbohydrates and excess consumption of fats in the U.S.A. (Permission from Medical Hair Research Inc. Reproduced from Inaba 1985)

Japanese are now consuming a satisfactory amount. In adults, the protein intake required per day is about 1 g/kg, body weight, i.e., approximately 12% of the total energy intake, although the figure may fluctuate according to the protein source.

Comparison of caloric intake between Japan and the U.S. is shown in Fig. 23.2. The Americans are trying to obtain their goal by reducing the consumption of fat and sugar while increasing that of grains and cereals. The national survey on nutritional intake in Japan in 1978 showed the average figures being fairly close to the ideal ratio for each nutritional element (Fig. 23.2). Currently, the increased use of vegetable fiber is being advocated. However, the Japanese are already consuming a satisfactory amount of fiber from various vegetables and seaweeds (reproduced from Inaba 1985).

Furthermore, it is important to take three meals per day, each at its regular time, as well as having proper exercise and rest. To keep ourselves fit we should: (a) eat well-balanced meals, which will maintain the average optimal weight, (b) refrain from excessive intake of animal fat, sugar, and salt, (c) control smoking and drinking habits, (d) exercise, and (e) get plenty of rest.

23.4 Relationship of Diet to Baldness and Hircismus (Offensive Body Odor)

Diet may influence both baldness and hircismus. The tendency toward hircismus and baldness is much higher among Caucasians than it is among Orientals. Caucasians typically take in great quantities of animal fats. It seems quite plausible to suggest that diet can influence body odor as well as baldness. The intake of animal fat in large quantities is common to both conditions.

The human skin contains two kinds of sweat glands for metabolic and thermoregulatory functions, the apocrine and eccrine glands (see Fig. 1.1). Eccrine glands (more than 2 000 000 in number) are found all over the body, while apocrine glands are localized around the armpit, nipples, vulva, anus, and navel. Apocrine glands are a degenerative form of aromatic glands and play an important role in bromidrosis. The perspiration secreted directly from the apocrine gland has a mild odor. The problem of offensive odor occurs after the perspiration has been secreted. Human perspiration contains fats, iron, fluorescent substances, and pigments. The fat component contains various kinds of fatty acids and cholesterol.

Fats and pigments play an important role in hircismus, and may cause soiled clothing (Hurley and Shelley 1960). Offensive odor is not due to the apocrine perspiration alone. Eccrine perspiration, sebum secretion from the sebaceous gland, and bacteria contribute to the characteristic odor of apocrine perspiration. In the perspiration secreted from the eccrine gland, the odor is actually diffused as the perspiration evaporates into the air.

In the fetal period, apocrine glands cover the entire body, gradually degenerating and localizing at specific sites in adult life. Apocrine gland localization in Caucasians develops again in puberty, whereas their degeneration continues in Orientals.

Figure 1.1 demonstrates that the apocrine gland is appended to the hair follicle in much the same way as the sebaceous gland. Perspiration secreted from the apocrine gland is high in lipid content. This indicates that the sebaceous gland may play a role in the metabolic activity and excretion of lipids. A reduction of lipid intake may cause diminution of the sebaceous gland and degeneration of the apocrine gland. This fact has been supported by the data that occurrence of androgenetic alopecia and bromidrosis can be observed much more often in Occidentals than in Orientals due to the difference in food intake, not to mention the hereditary factor. Occidentals who consume greater amounts of meat and dairy products than Orientals have comparatively large sebaceous glands, which may induce hypertrophy of the sebaceous gland. As a result, production of 5α-reductase is increased and development of apocrine gland is also accelerated. To the contrary, intake of animal fat has been low in Orientals and, therefore, development of the apocrine gland and production of 5α-reductase are moderate, resulting in low occurrence of androgenetic alopecia (see Section 19.4, Fig. 19.2).

A diet of ground/powdered foodstuffs that is also high in animal fats may induce an enlargement of the sebaceous gland, which in turn causes baldness and regeneration of the apocrine gland, which causes hircismus. A close relationship between baldness and hircismus can be postulated on that basis. People who have hircismus will not necessarily grow bald, but the risk of baldness is greatly increased.

In the past, cultural inheritance and traditional diet has caused various differences between Orientals and Occidentals in regard to baldness and hircismus. The changing Oriental diet may increase the incidence of baldness and hircismus in Oriental populations of the present and future.

23.5 Diet Therapy for Androgenetic Alopecia

23.5.1 Basis of Diet Therapy

The Japanese traditionally believe that certain seaweeds, such as *wakame* (*Undaria pinnatifida*) and sea tangle (*konbu*), enhance and protect the growth of luxuriant hair. These seaweeds have a high content of iodine and other minerals. Iodine is a component of thyroxine, the thyroid hormone. Intake of these seaweeds is believed to activate or enhance thyroid function. This has a positive effect on other endocrine organs and enhances the basal metabolic activity promoting the growth of hair.

The belief that hair growth or retardation in the occipital and temporal regions is related to sexual and thyroid hormones is based on dietary theories (see Section 15.6, Thyroid Hormone).

Diet can be a contributory factor in both the prevention and the treatment of baldness. A well-balanced diet supplies the essential nutrients needed for hair growth and health:

1. Protein builds up body tissue and is also utilized for energy as occasion demands. An adult requires 1 g of protein daily for each kilogram of body weight. It takes about 10 days to build up the protein in the liver and blood plasma and about 150 days to build it up in muscle tissue. Protein is broken down into amino acids by digestion and is thus absorbed by the body. Proteins are also synthesized in the body.

2. Carbohydrates are an important source of energy. In plants, carbohydrates are distributed throughout the plant as cellulose and starch bound by saccharide; however, in the human body, the amount of carbohydrates which builds up is quite small. Ingested carbohydrates are absorbed as glucose, carried in the circulatory system, and stored as glycogen in the liver and the muscle tissues.

3. Fats must be consumed in foodstuffs to build up fatty tissues. There are various fatty tissues containing large deposits of fat in the subcutaneous tissue, the intestinal mesenterium, and the muscle tissue. Fats can become a source of energy much like carbohydrates. Fats in their initial form are oxidized to fatty acid and glycerin, consisting of carbon, hydrogen, and oxygen. This perfect oxidation in the body produces twice the energy of other nutritive elements. Fats are a good source of energy.

4. Vitamins are essential organic compounds required for the growth and maintenance of the normal physiological condition in living organisms. Very small amounts of vitamins regulate physiological processes in the body. Vitamins in pure form cannot be synthesized in the body, so that materials containing these vitamins must be taken in as food. Liver, for example, contains vitamins A, B_2, B_6, K, nicotinic acid, pantothenic acid, and folic acid. High doses of vitamin A may affect hair growth. Vitamin A deficiency as a cause of hair abnormality, however, is more contentious. Hyperkeratosis due to vitamin A deficiency may result in plugging of the follicle, thereby preventing the emergence of the hair shaft from the follicular canal (Gummer 1985). High doses of vitamin A may cause dryness and itching of the skin, together with sparseness of most body hair, due to telogen effluvium (Soler-Bechara and Soscia 1963). Deficiency of vitamin B_1 causes beriberi and

neuritis. This vitamin is abundant in rice bran and beans. Lack of vitamin B_{12} may be associated with premature graying, although vitamin B_{12} supplements do not delay the process (Gummer 1985). Lack of vitamin C causes scurvy. Oranges and persimmons are high in vitamin C. Vitamin D, which prevents rickets and osteomalacia (softening of bones and teeth) is abundant in mushrooms and in cod liver oil and fish oils. In rickets (due to a deficiency of vitamin A) complete and persistent alopecia has been reported (Rosen et al. 1979). Vitamin P is needed to enhance the activity of the capillary vessels and to prevent subcutaneous hemorrhage; it is abundant in green peppers, lemons, and grapes.

5. Minerals are required for certain physiological processes and for the formation of tissues. Calcium, potassium, sodium, iron, magnesium, iodine, and other minerals are needed in very small quantities (Klevar 1978). The lack of even one of these minerals can cause an abnormal condition in the body. For example, a deficiency of potassium or sodium can cause digestive trouble, neuropathy, and spasms. Potassium is abundant in most foodstuffs, but there are few foods which contain sodium, so it is ordinarily supplied in table salt. Excessive intake of common table salt can cause hypertension.

6. Zinc is an important constituent of hair (Remedco 1978). Zinc deficiency produces diffuse alopecia in varying degrees. In a rare hereditary disorder of zinc metabolism, the hair may be sparse and dry and is sometimes completely shed (Remedco 1978; Comaish 1981). Copper is thought to be necessary in producing the resilient properties of keratin fibers in hair and wool (Gummer 1985). Iron deficiency may be accompanied by diffuse hair loss. Menorrhagia may cause anemia and diffuse hair loss, but symptoms may be corrected with dietary iron supplementation. Increasing the iron content of an already adequate diet does not, however, promote hair growth (Gummer 1985).

Hardness or softness of the hair and the tendency toward baldness are not always inherited, and can be influenced by the quality of the diet. Evidence is found in the increased tendency toward baldness in the postwar generation of Japanese men who have gravitated more and more toward a Western-style diet overly rich in animal fats. The Western-style diet may also contribute to an increase of cholesterol. This can lead to arteriosclerosis, which can trigger cerebral hemorrhage and cardiac disease.

Prevention or retardation of baldness must be based on a well-balanced diet containing fats, protein, carbohydrates, vitamins, minerals, and other nutrients.

23.5.2 Comparison of Dietary Habits

Typical and ideal caloric intake patterns in the diet in Japan and America are shown in Fig. 23.2. This figure shows that the ratio of animal fats, protein, and carbohydrate consumption is nearly ideal in the typical Japanese diet. In America, in contrast, it is clear that the ratio of animal fat is high enough to be considered excessive. In Americans, the ratio of glucide is lower and that of fat much greater than in the Japanese diet (Table 23.3). Suggested dietary guidelines for Americans are:

1. Increased consumption of fruits, vegetables, and cereals.
2. Decreased consumption of meat and increased consumption of fish.
3. Decreased consumption of fatty foods and a switch from the consumption of saturated to unsaturated fats.
4. Skim milk should be substituted for ordinary milk.
5. Dairy foods high in cholesterol, such as butter and eggs, should be decreased.
6. Sugar should be decreased.
7. Salt should be decreased.

Saturated fatty acids include palmitic and stearic acids abundant in animal fat. Unsaturated fatty acids are found mainly in plants, and include oleic acid in bean, cottonseed, and sesame oils.

Fish fat is quite different from beef and pork fat, and is quite similar to vegetable oil in that it contains much polyatomic unsaturated fatty acid. Linoleic acid is scant in fish fat, but eicosapentaenoic acid (EPA) and docosahexaenoic acid (DHEA) are abundant. Fish fat lowers cholesterol level. Recent studies reveal that fish fat inhibits blood coagulation and prevents coronary disease, which arises from clogged blood vessels. Eskimos, who subsist largely on fish, are noted for their lack of cardiovascular disease. The Eskimos resemble the Japanese both in physique and in their lack of a tendency toward baldness. The consumption of fish is thus highly recommended as it may help in the prevention of baldness.

23.5.3 The "Japanese Food Boom"

Americans, realizing the unhealthy aspects of a diet based mainly on animal protein and fat, have discovered the merits of the Japanese diet. Japanese food has now won widespread acceptance worldwide. Popular Japanese food items in America include sake (rice wine), soy sauce, misoshiru (soybean soup), and tofu (soybean curd). Tofu, with its odorless and naturally pleasant light taste, can be eaten like a steak or can be combined with sliced onion and eaten with a spoon. One popular dish is hiyayakko (soft tofu on a bed of ice). Gomatofu (soybean curd with powdered sesame seed) is also popular. Soy sauce is essential for teriyaki and sukiyaki beef dishes, which have gained great popularity. The low evaluation of the traditional Japanese diet in the immediate postwar period is in sharp contrast with the present popularity of the Japanese diet in the United States. In postwar Japan, the rice-based diet was denounced as unhealthy and a bread-based diet was recommended. It is a paradox that the Japanese people are now bound to a diet of bread, while a rice diet has won new acceptance in other countries.

23.5.4 Intake of Fats and Lipid Peroxide (Ochi 1989)

Needless to say, nutritive elements play a very important role in maintaining health. Of such elements, fats have been found to have an especially close relationship with adult diseases such as arteriosclerosis and with aging. Until now, the harmful influence of the excessive intake of animal fats has been the main focus of debate, and the necessity for a minimum intake and their importance seem to have been neglected. In contrast, for vegetable oils, only their advantages have been focused on, and any ill effects caused by excessive intake have been neglected.

It has been widely acknowledged that vegetable oils decrease the amount of LDL cholesterol and help to prevent the occurrence of arteriosclerosis or myocardial infarction. However, at the same time, they are the main ingredients of lipofuscin, and excessive intake of this must naturally be avoided, as the required amount is a mere 2–4g/day.

Arachidic acid is metabolized in the body to prostaglandin. From the arachidic acid cascade, lipid peroxide is produced. Because the content of W3 type (linoleic acid) and W6 type (linolic acid) lipids differs in various types of oil, it is necessary to take the ratio into consideration.

The excessive intake of di-saturated lipid acids induces the accumulation of lipid peroxide and leads to the development of arteriosclerosis and vascular trouble. Since EPA, contained in large amounts in fish oils, helps prevent blood coagulation, attention has been focused on it as being effective in preventing myocardial infarction. However, EPA is a di-saturated lipid acid, and excessive intake is naturally not recommended.

Since saturated lipid acids, contained in large amounts in animal fats, increase the amount of LDL cholesterol in the blood, their relationship with the development of arteriosclerosis has been mentioned; however, palmitolein acid, contained in animal fats, has been reported to be effective in strengthening blood vessels and preventing cerebral apoplexy.

The most notable element in fats is lipid peroxide, since, when it is produced in the body, it influences the aging process. Lipid in organic tissues produces lipid peroxide through the process of autoxidation and active oxygen reaction. In particular, the organic membrane often takes the form of a dual structure with phospholipid as the major element, and it abounds with multivalent di-saturated lipid acid, which makes it susceptible to peroxide reaction. The lipid composition of the organic membrane is largely influenced by the foods taken in; therefore, the lipid taken in from foods is of great significance.

Lipids containing a large amount of di-saturated lipid acid are easily oxidized, and this defective oxidized oil, which is offensive in taste and odor, may even be toxic after becoming polymerized. Another problem is that the excessive intake of fats affects the intestinal bacteria, and the excessive bile acid secretion thus produced is likely to contain carcinogenic substances.

As mentioned above, the points to be noted about lipid intake are caution, avoiding excessive intake of fats and fatty foods, care to avoid the danger of oxidation during food storage, and concern, taking in a well-balanced diet of saturated lipid and di-saturated lipid acids. The ideal ratio of animal fats: vegetable oils (fishery fats) is 1:1–2.

It is well known that the taste of processed foods deteriorates if the lipid contained in them is oxidized during storage. It is imperative, from the standpoint of preventing the process of aging in humans, to avoid oxidation of food during storage. With respect to this, a compound gas of nitrogen and carbon dioxide, produced from air, from which the oxygen has been easily and cheaply removed, is expected to become widely used in food packaging. It is also hoped that new cooking oil (salad oil) products containing an anti-oxidant will appear on the market (reviewed from Ochi 1989).

General Measures for Prevention of Baldness

24

Although many methods have been promoted to prevent baldness, there is still no foolproof method for the prevention and treatment of premature baldness.

However, the most important basic factor in the prevention of baldness is inhibiting enlargement of the sebaceous gland (Inaba 1985). It must be kept at a proper size by regular removal of the skin surface lipid membrane (sebum). Cleansing agents are useful for removing this lipid membrane from the scalp. However, insufficient washing and rinsing can leave accumulated residues in the pores.

A second important factor in the prevention of baldness is diet, which includes proper minerals and fats. An excess of animal fat should be avoided.

24.1 Prevention of Baldness by Measures That Promote Healthy Scalp Hygiene

24.1.1 Skin Condition

The skin covering the surface of the body cannot remain in good health in a condition of excessive dryness and bacterial invasion. Therefore, sebum is secreted from the sebaceous gland and conveyed to the skin surface to provide a proper degree of moisture and to prevent bacterial invasion. However, it is incorrect to suppose that the thicker the membrane, the better the condition of the skin. A very thick membrane collects more dust, with more noticeable dirt deposition. In that condition, bacterial growth and invasion can be aggravated rather than prevented.

From the standpoint of hair hygiene, enlargement of the sebaceous glands is undesirable. The sebaceous gland enlargement leads to greater secretion and accumulation of the enzyme 5α-reductase. The amount of male hormone (5α-DHT) is increased when the 5α-reductase enzyme level increases. The dihydrotestosterone exerts an inhibitory effect on the hair follicle (Steggerda 1940; Adachi 1973). Atrophy of the hair occurs, and baldness follows, according to the sebaceous gland hypothesis of Inaba (1985; Inaba and Inaba 1992a).

The sebaceous gland hypothesis is contrary to the seborrhea theory (Section 18.1) that has commonly been accepted. The seborrhea theory holds that dandruff and bacteria form deposits in the skin surface lipid membrane (sebum) constitute seborrhea, which occludes the hair canal and causes baldness. However, this explanation suggests only part of the overall cause and does not clarify the basic mechanism by which baldness begins.

It is important to keep the skin surface lipid membrane (sebum) in proper condition by keeping the surface of the skin clean. Fundamental prevention of baldness lies in reducing the size of the sebaceous gland (if enlarged) in order to inhibit the secretion and accumulation of the 5α-reductase enzyme.

When a cast is removed after a fracture has healed, the vellus hair at the cast site is often found to be replaced by terminal hair, an indication of the importance of sebaceous gland function. How can we account for this finding? The explanation most often offered is that the cotton bandage of the cast has a stimulative effect, improving blood circulation. This does not appear to be a satisfactory explanation. Not much stimulation can be expected beneath a cast which is dressed firmly to prevent movement. A more logical explanation is that the skin surface lipid membrane is constantly wiped off by the cotton bandage, which absorbs the sebum secreted from the sebaceous gland. It is considered that the frequent removal of lipids will lead to enhanced secretory activity by the sebaceous gland (Kligman et al. 1981a).

Probably due to the stimulation of sebum secretion, the upper isthmal portion and the sebaceous gland, the assumed center of hair regeneration, are stimulated, leading to the phenomenon of coarsening of the vellus hair.

24.1.2 Importance of Cleanliness

Some people may avoid washing the hair because of fear of hair loss due to washing; however, if the number of lost hairs is generally within 100 per day, there is no need for concern. Moderate washing is recommended two or three times a week. Lost hairs in the natural resting telogen stage will be replaced by the next generation of healthy hairs (Section 6.4.2). A cleansing agent should foam sufficiently. Vigorous shampooing massages the skin and removes fatty and other deposits accumulated in the pores.

24.1.3 Soap

It is sometimes claimed that soap does no actual harm to the hair because it is alkaline. This seems to be true. However, this alkalinity is neutralized by acidic body fat or perspiration within 30 min after washing; thus, its long-term effect is negligible. The real problem is excessive removal of hair oil. If this is the case, the hair after washing will be stiff and hard to the touch. The same condition can occur with insufficient rinsing, which will also leave washing scum in the pores, especially when hard water (containing much calcium) is used. This is because the soap will combine with the calcium to form a water-insoluble calcinated substance. This substance will occasionally cause eruptions because it also occludes the sweat glands to inhibit secretion and is decomposed to a noxious substance by the action of oxygen or ultraviolet rays that stimulate the skin. This problem can occur in areas where water is conveyed underground through water pipes made of iron, or in areas of hard water.

24.1.4 Shampoo

Shampoos consist mainly of a surfactant, together with a smaller amount of fatty substance. Shampoo surfactants are usually anionic, and are seldom cationic, whereas the reverse applies to conditioners; shampoos are microemulsions and are clear, unless specially opacified (Hunting 1988). The original shampoos were saponified fatty acids of plant and animal origin. The C_{10-12} acids are better foaming agents, C_{14-16} clean better, and the C_{16-18} work better at a high temperature (Fox 1985).

Over the years, shampoo composition has changed, from being based on straight anionic surfactant/fatty amide components, to mixtures of these materials with amphoteric surfactants for better hair conditioning and manageability (Fox 1986).

Although common soap is useful for removing deposits on the hair and scalp without irritating the skin, the best shampoo product should have the following properties:

1. It does not remove too much oil from the hair.
2. It must dissolve readily in any kind of water, hard or soft, and foam well.
3. It must rinse away readily and leave no residue.

Washing agents developed to satisfy these requirements are called shampoos. They are more suitable than common soap for washing the hair.

The detergency of shampoos should be moderate (Sorkin et al. 1966). If the cleaning action is too strong, it will snarl or tangle the hair and make it difficult to comb and brush. If this action is too weak, oily dirt and soil will not be sufficiently removed from the hair and scalp. The shampooing of scalp hair, if performed with mild commercially available shampoos at regular intervals, has only a minor influence on the structure of the hair shaft, but transitory dissolving of the extractable fatty material does take place (Brasch and Amoore 1967). Mild changes due to alkali can be reversed with an acid rinse. It has been suggested that shampoos may also occasionally influence hair growth by producing auto-oxidation products of hair surface lipids (Thiele 1975). Lipoperoxides were once thought to block or inhibit mitotic activity and the activity of certain enzymes in the matrix cells; this would reduce the growth of new hair and cause increased telogen effluvium. Today, however, most investigators agree that seborrhea has no influence on the growth of scalp hair.

24.1.5 Rinsing Agents (Hair Conditioners)

Even though the hair is properly washed with shampoo, excessive hair oil may be removed. The hair after washing may be quite naked, without any coating of oil. To replace this oil after washing it is necessary to use an agent that restores manageability and soft texture and minimizes fly-away (Spoor and Linds 1973). This is the role of the rinsing agent (hair conditioner). A proper rinsing agent assists the polypeptide substance adhering to the hair to form a film. Hair conditioners may be in the form of oil rinses, cream rinses, and cation rinses. The oil rinse is almost neutral in its effect. The cream rinse is weakly acidic and the cation rinse slightly alkaline. Specific formulations are available to suit any type of hair, from very oily to very dry.

24.1.6 Shampooing Frequency

How often should shampooing and rinsing be done? There is no absolute standard because it depends on the condition of the hair and the scalp, whether the hair is soft or hard, and whether the dandruff is oily or dry. But it is still best to keep the hair and scalp clean, and to use a shampoo two to three times a week to enhance sebum secretion (Archibald and Shuster 1970).

Eberhardt (1978) asserts that frequent shampooing stimulates sebaceous gland secretion in humans, in contrast to the belief of Leonhardi (1973). Kligman and Shelley (1958) conclude that the production of sebum is constant regardless of whether or not oil is removed. According to Kligman et al. (1981a), daily shampooing had no effect on dandruff, merely making it nonvisible. It is considered that the frequent removal of lipids will lead to enhanced secretory activity by the sebaceous glands.

Wirth et al. (1982) studied the mitotic activity of sebaceous glands after infrequent and after frequent shampooing, and showed that the latter actually led to sebocyte proliferation. On the other hand, they found that the amount of scalp and hair lipids was not increased by frequent shampooing. When no shampooing was done for 1 month, the only noteworthy finding was that dandruff became worse and more oil accumulated, evidently being soaked up by a thick mat of surface scales. However, the health of the scalp was not affected.

The hairs become greased by mechanical transfer, from the scalp surface to the hairs, and from hair to hair. The hair acquires sebum by direct contact. The dispersal of sebum from the surface is facilitated by combing and brushing, by wearing a hat, and by rubbing the fingers through the hair (Kligman et al. 1981a).

Young people with healthy hair do not necessarily need to shampoo every day or every other day. What is most important is complete rinsing to remove the unwanted substances contained in washing agents. Shampooing appears to be necessary at intervals of 2 or 3 days. Especially in the case of fragile hair, strong detergents should not be used daily, and the shampoo should be applied only once each time.

People who dislike or cannot use shampoo should remove the skin surface lipid membrane from the scalp with a hot, wet towel. This has a positive effect on the sebaceous gland by inhibiting its enlargement.

24.1.7 Brushing of Hair

Brushing can cause the sebum at the base of the hair shaft at the scalp surface to slide upward on the hair. The decrease of oil on the scalp surface and the consequent secretion of more sebum can help prevent enlargement of the sebaceous gland. Accordingly, brushing can be effective. A proper hair brush will not damage the scalp, and will bring the sebum smoothly to the tip of the hair shaft.

Japanese women of old times combed their long black hair with boxwood combs. The secret of their copious raven-black hair may have been due to the secretory activity of the sebaceous gland.

Nylon brushes are known to generate static electricity, which causes hair to twist and coil, and can lead to alopecia. Brushes made of stiff pig or boar bristles do not create static and are recommended.

Therapy for Androgenetic Alopecia

25

25.1 Increased Massage and Circulation

Why do men go bald with age? In normal men, advancing age is accompanied by an increase in the incidence and extent of baldness. In eunuchs castrated prepubertally and given androgen treatment in the second decade of life, hair was lost slowly over a period of years, resulting in hair loss similar to noncastrated men of the same age. In contrast, the eunuchs who had reached the sixth decade of life before receiving androgens lost hair within a few months after beginning the treatment. Evidently the susceptibility to alopecia increases with age but is not expressed in the absence of inciting agents such as androgens (Hamilton 1942).

Improvement of scalp circulation through massage or other means may not regenerate scalp hair or prevent male pattern baldness. Vigorous massaging may, rather, result in accelerating the loss of resting telogen hairs, causing male pattern baldness. However, since improvement of the blood circulation in the scalp has been the major treatment method up to the present, the following is a description of how it might work, according to Margot (1980). If one does not regularly rub or massage the scalp, the circulatory system gradually deteriorates.

Rub where the hair is thinning and more hair is desired. Rub the naked areas of the scalp and concentrate on areas where there is some hair. The purpose of rubbing is the gradual resupply of the capillary network of the scalp. The rubbing stimulates the furthest points the blood reaches, the leading edge hairline, the upper edge of the horseshoe, and the inner circumference of the crown over the top of a thinning pate. Margot (1980) claims that it takes 3–4 months from the time that rubbing is begun for the first new hair to grow on the scalp. The precise amount of time seems to depend on the circulatory system. The time required for the new growth appears to conform with what we know about the hair cycle. The resting stage, when the hair stops growing, lasts for 3 months. During this time, the papilla undergoes certain chemical processes that prepare it to send forth the new hair. It is after the resting stage that old hair is pushed out of the follicle by new hair.

By extending the reach of the blood in the scalp, Margot (1980) declares, rubbing seems to put a newly revived papilla in the resting stage, during which it assembles the raw materials to build a new hair. After 3 months, a new hair shaft begins to emerge. A month or so later, a little less than half of the anagen hair follicle is noticeable. The hair that falls out when rubbing is hair that is naturally shedding. Hair that is not ready to shed cannot be pulled out even with the most vigorous rubbing. In the normal course of replenishment, one hair grows back for every hair that is shed. When rubbing, two hairs grow in for every hair that is shed. After 3 months, the shaft sends forth reviving papillae and starts to break through the surface. The scalp feels rough, as though a beard were growing on the top of the head. The new growth will be noticeable more quickly if the hair is coarse and dark. If the hair is light, new growth will be less noticeable. Margot recommends that vigorous rubbing be made a regular part of the daily shampooing routine. Rubbing the scalp while shampooing will restore blood supply and nurture hair growth and replenishment. Towel drying to remove excess moisture will also polish the shafts and give them a high gloss. Caring this way for the hair and scalp will eliminate a significant part of the problem.

25.2 Diet Therapy

As described in Chapter 23, it is important to reduce the consumption of high-calorie or high-lipid foodstuffs which cause excessive secretion of sebum. The intake of animal fats or high-calorie foods may bring about an enlargement of sebaceous glands, leading to an increase in 5α-reductase. As a result of increased formation of the male hormone (5α-DHT), mature hair follicles produce downy hairs (balding). Therefore, the first step in the prevention of balding is control of diet, minimizing foodstuffs that contain animal lipids. The more traditional Japanese diet, well-balanced in protein, carbohydrates, and fats, is encouraged to restrict the ingestion of animal fats (see Section 23.5).

25.3 Conventional Treatment

Once baldness begins, the most common reaction is to accept it as inevitable. This has changed, however, in recent years, with new developments in treatment procedures that have been effective to some extent.

Behind the most common treatment approach is the notion that improvement of blood circulation in the hair roots will relieve the condition. Circulation-stimulating massages and hair tonics have been developed as a direct result of that assumption. Formulas for such preparations have been classified according to their mechanisms of action (Watanabe and Nagashima 1984; Hara 1987; Oba 1988):

a. Vasodilation of peripheral vessels: acetylcholine, carprinoyl chloride, vitamins, capsium extract, and tocopherol acetate
b. Stimulation of blood circulation for local irritation: red pepper tincture (capsicum tincture), cantharides tincture, and methyl nicotinate
c. Nutrients and agents to improve the matrix cells: vitamins, amino acids, (pantothenic acid, cystine, methionine), and placenta extract
d. Hormonal action (steroidal antiandrogen): estrogen, progesterone, spironolactone, androgen, thyroxine, and cyproterone acetate (CPA)
e. Antiphlogistic agents: guaiacol and hinokitiol
f. Antiseptic agents: salicylic acid, resorcin, sodium hydrochloride, diphenylhydramine
g. Cooling substances and fragrances: menthol, alcohol

Most of the products now used may be regarded as second generation; however, they have had little effect on the retardation or prevention of hair loss due to male pattern baldness.

The use of antiandrogens (steroidal antiandrogens) and other treatment modalities is discussed in the next chapter (Chapter 26).

Agents Used for the Treatment of Androgenetic Alopecia

26

26.1 Background and Historical Aspects of Agents Used for the Treatment of Androgenetic Alopecia

The Ebers Papyrus, a document written in about the year 1550 B.C., found in the tomb of an Egyptian mummy, provided a prescription for baldness (Vath 1963; Gerstein 1986). The prescription called for taking equal parts of fat from a lion, a hippopotamus, a crocodile, a goose, a snake, and a goat, mixing, and applying liberally to the bald pate.

The latter half of the twentieth century has seen great progress in the field of medicine and pharmacology, and maladies once incurable have become almost curable. However, studies of male pattern baldness have fallen far behind others due to their extreme difficulty, and truly effective treatment agents are yet to be developed. Because the causative mechanisms of male pattern baldness are yet to be clearly elucidated, no effective treatments for it have been developed.

Up to the present, the treatment of male pattern baldness has been based on the causal mechanism related to male hormones. Such treatment has consisted of the application of various agents, such as antiandrogens, cyproterone, and cyproterone acetate or antagonizing materials with steroidal structures, known by the acronyms 17BC and 17BME. To be effective, however, the agent should be either an inhibitor of 5α-reductase or a receptor competitor. Such agents (nonsteroidal antiandrogen), are preferable for external application, as they have neither a steroidal structure nor hormonal effects. These agents are used to reverse or halt a physiological phenomenon.

26.2 Treatment of Androgenetic Alopecia with Steroidal Antiandrogens

26.2.1 Antagonist Hormones

Another approach to the treatment of androgenetic alopecia is the systemic or local administration of estradiol, a male hormone antagonist; however, the effect of this treatment is, again, insufficient. Funk (1951) and Gloor et al. (1974) reported that, while systemic administration of estradiol was effective in decreasing the size of the sebaceous glands, the effect was doubtful with only local topical administration. Orfanos and Vogels (1980), in pursuit of hair regeneration, reported that the local administration of 0.025% solution of 17α-estradiol decreased the numbers of telogen stage hairs. Watanabe and Nagashima (1984) have reported good results with higher concentrations of estradiol for local topical administration. However, in Japan, only a very low concentration of estradiol is permitted for topical use, and thus these results cannot be confirmed in tests in Japan.

Another male hormone antagonist, progesterone, has been effective, to some degree, in preventing further hair loss, but has not led to regeneration of new hairs (Frost and Gomez 1972; Voigt and Hsia 1973). Natural steroids, such as progesterone, safely reduce the production of dihydrotestosterone (DHT) from testosterone. Because both testosterone and progesterone contain a 4-5 double bond in the steroid A ring, in vitro and in vivo studies have shown that they compete with each other for the 5α-reductase enzyme that converts testosterone to DHT. Tinctures and locally injected aqueous suspensions of progesterone have been used safely for 20 years (Orentreich 1978). Mauvais-Jarvis et al. (1974) observed beneficial effects of the local administration of progesterone on seborrhea in 23% to 55% of their patients, and found an improved ratio of anagen to telogen hairs in 22% of the patients. However, the effect of local progesterone treatment, when administered percutaneously, on hair follicles and sebaceous glands was not reported.

Certain competitive antagonists (steroidal antiandrogen agents) have been used to disrupt the formation of DHT by combining 5α-reductase in the hair matrices with other male hormone derivatives (Price 1975). Steroid formulations containing progesterone hormones, 4-androstene-3-one-17-carboxylic acid, androstenedione, and deoxycorticosterone have been tested; however they were not truly effective and had strong negative side effects.

The agent 11α-hydroxyprogesterone has an antiandrogen effect and leads to the reduction of sebaceous gland secretion when applied appropriately (Tamm et al. 1982; Simpson and Martin 1983).

Glucocorticoids are effective in suppressing androgens in many women whose levels of these steroids are elevated. Redmond et al. (1990) reported the use of dexamethasone as a safe agent for the suppression of elevated levels of dehydroepiandrosterone sulfate (DHEAS) when the dose was carefully titrated and patients were closely monitored.

26.2.2 Antiandrogens

Antiandrogens are compounds which block the action of androgens, and are thus of potential use in the alleviation of skin conditions such as acne vulgaris, hirsutism, and those MPB-type alopecia conditions which are androgen activated. All of the antiandrogens are synthetic compounds, since none occur in nature.

The current hypothesis of androgen action, based on studies of the ventral prostate gland in rats (Dorfman and Dorfman 1962), is that free testosterone in the plasma enters the cell and is rapidly reduced by 5α-reductase and cofactor NADPH, and is then bound to a highly specific receptor protein in the cytoplasm. The steroid-receptor complex is converted to an activated form. It is then translocated into the unclear chromatin. Once inside the nucleus, the testosterone-receptor complex is believed to combine with sites on chromatin binding which in turn results in transcription of specific DNA sequences to form messenger RNA, and ultimately results in synthesis of new proteins necessary for the expression of virilizing activities by the cell (Williams-Ashman 1975).

The mechanism of action of androgens is complex and not well understood. However, in the past decade, progress has been made in identifying and studying the initial steps of the interaction of androgens with their target organs. The first step in some target organs is the metabolic transformation of circulating androgens into the more active forms. The most extensively studied reaction of this type is the 5α-reductase transformation of testosterone to DHT. The second involves the binding of active androgens to a receptor protein present in the target cell cytoplasm (Fig. 15.2).

Two classes of antiandrogens are known. Antiandrogens of one class inhibit the androgen reduction of testosterone to DHT, while antiandrogens of the other class inhibit the binding of active androgens to the cytoplasmic receptor (Fig. 15.2). Neumann (1977) outlined the nature and possible modes of action of antiandrogens and the clinical indications for their use.

26.2.3 Cyproterone Acetate (CPA)

Cyproterone acetate (a hydroxyprogesterone derivative) blocks the action of testosterone on target organs, including the human sebaceous gland. A similar local inhibition of testosterone action in the hair follicle seems possible. The binding of cyproterone acetate to the androgen receptor competitively inhibits the intracellular binding of DHT and decreases its nuclear uptake. Cyproterone acetate competes for androgen receptor sites and inhibits the translocation of the hormone-receptor complex into the nucleus. To obtain a 50% inhibition, a three- to tenfold excess is required; 15-OH cyproterone acetate is even more active than the parent compound. This drug has been used extensively in the treatment of androgenic cutaneous changes, for example, in idiopathic hirsutism in women (Hammerstein and Cupceancu 1969). Cyclic antiandrogen therapy has been conducted with cyproterone acetate and ethinylestradiol. Cyproterone acetate, however, is an extremely potent drug which can produce unwanted systemic and mental side effects. It is unsuitable for use in men and its use in women is limited (Hammerstein et al. 1975).

Some trials with cyproterone acetate, however, have confirmed high success rates in acne and hirsutism, and the response to androgenetic alopecia was also great enough in many women to give marked clinical benefit. The rate of telogen shedding was reduced, and in some patients there was some regrowth of terminal hair (Peereboom-Wynia and Bockhurst 1980; Ekoe et al. 1980). The difference noted between sexes was a considerably lower half-life of the distribution phase III, with 3.17 ± 0.96 and 3.22 ± 0.6 days in normal and androgenized women, respectively, as compared to 1.6 ± 0.2 days in normal men. Variously sized compartments of body fat may be responsible for the sex difference.

Zaun (1986) discussed the use of antiandrogens for androgen-potentiated alopecia. In females, reverse sequential therapy resulted in a decrease in the proportion of scalp follicles in the telogen stage, as determined from plucked hairs. Similar changes were detectable in patients under the Diane regimen (1977) (which contains 2 mg cyproterone acetate and 50 μg ethinyloestradial per tablet throughout the package made in Germany), in which of a group of 25 sexually delinquent men receiving 100–200 mg cyproterone acetate over a period of 3–30 months, 9 shared a similar decrease in telogen stage hair count.

In an in vitro study, low doses of either cyproterone acetate (24 n*M*) and 17α-propylmesterolone (29 n*M*) induced growth enhancement, especially of papilla cell and outer root sheath keratinocytes, whereas high doses of cyproterone (1.20 μ*M*) and 17α-propylmesterolone (1.45 μ*M*) had opposite effects. Applying increasing doses of androgens to cyproterone acetate (24 n*M*)- or 17α-propylmesterolone (29 n*M*)-containing media neutralized the growth-stimulating effect of antiandrogens, particularly in papilla cells and outer root sheath keratinocytes. However, minor differences between the effects of testosterone and dihydrotestosterone on cell growth were found (Kiesewetter 1992).

26.2.4 Spironolactone

Experimental treatments of male pattern baldness and acne vulgaris have been conducted with various preparations containing a substance thought to contain an inhibitor for 5α-reductase; however, no successful results were achieved although the preparation was obviously effective in blocking the receptor (Loriaux et al. 1976; Levy et al. 1980; Evron et al. 1981; Barth et al. 1989). This result suggests that spironolactone, which is thought to exhibit similar action to that of the above inhibitor, could be very effective. Spironolactone was originally developed as a diuretic, an antagonist of aldosterone. It inhibits the activity of aldosterone by making it compete with the mineral corticoid receptor, thus suppressing sodium resorption in the renal tubules by inducing sodium discharge. It has been used for the treatment of hirsutism and the improvement of acne (Shapiro and Evron 1980) and when used for androgenetic alopecia, subjective improvement was shown by the end of 6 months (Burk and Cunliffe 1985). Gynecomastia may occur as a side effect. The occurrence of gynecomastia with this treatment is thought to be induced by antiandrogen activity, since, during the process of elucidating the mechanism of action of spironolactone, it was found to bind with the 5α-reductase receptor (Loriaux et al. 1976; Rose et al. 1977). Unlike cyoctol (a synthetic nonsteroidal drug), spironolactone is a steroidal drug, but if it has the same mechanism as the inhibitor noted above, it may also be effective in treating male pattern baldness and acne vulgaris. As a matter of fact, both oral and parenteral spironolactone have often been reported to be effective in the treatment of acne vulgaris but there is no reported experience in androgenetic alopecia (Nielsen 1982).

Other Products Being Developed by Pharmaceutical and Cosmetic Companies

27

27.1 Treatment of Androgenetic Alopecia with Chemical Products

27.1.1 Minoxidil

Minoxidil is a piperidenopyrimidine derivative and a potent peripheral arteriolar vasodilator used in the treatment of resistant hypertension (Ducharme et al. 1973; Mehta et al. 1975; Novak et al. 1985). It is marketed by the Upjohn Pharmaceutical Company (MI, USA) under the trade name Loniten. The drug has several side effects. On the negative side, it may cause edema, reduced blood pressure, tachycardia, nausea, dyspnea, and anemia (Mehta et al. 1975; Devine et al. 1977). The positive side effect of Loniten, however, is regeneration of hair growth in the temporal area (Burton and Marshall 1979b; Seidman et al. 1981; Fiedler-Weiss 1987). Hypertrichosis is a frequent (30%–100% in different reports) side effect of oral therapy in adults (Burton and Marshall 1979b; Seidman et al. 1981).

Upjohn hoped to refine the hair-growing aspects of the drug and to eliminate the negative side effects by administering the medication topically rather than orally. They used a 3% minoxidil solution and started their studies on 2000 volunteer patients, beginning in July 1983. Of the 2000 volunteers who participated in the testing program, 1800 completed it. Forty percent of the volunteers who used the product on an experimental basis claimed moderate to dense hair growth. When minoxidil is discontinued, the new hair growth ceases abruptly and shedding occurs in a few months (Fenton and Wilkinson 1983; Sansing 1987).

In the minoxidil studies, it was found that cosmetically adequate hair regrowth could be expected in up to 25% or 30% of men treated with a topical 2% or 3% minoxidil solution for androgenic alopecia. No significant differences in efficacy were seen between the two solutions. The hair regrowth response was most likely to be favorable at the vertex in a patch of baldness less than 10 cm in diameter that contained more than 100 indeterminate hairs. Hair regrowth was most likely to appear in those who had had the hair loss for less than 10 years. The evidence suggests that hair loss, at least at the vertex, may be retarded by topical minoxidil.

Studies of an extemporaneous topical formulation compounded from crushed tablets of minoxidil are difficult to interpret. Assays have shown that filtered and unfiltered preparations contain different concentrations of minoxidil. The unfiltered preparation contained 36.2 mg minoxidil per ml, whereas the filtered preparation contained 6.3 mg per ml. Reports of studies in which extemporaneous preparations were used are very difficult to interpret because of this variation in concentration. With the poor percutaneous absorption of minoxidil, these differences in formulation are relevant.

Minoxidil is clearly better for retarding hair loss than for growing new hair. The drug works best on men younger than 30 whose hair loss is not extensive and has started within the last 5 years. In this particular group of men under 30, only one-third can expect a good result (a doubling of hair density) and about 40% can expect fair results (Burton and Marshall 1979b).

According to Tromovitch et al. (1985), regardless of minoxidil therapy, no treatment has been successful in men with far-advanced baldness.

Merk (1990) reported that regrowth of short fine hairs was observed in androgenetic alopecia after treatment with topical minoxidil, but the regrowth of normal terminal hair seemed to be a rare event.

27.1.2 Diazoxide

Diazoxide (Schering: Baker Norton Pharmaceuticals, FL, USA), like minoxidil, is a potent vasodilator, although the drugs are not chemically related. It was previously suggested that diazoxide could cause hypertrichosis, either by increasing cutaneous perfusion or by its known effect in increasing intracellular cAMP levels (Burton et al. 1975); minoxidil is not thought to increase cAMP, and it now seems more likely that both drugs act by increasing the blood flow to the hair follicles. Moore (1968) suggested that diazoxide was an inhibitor of the enzyme phosphodiesterase, which breaks down cAMP, and that the resulting increase in intracellular cAMP levels could stimulate hair growth. Uno et al. (1990) confirmed that diazoxide (5% solution) was effective in topical use.

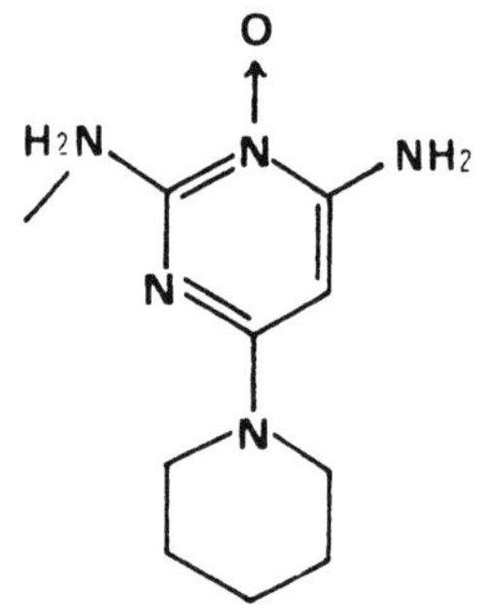

2,4-diamino-6-piperidinopyrimidine-3-oxide

Fig. 27.1. Minoxidil (Loniten, Upjohn)

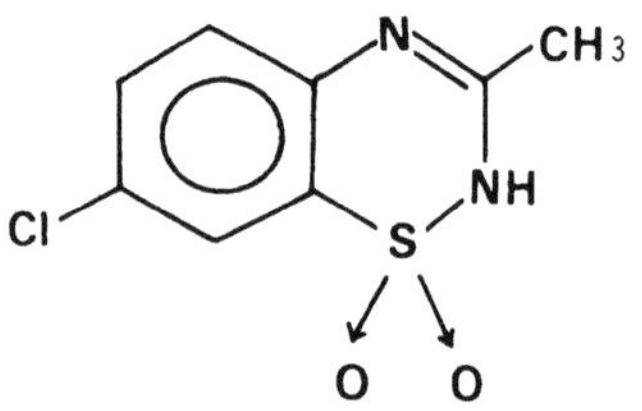

7 chloro-3-methyl-2H-1,
2, 4-benzothiadiazine -1, 1-dioxide

Fig. 27.2. Diazoxide (Schering, Baker Norton Pharmaceuticals, FL, USA), a benzothiadiazine derivative

27.2 Chemical Structure of These Products

Minoxidil is 2,4-diamino-6-piperidinopyrimidine-3-oxide. Its chemical structure is shown in Fig. 27.1. It dissolves well in ethanol and propylene glycol and is stable in solutions prepared for topical application.

Diazoxide, 7-chloro-3-methyl-2H-1,2,4-benzothiadiazine-1,1-dioxide ($C_8H_7Cl\text{-}N_2O_2S$), is an anti-hypertensive, structurally related to chlorothiazide but having no diuretic properties. It occurs as white or cream-colored crystals or a crystalline powder (Fig. 27.2). It is usually administered intravenously. Interestingly, both minoxidil and diazoxide are oxidizing agents.

27.3 Mechanism of Hair Growth in Relation to New Drugs

Minoxidil and diazoxide when used for the treatment of hypertension have the unique side effect of increasing the growth of vellus hairs. The precise mechanism for this stimulation of hair growth is still unknown, but it has been postulated that vasodilation of dermal blood vessels could be responsible. Using a laser Doppler technique, Burton and Marshall (1979b) and Wester et al. (1984) demonstrated increased blood flow following the topical application of minoxidil to the bald scalp of men. Although the mechanism of action by which this hair growth is stimulated has not yet been established, minoxidil, whether taken orally or applied topically, presumably works in MPB by increasing local cutaneous perfusion in the scalp, thereby reducing the difference between core and skin temperature. The rate of hair growth is increased by this raising of skin temperature.

Baden and Kubilus (1983) considered that, since vasodilatation of the skin was not consistently associated with enhanced hair growth, minoxidil may stimulate hair matrix cells directly.

Daigie et al. (1977), and Devine et al. (1977) have reported that patients receiving these agents systemically for periods of more than 1 month to control severe hypertension were also found to have generalized, reversible hypertrichosis. However, Koperski et al. (1987), and Olsen et al. (1990), found that hair regrowth with topical minoxidil tended to plateau at about 12 months of treatment, with a slight decline in this new growth by 2½–2¾ years. With follow-up at 4½–5 years (Olsen et al. 1990), it was found that continued use of topical minoxidil was associated with a slow decline in the 12-month hair counts. However, continued maintenance of nonvellus hair regrowth was well beyond baseline levels. No noticeable systemic side effects were observed after the topical application of minoxidil for considerably long periods (approximately 5 years) (Uno et al. 1987; De Villez 1990; Olsen et al. 1990).

Baden and Kubilus (1983), however, indicated that minoxidil had a rather characteristic effect on cultured epidermal cells in that it control cultures. Cultures of human epidermal cells were treated with minoxidil and it was found that they survived longer than control cells. In addition, minoxidil prolonged the time that cells could be passed after reacting confluence. A better explanation for his findings is that minoxidil has an epidermal growth factor (EGF)-like action in that it delays senescence of cells.

27.4 Mechanism of Action of New Drugs on Target Tissue

As stated above, the mechanism of minoxidil-induced hair regrowth is not fully understood. It may involve the synergistic effect of minoxidil on a variety of cell types. According to Cohen et al. (1984), a possible mechanism of action is that minoxidil has a direct effect on hair itself. Minoxidil slows the senescence of human epidermal keratinocytes similarly to the action of epidermal growth factor.

Uno et al. (1987) reported no increase in hair density with the passage of time after the topical application of minoxidil. Also, there seems to be no evidence that minoxidil was selectively taken into the hair follicle after it was observed subcutaneously (Zelei et al. 1990).

Experiments on the sulfotransferase activity of minoxidil in epithelium, hair follicle, and connective tissue of the scalp revealed that more than 60% of this activity was observed in the hair follicle. This finding suggests that minoxidil-induced enlargement of subcutaneous blood vessels enhances the proliferation of hair follicle tissue (Uno et al. 1985; Baker et al. 1991).

According to Buhl et al. (1992), a group of drugs that includes minoxidil and diazoxide functions in other target tissues as potassium channel openers. Weston et al. (1990) and Robertson and Steinberg (1990) have also described potassium channel openers in the context of controlling the matrix. The hypothesis has been proposed that the potassium channel opening is a common and important mechanism for drugs that stimulate hair follicles (Cook 1988).

The potassium channel modulators have been reported to have antihypertensive effects through exerting a direct action on vascular smooth muscle (Weston et al. 1990; Robertson and Steinberg 1990). Although minoxidil increases cutaneous blood flow (Wester et al. 1984), it also exerts direct effects in cultured follicles on both the proliferation and differentiation of the epithelial cells that comprise the hair shaft (Buhl et al. 1989). Buhl et al. (1992) provide the best evidence to date that the opening of potassium channels is an important regulatory mechanism for hair growth. In one report (Ryan 1973), the most interesting finding was that both minoxidil and diazoxide are oxidizing agents. It has been postulated that vasodilatation of dermal blood vessels could be responsible for the side effect of both these agents in stimulating hair growth.

Since vasodilatation of skin and skin appendages is not consistently associated with enhanced hair growth, it is also quite possible that minoxidil and diazoxide may stimulate the hair matrix cells directly. The authors suggest that both these agents may act as oxidizing agents, inactivating 5-α-reductase in the sebaceous glands and the matrix cells (Inaba 1985) (see Chapter 15 and Section 28.5.1).

27.5 Viprostol

Viprostol, manufactured by American Cyanamid (Lederle Laboratories, Pearl River, NY, USA) is also undergoing clinical examination to determine its capacity for promoting hair growth. An analogue of prostaglandin (PGE_2), viprostol is a topically effective antihypertensive agent that has been found useful in treating vascular disorders of the extremities. Similar to minoxidil and diazoxide, viprostol is a vasodilator, expanding blood vessels and facilitating blood flow (Olsen and Delong 1990). Although news reports have told of promising hair growing effects, Olsen and Delong (1990) reported that viprostol was not an effective hair growth promoter in androgenetic alopecia.

27.6 Other Products in Development

27.6.1 Cyoctol

A Los Angeles company, Chantel Pharmaceuticals (Los Angeles, CA, USA), obtained permission from the Food and Drug Administration (FDA) to begin testing on Cyoctol (a synthetic nonsteroid drug) in December 1986. This drug, a nonsteroidal androgen receptor blocker, 6-(5-methoxy-1-heptyl) bicyclo (3,3,0) octan-3-one (Fig. 27.3), supposedly blocks the androgenic hormones that are thought to cause male pattern baldness. Steroidal hormone blockers are used in Europe, but produce feminizing side effects such as breast growth and loss of facial hair. Cyoctol is also being tested for the treatment of acne and has shown none

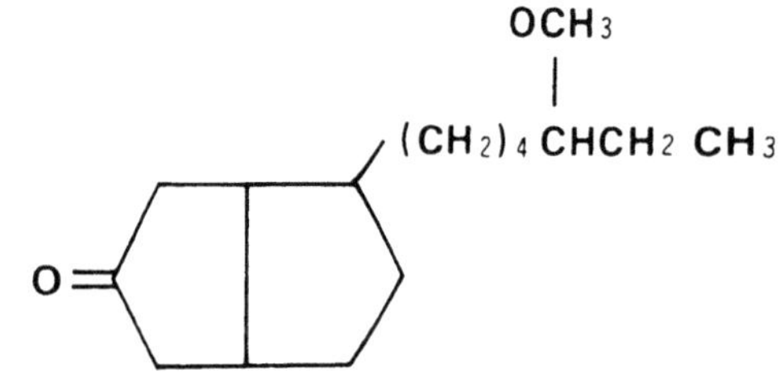

Fig. 27.3. Cyoctol, a nonsteroidal androgen-receptor blocker, 6-(5-methoxy-1-heptyl) bicyclo [3,3,0] octan-3-one

of these side effects. Testing for the prevention of male baldness is being done in Los Angeles and Japan.

27.6.2 Cyclosporine A

Cyclosporine A is a potent cytostatic drug with apparent specificity for the immune system. Therefore, it is now widely used as a potent immunosuppressive agent in organ transplantation and in disorders predominantly affecting the immune system, such as pemphigus vulgaris and bullous pemphigoid (Biren and Baar 1986). It enhances the T suppressor cell activity and depresses both the amount and the function of T helper cells. Therefore, cyclosporin A should be effective in alopecia areata (Kahan 1982).

One clinical complication of immunosuppressive therapy with cyclosporine A (CsA) is the stimulation of hair growth. Previous investigators have shown that CsA affects hair growth in humans (Wysiocki and Daley 1987) and in laboratory rats with several genetic variants of acne, and they have concluded that CsA predominantly influences keratinization (Pauss et al. 1989).

CsA stimulates hair growth in athymic nude mice (Sawada et al. 1987). A stimulatory effect on nude mouse cultured vibrissa follicle has also been observed (Buhl et al. 1990). Evidence from animal studies suggests that CsA causes premature entry of follicles into anagen (Pauss et al. 1989), but this alone would be insufficient to account for the hypertrichosis in humans, where there is an increase in the length of the hair fiber. According to Taylor et al. (1993), the hypertrichotic action of CsA may be due to the prolongation of the anagen phase of the hair growth cycle.

27.6.3 Aramis Nutriplexx

Besides the pharmaceutical companies, a number of cosmetic companies are manufacturing products which have similar effects on hair growth. These products are marketed under different names and are based on mucopolysaccharide, a natural sugar compound. Aramis' (New York, NY, USA) Nutriplexx is touted as a thinning hair supplement. The fine print admits that it does not cure or prevent baldness. Nutriplexx supposedly penetrates the hair to make it look fuller.

27.6.4 Foltene and Flowlin

Nutriplexx and other products such as Foltene and Flowlin (Shiseido Co., Tokyo, Japan) differentiate themselves from conditioners that merely coat the hair. The package often simulates that of a prescription drug. Cosmetically they may do some good, though claims that they enlarge the follicles, thus allowing each hair shaft to become fatter, are dubious. The products are marketed as "hair restorers" in other countries without the stringent requirements imposed by the FDA. In November 1980, the FDA published in the Federal Register the panel's proposal to remove this type of hair products from the market (FDA 1980).

Shiseido continues to study materials for promoting hair growth; its Japanese Patent JP 60 054 310 discloses the use of 4-estren-3-one-17β ethoxy derivatives for the stimulation of hair growth (and also for the treatment of acne). These constituents are said to have no undesirable side effects such as hormonal action. They inhibit reductase activity as well as the combination of 5-α-dihydroxy testosterone with receptor proteins. The preferred preparation contains 0.02% of 17-β-(2-hydroxyethoxy)-4-estren-3-one or 0.2% of 17-β-(2-hydroxyethoxy)-4-estren-3-one acetate in a hydroalcoholic vehicle (Fox 1986).

According to Orentreich and Orentreich (1988), new horizons in the treatment of androgenetic alopecia have been reported, as follows:

1. *5α-reductase inhibitors*
   a. A steroid, 4-androsten-3-one-17β-carboxylic acid (Voigt and Hsia 1973)
   b. Secosteroids. The allenic ketone group (Rando 1974)
   c. Allenic 3-keto-5,10-secosteroids (Robaire et al. 1977)
   d. Allenic 3-keto-5,10-secosteroids (Voigt et al. 1978)
   e. 5α-Reductase inhibitor (Brooks et al. 1981)
   f. N,N-Diethyl-4-methyl-3-oxo-4-aza-5α-androstane-17β-carboxamide (4-MA) (Rittmaster et al. 1987)
2. *Inhibitors of testosterone to DHT conversion*
   a. Antiandrogen, 17α-β-nortestosterone (Zarate et al. 1966)
   b. 17α-Methyl-β-nortestosterone (Strauss and Pochi 1970)

c. Trimethyltrienolone (R-2956: 17β-hydroxy-2,2,17α-methylestra-4,9,11-trien-3-one) (Boulanger et al. 1974; Bonne and Raynaud 1974; Takayasu 1979)
d. 17α-Propyltestosterone (WIN-17665) (Ferrari et al. 1978; Chakrabarty et al. 1980)
e. Antiandrogen (TSAA-291) (16β-ethyl-17β-hydroxy-4-estren-3-one) (Sudo et al. 1979)

3. *Nonsteroidal antiandrogens*
a. Nonsteroidal antiandrogen (RU-22930) (Raynaud and Boone 1977)
b. Synthetic antiandrogen (11α-hydroxy-progesterone) (Tamm et al. 1982; Matias et al. 1984; Luderschmidt et al. 1983)
c Ketoconazole (treatment of mycoses) (Pont et al. 1982 noticed no growth of scalp hair when this drug was administered)

4. *Other drugs causing hypertrichosis*
a. Hexachlorobenzene (Cam and Nigogosyan 1963)
b. Phenytoin (Bray 1959)
c. Glucocorticoids (Rook 1972)
d. Psoralen (Singh and Lal 1966)
e. Streptomycin (Fono 1950)
f. Nicotinic acid (Setala et al. 1972)
g. Biotin (Vitamin H) (Settel 1977)
h. Mineral oil, marrow, and sulfur, etc. (Alfonsi 1985)
i. Horseradish and mustard seed extracts (Banfi 1985)

Trial Treatment of Androgenetic Alopecia with Oxidizing Agents (Inaba and Inaba 1984)

28

28.1 The Hair Growth-Stimulating (Trichogenous) Effect of Cold Wave Hair Styling

Inaba presented his original hypothesis of how hair is generated in *Science*, the Japanese-language edition of *Scientific American* (Inaba 1981). One physician informed him that new growth of hair had been observed after permanent waving. The reader reported new hair generating between thin hairs when the scalp hair was permed directly and lightly. Later, Inaba found that treatment of baldness has been carried out at a few research centers using this method.

Investigating the phenomenon, Inaba found that cold wave permanents had a trichogenous effect on complete baldness patients. However, cold wave permanents also damage the hair. The new hairs may be damaged by further treatment and fall out. Inaba took great interest in the underlying reason why the cold wave permanent induced new hair growth.

28.2 The Cold Wave Principle

Human hair keratin is a high molecular weight protein with large amounts of cystine; hydrogen bonds, salt bonds, and numerous disulfide cross-links provide the enormous physical strength of the macromolecule.

Hair consists of a hard protein called keratin. Proteins are compound amino acids, especially those containing sulfur, cystine, and methionine. The sulfur in each of these amino acids combines to form an S–S bond, which creates the hardness of hair (Fig. 28.1).

The bonding of the sulfur atoms must be blocked in order to soften the hair sufficiently for free styling. The primary chemical agent used for this purpose is thioglycolic acid. The reductive effect of this acid blocks the S–S bond. Softened hair containing cysteine may be wound on curlers and set for the desired styling. Secondary solutions such as sodium bromide, which has an oxidative effect, are used in recombining the blocked S–S bond to harden the hair once it is set in the new style.

28.3 Basis of Hair Regeneration

Even though hair growth using the cold wave was only temporary, its effect was thoroughly examined. Controlled experiments were conducted using thioglycolic acid, sodium bromide, etc., under safe conditions. Hard hairs regenerated in the bald areas. This discovery toppled the notion that baldness is caused by the loss of the hair roots. Obviously, with these new hairs emerging, the hair roots had not died. These experiments suggested a possible route to a new treatment procedure for baldness. Considering the respective effects of the primary and secondary agents, the secondary agent was probably the prime mover.

The first agent, thioglycolic acid, is a reductant. The effect of the 5α-reductase enzyme in the sebaceous gland is also reductive. Both are active at a pH of 8.0–9.0, so that chemical interaction between them did not seem feasible.

To clarify this point, please recall the effect on the 5α-reductase enzyme secreted from the sebaceous gland. The male hormone, testosterone, secreted from the testes and carried to the sebaceous gland in the bloodstream, is converted into the more potent androgen 5α-dihydrotestosterone

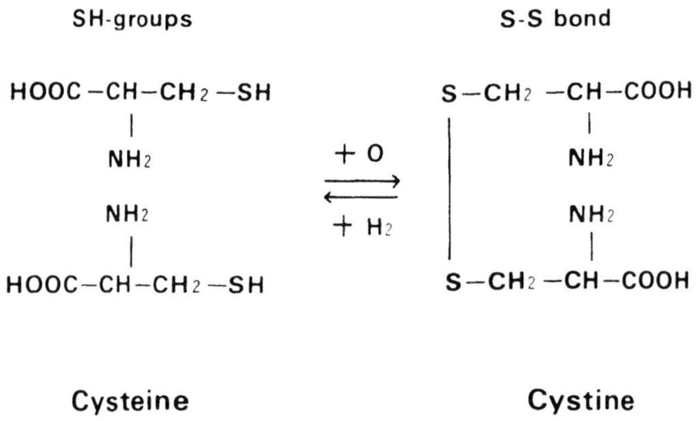

Fig. 28.1. Cold wave principle. Cold wave permanents have a trichogenous effect on complete baldness patients

(5α-DHT) by the action of 5α-reductase. This androgen agent is circulated through the blood vessels surrounding the hair follicle inside the connective tissue sheath to the dermal papilla and then its matrix (Fig. 19.1). In excessive amounts, it can cause atrophy of the hair follicle due to inhibition of hair matrix activity, which leads to deterioration of vigorous hair growth and brings with it the onset of baldness (Adachi and Kano 1970; Adachi 1973).

The experiments noted above suggested that, by depressing excess production of the 5α-reductase enzyme, its negative effect on hair growth could be inhibited sufficiently to prevent, or at least retard, baldness.

Since it was evident that the primary agent of the cold wave permanent, thioglycolic acid, did not counteract 5α-reductase, attention was then redirected to the secondary oxidizing agent. However, the secondary agent, in the form of sodium bromide, also showed little detectable effect, and there was the continual risk that too-frequent application of the cold wave treatment could be destructive to the hair.

28.4 Discovery of an Effective Trichogen

Research studies of the cold wave treatment supported the basic sebaceous gland hypothesis. The next step was to discover a chemical agent capable of blocking production of the 5α-reductase enzyme or inhibiting its impact on hair matrix activity.

Inaba began to ask various informed sources, "Is there any chemical agent capable of counteracting 5α-reductase?" It was in the field of cosmetic products that he found his initial lead. He investigated the claim that Paddy Leaf Shampoo and Tonic (Medical Hair Research [MHR], Tokyo, Japan) was effective in retarding hair loss by removing the skin surface lipid membrane (sebum) of the scalp, while having a somewhat trichogenous effect. The shampoo contained Water Gel (MHR), a polysaccharide that is a pure natural vegetable polymer. The chemical structure of Water Gel is a complicated combination of a chemical chain specific to natural polymer groups and a branch-like configuration spreading outward from the basic chain; the molecule absorbs as much as 20 times its own weight of water. It then expands and produces moisture for a proper shampoo viscosity.

The shampoo cleanses the scalp by removing surface deposits. It penetrates beneath the skin surface down to the pore of the hair canal and its cleansing effect is excellent. Water Gel has a "conveyer system" effect that assists the transfer of a substance somewhat in the manner of a waterway. It carries substances needed for healthy metabolic activity in the skin as well as permeating the pores to carry off waste material and excessive sebum. Quite possibly, it could prevent the enlargement of the sebaceous gland or reduce its size if already enlarged. This would reduce the effect of testosterone by suppressing the amount of 5α-reductase secreted from the sebaceous gland.

The shampoo alone, however, could not have a great trichogenous effect. Attention then shifted to the hair tonic. No matter how thoroughly the constituents of the hair tonic were scrutinized, none of the principal chemical agents could be identified as an active trichogenous agent.

The tonic contained capsicum tincture, cantharides, alcohol, and other skin stimulants, as well as a few oxidizing agents used as antiseptic bactericides. The inhibition and reduction of 5α-reductase by these oxidants ultimately caused the trichogenous effect. Long-term application of the hair tonic was reported to have a trichogenous effect.

28.5 Development of New Tonic Formulation

Convinced that more effective and reliable chemical agents were available, a joint study between Inaba's research center resources and a pharmaceutical manufacturer was launched. The goal was to find an oxidative and reductive agent capable of counteracting 5α-reductase, such as a nonsteroidal antiandrogen agent, thus avoiding the undesirable side effect that steroid agents can cause.

Many substances, including an American cosmetic agent, e.g., commercial perfumes (Guin 1982), face creams (Cronin 1980), hair dyes (Cronin 1980), and hair lotions (Dooms-Goossents et al. 1989) containing an oxide compound similar to the chemical agent used to suppress the blooming of flower buds during long-distance shipment, were studied. This compound worked by suppressing various kinds of enzyme activities. The connection became clear; since the oxidant suppressed enzyme activity under other conditions, it could possibly be used to suppress the enzyme 5α-reductase as well.

28.5.1 Oxidizing Agents for the Treatment of Baldness (Inaba and Inaba 1984; Inaba 1985)

Various oxidizing agents for inactivating 5α-reductase were investigated. Of these, potassium bromide ($KBrO_3$), sodium bromide ($NaBrO_3$), and chloramine T are used in cosmetics, and sodium hypochlorite ($NaClO$), sodium chlorite ($NaClO_2$), and stabilized chlorine dioxide (ClO_2) are used as food additives in Japan.

The studies finally came to focus on stabilized chlorine dioxide (ClO_2), which has the most potent oxidizing action for enzyme suppression. Trial use of a treatment formula containing this agent was conducted for clinical observation. The first step in preparing the formulation was a study of the properties of this agent. This potent oxidizing agent is widely used as a disinfectant, antiseptic, deodorant, and bleaching agent (Magara 1982). However, ClO_2 above the concentration of 8 g/l is explosive when it comes in contact with sulfur, phosphorus, or phosphide. Because of this instability, the manufacturing process is difficult.

Studies were conducted to produce stabilized chlorine dioxide in a safe and storable substance. This stabilized agent has an oxidizing power 2.5 times as strong as that of pure chlorine and is stable for more than 1 year at pH 8.0–8.6. The stabilized ClO_2 is used as a bleach, bactericide, and deseasoner for wheat flour, in the same manner as unstabilized ClO_2. It is also used as a disinfectant for tap water and as an antiseptic bactericide for cosmetics. The disinfectant and bactericidal actions of this chemical agent are based on the inactivation of enzymes or on the direct denaturation of cytoplasm by oxidation, thus occurring in the same manner as with ozone and chlorine.

Chlorine and hypochlorite used as disinfectants react with organisms, producing chlorinated products. One representative product is a trihalomethane such as chloroform, whose concentration in drinking water is regulated because it is carcinogenic. Stabilized chlorine dioxide does not produce trihalomethane because it also oxidizes organisms that may produce chlorinated products.

The discovery of the formation of trihalomethanes in the disinfection of drinking water with chlorine focused attention on health effects that might arise indirectly from its use. Results released by the National Cancer Institute (NCI) have shown at least one of the trihalomethanes, chloroform, to be carcinogenic in both rats and mice.

Bull (1980) stated that chlorine dioxide and its organic reaction products may present a higher risk of acute toxicity than chlorine, combined chlorine, or ozone in the disinfection of drinking water. However, the use of chlorine dioxide may be advantageous when the generation of possibly carcinogenic byproducts by other disinfectants is considered.

The authors considered this substance the best agent for inactivating 5α-reductase in the sebaceous gland because safe inactivation of enzymes by oxidation, without any problematical side effects, could be expected. Clinical observation of the trial use of a hair treatment formula containing this agent has been conducted with marked success.

Supporting findings include studies on the use of benzoyl peroxide in a gel base on hairless skin (Fanta 1978; Fulton et al. 1974). It was shown that the amount of skin surface lipids was appreciably reduced by benzoyl peroxide. Benzoyl peroxide does lead to a reduction in the proliferation of cells in the sebaceous gland. It was also shown autoradiographically, by an in vitro technique, that in humans, the ^3H-thymidine labeling index in the sebaceous gland was reduced by benzoyl peroxide (Fanta 1978; Gloor et al. 1980; Wirth et al. 1983). Gloor et al. (1980) found, in the Syrian hamster ear model, a decrease in mitosis, a reduction in sebaceous gland size, an increase in the duration of the synthesis phase (S-phase) of the cell cycle, and a shortening of the time to detachment of the cells from the basal lamina of the sebaceous gland.

Chlorine itself, on the other hand, is capable of reacting with all amino acids present in keratin fibers; cystine and tyrosine are found to be particularly susceptible to attack (Kantouch and Abdel-Fattah 1972). According to Fair and Guptar (1987), in the shrink-proofing treatment of wool, chlorination has been shown to alter the surface morphology, primarily through breaking the disulfide and peptide bonds in the proteinous material of the fiber.

28.6 Treatment of Androgenetic Alopecia with Stabilized Chlorine Dioxide (Inaba 1985)

The formula used in the treatment program included glycerin, alcohol, and fragrance, in addition to 250 ppm stabilized ClO_2, whose inactivating effect on 5α-reductase was studied. In liquid form, the preparation was applied to the scalp two to three times daily, treating some 100 test patients. Results were obtained by questionnaire 10 months later.

Conditions of dandruff, itching, and sebum in the scalp after the 10-month treatment period are shown in Tables 28.1, 28.2, and 28.3. Dandruff produced when sebum excreted from the sebaceous gland is mixed with the corneal layer exfoliated from the scalp is classified as soft or dry type. Increased sebum stimulates and enhances cornification, and therefore increases dandruff in a vicious cycle.

In the test subjects, this condition generally improved 1 month after they began topical application of the formula, and was eventually better in about 68% of the patients.

Sebum plus bacteria in the scalp can cause inflammation. This condition (itchiness), if present, improved in 63% of the respondents (Table 28.2). The sebum condition alone was improved in 59% (Table 28.3). It is presumed that the improvement of this condition, which is basically attributable to hypertrophy of the sebaceous gland, was the result of a diminution in the size of the sebaceous gland effected by the agent used for inactivating 5α-reductase.

Decreased loss of hair was noticeable about 2 months after application began (Table 28.4). This was due to improvement of the ratio of hairs in anagen stage to those in telogen stage. About 53% of the patients showed this improvement. This decrease in hair loss, the first stage in treatment of hair in the anagen stage, suggested that the amount of dihydrotestosterone produced by the sebaceous gland had declined below the level at which normal hair matrix activity would be suppressed.

The development and growth of hair are shown in Table 28.5. Completely bald areas were darkened by new growth of vellus hair to some degree in 30% of the test subjects. This vellus hair then became thicker and harder in 24% of the patients. An especially marked degree of hair growth was

Table 28.1. Dandruff

Dandruff	%
a. Disappeared	38
b. Decreased	30
c. No change	25
d. Increased	1
e. Uncertain	6
Total no. of patients	100

Table 28.2. Itchiness

Itchiness	%
a. Disappeared	30
b. Decreased	33
c. No change	31
d. Increased	1
e. Uncertain	5
Total no. of patients	100

Table 28.3. Sebum

Sebum	%
a. Disappeared	20
b. Decreased	39
c. No change	35
d. Uncertain	6
Total no. of patients	100

Table 28.4. Loss of hair

Loss of hair	%
a. None	13
b. Decreased	40
c. No change	40
d. Increased	1
e. Uncertain	6
Total no. of patients	100

Table 28.5. Development of hair

Development of hair	%
a. Hair generated	30
b. Vellus hair became harder	13
c. Vellus hair became thicker	11
d. No change	34
e. Uncertain	12
Total no. of patients	100

Table 28.6. Hair growth

Degree of hair growth	%
a. Marked	13
b. Mild	34
c. Very slight	12
d. No change	29
e. Uncertain	12
Total no. of patients	100

Table 28.7. Hair color change

Change of hair color	%
a. No change	90
b. Change to brown	7
c. Change to black	3
Total no. of patients	100

Table 28.8. Effect of Inaba reagent on baldness preceding forehead (100 patients)

Status of hair growth	No. of patients	%
Hair growth visualized	28	28
Thickness of already fine hair increased	22	22
Retardation of hair loss	30	30
No change	20	20

With permission from T.H. Chung, personal communication, 1984.

found in 13% and slight growth in 34%. The results were even more favorable when the period of application was prolonged (Table 28.6).

The finding that vellus hairs were eventually replaced by terminal hairs indicates that testosterone transported directly from the testes to the hair matrices is converted in small amounts to dihydrotestosterone by the 5α-reductase present. This promotes regeneration of hair once the excessive amount of dihydrotestosterone secreted from the sebaceous gland has been suppressed.

Change of hair color and other side effects are shown in Table 28.7. While 90% of the test subjects reported no change in hair color, 7% experienced change in coloration from black to brown. This shows that hair became somewhat bleached if the oxidizing agent was too strong (500 ppm in some cases). Perspiration may also have contributed to the oxidizing strength by decreasing the pH level. In 3% of the subjects, black terminal hairs were regenerated in a region of white hairs. Almost all terminal hairs that replaced vellus hairs were black. The change to black hair suggests that tyrosinase, an oxidase required for the production of melanosomes, was enhanced in strength by the oxidizing agent in the formula. This finding may prove useful in future treatment of white hair. No other side effects, such as dermatitis, were observed in any of the test subjects.

The findings in this trial treatment of male pattern baldness with the nonsteroidal hair tonic (Inaba reagent) may provide some insight into the treatment of this disease, and, on the basis of this insight, a better formula may be developed in the near future.

Male pattern baldness is not solely a hereditary disease. The main factor is hormone activity, although hereditary and dietary factors may trigger the onset of this condition.

28.7 Supporting Findings

The effect of the nonsteroidal hair tonic (Inaba reagent) was investigated by Prof. T.H. Chung (Biomedical Research Laboratories of Kyungpook National University) in Korea. The agent was applied to 100 baldness patients, aged from 18 to 55, at their laboratories from July 1984 (personal communication, T.H. Chung 1984). The results are shown in Table 28.8.

We have applied for patents on this formulation and have patents issued in 16 countries, including the seven European Community (EC) countries (European patent No. 0067159); Canada (Canadian patent No. 1232545); Australia (Australian patent No. 566402); and Japan (Japanese patent No. 1562459). Paddy Leaf Hair Tonic is formulated on the basis of a new concept of the hair-growing mechanism. In this formulation, the active ingredient, which has an oxidative effect, stimulates the circulation of the blood, thereby controlling the negative influence of 5α-reductase, thus lowering the level of sebum secretion and stimulating healthy hair growth. In addition, it acts to control dandruff, itchiness, and the splitting, falling out, and breaking of hair. As a result of elevated hair metabolism, both the scalp and hair are kept healthy.

It has been 12 years since MHR Co. introduced Paddy Leaf Shampoo and Tonic to the world. Growing demand from the customers indicates the effectiveness of the formula, and it is hoped that this will provide the base for a better formula to be developed in the future.

28.8 Individual Case Reports of Patients with Androgenetic Alopecia Treated with the Inaba Reagent

28.8.1 Experience Using 5α-Reductase Inhibitor (Stabilized ClO_2)

In patients in whom the baldness was of more than 20 years duration, hair growth took somewhat longer to appear, but some degree of growth was observed. This test formula is not considered to be completely satisfactory, although comparisons with less effective treatment formulas give it the status of a breakthrough in new treatment techniques for baldness. The turning point for the development of a universally effective treatment has been reached.

28.8.1.1 Case 1

This patient was a 59-year-old male. He had begun to grow bald in his twenties, and had only a scant number of long hairs remaining in the frontal region. In the occipital region no vellus hairs were visible. The borderline of hair in the occipital re-

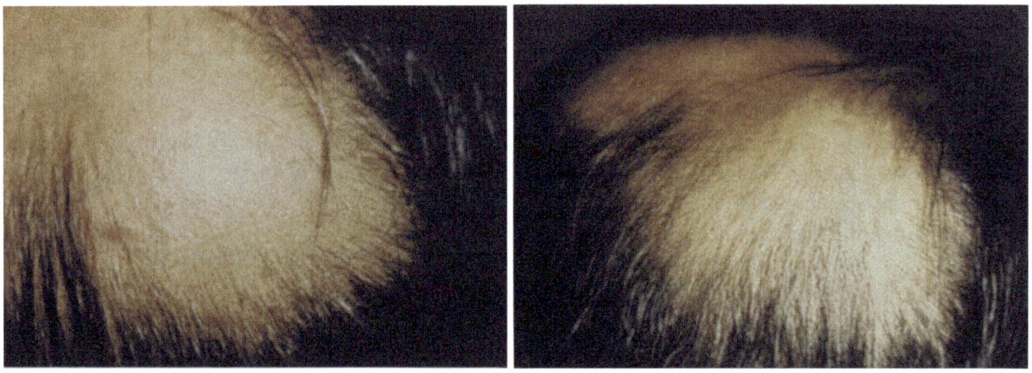

a b

Fig. 28.2a,b. Case 1, 59-year-old male. The borderline of hair in the occipital region was hyperbolic in outline, and completely bereft of visible vellus hair in the central portion. Pores in the occipital region began to open 2 months after test applications began. The pore area turned blue and the texture of the scalp became roughened, like an orange rind. **b** Ten months later, the vellus hairs which remained had become hardened and the bald area had become smaller in size

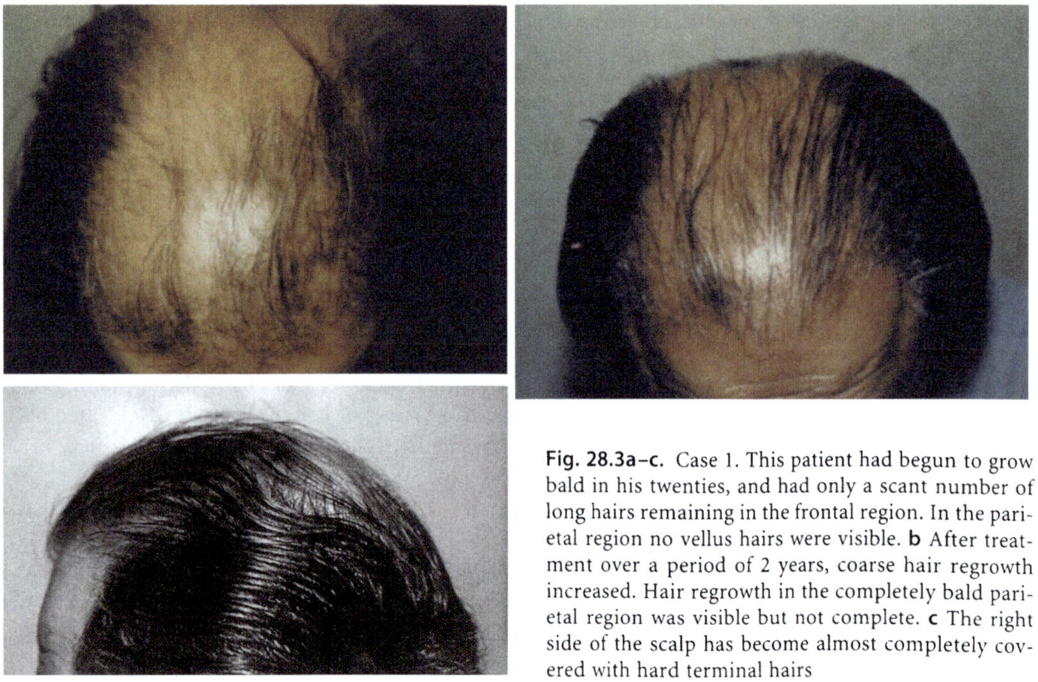

a b c

Fig. 28.3a–c. Case 1. This patient had begun to grow bald in his twenties, and had only a scant number of long hairs remaining in the frontal region. In the parietal region no vellus hairs were visible. **b** After treatment over a period of 2 years, coarse hair regrowth increased. Hair regrowth in the completely bald parietal region was visible but not complete. **c** The right side of the scalp has become almost completely covered with hard terminal hairs

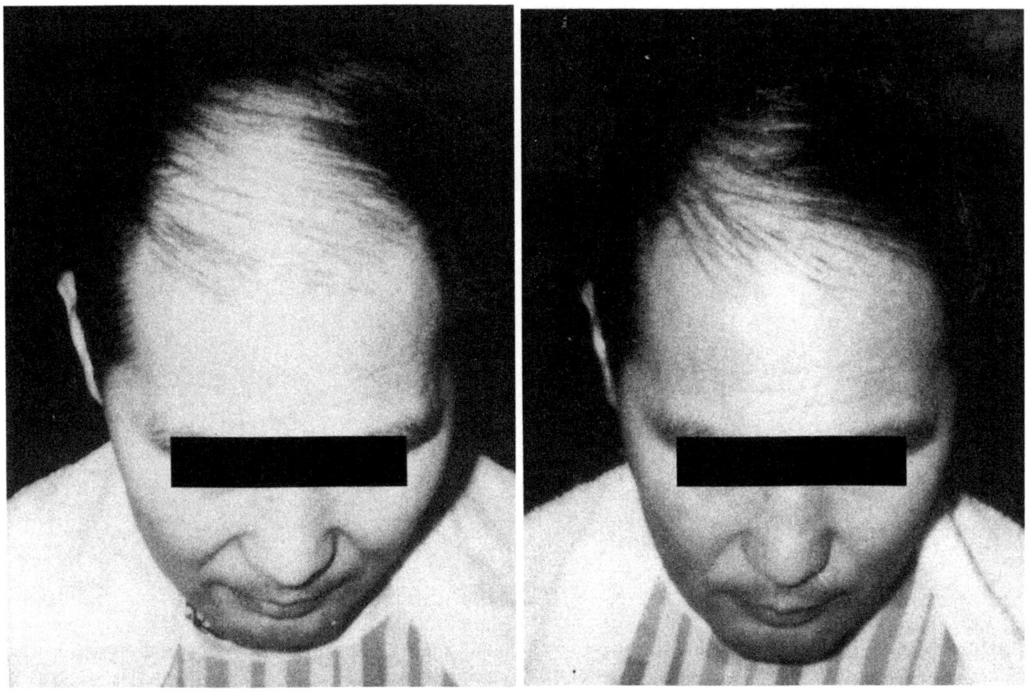

Fig. 28.4a,b. Case 2. Before treatment. Typical male pattern baldness. New hairs did not grow. **b** Existing hairs have become longer after 1-year treatment

gion was hyperbolic in outline, and completely bereft of visible vellus hair in the central portion (Fig. 28.2a).

The pores of the occipital region began to open 2 months after the test applications began. The texture of the scalp became roughened like that of an orange rind. Ten months later, the vellus hairs which remained had become hardened and the bald area had become smaller in size. The left side of the scalp had become completely covered by hard terminal hairs (Fig. 28.2b). In the parietal region, where originally no vellus hairs were visible (Fig. 28.3a), the bald scalp color gradually began to fade and vellus hair growth was quite noticeable.

Vigorous new hair growth was thick among the longer hairs, and the growth rate thereafter did not slow down. After 2 years, coarse hair regrowth continued to increase. Hair regrowth in the completely bald parietal region was visible but not complete (Fig. 28.3b). Eventually, the right side of the scalp became almost completely covered with hard terminal hairs (Fig. 28.3c).

28.8.1.2 Case 2

This patient was a 50-year-old male with typical male pattern baldness. New hairs did not grow, but existing hairs became longer after a treatment period of 1 year (Fig. 28.4a,b).

28.8.1.3 Case 3

This patient was a 36-year-old male who had experienced typical male pattern baldness in the parietal and occipital region for about 5 years (Fig. 28.5a). Generation of other new hairs was found among the longer hairs after a treatment period of about 18 months, although this growth was considered insufficient (Fig. 28.5b).

28.8.1.4 Case 4

This patient was a 30-year-old male whose hair had gradually receded from the parietal region in a pattern of premature baldness since his twenties (Fig. 28.6a). Although no tendency toward baldness was observed in his father, his brother showed almost the same bald condition. For occupational reasons, he had covered the bald region with a hairpiece. His experience in using the test formula was extremely favorable. Hair loss, dandruff, and itching ceased after 2 weeks. Short hairs, about 5 cm in length, grew longer, to as much as 10 cm over the period of 1 year after beginning the treatment. Further generation of new hair was observed (Fig. 28.6b).

28.8.1.5 Case 5

This patient was a 56-year-old male, with typical male pattern baldness. The hair had receded com-

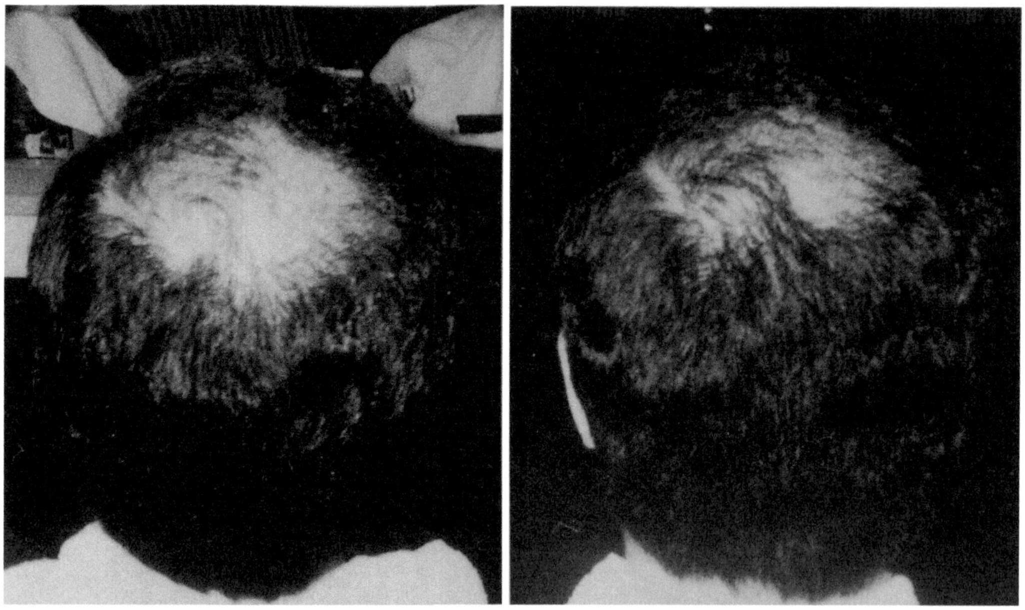

Fig. 28.5a,b. Case 3. Thirty-six-year-old male. **a** Before treatment. Typical male pattern baldness. **b** After 18-month treatment. Generation of other new hairs is found among the long hairs, although the growth was insufficient

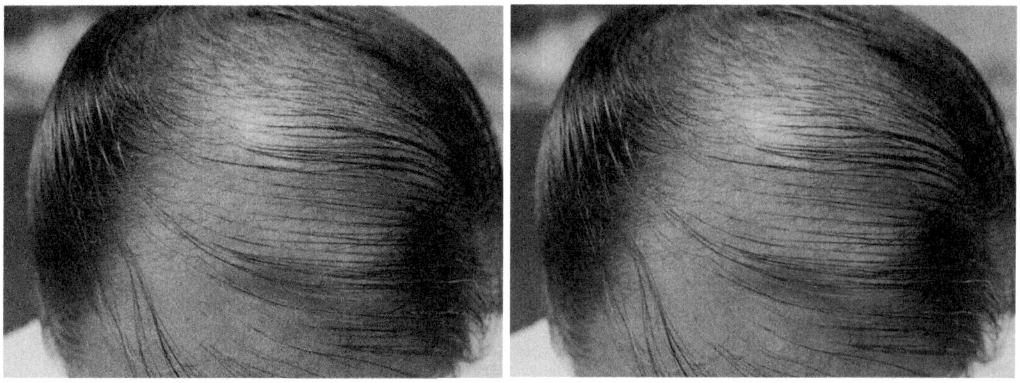

Fig. 28.6a,b. Case 4. Thirty-year-old male. **a** Typical androgenetic alopecia. **b** After 1-year treatment. Short hairs of about 5 cm in length have grown longer, to as long as 10 cm

pletely, except for the temporal region, by the age of 30 (Fig. 28.7a). After 10 months of treatment, regeneration of hair was noticeable in the parietal region. Gradual growth of hair moved forward over the scalp toward the frontal region (Fig. 28.7b). The vigorous regeneration of hair growth in the parietal region was apparently due, essentially, to the presence of vellus hairs. The slower rate of regeneration observed in the frontal region was due to the extreme atrophy of this completely bald region.

28.8.2 Experience Using Paddy Leaf Shampoo and Tonic

It has been over 10 years since Paddy Leaf Shampoo and Tonic appeared on the market (Fig.28.8). Because they are OTC products, they are manufactured to meet requirements that they are safe and have no side effects. For all that, their efficacy in preventing hair loss and promoting hair growth to a certain degree have been recognized, while no claims on side effects have been raised to date, which testifies to their good quality.

The following is a case in which their efficacy was noticeable.

a 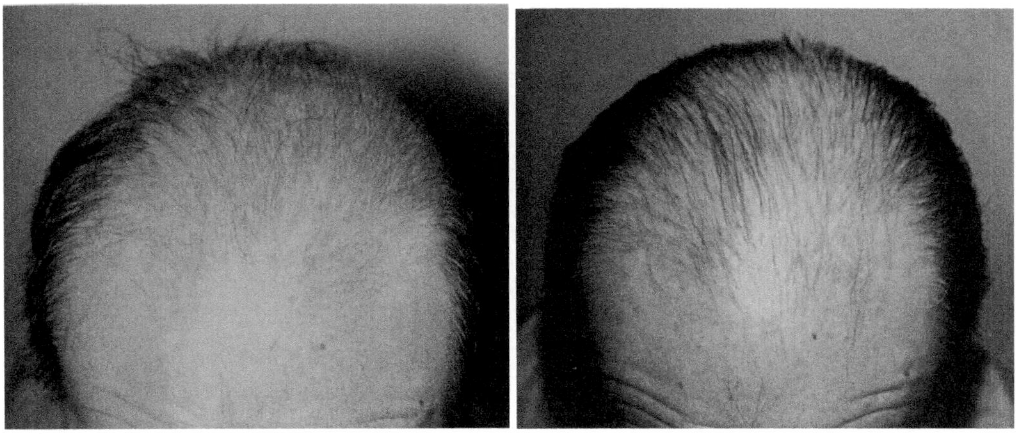 b

Fig. 28.7a,b. Case 5. Typical androgenetic alopecia. **b** After 10-month treatment, regeneration of scalp hair was noticeable in the parietal region

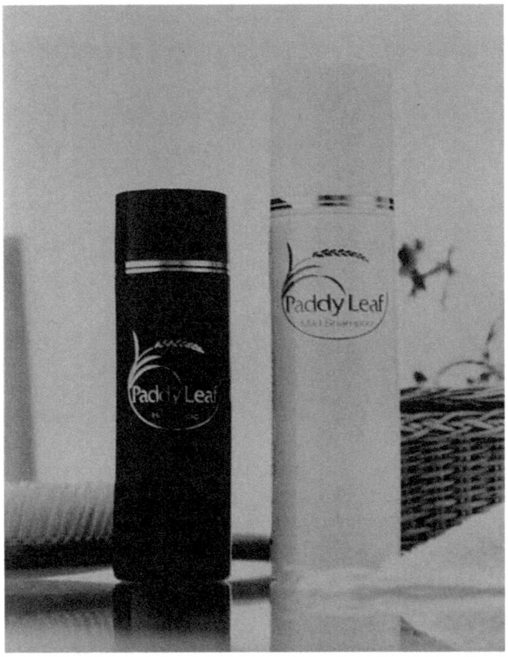

Fig. 28.8. Paddy Leaf hair tonic, manufactured by Medical Hair Research, Tokyo, Japan

Case 1. Male, 23 years old. His father had experienced typical male pattern baldness. Hair loss started when the son was about 20 years old and progressed until he fell into Norwood's classification III type. His hairline receded in the M shape and he had begun to suffer from neurosis because of this (Fig. 28.9a). We advised him to apply Paddy Leaf Hair Tonic at three times the normal frequency.

After 4 months of application, hair loss decreased and hair generation in the bald M-shaped region was recognized. Vellus hairs turned into coarse hairs and grew to a length of about 1.5 cm. The bald area was greatly improved, and a hairline was formed (Fig. 28.9c,d).

After 6 months, remarkable hair growth in the frontal region was recognized (Fig. 28.9e,f).

The above case suggests that oxidative agents are effective in counteracting 5α-reductase, which lends validity to our sebaceous gland hypothesis.

Case 2. Male, 35 years old. Showing symptoms of typical androgenetic alopecia, his hair curled and did not grow longer. However, 4 months after he had started to use Paddy Leaf Shampoo, and Hair Tonic at three times the normal amount, the short curly hair began to grow longer (Fig. 28.10a,b).

28.9 Classification of Active Principles of Hair Tonics by Mechanism of Action (Reviewed by Imada 1983)

Classification of the active principles of hair tonics and trichogenous agents according to content, e.g., vitamins, amino acids, organic compounds, minerals, and medications is already available. Imada (1983) has classified these constituents of hair tonics and trichogenous agents by their mechanisms of action, namely:

- Nutritional supply
- Telangiectasis activity
- Enhancement of enzymatic activity
- Other (overall actions of natural and other substances)

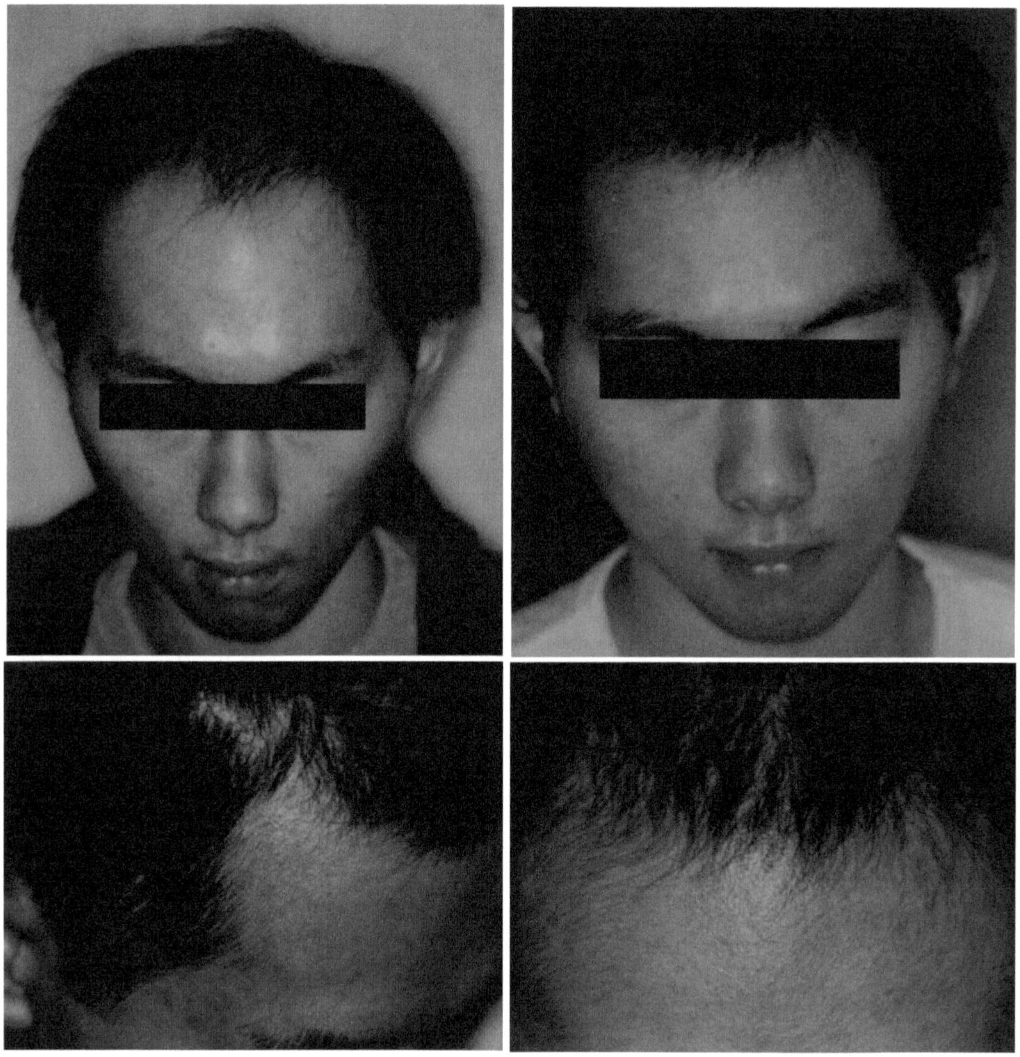
a c b d

Fig. 28.9. **a** A 23-year-old male. Hairline receded in the M shape (Norwood's classification III type.) **b** Recession of the apex can be seen clearly. **c** After 4 months of application of Paddy Leaf Shampoo and Tonic the bald area was greatly improved, and a hairline was formed. **d** Vellus hairs turned into coarse hairs. **e** After about 6 months, remarkable hair growth in the frontal region can be seen. **f** The hair growth in the apex is conspicuous

The following are examples of this classification:

1. Nutritional Supply

Vitamins, amino acids, minerals, and hormones fall into this category.

(a) Vitamin Group. The vitamin group contains derivatives which are used in combination with various other vitamins or with various other substances besides being used alone. They are utilized in preventing dermatitis caused by avitaminosis, dryness, loss of luster, and growth inhibition of scalp hair. Because of their comparatively mild action and safeness, they have been used in a wide range of products, from quasidrugs to medications.

Vitamins A, B_1, B_2, B_6, B_{12}, C, pantothenic acid, nicotinic acid, the K group (including ubiquinone), etc., PABA, biotins, inositol, choline, and vitamin D are also used.

(b) Amino Acid Group. Cystine, tryptophan, leucine, serine, methionine, methione, as well as collagen, peptides, and hydrolyte keratin are said to be active.

(c) Minerals. Iodine and its compounds, and P, S, and inorganic compounds containing S (e.g., K_2SO_4, $FeSO_4$, K_2S) have been combined. Fe, Mn, Cu, etc., as well as P and S are contained in scalp hair as microelements; however, the relation between these microelements and hair growth or between lack of these microelements and hair loss

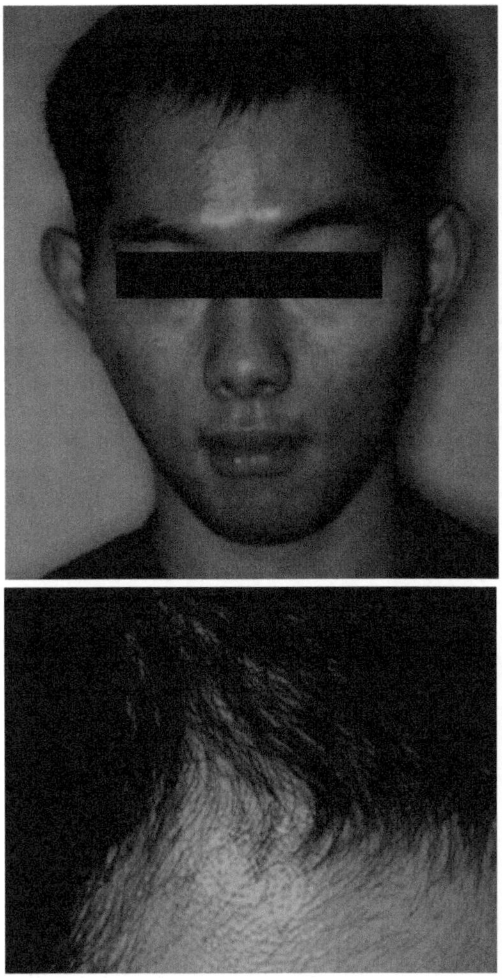

e

f

Fig. 28.9. *Continued*

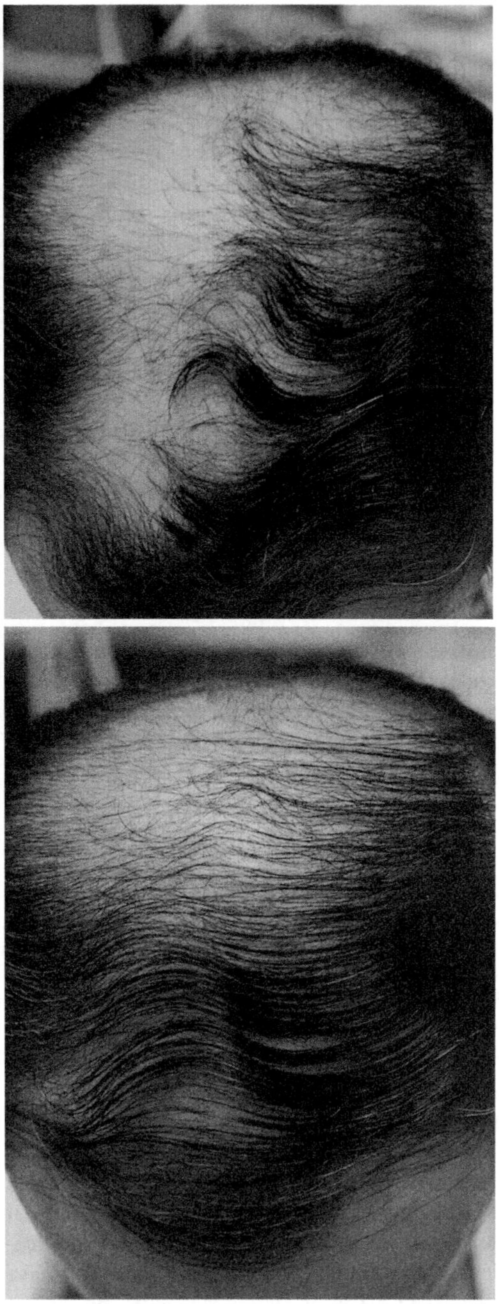

a

b

Fig. 28.10. **a** The hair curls and does not grow. **b** The patient was advised to use Paddy Leaf Shampoo and Hair Tonic at three times the normal rate. Remarkable hair growth can be observed after 4 months

has not been elucidated. Further studies on this are encouraged.

(d) Hormones. Studies of estrogen, androgen, estradiol, and ethylestradiol as well as thyroxine, pituitary hormone, posthypophysis extract, thymus hormone, and placental gonadotrophin have been reported.

(e) Others. Mucopolysaccharides such as hyaluronic acid, chondroitin sulfate, and placental extract are active.

(2) Telangiectasis Activity

When classifying active principles by their mechanisms of action, some authors may mention the activation of blood circulation, a rise in dermal temperature, or the action of dermal irriation. However, in a broad sense, all these actions may be considered to constitute a part of the telangiectasis activity. Substances which belong to this category include acetylcholine, vitamin E, and extracts of capsicum, cantharides, cinchona, garlic, and gentian. Salicyclic acid and aspirin may also be included in this category although these two agents also have a keratolytic action. While the vitamin group is widely used, substances in this category are generally used in medications.

(3) Enhancement of Enzymatic Activity (Enhancement of Enzymatic Activity Around Hair Follicles)

Porphyrin derivatives (protoporphyrin, hematin, iron chlorophyll, etc.) are thought to enhance peroxidase activity, melanin formation, and hair growth (Ando 1978). Adenosine triphosphate (ATP) is believed to be effective in treating alopecia areata, from a mechanical standpoint, since it enhances phosphorylase activity and increases glycogen productivity. ATP increases glycogen productivity by activating the weakened phosphorylase activity in the hair bulb portion in the balding area, and it restores choline isolated from the distal parasympathetic nerve due to stimulation to acetylcholine under the influence of enzymatic reaction.

(4) Other (Overall Actions of Natural and Other Substances)

This mechanism may be classified as the overall actions of agents of natural origin such as the vitamin group, amino acid group, and mineral groups. Carrot, gentian, aloe, honey, vegetable oil, hydrolytic residues of scalp hair, and bovine skin collagen may be included in this category.

28.10 Future Aspects of Hair Care Products

Hair tonics and trichogenous agents hold a unique position in the cosmetic market due to their positive effects in enhancing and stimulating hair growth. It is interesting to note that although a great number of such products have appeared on the market, only a few of them contain active principles developed after going through the process of drug design, first screening tests, and animal experiments, the basic requirements for medications today. Instead, most of these products have been taken from medications, including herbal medications. That is, among the comparatively safe substances such as the amino acid group, the vitamin group, extracts of natural substances, organic components, and agents used for ameliorating enterogastric function, more than a few substances have been selected and developed after going through clinical tests in Departments of Dermatology, only because they possessed telangiectasis activity or because they were presumed to have some trichogenous effects, due to their nutritional action on the skin. Although this tendency may continue, variations in combinations of vitamin group and amino acid group and further studies on the dosage may be expected, and derivatives of these substances, designed for improved solubility, diadermic absorption, and stability may appear on the market. Furthermore, more detailed studies on as yet unused natural substances may also be encouraged (reviewed from Imada 1983).

28.11 Trichogenous Agents in the United States

In 1980, the Food and Drug Administration (FDA) of the United States announced that a thorough review must be conducted on trichogenous agents assumed to be topically effective (FDA 1980). As a result of wide research, they concluded that topical trichogenous agents were by no means effective (FDA 1985).

The standards for Trichogenous Agents now set forth by the FDA (FDA 1985) state that: "Any substance claiming to have influence on hair regeneration must work effectively on the hair bulb. Therefore, clinical data will be required as to the process through which the substance enters the hair bulb and induces hair growth." These standards also mandate that the half-side method, in which the scalp is divided into two sections, should be adopted in indicating quantitatively (1) the increase of hair growth rate, (2) the increase of the diameter of the hair shaft, and (3) the duration of anagen stage.

Operative Treatment for Androgenetic Alopecia

29

29.1 Punch Graft Method

29.1.1 Concept of the Punch Graft Method

Autografts for the correction of traumatic alopecia have been carried out with varying degrees of success since 1893 (Davis 1911) at the earliest.

Many patients in Japan are deeply conscious of hair defects on various areas of the skin, and various methods of hair grafting have been practiced in order to repair the defects. Methods of small-piece grafting in particular have been developed in Japan. For instance, the hair shaft insertion method was reported by Sasagawa in 1930 and punch hair grafting by Okuda (1939); the latter, in a report virtually unrecognized in the English-speaking world, described the use of small full-thickness homografts of hair-bearing skin for the correction of alopecia of the scalp, eyebrows, and moustache area. He constructed special metal trephines (circular punches) with diameters of 2–4 mm and used these to bore out grafts from hair-bearing areas of the scalp. A similar instrument was used to prepare recipient sites in the area of alopecia into which grafts were placed. He noted that better cosmetic results were achieved if slightly smaller trephines were used for the recipient holes. Two patients who had cicatricial alopecia were successfully treated in this fashion. Okuda did not, however, specifically note its use in patients with androgenetic alopecia.

Tamura (1943) reported pubic hair reconstruction in women by means of single hair grafting and Fujita (1953) reported eyebrow reconstruction in leprosy patients by means of punctiform hair grafting. Fujita (1953) reported (in Japanese) punch hair grafting, in which a free skin graft with hairs was divided into small pieces, each containing two to three or four hairs, using a scalpel or a pair of scissors. These pieces were inserted separately into many holes, which were prepared in the recipient site utilizing a thick injection needle or a slender scalpel.

Orentreich (1959) reported on the use of autografts for the investigation of various types of alopecia and other dermatological conditions. This report is quite similar to Okuda's. Orentreich's first patients were operated on in 1955 and, to date, the procedures have been proven to be valid.

Unfortunately, because of World War II, Okuda's work was not recognized outside Japan until many years later. Knowledge and trial of these techniques outside Japan were long delayed (Kobori and Montagna 1976). This free punch graft was named by Friederich (1970) the Okuda-Orentreich technique.

29.1.2 Punch Graft Method in Practice

A brief outline of the punch graft method follows:

(1) Preanesthesia. The operation is performed under local anesthesia and sedation. One hour before the operation the patient should be given diazepam (15–20 mg) and antibiotics. Nitrous oxide and methoxyflurane (Penthrane) have been employed by some practitioners to minimize trauma caused by anesthesia (Lewis 1979).

(2) Anesthesia. Most physicians use 0.5% lidocaine with 1:2 000 000 epinephrine. Allergic reaction to lidocaine has not been reported, but overdosing can produce toxic effects. We have used more dilute lidocaine for anesthesia in the treatment of bromidrosis. Considering its toxicity, we use very dilute lidocaine (1% in eightfold dilu-

tion, i.e., 0.14%) with epinephrine (1:100 000). We obtain good results without pain or side effects (Inaba 1983c; Inaba and Inaba 1992a). Adding epinephrine reduces local bleeding, prolongs anesthesia, and helps reduce vaso-vagal syncope. However, excessive epinephrine will produce anxiety and tachycardia. Coiffman (1977) recommended the use of blocking anesthesia. The anesthesia is aimed at blocking the supraorbital and supratrochlear nerves, because the central zone of the forehead is very difficult to anesthetize.

(3) Taking the Grafts. During the first session, grafts are usually taken from the lateral inferior occipital area, and during the second session, usually from the superior occipital area (Fig. 29.1c). The donor site hair should be clipped short, not shaved, to allow visualization of the angle and direction of the hair. This will prevent an improper angle of the punch when cutting the plugs. The standard size punches used in the donor area are 4.0 and 4.5 mm. Donor punches must have a larger diameter than recipient punches to compensate for the tendency of the grafts to shrink to a variable degree after they have been cut (Fig. 29.1a,b).

Coiffman (1977) reported the use of square scalp grafts rather than circular ones, constituting an important innovation in this surgical field, using a corresponding parallel scalpel 0.3–0.5 mm wider than the square one.

Cutting of scalp plugs across hair follicles distorts them and reduces the number of hairs that will grow from each plug. The scalp plugs should be removed gently and be parallel to the hair direction. If it is necessary to cut the donor graft free of its fibrous band attachment, care should be taken to cut below the dermal papillae. Cutting through or above the dermal papillae will destroy hair growth potential.

Even if the lower portion of the plugs, including the dermal papilla, is cut obliquely, this plug must be transplanted in the recipient area. This transplanted hair seems to regenerate (see Section 29.5.2.2).

The scalp plugs should be immediately placed in physiologic solution. The donor scalp plugs should be trimmed of excess fat, since the donor site skin is 0.5–1.0 mm thicker than the recipient skin. Bleeding sites are sutured with 2.0-mm supramid thread (Jackson, Alexandria, VA, USA). Unger (1990) states that most suturing produced scars that were no better and were sometimes worse than the former scars. This problem will be examined later (see Chapter 32).

(4) Transplanting to the Recipient Area. The art of properly placing the frontal hairline is essential to prevent an unnatural appearance. It is important that the position be carefully planned and designed. To avoid hairs growing awry, all plugs in the recipient area should follow a constant directional pattern. This is usually centripetal on the dome of the scalp and invariably frontal in the anterior scalp.

Unger (1979) pointed out the importance of the hairline. A low "youthful" hairline often looks less natural as the individual gets older, and the hairline can never be moved more posteriorly. Normally the face is divided into equal segments: hairline to glabella, glabella to columellar-labial angle, and columella-labial angle to the chin. Hairlines may be placed higher than the superior line in order to conserve grafts for use more posteriorly, but should never be placed lower. One should never attempt to move the temples more anteriorly (Fig. 1.14).

Ayres (1964) described a series of punches placed side-by-side to create a new frontal hairline. According to Unger and Maritt (1988), the pattern that is generally used in punch transplanting is one that is U-shaped and four or five rows wide. Ohmori (1988) states that the hairline runs horizontally across the forehead. However, when the hairline is looked at from above the conventional hairline, it forms a crescent shape conforming to the shape of the skull.

Recipient holes should be large enough to accept the donor plugs. Whenever the recipient plug fits into a hole 1 mm smaller than the donor plug without bulging, this size difference is obviously the best one from an esthetic point of view.

In regard to hair direction, in most patients the natural direction is anterior and slightly away from the side of the scalp on which the part is made. Hair should never be directed posteriorly, even if the ultimate intention of the patient is to comb it posteriorly.

A natural hairline consists of a moderately spaced growth of fine hairs arranged in a ragged or random fashion, gradually becoming coarse and denser as one moves more posteriorly. The grafts are inserted into recipient holes with nontoothed forceps and are oriented in the original hair direction. A standard turban-like bandage is applied overnight.

There are as many variations to bandaging as there are surgeons. The purpose is to protect the grafts for the first 24 h to prevent and absorb any oozing or bleeding. Occasionally, some pressure can be applied with bandaging, if grafts are particularly stubborn about staying flat.

Since the recipient holes are 0.5–1.0 mm shallower than the donor plug, care should be taken to remove, with forceps and scissors, any fibrous tissue at the base of the hole. The recipient holes can be made with a punch 0.25–0.5 mm smaller in diameter (3.5–2.75 mm for a 4.0-mm donor plug) to insure a better fit.

Cutting the recipient holes one punch diameter apart permits adequate blood supply for good graft takes and optimal hair growth and also prevents avascular necrosis. If too large a punch (exceeding 5 mm) is used, there is invariably central hair loss, with growth only at the periphery of the plug (see Section 29.5).

29.1.3 Advantages of the Punch Graft Method (with Reference to Unger and Nordström 1988)

Two advantages of the punch graft method are:

(1) Donor Dominance. The designation "donor dominance" is used to describe the maintenance of the integrity and characteristics of transposed

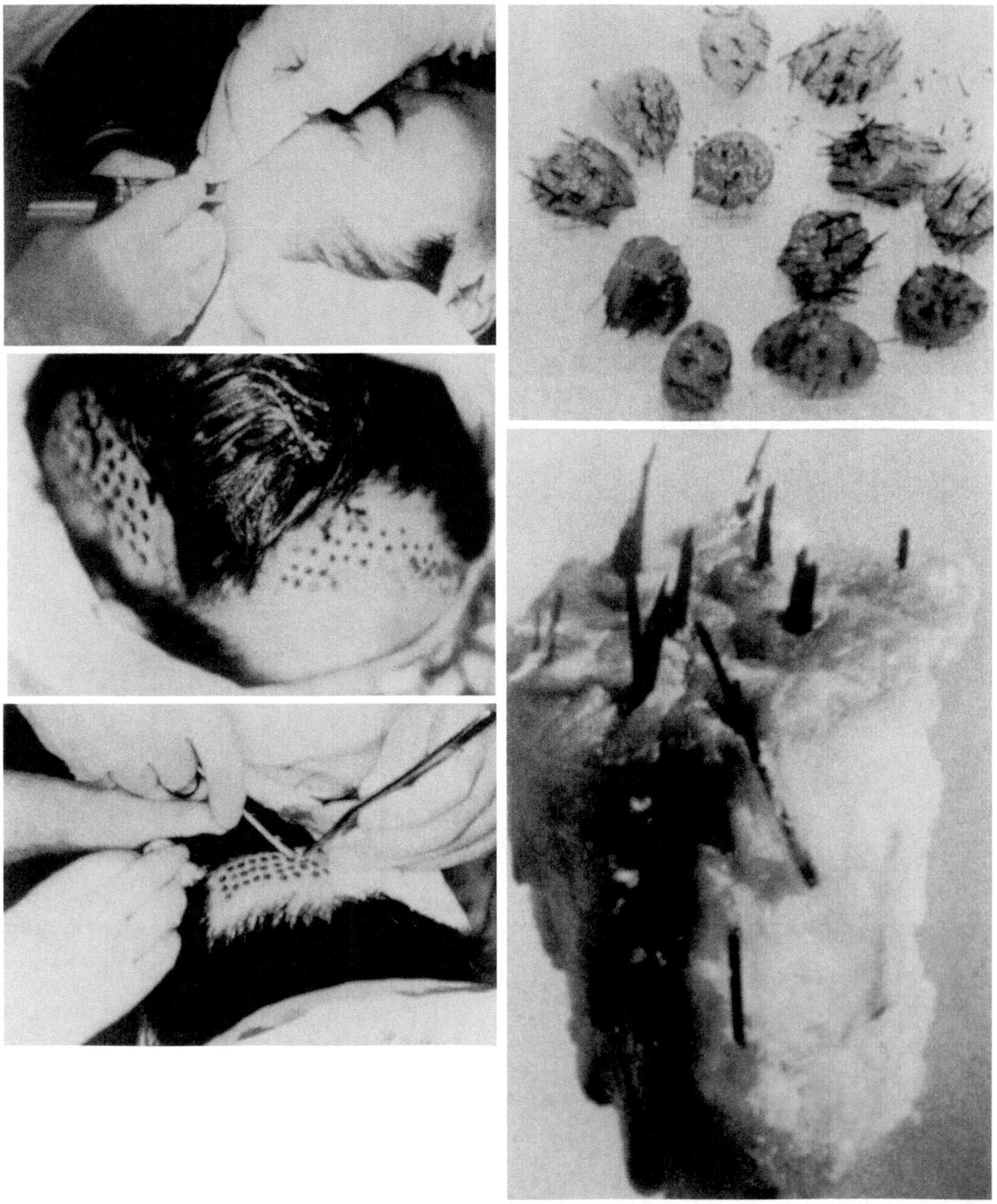

Fig. 29.1a–i. Punch graft method. (**a–g** Courtesy of Ezaki 1990). **a** The punch (3.5 mm wide) entering the recipient site. **b** The left sides (donor site) are removed with a 4-mm punch. The right sides (recipient site) are removed with a 3.5-mm punch. **c** Graft is removed from donor site. **d** Four-mm punch graft specimens. **e** High-power view of column specimen. **f** *Left*, before treatment. *Right*, follow-up result 1 year postoperatively. **g** *Left*, before treatment. *Middle*, secondary repunch transplantation 8 months postoperatively. *Right*, follow-up result 17 months postoperatively. **h** Punch grafting 2 months postoperatively. **i** Sporadic punch grafting

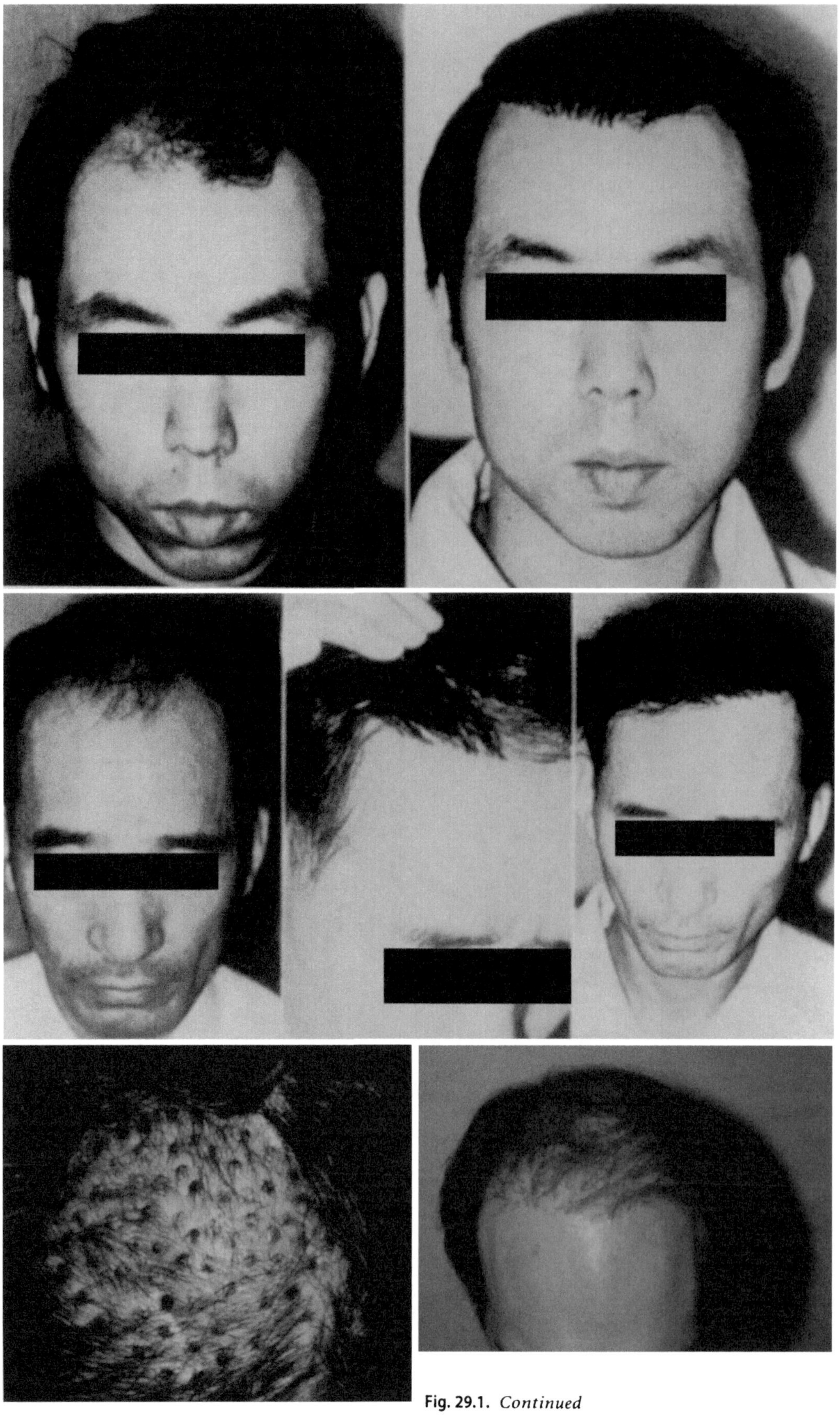

Fig. 29.1. *Continued*

grafted skin independent of the characteristics of the recipient site. Grafts from the hair-bearing rim of scalp were donor dominant and continued to grow hair when implanted in areas of androgenetic alopecia (Orentreich 1959).

(2) Fairly Easy Procedures. Pedicle flaps (temporo-parieto-occipital pedicle flaps to treat alopecia—"Juri method," "bitemporal flap") are esthetically superior to other methods in regard to hairline refinement. However, the wider the flap, the more likely it is that necrosis will occur in the frontal region, and much experience is required to perform this method. In view of this, the punch graft method is superb, in that it is comparatively easy to perform and the risk is low (Fig. 29.1a–c).

29.1.4 Disadvantages of the Punch Graft Method (with Reference to Norwood et al. 1984)

Disadvantages of the punch graft method are:

(1) Bleeding. Two types of bleeding occur both during and after surgery:

a. Arterial spurting or pumping that actually requires homeostasis, needing sutures or very protracted pressure.
b. Steady excessive oozing that eventually stops with pressure and time but can be a nuisance. However, with experience, bleeding becomes less of a problem.

(2) Syncope. Anything that can be done to reduce the patient's anxiety will reduce the incidence of syncope. The use of preoperative medication, e.g., diazepam, is of utmost importance. Diazepam not only reduces syncope but also seems to elevate the tolerance for pain.

(3) Poor Design, Planning, and Timing of Procedure. Improper hairline placement is one of the most common errors and is definitely the most conspicuous mistake made by the inexperienced operator. Special attention should be given to the shape and size of the patient's head, and improper angle and direction of hair growth must be considered.

(4) Transitional Epilation. The worst drawback of this method is that the scars left by the operation are overly conspicuous before they become camouflaged by the postoperative hair regeneration. The transplanted hair starts to fall out about 3 weeks after surgery by telogen effluvium and it will take approximately 5–6 months before hair regeneration begins. Again, the round scars left in the frontal bald region are extremely unsightly (Fig. 29.1h,i). Especially in Japan, it would be unbearably embarrassing for office workers to have to contend with any such condition for a long period (Fig. 29.1i).

(5) Poor Hair Growth (Fig. 29.1h,i). Poor hair growth can be caused by the following: (a) Dull punches cause grafts to be coned, bevelled, and lipped. (b) Cutting the grafts at the wrong angle results in bevelling of grafts, usually on one side. (c) The sharper the punch the less saline edematization will be required. (d) Crowding of the grafts in the recipient area without regard for the blood supply can reduce hair growth. The grafts should always be separated by at least the width of a graft. (e) Grafts must fit in the recipient sites comfortably without repeated adjustment or pressure. If grafts are elevated, they become desiccated and will not produce hair. (f) Poor growth may result from grafting thin recipient areas (see Section 29.1.2, Fig. 29.1i).

29.2 Minigrafts

Many hair transplantation surgeons (Tamura 1943; Fujita 1953; Marritt 1980; Nordström 1981) have advocated the use of small grafts for filling small spaces, softening the hairline, and replacing eyebrows. In most operations difficulty is experienced in cutting these small plugs with conventional power or hand punches.

Shiell and Norwood (1984) reported the advantages of minigrafts: (1) for softening the established graft line; (2) for filling gaps too small for conventional grafts; (3) as a means of gaining time while waiting for full development of earlier graft sessions; and (4) as hair replacement in other areas.

Shiell (1972) developed a technique of dissecting 4.0-mm grafts into smaller pieces. Using a scalpel and low-power magnification, he found that these plugs could readily be divided into units of one to two hairs. The graft is firmly grasped with a fine-toothed forceps and sliced parallel to the hair shafts, using a sharp scalpel. A No. 15 blade is usually still sharp enough to produce tiny grafts containing the required number of hairs. The so-called micrografts are kept in physiological saline. The minigrafts are picked up with five dissectors and inserted firmly into scalpel slits in the recipient zone (made with a No. 15 blade). Once the graft is in place, gentle pressure is applied with a swab while adjacent micrografts are inserted (reviewed from Shiell and Norwood 1984).

Since inexperienced operators experienced considerable difficulty at first, a new instrument was developed for inserting the micrograft. As described later, this was developed by the authors and by Choi et al. (1990b) (see Section 29.3.1).

Bradshaw (1988a) recently modified the technique and uses larger units of three to eight hairs (minigrafts) (Shiell and Norwood 1984).

29.3 Single Hair Graft Transplantation

Excision or damage to the scalp, even if sutured esthetically, will gradually expand and appear unsightly, especially when the scar runs parallel to the hair stream.

For the improvement of large scars in the bald scalp caused by burns, the suture method, composite pedicle flap method, or tissue expansion method has been adopted; however, ugly scars are left after the operation.

For the treatment of male pattern baldness, the punch method or flap method is generally employed, but neither is truly effective in terms of hairline refinement. The abrupt "edged-lawn" appearance of the traditional transplanted hairline has been a constant source of apprehension and dissatisfaction, not only to the patient, but to the frustrated surgeon as well. It has always been apparent to even the most casual observer that the natural, mature hairline consisted not of a line of hair, but of an area in which isolated, randomly growing individual hairs gradually increased in density to blend with the main body of the frontal forelock. Though relatively few in number, these scattered single hairs are the cosmetically critical ingredient for softening the transition from the bald forehead to the hairy scalp. Therefore, the failure of transplant surgeons to consistently reconstruct an undetectable hairline cannot be traced to an esthetic myopia, but, rather, to the technical difficulties and time-consuming tedium of single hair transplanting.

For hairline refinement, single hair-bearing grafting is superior to other methods from the esthetic standpoint, although it has some drawbacks in that it requires great patience and scar formation in the donor site is unavoidable.

As described in Section 29.1.1, the single hair-bearing graft or micrograft was first developed in Japan.

In 1980, Marritt reported a simple method of harvesting single hairs from the periphery of standard grafts. These small grafts are removed from a standard size graft by carefully incising the standard graft with a very sharp scalpel. Tenotomy scissors are then used to cut the small piece of tissue containing the single hairs from the larger graft.

Nordström (1981) reported micrografts for improvement of the frontal hairline after hair transplant. Shiell and Norwood (1984) used a No. 11 blade to cut single hairs from a standard 4-mm graft, and Unger and Nordström (1988) described a process in which individual hairs are stripped from the periphery of standard grafts by using forceps, thus not cutting or removing any of the skin or subcutaneous tissue.

Marritt (1988) introduced a method in which the recipient site was expanded with a metal expander and the coarse hair-bearing grafts, 4 mm in diameter, collected by the punch method were inserted into the recipient site after they had been dissected into smaller pieces. This method is excellent, since, when new recipient sites are created close (3–4 mm) to previously implanted micrografts, the downward pressure of the needle on the skin almost always forces the previously placed micrograft to pop out of its site. Popping could be avoided only by increasing the distance between micrograft recipient sites, which then actually decreased the number of micrografts that could be transplanted in each session.

Bradshaw (1988a) divided the 4.5-mm punched graft into four pieces (minigrafts), transplanted them into the previously made slit, and fixed them with a nylon ligature. He used a No. 20 blade to separate individual hairs from the strip of hair-bearing scalp. Recipient sites for single hair grafts were made with large-bore needles (No. 16 or 18), surgical blades (No. 11 or 15), and Marritt micrograft dilators. However, it requires painstaking effort to obtain single hair-bearing grafts suitable for placement inside the extremely thin inserting needle. Furthermore, complete training in this method is mandatory in order to prevent the formation of large scars at the donor site.

Choi et al. (1990b) and Choi and Kim (1992) have developed an insertion needle capable of easy insertion of single hair-bearing grafts.

29.3.1 Development of Inaba Method for the Micrograft or Single Hair-Bearing Graft Transplantation

To solve such problems, we have developed a completely new method in which our 1-mm micropunch is employed in collecting single hairs sporadically from the occipital region, and a specially devised insertion needle is used for easy insertion.

29.3.1.1 Inaba Method for Collection of Single Hair Grafts or Micrografts (Inaba and Inaba 1993a)

Inconspicuous sites in the occipital area are selected for the collection of single hairs. Hair clippers are employed to trim the hairs down to a length of about 2 mm, after which they are punched down to the level of the dermal layer while due attention is paid to the direction of hair growth. This method is ideal for preventing the hair roots from being cut apart (Fig. 29.2a).

Next, the free composite hair is lifted with a pincette (Fig. 29.2b) and its root is nipped with very thin Pean's forceps for easy collection of the compound hair covered by the connective hair follicle (Fig. 29.2c). In performing this method, it is essential to preserve the whitish, transparent connective hair follicle. Utmost care must be taken in pulling out the hair root because the blood plexus is present, surrounding the hair connective follicle in the hair root (Fig. 29.3a–d).

Both a hair containing only the upper hair follicle, if the lower follicle has been cut apart during the process of collection, and a hair with its root exposed, if the connective hair follicle has been erroneously removed, are acceptable for transplantation, in the light of the possibility that hair regeneration can be expected if the upper isthmal portion of the hair follicle remains intact (see Section 29.5.2.2).

29.3.1.2 Single Hair Graft Transplantation Method

(a) Development of Hair-Inserting Needle. It was extremely painstaking and time-consuming to insert micrografts into a small slit made with a thick needle by employing a micro-pincette.

To solve this problem, we developed an insertion needle (partially coated needle) with which single hair-bearing graft transplantation can be performed easily. This needle, 18 gauge in size, has a coated portion (A) of approximately 20% and a 50% uncoated portion (B) in the tip (Fig. 29.4a). First, the hair root of the collected single hair-

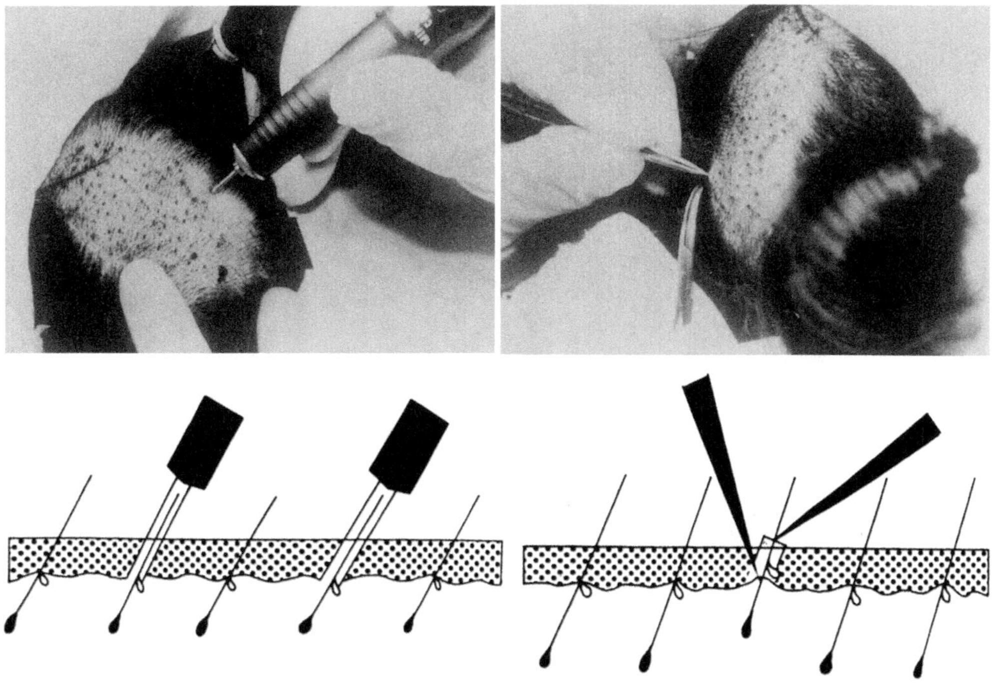

a

b

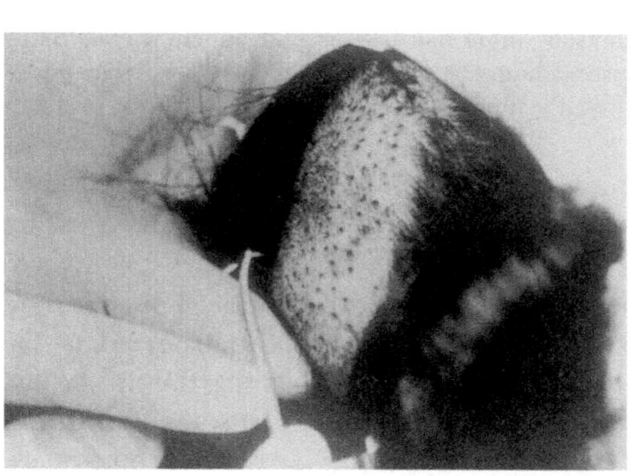

c

Fig. 29.2a–c. Single hair transplantation method. **a** The micro-punch instrument is used to punch the scalp parallel with each hair to be collected. *Below*: schema of **a**. **b** A pincette is used to hold the punched micrograft and lift the hair root for single hair collection, using Pean's forceps. *Below*: schema of **b**. **c** Micrograft is pulled up from the recipient area

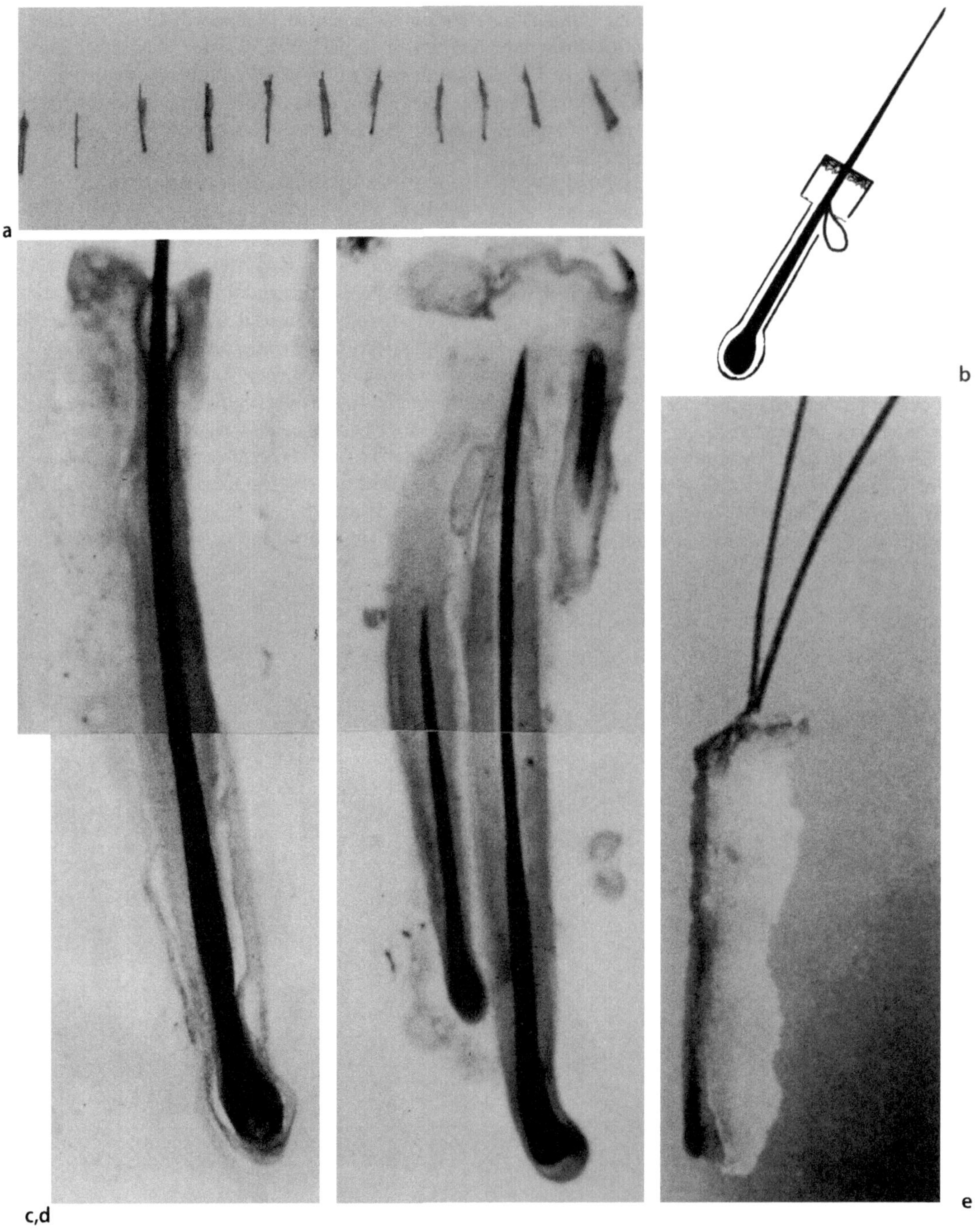

Fig. 29.3. **a** Collected single and micro hair-bearing grafts. **b** Single hair-bearing graft. Subcutaneous tissue surrounding the hair root is removed. **c** High-power view of a single hair-bearing skin graft 1 mm in diameter, with dermal tissue and hair root and without fatty tissue. **d** Micrograft including two or three hair roots; surrounding fatty tissue is removed. **e** Conventional micrograft. Hair root is surrounded by thick fatty tissue

bearing graft, or micrograft, is placed over portion B (Fig. 29.4b) and then it is transferred to the coated portion A (Fig. 29.4b), using the tip of a fine needle. Since the punched grafts are uniform in size, transfer to portion A can be performed easily.

(b) Insertion. The single hair-bearing graft or micrograft is placed inside the insertion needle after collection. It is then inserted into the recipient site in harmony with the hair stream. The hair placed over the upper part of portion A (Fig. 29.4a)

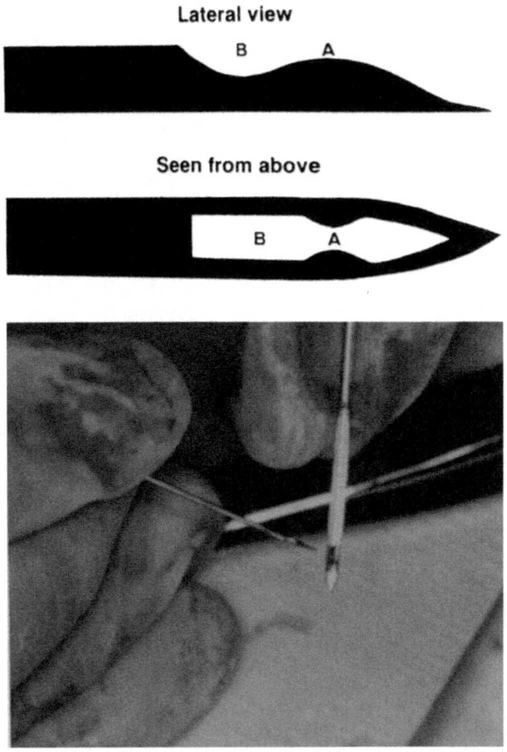

a

b

Fig. 29.4. a Insertion needle (partially coated). *A*, coated portion; *B*, uncoated portion. **b** The hair root of the collected hair graft is placed on portion *B* and then transferred to the coated portion, *A*

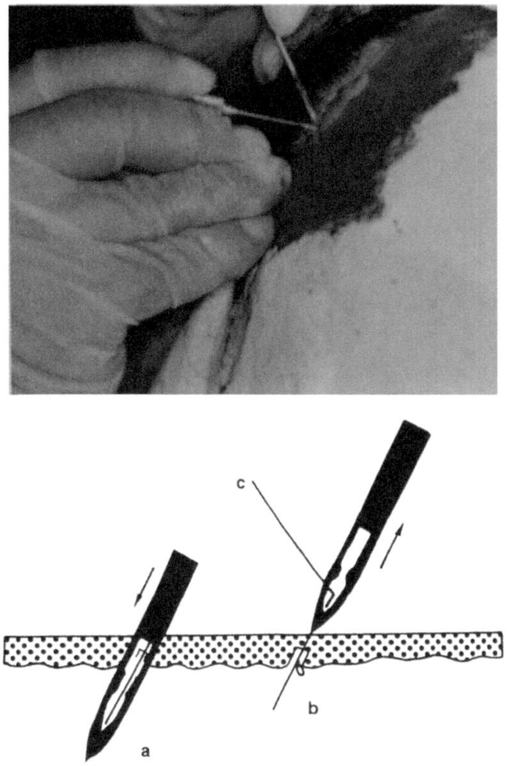

a

b

Fig. 29.5. a A single hair is held inside the partially coated needle. **b** Schema of **a**. A single hair is held inside the specially devised needle (*a*). Implantation can then be performed comparatively easily by pulling up the needle (*b*) with the hair being pressed down with another needle (*c*)

of the insertion needle is held with the tip of a thin needle while the insertion needle is being pulled out. In this way, single hair transplantation can be performed quite easily (Fig. 29.5b).

(c) Prevention of Jumping Up or Popping Out Phenomenon. The phenomenon of jumping up or popping out caused by pressure often occurs when hairs are transplanted in close proximity. When we created new recipient sites close (3–4 mm) to previously planted micrografts, the downward pressure of the needle on the skin almost always forced the previously placed micrograft to pop out of its site. Popping could be avoided only by increasing the distance between micrograft recipient sites, which then actually decreased the number of micrografts that could be transplanted in each session. To prevent this, we have used the Marritt method (Marritt 1988), in which the recipient site is expanded with multiple dilators (No. 20 needle) to prevent popping out. The micrograft dilator transforms micrografting into a rapid, highly efficient follicular assembly line (Fig. 29.6).

Antibiotic ointment and light pressure are applied over the recipient site for 1 day after transplantation. An expert can punch out and transplant approximately 50 hairs in about 1 h. This

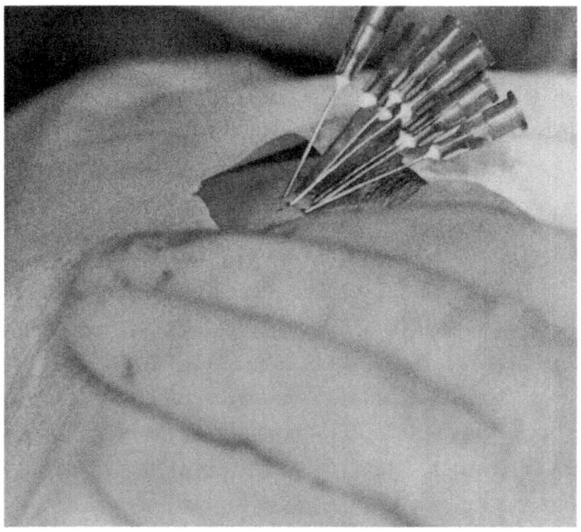

Fig. 29.6. Prevention of jumping up or popping by the Marritt method (Marritt 1988) is useful

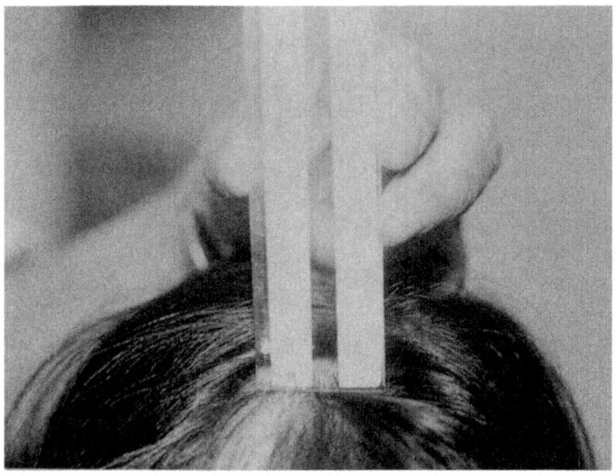

Fig. 29.7. Blood circulation for the transplanted single hair is superb, so the transplanted hair will start to grow well.

method is superb, in that it can be performed very easily and almost no scars are left at the donor site.

(d) Hair Growth After Transplantation. In general punch methods, hairs within the plugs initially appear to be growing but are, in reality, slowly being extruded. In 2–8 weeks, virtually all of them have been shed, although occasionally some hairs start growing without prior loss. From 8 to 16 weeks (average 3 months) after the procedure, new hair growth begins. However Inaba's single hair graft or micrograft transplantation is superb, in that blood circulation for the hair follicle is resumed immediately (Fig. 29.7), so that transplanted hairs start to grow well. Although no accurate data have been obtained on the rate of regrowth, it can be assumed that more than 80%–90% of transplanted hairs take well.

29.3.1.3 Advantages of Inaba's Method for Micrograft and Single Hair Transplantation

The advantages of Inaba's method are:

(1) Hair Plugs Can Be Obtained Easily. Many physicians have successfully collected occipital donor grafts and divided them into single hair grafts to be transplanted in various regions. However, this process was extremely painstaking and left scars at the donor site (Unger and Nordström 1988; Norwood et al. 1984; Choi et al. 1990b).

In the 1-mm punch method, on the other hand, the scalp is punched only down to the dermis toward the same direction as the hair stream, leaving the subcutaneous tissue untouched, thus avoiding damage to the lower follicle. The collection of hairs can then be performed comparatively easily by plucking out the follicle, enveloped by the connective tissue, after punching.

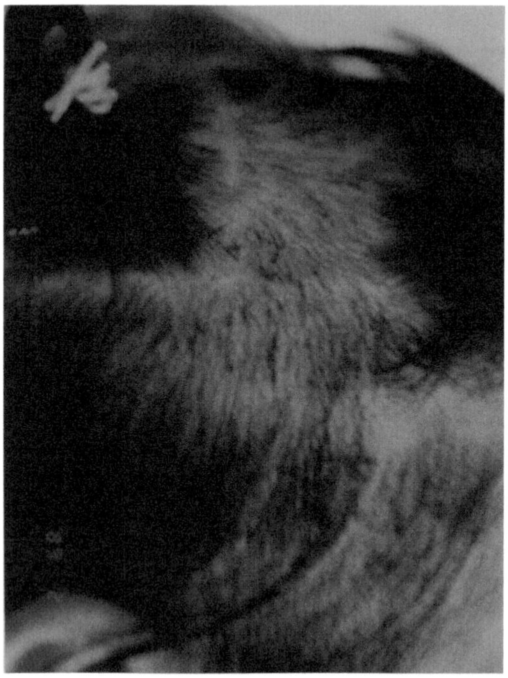

Fig. 29.8. Inaba method. After the 1-mm punch method is used, no scar remains. The *upper portion* is the area from which hairs were removed 1 month earlier. No scar remains

(2) No Scars Are Left at the Donor Site. The conventional punch method has a drawback in that it leaves scars at the donor site, since grafts are collected from the occipital region by punching large areas (4 mm), or by scalp excision. Compared to this, scars left by the 1-mm punch method are almost invisible, since single or compound hairs are collected sporadically across the scalp (Fig. 29.8).

(3) Hair Growth After Transplantation. Hair transplantation by the conventional punch method has a drawback in that the transplanted hairs begin to fall out after about 3 weeks, on the average, and it takes about 3 months before regeneration begins. In contrast, most single grafted hairs enter anagen immediately after transplantation, without the occurrence of telogen effluvium, this being ideal from an esthetic standpoint. This aspect is discussed in depth in Section 29.5.1 regarding the histological study of the grafts.

29.3.1.4 Disadvantages of Micrograft and Single Hair Transplantation

(1) The Number of Hairs That Can Be Collected Is Limited. In the conventional punch (4-mm) or scalp excision methods, a greater number of hairs can be obtained than with the 1-mm punch

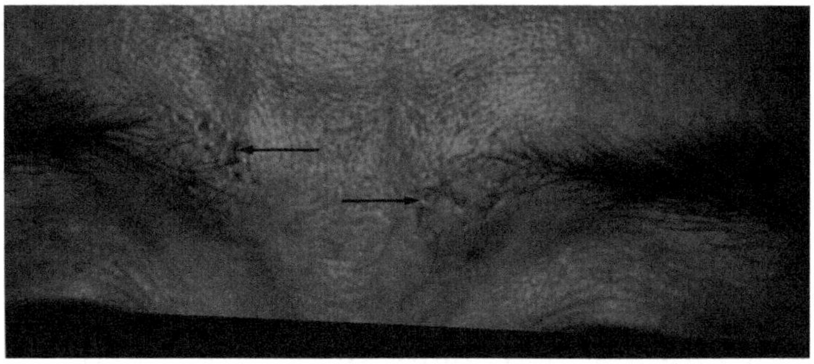

Fig. 29.9. Inverted epidermis (*arrow*) after single hair-bearing skin graft (1-mm)

method, although the problem of scars remains unsolved. In the single hair method developed by Inaba in comparison, hairs are collected sporadically from the entire scalp, which makes it ideal from an esthetic viewpoint. However, hairs have to be collected from a much wider area compared to the conventional punch method, and the number of hairs that can be collected is naturally limited, which makes it particularly applicable for transplantation in small areas (Fig. 29.8).

(2) The Areas Suited for Transplantation Are Limited. This single hair or micrograft method has been used only for the reconstruction of eyebrows and eyelashes, and for hairline refinement after hair transplantation. A tense area such as the scalp is suited for transplantation; however, in areas composed of soft tissue such as the eyebrow, epidermal constriction or depression, such as ingrowing epidermis (comedo) may occur, resulting in inflammation (Fig. 29.9).

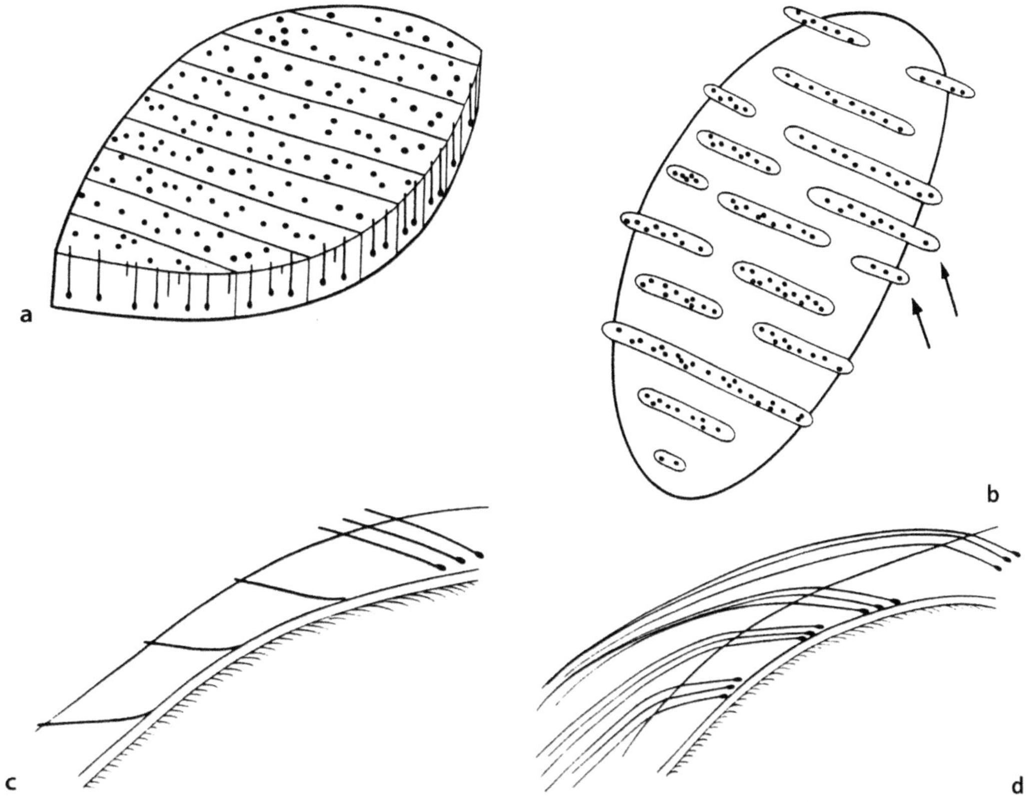

Fig. 29.10a–d. Multiple strip composite graft (Ariga 1989). **a** Hair-bearing scalp is excised in a spindle-shaped piece which is then cut into long strips, 2–3 mm in width. **b** Care must be taken that the gaps between the grafts are not symmetrical. In order to make the hair-bearing scalp region and the transplanted region inconspicuous, multiple strip composite grafts are inserted across the border, as indicated by the *arrows*. **c** The incision has to be made perpendicular to the hair stream at a proper angle in order to produce a natural-looking hair stream. **d** The transplanted hairs appear thick in layers. (With permission from Ariga 1989)

(3) Hairs Transplanted in the Scar Region Do Not Take Well. Because the blood circulation to the hair plug is disturbed by pressure, the sebaceous gland and the upper isthmal portion of the hair follicle begin to atrophy after transpxlantation and no regeneration can be expected. For improvement of the scar, the excision method or punch graft may be recommended.

29.4 Multiple Strip Composite Graft

Ariga (1989) reported this method and obtained good results (Fig. 29.10). The hair-containing scalp skin should be excised as a spindle-shaped block, which is then cut into long strips. Prepare pockets on the cranial periosteum, using incisions across the hair stream. Be careful not to damage the cranial periosteum, and not to connect to the next pocket.

Strips of the hair-containing scalp skin are grafted in the prepared pockets on the cranial periosteum. One must be careful that the gaps between the grafts are not symmetrical, to prevent creating a long space parallel to the hair stream. Since the hairs grow one on top of another, the hair is piled up and appears very thick; the operated area can thus be easily covered by using an ordinary hair-brushing technique.

29.5 Histological Findings After Transplantation of Single Hair-Bearing Graft or Micrograft

As reported above, single or micro hair-bearing graft transplantation can be performed comparatively easily, so we often apply this method in hair transplantation. We conducted a histological study on how this single hair-bearing graft grows without causing telogen hair loss.

As described later in Section 29.5.4, since dermal tissue was contained in this single hair-bearing graft, microcirculation between the papillary blood plexus beneath the epidermis in the peripheral recipient site and the pilosebaceous apparatus began at an early stage after transplantation, thus supplying nutrition to the hair matrix (see Chapter 5).

29.5.1 Histological Follow-Up of Inaba's Single Hair-Bearing Graft Transplantation

First, the skin is punched down only to the epidermal and dermal layers with a 1-mm punch, preserving the hair bulb and the surrounding connective hair follicle in the lower hair follicle. The lower hair follicle is then pulled out. It is inserted into the recipient site with a specially devised insertion needle for transplantation (Fig. 29.5b).

We performed Inaba's single hair-bearing graft transplantation, and on the 7th postoperative day, in two patients, we collected the hairs transplanted by the punch method for histological study.

29.5.1.1 Case 1

We collected the transplanted hairs, by using the punch method, and prepared a thick tissue specimen (Fig. 29.11a–c). The lower hair bulb portion has been lost, probably because the hair root had taken so well after transplantation that it could not be pulled out with the punch. However, observation of the well-preserved melanin granules in the hair root indicates that the hair bulb portion is functioning in the same manner as in the normal state. This assumption is substantiated by the observation that the exfoliated skin is attached to the hair shaft protruding from the skin surface, the epidermis is fixed in place surrounding the hair, and a gap has formed between the exfoliated skin and the skin surface (Fig. 29.11b,c). These findings indicate that the hair has started to grow from the matrix of the hair bulb immediately after transplantation.

29.5.1.2 Case 2

Likewise, in this case, the epidermal skin was attached to the hair shaft, which protruded from the skin surface (Fig. 29.12a,b). As in case 1, the hair bulb in the hair root could not be collected because it had fitted firmly into the recipient tissue. Hair matrix and melanocyte activities presumably take place, as melanin granules in the hair root are present in great numbers and there is no evidence of any telogen hair follicle.

These findings indicate that Inaba's single hair-bearing graft transplantation assures hair growth immediately after transplantation and it works well from both the clinical and histological standpoints.

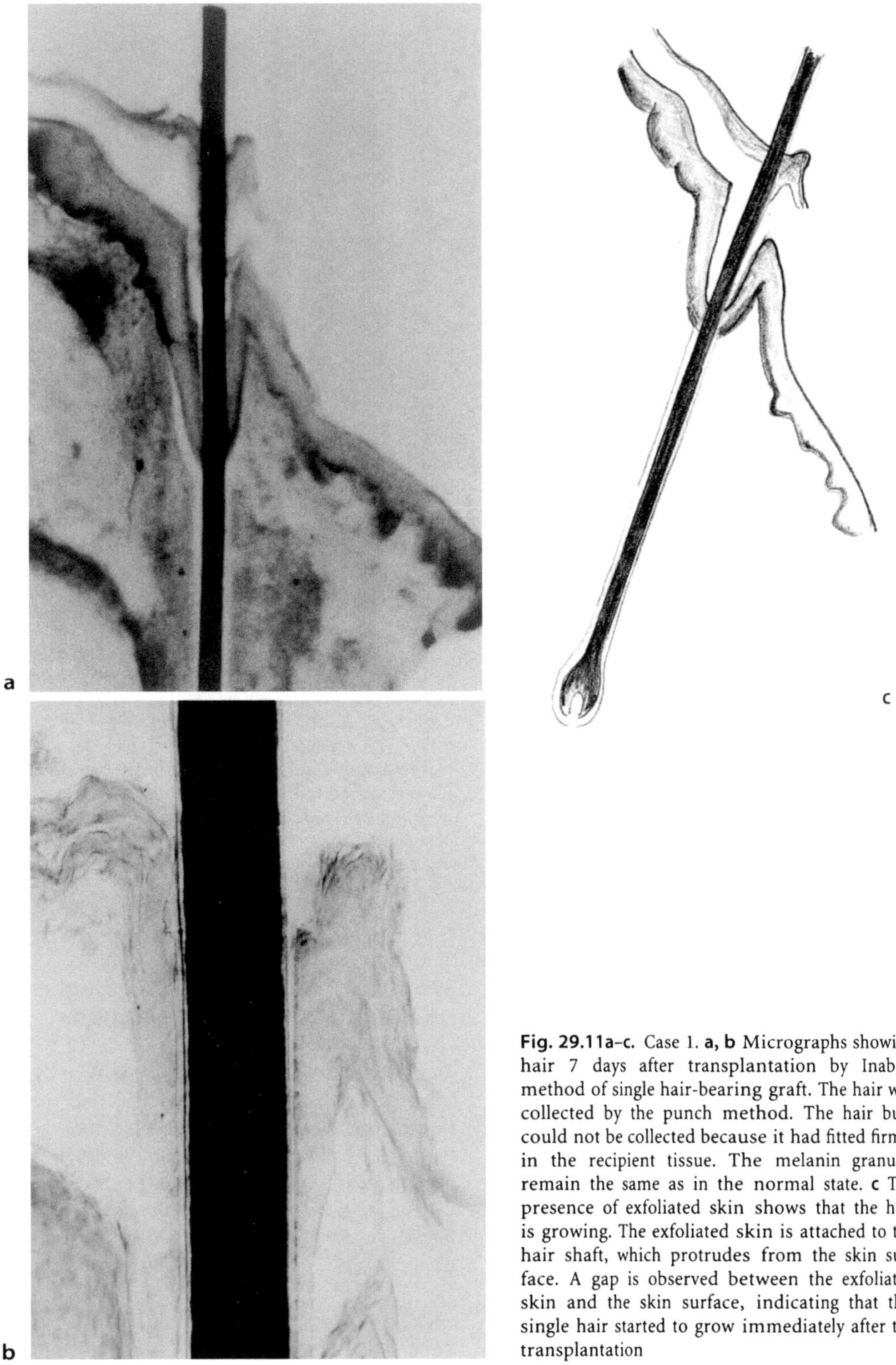

Fig. 29.11a–c. Case 1. **a, b** Micrographs showing hair 7 days after transplantation by Inaba's method of single hair-bearing graft. The hair was collected by the punch method. The hair bulb could not be collected because it had fitted firmly in the recipient tissue. The melanin granules remain the same as in the normal state. **c** The presence of exfoliated skin shows that the hair is growing. The exfoliated skin is attached to the hair shaft, which protrudes from the skin surface. A gap is observed between the exfoliated skin and the skin surface, indicating that this single hair started to grow immediately after the transplantation

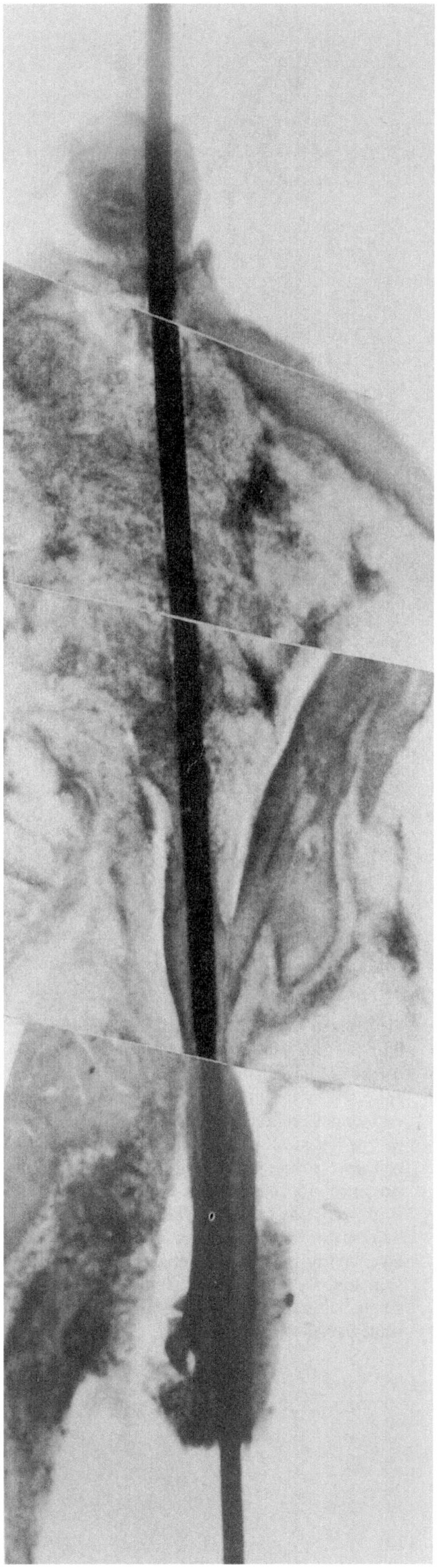

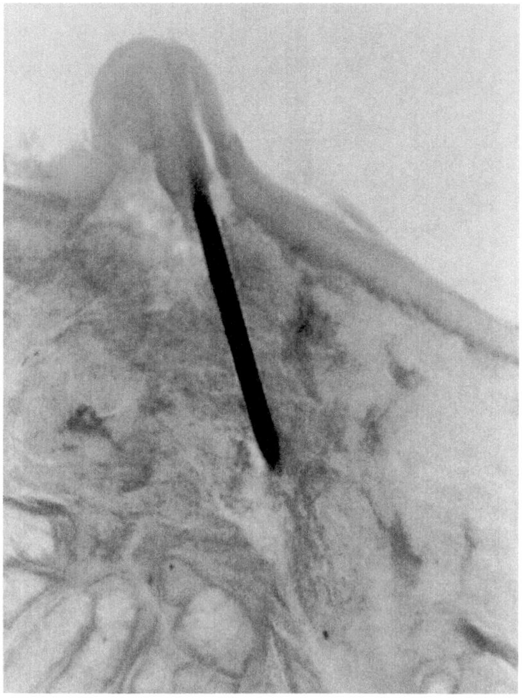

b

a

Fig. 29.12a,b. Case 2. **a** Microscopic view of the hair 7 days after transplantation by Inaba's method of single hair-bearing graft. The hair was collected by the punch method. The hair bulb could not be collected for the same reason as stated in regard to case 1. The exfoliated skin is attached to the hair shaft, which protrudes from the skin surface. This indicates that the hair started to grow immediately after transplantation. **b** Skin surface protrudes due to the growing hair

29.5.2 Experiment with Choi's Single Hair-Bearing Graft Transplantation

An elliptical graft was collected from the occipital region of a volunteer subject and dissected into the smaller pieces used in Choi's single hair grafts (Fig. 29.13). Then various levels of single hair-bearing grafts were transplanted in the balding parietal region, and tissue biopsies were conducted on the 7th and 30th post-transplantational days.

29.5.2.1 Composite Hair Follicle Transplantation

In Choi's single hair transplantation, as much as possible of the tissue surrounding the follicle is removed to allow easy insertion into Choi's insertion needle. To be more precise, most of the skin and the sebaceous gland are removed. The condition after Choi's transplantation is similar to that of Inaba's. It may seem slightly inferior to Inaba's with respect to ideal fitness, while in the eyebrow

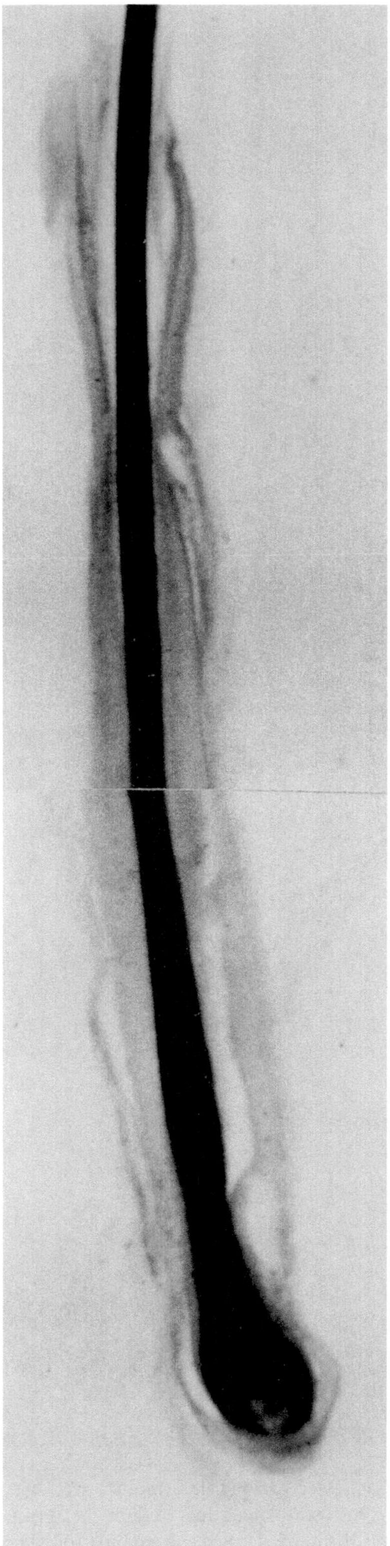

Fig. 29.13. Choi's single hair graft. Most of the skin and the sebaceous gland are removed

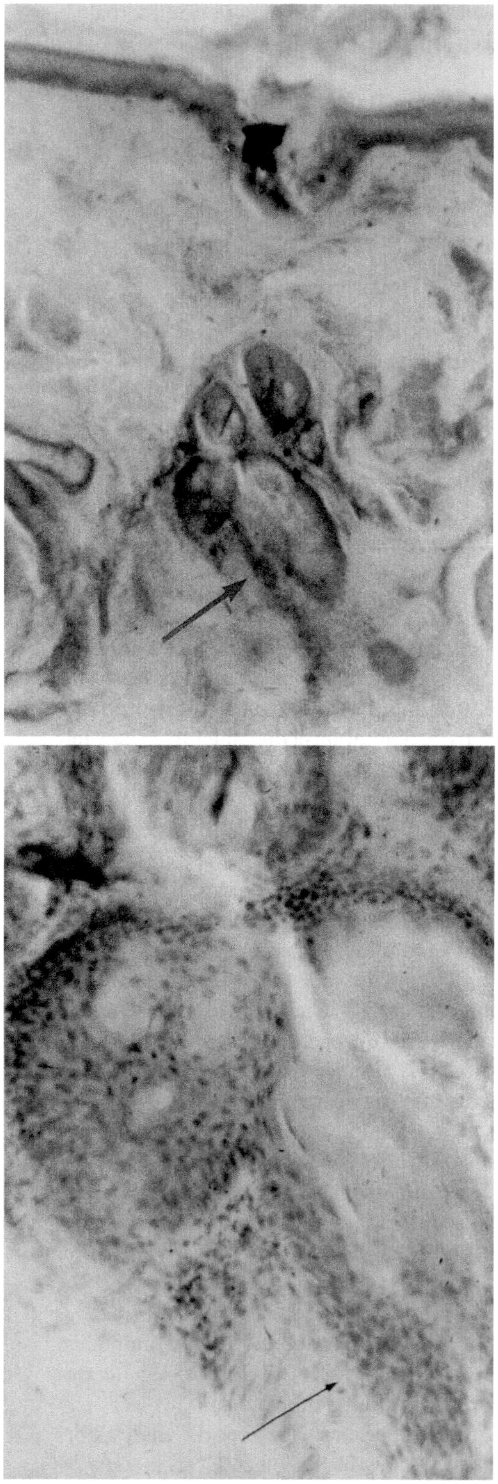

a

b

Fig. 29.14. a View of the upper hair follicle 1 month after transplantation. The hair root has prolapsed and only a few acinous cells can be observed in the sebaceous gland. A hair germ has formed in the peripheral region (*arrow*). b High-power view of a. Few acinous cells remain in the sebaceous gland. The hair germ is formed from the epithelial cells surrounding the acinous cells (*arrow*) and pubic regions it appears superior to Inaba's from the esthetic standpoint.

29.5.2.2 Upper Hair Follicle Transplantation

The lower hair follicle of Choi's single hair graft was removed and only the upper follicle, i.e., the portion including the skin, the sebaceous gland, and the upper isthmal portion, was transplanted. The transplanted graft was collected 1 month later for histological observation (Fig. 29.14a). The hair root in the follicle had prolapsed and only a few acinous lipocyte cells were observed in the sebaceous gland. The peripheral epithelial cell layer surrounding the sebaceous gland had become thicker, and a hair germ had formed in the peripheral region (Fig. 29.14a,b).

29.5.2.3 Lower Hair Follicle Transplantation

Only the lower portion of the hair follicle was transplanted. The hair was about to prolapse from the follicular orifice (Fig. 29.15a). Since the hair matrix is present in the hair bulb portion, this transplanted hair becomes typical telogen phase.

Thus, transplantation of only the lower hair follicle in the telogen stage does not assure a secure fit (Fig. 29.15b), but newly-formed connective tissue is formed in the lower telogen hair follicle and it then appears as if the top of the anagen hair pushes the transplanted hair (Fig. 29.15c). However, it cannot be ascertained whether this new young hair regenerates from the remaining hair matrix in the transplanted single hair. However, according to Philpott et al. (1990), if hair growth is observed in hair follicle culture and the lower follicle is not eliminated, it is possible that hair regeneration can occur from the matrix cell.

In a recent study carried out to assess the regenerative capacity of human hair, Kim (1993) isolated individual anagen hair follicles from the occipital scalp and grafted them onto the leg after cutting the follicles at the lower one-third. Two of ten grafted lower thirds were regenerated. The lower one-third follicle implants formed a follicular base and produced a curled hair fiber. The lower follicle implants were not regenerated until 8 months after grafting.

This finding supports the reports that, as described in Section 14.1.2, follicular stem cells reside in the lower one-third of rat vibrissa hair follicles (Oliver 1966a, 1967a,b; Inaba and Inaba 1992a).

According to Reynolds and Jahoda (1991b), if germinative cells, including the tip area of telogen phase follicles (secondary hair germ), are lost or cut off toward the end of each cycle, they are replaced by outer root sheath cells at the initiation of the next regeneration.

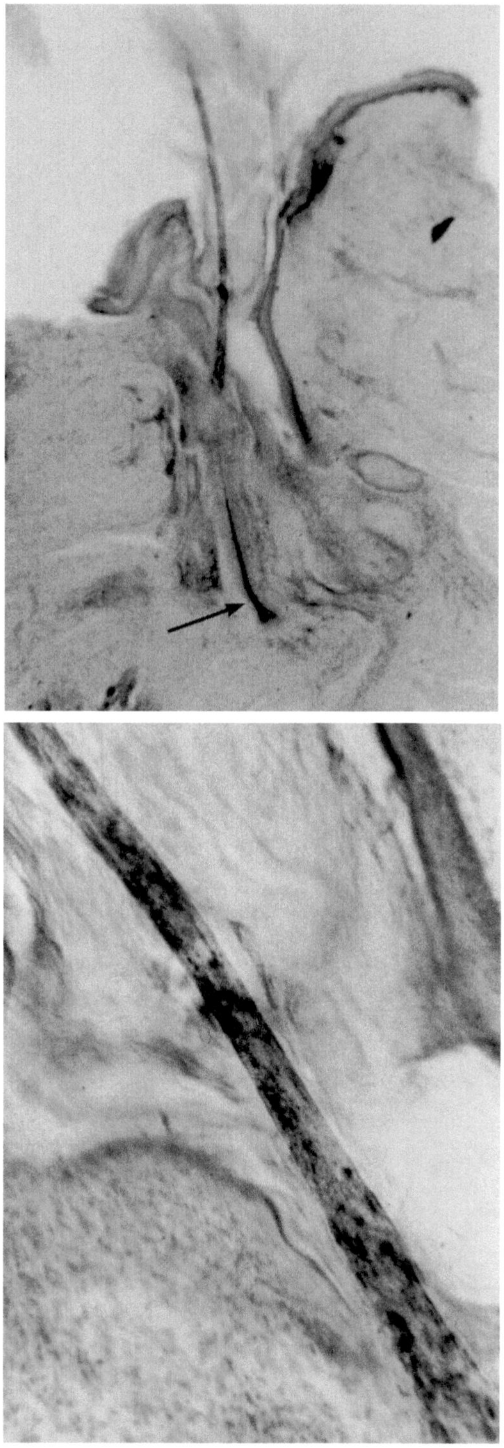

a

b

Fig. 29.15. **a** Lower hair follicle 1 month after transplantation. The transplanted hair follicle is about to come out, but the newly-formed anagen hair follicle can be seen (*arrow*). **b** The hair follicle is in the telogen stage. **c** High-power view of **a**. A new hair follicle has formed in the lower telogen hair follicle; it appears as if the top of the anagen hair (*arrow*) is pushing the transplanted hair

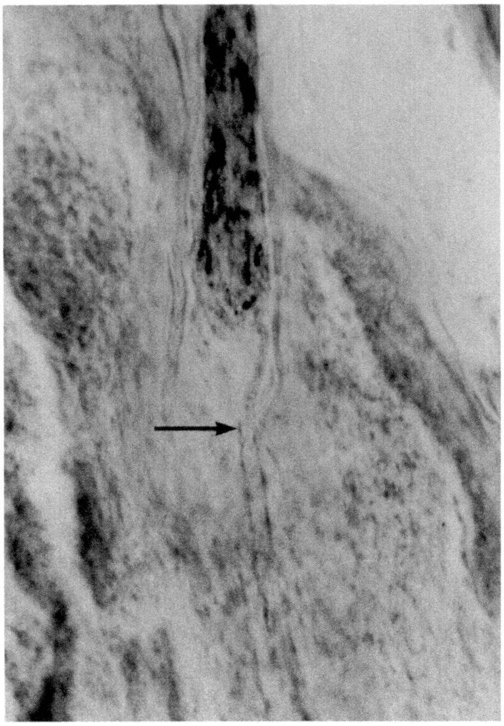

c

Fig. 29.15. *Continued*

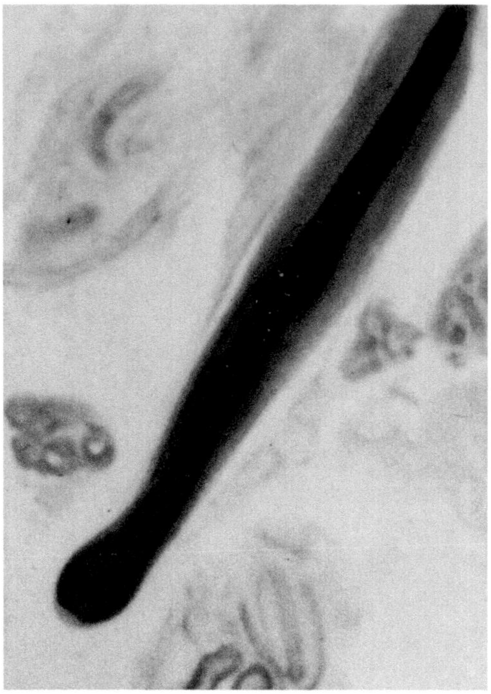

a

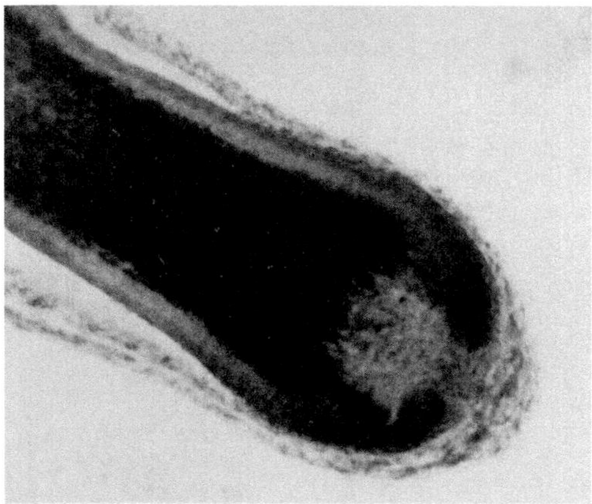

b

Fig. 29.16. a Subcutaneous tissue layer after transplantation. This hair follicle appears to be in the anagen stage. **b** High-power view of the lower portion of the hair follicle in **a**. Retrograde metamorphosis is observed in the hair matrix cell at *left*

Oliver (1970) and Reynolds and Jahoda (1990) have reported that the dermal papilla component of the follicle can induce the formation of hair-producing follicles containing germinative and outer root sheath epidermis.

In turn, Kim's (1993) findings indicate that the follicular stem cells reside in the secondary hair germ of the outer rooth sheath.

29.5.3 Experiment with Shaved Hair Root Transplantation

As stated earlier, the authors have developed a subcutaneous tissue-shaving method, in which both the sweat glands and the lower hair root are shaved and removed, for the radical treatment of bromidrosis; results have been successful. We conducted an experiment utilizing part of the tissue removed by this method, which we transplanted in the unshaved, obverse side of the axillary skin. We then collected the transplanted graft after 1 week to study the hair root portion. Some of the hair roots were in the anagen stage, with the functions of the hair matrix well preserved (Fig. 29.16a,b), but most were in the phase of retrograde metamorphosis (Fig. 29.17a,b). However, the hair matrix in the left portion of the hair bulb was observed to have atrophied (Fig. 29.16b), and this could lead to atrophy of the hair itself. These above findings indicate that in the experimental transplantation of only the lower hair follicle, no hair regeneration can be expected from the transplanted hair matrix. However, hair regeneration can be expected over a long period (Kim 1993).

29.5.4 Mechanisms of Hair Generation Without Temporary Hair Loss

The authors have reported that retrograde metamorphosis was induced by blood stagnation in the dermal papilla, the nutritional base for the hair

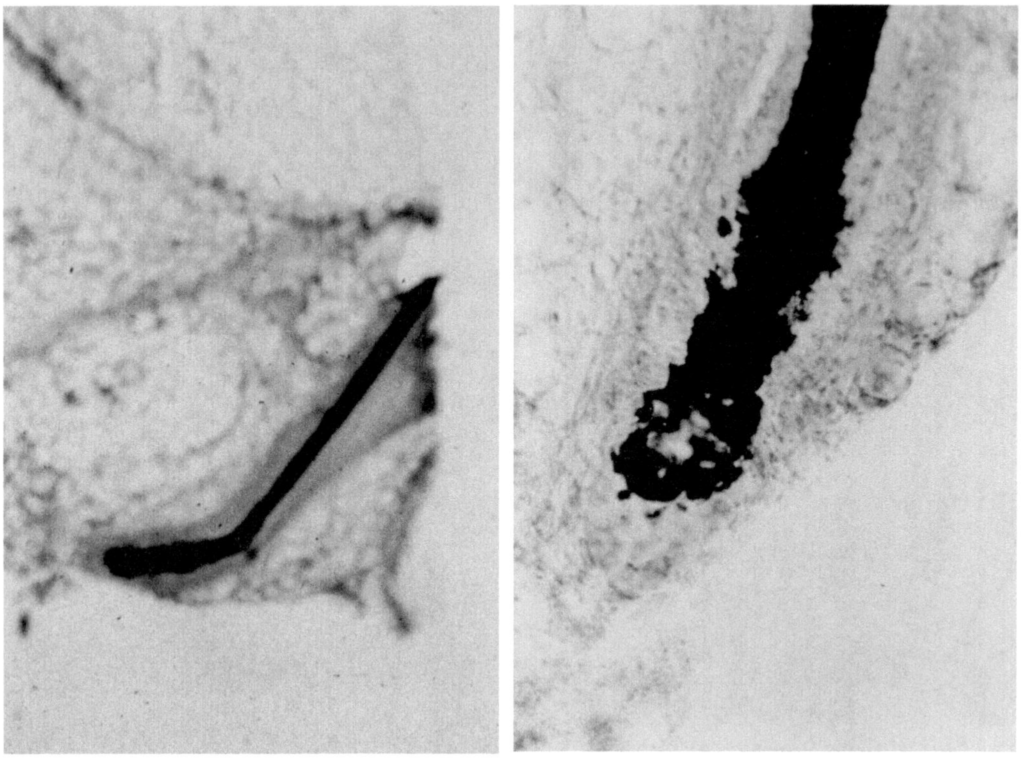

a b

Fig. 29.17. **a** Subcutaneous tissue layer, removed by Inaba's subcutaneous tissue shaving method, 7 days after transplantation. The shaved lower hair follicle has atrophied. **b** High-power view of **a**. The hair bulb in the lower hair follicle has disappeared and become a club hair

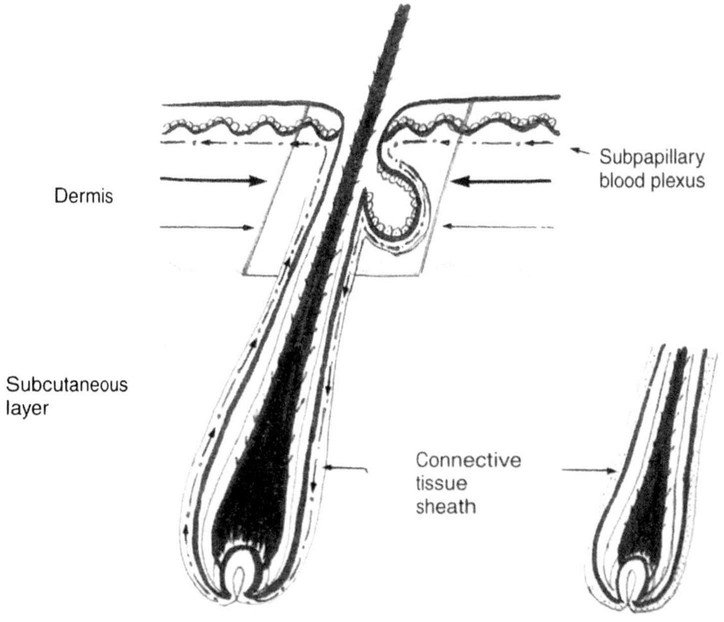

a b

Fig. 29.18. **a** Inaba's single hair transplantation. The dermal tissue (epidermis) contained in the coarse hair-bearing graft acts as a pump in blood circulation soon after it has fitted in well with the recipient tissue. The microcirculation is started from the subpapillary blood plexus beneath the epidermis to the blood vessels inside the connective tissue sheath of the transplanted hair follicle, supplying nutrition (blood cells) to the pilosebaceous unit. **b** Lower hair follicle transplantation. Blood congestion is observed inside the blood vessel inside the connective tissue sheath, resulting in degeneration matrix; in coarse hair-bearing graft transplantation, since the dermal tissue was contained in the graft, microcirculation, between the papillary blood plexus beneath the epidermis in the peripheral recipient site and the pilosebaceous apparatus, began at an early stage after transplantation, thus supplying nutrition to the hair matrix (see Chapter 5).

With regard to the mechanism of a good fit for transplanted grafts, Okada (1987) reported that, during some 48 h before blood circulation is resumed in the transplanted graft, plasma circulation is started first, followed by blood circulation starting from the recipient site (revascularization).

In single-hair transplantation (Inaba method), first the dermal tissue of the pilosebaceous hair follicle fits into the recipient site, and, after the plasma circulation phase, blood circulation is readily started (Fig. 29.18a). This indicates that the dermal tissue (epidermis) contained in the coarse hair-bearing graft acts as a pump in blood circulation, and that soon after the follicle has fitted in well with the recipient tissue, the microcirculation is started from the dermal subpapillary blood plexus beneath the epidermis, supplying nutrition (blood cells) to the pilosebaceous unit (see Chapter 5). Thus, it can be well understood that it is very important to preserve the connective tissue sheath surrounding the hair follicle (Fig. 29.18).

Contrary to the above finding, Nordström (1981) reported better results when the epidermis of the transplanted specimen was removed with a small amount of the dermal layer. However, Brandy (1987) and Bradshaw (1988b) suggested that the removal of the epidermis was not absolutely necessary, pointing out the drawback that hair direction cannot be determined if both the epidermis and the coarse hair are removed. In single hair-bearing grafting with the 1-mm punch, for tensionless regions such as the eyebrow region, unlike the tense parietal region, almost complete removal of the epidermis is recommended. Otherwise, scarring (ingrowing (inverted) epidermis) may occur in the follicular orifice (Fig. 29.9).

29.6 Flap Procedures

29.6.1 Juri Flap: Temporal-Parietal-Occipital (TPO) Method

Since 1975, Juri has been using TPO pedicle flaps to treat alopecia. Juri (1975) described a lengthy series of cases wherein long, delayed pedicle flaps were used. The superficial temporal artery on one side is palpated and marked by palpation or by the use of a Doppler flow detector. This will be the center of the base of the pedicle. A Doppler flowmeter may be used to help trace the course of this artery for usually at least half the length of the proposed flap (Kabaker 1988). The width of the Juri flap is approximately 4 cm wide. The flap must be carefully designed so as to produce a sufficient length, the length depending on the length and curvature of the frontal hairline design. Ezaki, a well-known hair surgeon in Japan, has designed a flap, shown in Fig. 29.19 (Ezaki 1993). The areas A and B in this figure, which are about 7–8 cm in length, are in the TPO region, and C is designed to

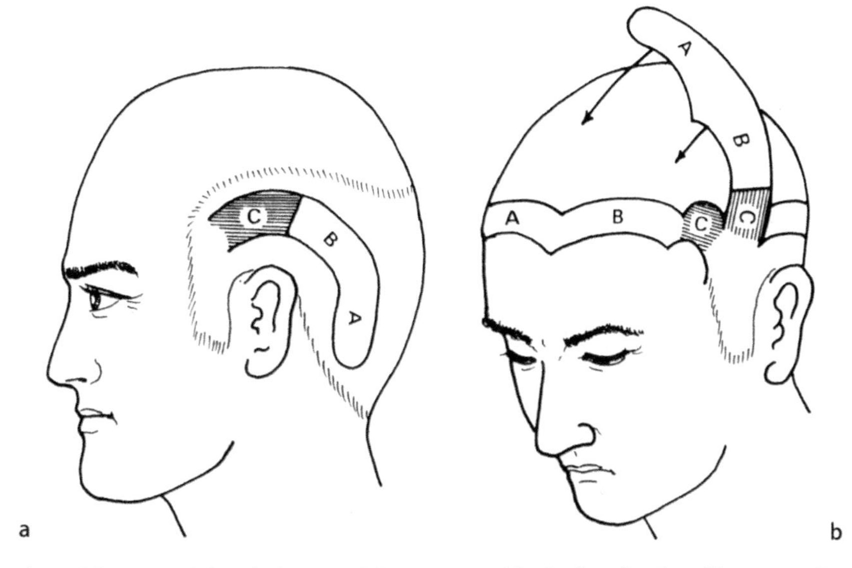

Fig. 29.19a,b. Ezaki's proposed flap design. *A* and *B* are proposed in the frontal region; *C* is proposed as a dog-ear portion. (Courtesy of Ezaki 1993)

avoid insufficient blood circulation in the future balding area, forming a dog-ear portion.

Two delays must be employed. The need for delay with these large flaps, which have a 7:1 length-to-width ratio, has been challenged. However, the procedure is carried out in two stages. In the first stage, the borders of the proximal three-quarters of the flap are incised down to the galea and the incision is closed with a running suture. One week later, the second stage is carried out, during which the distal 6–8 cm of the flaps is incised and undermined. After a further week, in the third stage, the flap is lifted up from its bed and moved into position in the recipient area, and the donor area is closed. Two delay procedures are required before going on to skin flap operation.

29.6.2 Ezaki Technique (Ezaki 1986; Inaba et al. 1989)

29.6.2.1 Decision on Hairline

Ezaki has used an incision that corresponds to the proposed anterior hairline. This incision, down to the galea aponeurotica, is made under local anesthesia 2 weeks preoperatively to prevent blood loss as far as is possible and to obtain good circulation (Fig. 29.20a–c).

29.6.2.2 Flap Transfer

The major procedure of moving the flap into the proposed position is performed in a hospital with a fully equipped operating room under sterile conditions. Local anesthesia with a vasoconstrictor is used.

The flap is elevated by sharp and blunt dissection deep to the galea (Fig. 29.20d) and is carefully wrapped in saline-soaked gauze. The sutures in the incision corresponding to the proposed hairline are removed and then the proposed frontal area is removed to a depth equal to that of the flap. This removed skin is stored in saline solution and is used for transplantation of the donor site. If it is expected that the donor site is to be completely sutured, the parietal scalp must be undermined in the subgaleal space to the nape and the posterior rim of the ear. However, the occipital scalp is undermined in the supramuscular plane. The postauricular skin is undermined to the helical rim to close the donor wound without tension. It is necessary to perform a deep undermining of the retroauricular area. The aponeuroses is sutured with 3-0 interrupted buried Dexon sutures and the skin with 5-0 interrupted nylon. Ezaki does not undermine up to the neck and helical rim and does not suture the donor defect, to avoid blood loss

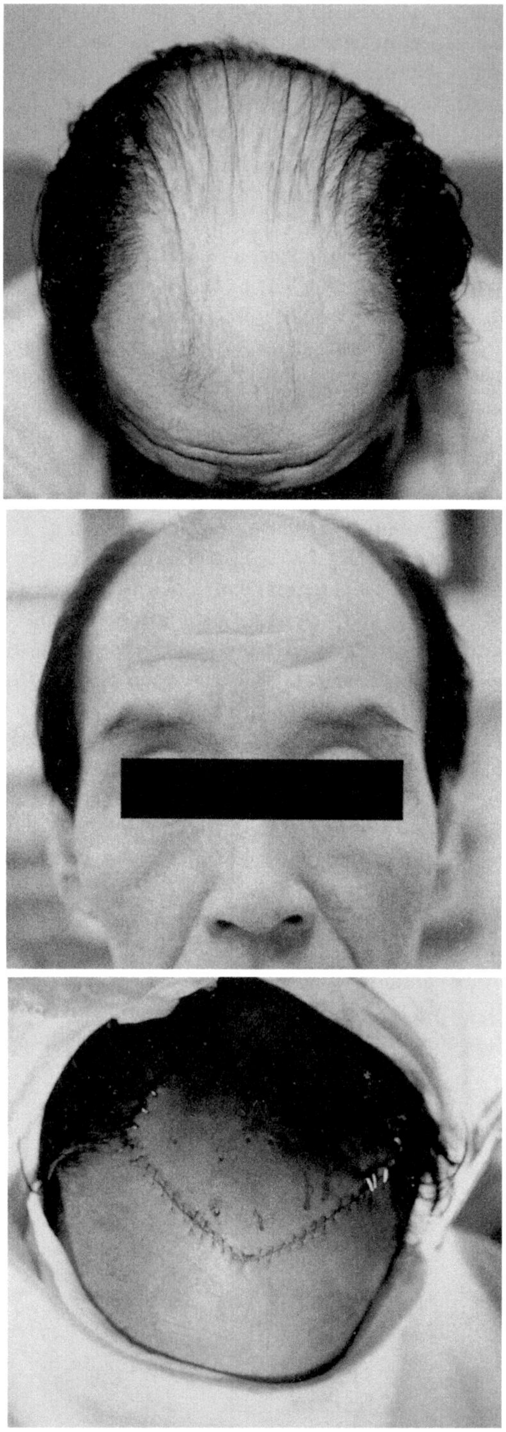

a

b

c

Fig. 29.20a–n. Typical androgenetic alopecia; (40-year-old). **c** Two weeks before operation. Incision corresponds to proposed hairline

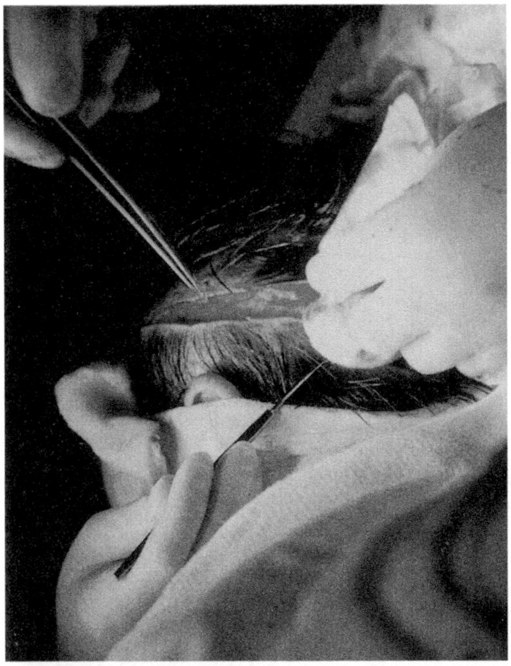

d

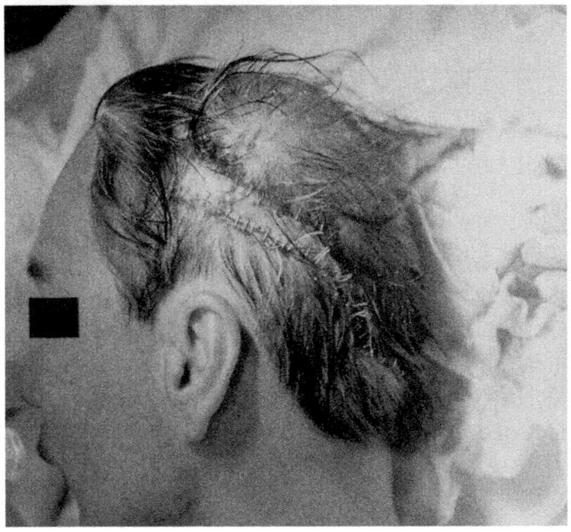

e

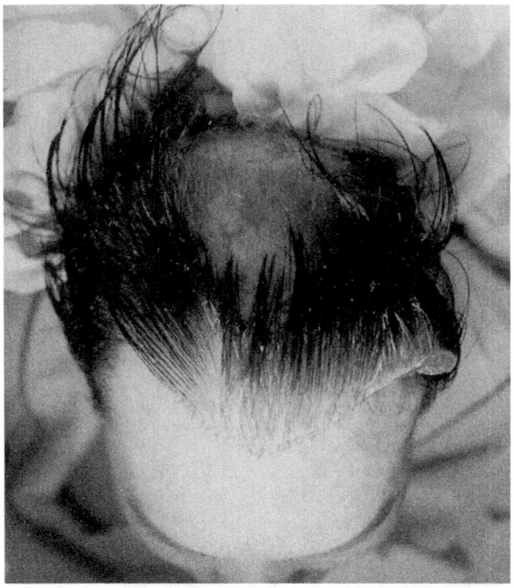

f

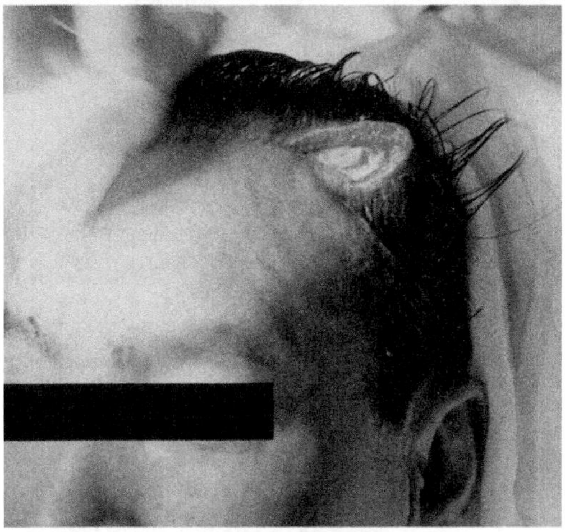

g

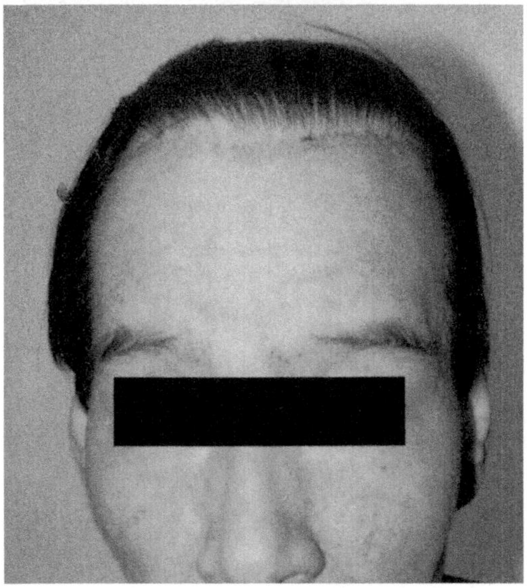

h

Fig. 29.20. **d** Pedicle flap is resected. Usually, undermining of surrounding region is not done. **e** With the Ezaki technique, the donor defect is not sutured. The bald frontal skin is transplanted to the donor site. **f** Pedicle flap is transplanted to the hairline. Dog-ear at the rotation point can clearly be seen. **g** Sofratulle gauze is thoroughly packed inside the dog-ear to prevent inflammation. **h** One year after operation. Scalp hair in the rotated flap has regenerated, but the scar remains visible. **i** Magnified view of **h**. The margin of the flap (about 1-cm-wide) shows temporary hair loss. **j** At the resected donor site, the scar clearly remains. In the near future, scar resection will be performed. **k** The scar area, covered with long hairs by the use of styling mousse. **l** After reduction of scar, the scar area is covered by long hairs. **m** Scar in hairline clearly remains. **n** Hairline is concealed by single hair transplantation

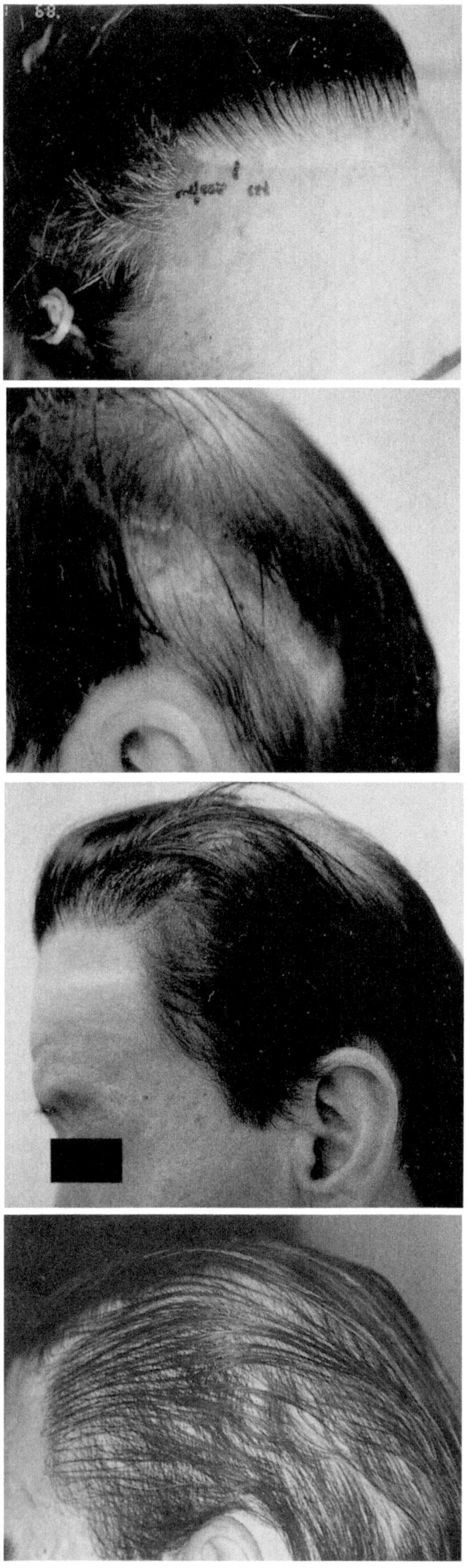

i j k l

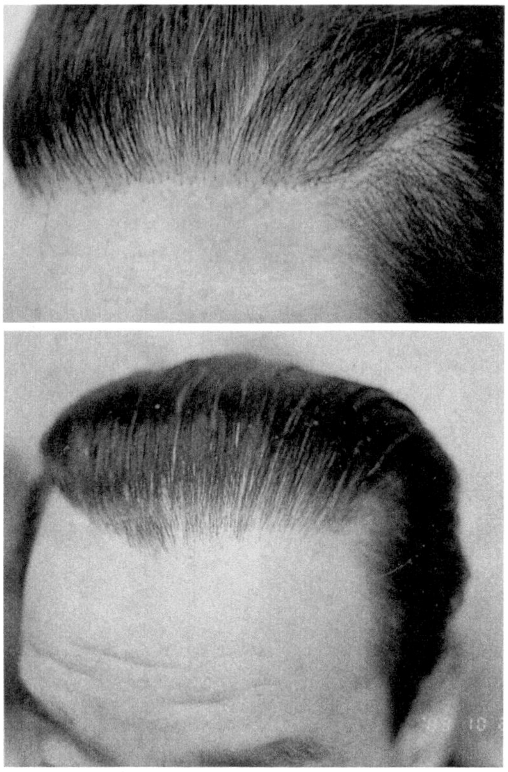

m n

Fig. 29.20. *Continued*

and to shorten the operation time. The already resected bald frontal scalp skin is transplanted to the donor site (Fig. 29.20e). At this transplanted area there will be a scar (Fig. 29.20j), but this scar will be resected in future. Until such time, the scar is concealed with long hair, by the use of styling mousse (Fig. 29.20k).

29.6.2.3 Flap Suture

Extensive undermining of the skin of the anterior scalp helps to avoid a dog-ear. The pedicle flap is sutured to the recipient site (Fig. 29.20f). To preserve blood circulation, the base of the pedicle flap must not be subjected to too much tension and then a dog-ear can be formed (Fig. 29.20f). The inside of the lateral protruding scalp skin (dog-ear) must be completely packed with Sofratulle gauze to prevent inflammation (Fig. 29.20g). The pedicle flap is sutured to the preformed hairline (Fig. 29.20c). Two weeks later, the excess scalp skin in the dog-ear is resected and sutured to the parietal site.

29.6.2.4 Follow-Up Results

After 1 year, the pedicle flap is transplanted in good condition. However, the margin of the flap (about 1-cm wide) shows temporary hair loss (Fig. 29.20i). Using single hair transplantation or artificial hair implantation, the hairline is concealed and a natural appearance is obtained with the passage of time (Fig. 29.20n).

The use of larger delays flaps, described by Juri (1975) and modified by others (Kabaker 1979; Fleming and Mayer 1984), is more often the flap operation of choice for male pattern baldness. Kabaker (1988) has found the larger delayed flap operations no more difficult to perform, and the cosmetic results seen are better.

29.6.3 Parietal or Lateral Flaps

29.6.3.1. Elliott's Technique

Small parietal or lateral flaps, first described by Elliott (1979), may also be used to produce a hairline in two operations. These smaller flaps do not require the delays of the larger Juri flaps and the operation may be performed in the surgery room of a properly equipped office.

A flap beneath and paralleling the hair-bearing fringe on the side of the scalp is designed, usually 3 cm wide at its base; the anterior superior limit of the flap is at a joint just on the temporal hairline. As the flap curves backward, it usually quickly tapers to 2.5 cm in width. The flap is usually between 12 and 15 cm long and is designed to stay well within the permanent fringe hair. A branch of the superficial temporal artery is not identified, but is presumed to enter the base of the flap for a short course. The flap is incised with cuts paralleling the hair shafts and is rotated into a previously designed and drawn half-hairline to make up a frontal hairline. The operation with the initial flap is performed 3-4 months prior to that for the second flap, which flap is taken from the contralateral area, and is designed so as to overlap slightly and fit into the first flap in the midline.

The bilateral flap is useful in those patients in whom the baldness at the front has not extended to the occipital region. This method is suitable for Type II and Type III baldness, which is, according to the so-called Hamilton's classification, a mild baldness where the hairline retreats in the front and temporal region in a triangle; this procedure is also applicable to Type IV and V baldness, when a second hair transplantation is made in the occipital region.

29.6.3.2 Ezaki's Technique (Bilateral-Temporal-Parietal Flap Method)

29.6.3.2.1 Design of the Donor and Recipient Regions in the Temporal-Parietal Flap Method. Firstly, the position and type of the proposed hairline on the forehead and parietal region are both determined. The type of hairline should be carefully considered to maintain the balance and the contours of the face (Fig. 29.21a). As shown in Fig. 29.21a, it is preferable to make the frontoparietal angle between 80° and 90°, and the flaps should be designed so that BE = AB + DE + 1.5 cm.

An angle of more than 90° gives a somewhat unnatural image. The width of the flap is usually between 2.0 and 3.0 cm, depending on the severity of the baldness, but sometimes a flap of 3.5 cm width is prepared. The width of the flap is the same from the starting point to the end. The ratio of length to width is 4:1 to 5:1.

When normal hairs remain at the center of the frontal region, it is not recommended to utilize these by bringing the ends of the flaps on both sides of the hair. In fact, it is preferable to ignore the preservation of the original hairs when applying the flaps. Otherwise, as baldness progresses, the natural hairs fall out, giving rise to a greater area of baldness between the left and the right flaps. This area would contrast unnaturally with the profuse hair of the flaps.

A Doppler flowmeter has been used to search for an artery and then to design the procedure so as to keep the artery on the starting points of the flaps. In this technique, delay procedure is not necessary. However, if the flaps have any previous scarring or a punch donor scar, they are given a week's delay.

29.6.3.2.2 Operative Technique. Before the operation, the scalp hair should be well shampooed and the operative region disinfected. The hair, which is not trimmed, is treated with an antibiotic ointment, used as a pomade, as a premedication. Diazepam (10 mg) is used preoperatively.

Sufficient local anesthesia is induced in the area around the flap. The flap and the recipient frontal region are injected with 0.5% xylocaine containing 1:100 000 epinephrine. Injection into the muscle should be avoided. As the frontal region is relatively sensitive, 1% xylocaine is sometimes used. In principle, epinephrine in xylocaine is not used in the flap operation when obtaining the donor region, but since the blood circulation in the scalp is extensive and hemorrhaging occurs, epinephrine seems to give better results in preventing hematoma. In terms of the patients so far observed there has been no blood flow disorder in the flaps.

In the donor region, using the scalp along the hair direction, the flap is elevated at the subgalea (Fig. 29.21B). In order to secure the flap on the recipient area, a fibrin adhesive system (Tisseel Kit, Immunology Co., Tokyo, Japan), is sometimes used. This has good binding power and is very useful for the prevention of hemorrhage or the occurrence of hematoma under the flaps (some-

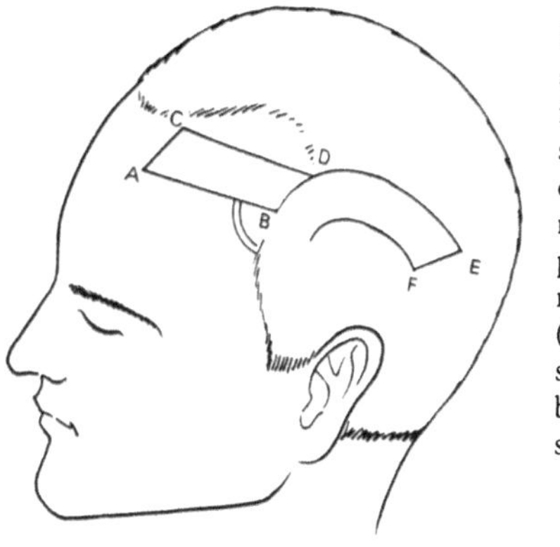

a

Fig. 29.21. **a** Ezaki's design (temporal-parietal flap method). In designing the flap, the formula should be $BE = AB + DE + 1.5$ cm, and the frontoparietal angle (B) should be between 80° and 90°. (With permission from Ezaki 1986). **b** Ezaki's operation technique (temporal-parietal flap method). When the flap is moved to the frontal region (B), a rotation of about 130° is made. This results in a dog-ear at the rotation point; the dog-ear should be removed 14 days later (C, D). The donor region is sutured after extensive undermining of the surrounding scalp (B) (with permission from Ezaki 1986). **c** Case 1. Before surgery. **d** After surgery. **e** Case 2. Before surgery. **f** After surgery. In cases 1 and 2 the bilateral flaps are connected at the center, and the joint line has become so natural as to be almost indiscernible (courtesy of Ezaki 1993)

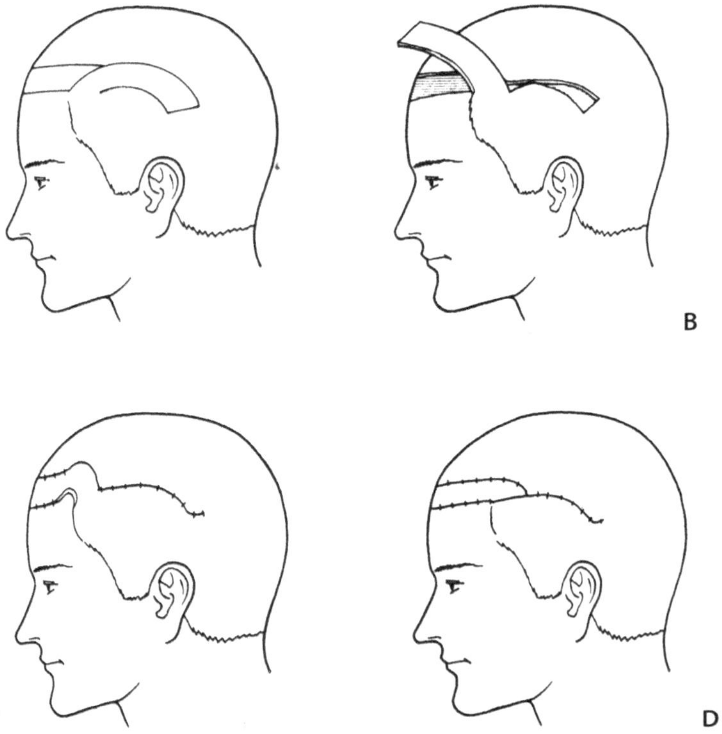

b

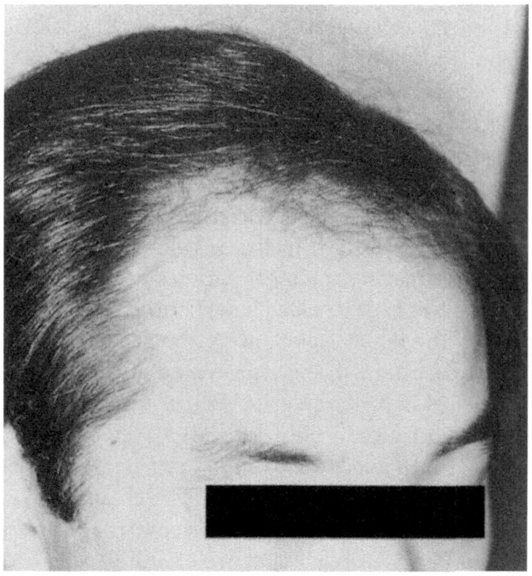

c

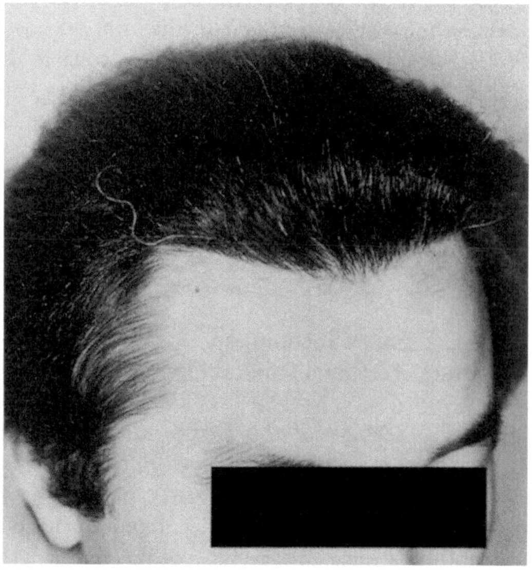

d

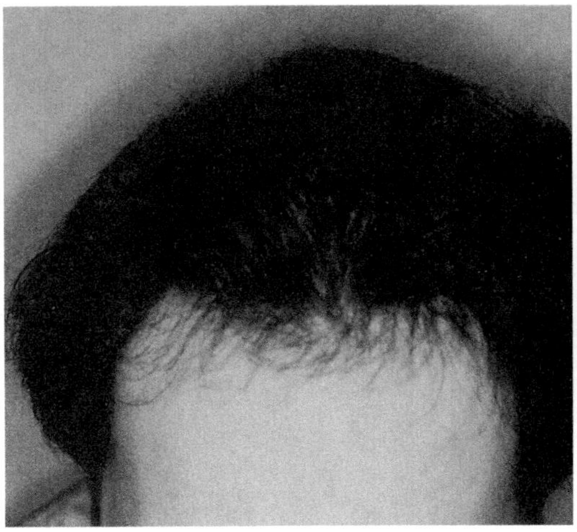

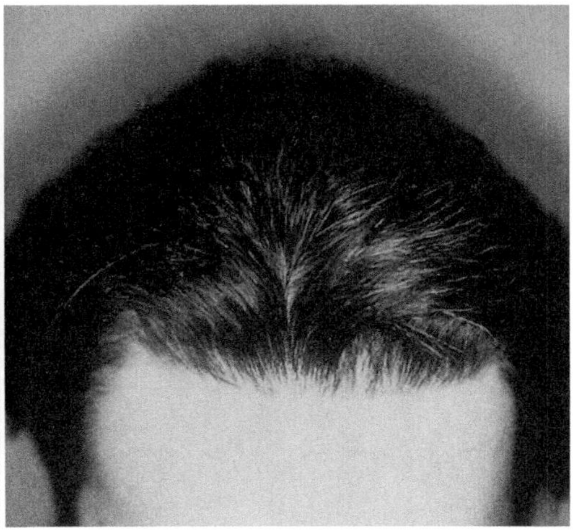

e f

Fig. 29.21. *Continued*

times a light tie-over dressing will be used on the flaps).

In the flap technique there have been cases of flap compression by hematoma, giving rise to blood flow disorder or infection. Therefore the prevention of hematoma is also a key to successful transplantation.

The donor region is sutured by pulling the upper and lower scalps together after extensive undermining of the surrounding scalp. When the flap is moved to the frontal region a rotation of about 130° is made. This results in a dog-ear at the rotation point which should be removed 14 days later.

A frontotemporal angle is made by using the dog-ear skin. The extra skin should be returned to cover any laterally exposed defect. The flap is sutured with 5.0-6.0 nylon. The bilateral flaps are connected at the center, and there should not be any tension between the two flaps. The joint line becomes so natural as to be almost indiscernible (Fig. 29.21c-f).

With this technique, both bilateral flaps can be transferred at one time; however, if the patient has enough time, the operations can be performed one after the other at intervals of 4-7 days, which is less unpleasant for the patient. It is imperative not to put too much pressure on the dog-ear while a dressing is used in the operated region.

29.6.4 Pre-Auricular and Post-Auricular Flaps (Reviewed from Unger 1990)

Nataf and Dardour (1988) have described very narrow pre-auricular or post-auricular flaps based superiorly and employed to obtain a dense frontal hairline. A great advantage of these flaps is that the hair within them grows anteriorly in the normal direction of hair growth. Since these flaps are based opposite to the circulation of the scalp, this type of flap has several problems, including the necessity of a delay procedure, a less than optimal survival rate, and a length which rarely would be long enough to produce even half a hairline. When expertly carried out, however, such flaps can produce cosmetically excellent results for a good portion of the part side hairline. Marzola (1984) advocates the use of the pre-auricular flap in conjunction with extensive scalp reductions and has presented some exemplary results.

29.6.5 Occipital-Parietal Long Flap Method (Ezaki 1993) (Fig. 29.22.1)

This method is applicable to the improvement of horseshoe-shaped baldness occurring in the region from the frontal and parietal scalp (Hamilton classification, Types IV and V). As shown for case 1 in Fig. 29.22.1A, Fig. 29.22.2a, an incision is made over the site of the donor flap in the occipital area after local anesthesia is performed. After a delay of 1 week, the flap is collected (Fig. 29.22.2a) and the donor site is sutured after extensive undermining in the peripheral region (Fig. 29.22.1B, Fig. 29.22.2b). The flap is rotated 90° and sufficient blood circulation is assured by dilating the area with a dog-ear; the scheduled frontal line is then drawn (Fig. 29.22.1C, Fig. 29.22.2c). The scalp on the recipient site is then removed and the flap is transplanted (Fig. 29.22.1D, Fig. 29.22.2d). A tie-over dressing is applied to the site Fig. 29.22.2e. The swollen portion of the dog-ear is improved after 2-3 weeks by removing excessive skin (Fig. 29.22.1D).

The patient, case 2, was treated as shown in Fig. 29.22.3a-c with a satisfactory result.

The hairstream may flow toward the frontal region and cover the balding area, as shown in Fig. 29.22.3C, 29.22.4b. The baldness on the left side, which cannot be covered, may be improved by scalp reduction (Ezaki 1993).

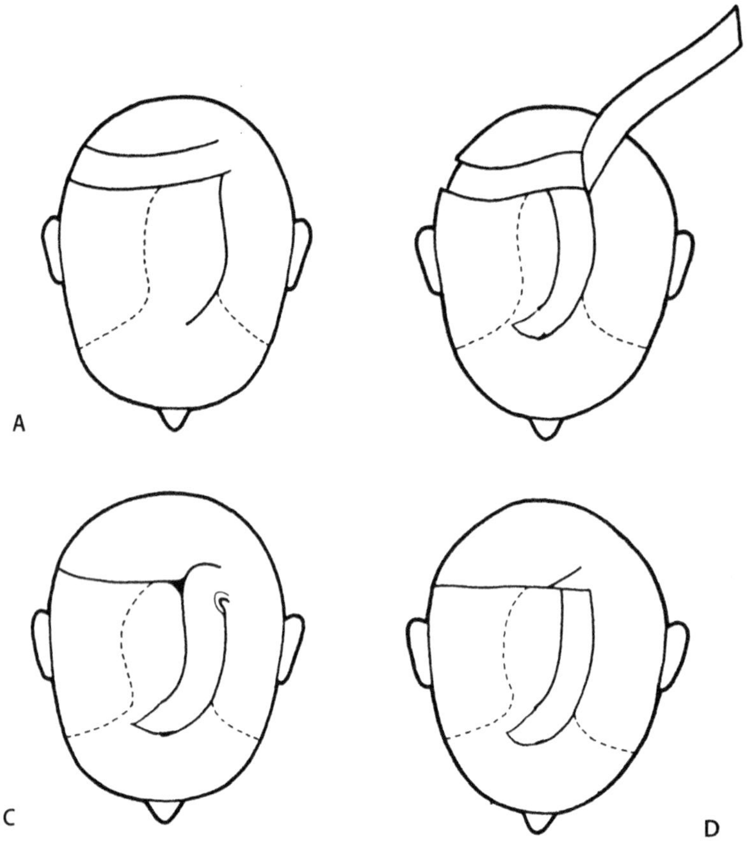

Fig. 29.22. 1 Occipital flap method. (Courtesy of Ezaki 1993)

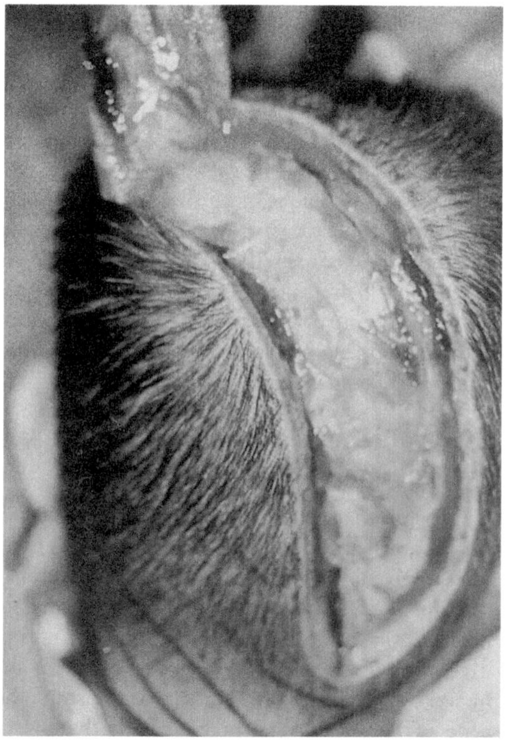

2a

Fig. 29.22. 2a Case 1. Collection of donor flap, 3–4 cm in width, from the occipital region. **2b** Reduction suturing of the donor site. **2c** A rotation is made to move the occipital flap to the frontal region, and the scheduled line is drawn in the balding area. **2d** The flap is fixed to the recipient site by suturing. **2e** A tie-over dressing is placed over the operated area

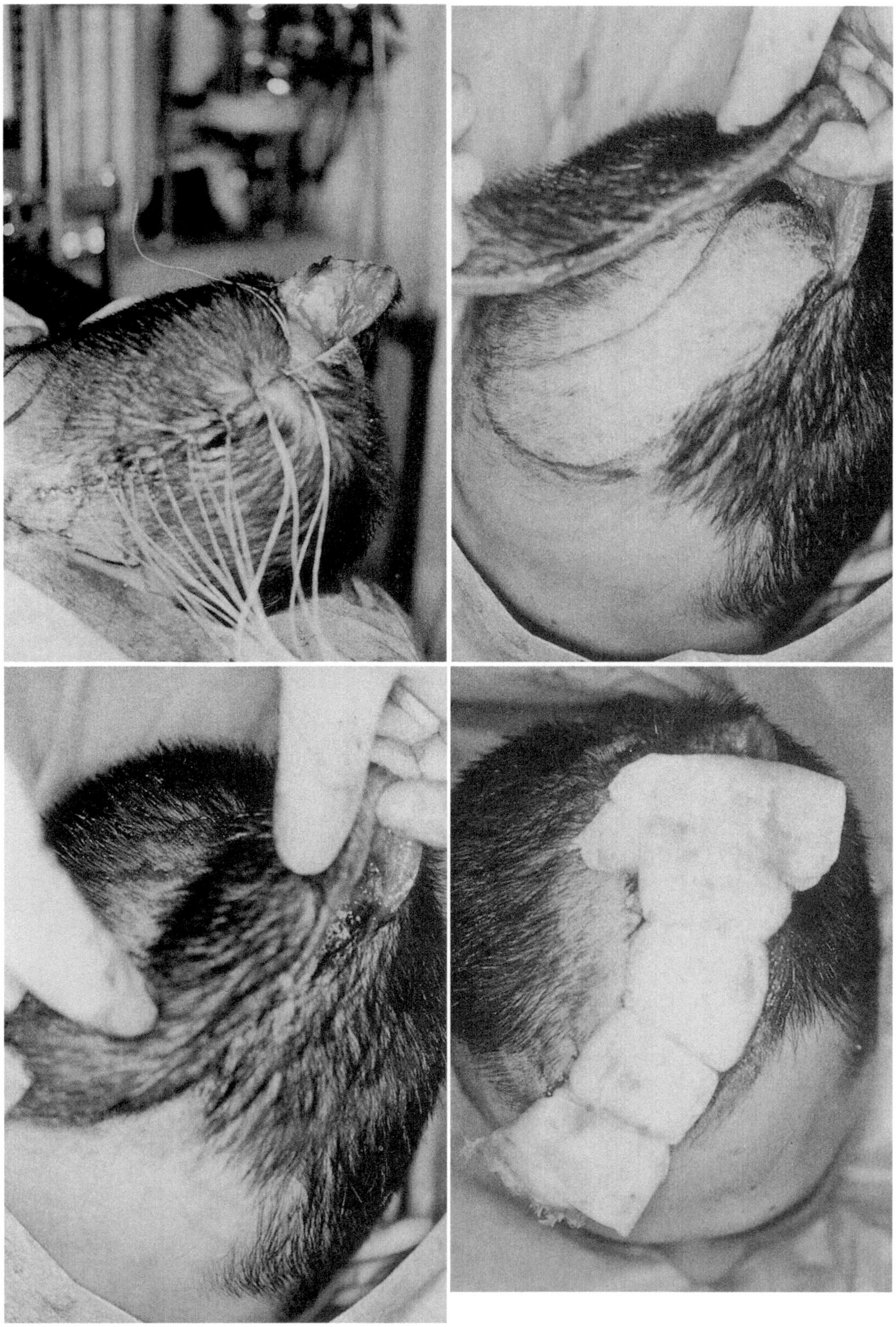

2b 2c 2d 2e

Fig. 29.22.2. *Continued*

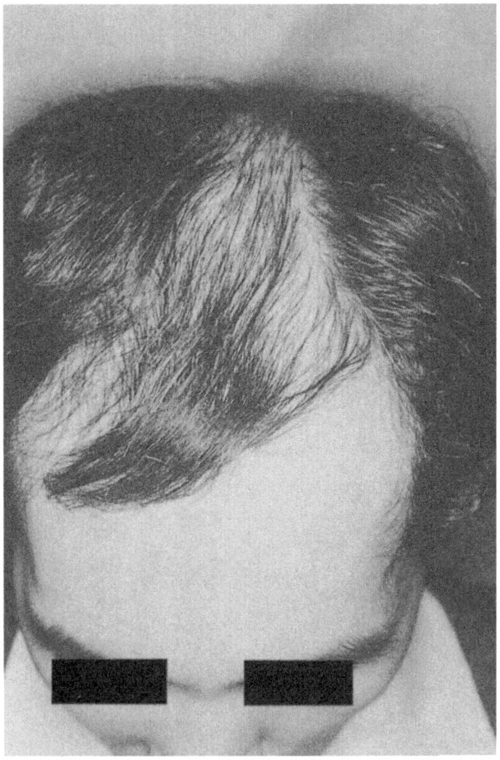

3a

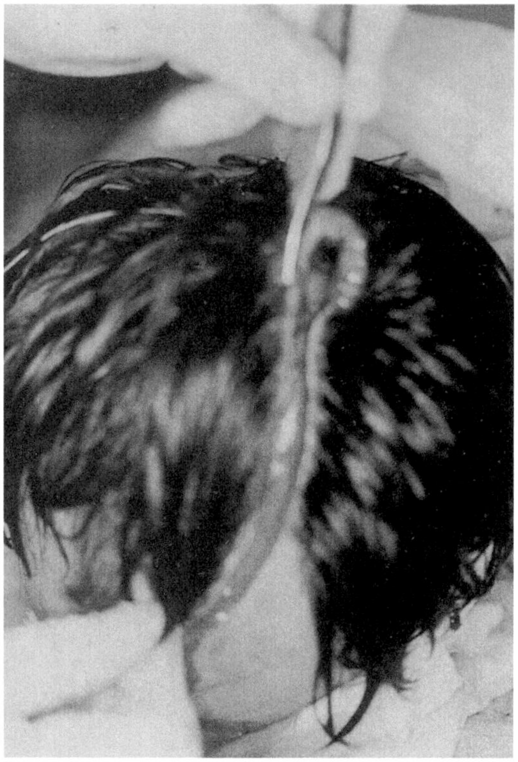

3b

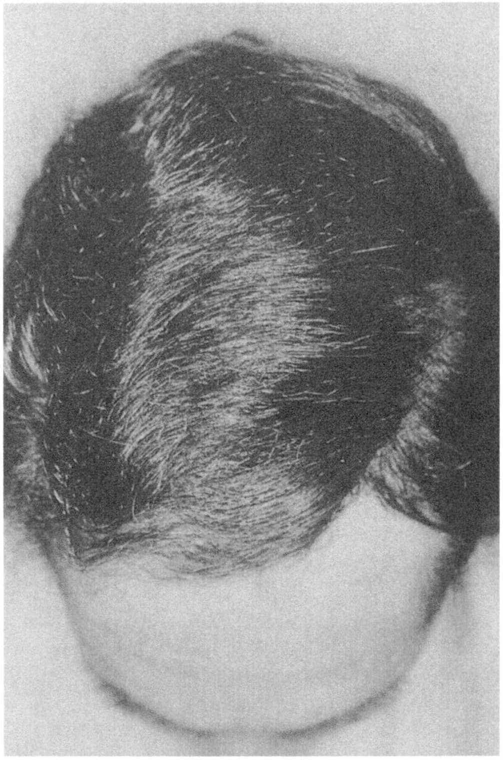

3c

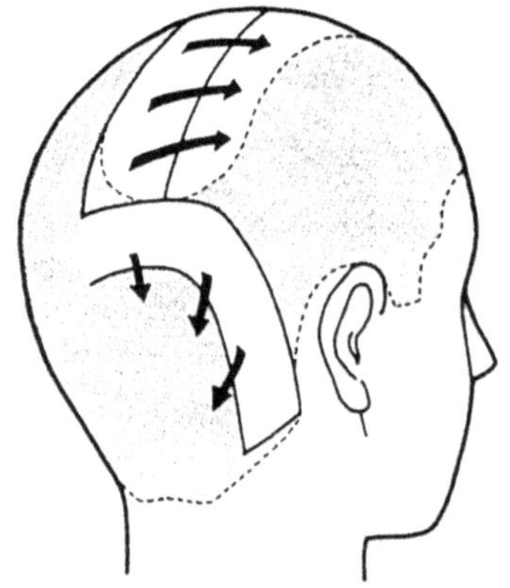

4a

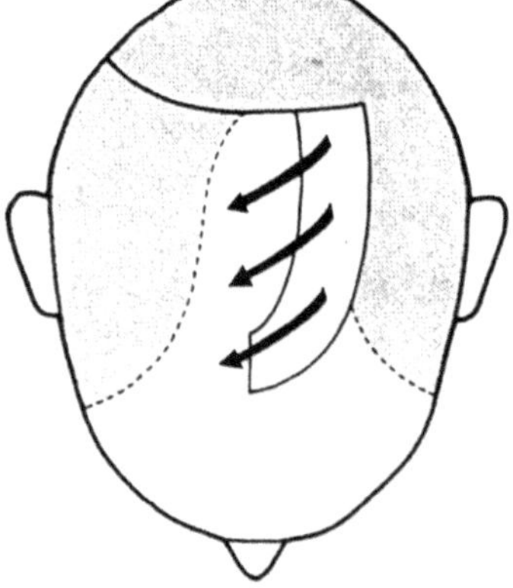

4b

Fig. 29.22. **3a** Case 2. Before surgery. **3b** The occipital flap is adapted to the balding area. **3c** Postoperative view. **4a,b** Hairstream

Fig. 29.23. **a** (*A–G*) Basic patterns for excision; *dots* indicate areas to be excised, *shading* shows punch-transplanted areas. **b** Dorsal schematic demonstrating the large horseshoe-shaped area removed with the bilateral occipital-parietal flap. **c** The four primary lines of incision. **d** Distances between incision lines and the direction of shift. **e** Extent of undermining. (Courtesy of Brandy 1986a)

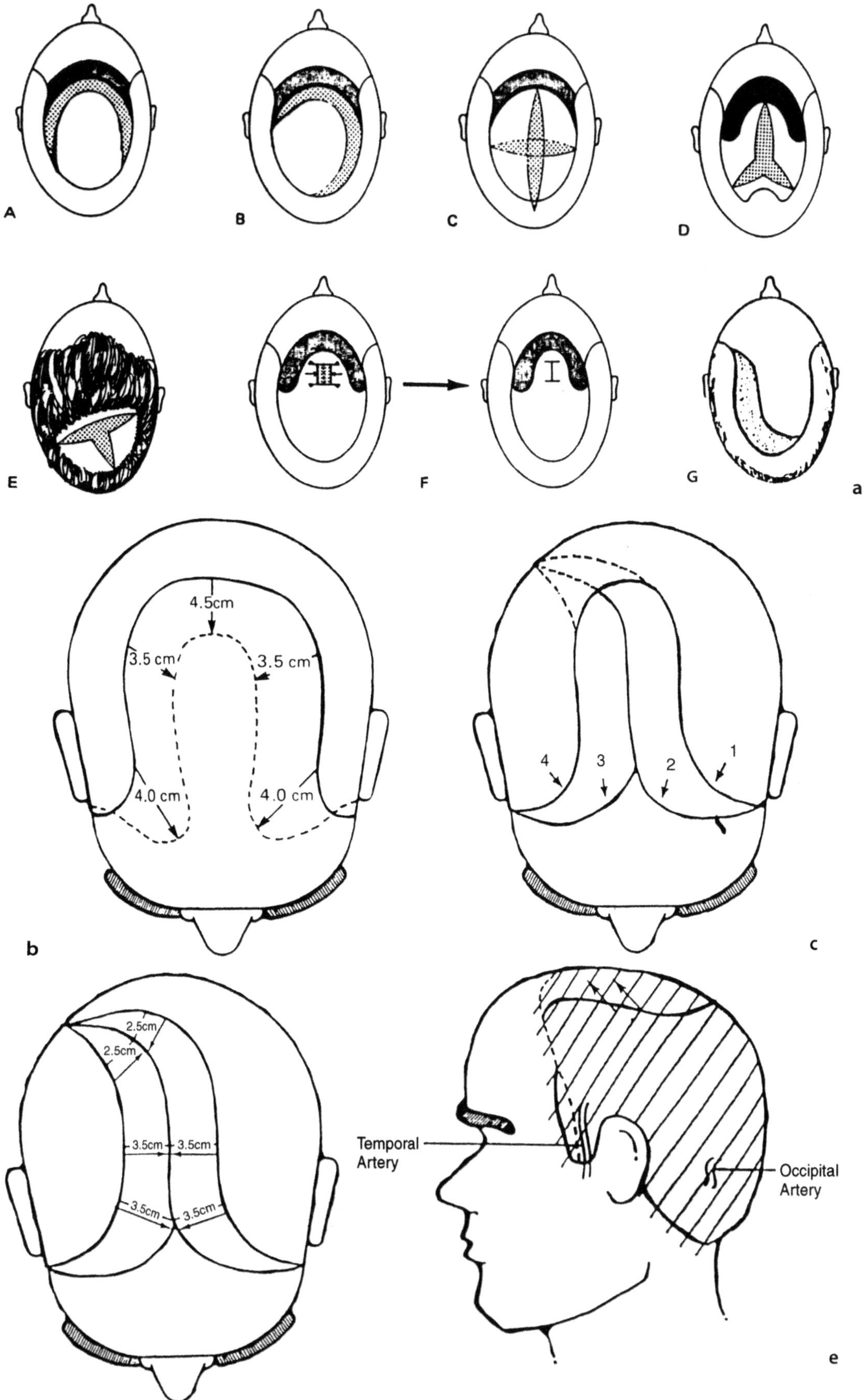
A
B
C
D
E
F
G
a
4.5cm
3.5 cm
3.5 cm
4.0 cm
4.0 cm
b
1
2
3
4
c
2.5cm
2.5cm
3.5cm
3.5cm
3.5cm
3.5cm
d
Temporal Artery
Occipital Artery
e

29.7 Scalp Reduction Procedures

29.7.1 Scalp Reduction

Alopecia reduction has been used for many years on patients with cicatricial alopecia (Oericcochea 1971; Huang et al. 1977) but it was not incorporated into the treatment of male pattern baldness until the mid-1970s. Unger and Unger (1978) neglected to give these authors due credit. New procedures which incorporate soft tissue expansion prior to alopecia reduction and/or extensive undermining are making this procedure progressively more important.

Brandy (1986a) began to perform scalp reduction experimentally in 1985 with a new approach to the bitemporal flap, which is an offshoot of the Marzola (1984) lateral scalp reduction.

Unger (1990) divided this alopecia reduction into seven common patterns. These are shown in Fig. 29.23a as: A, Sagittal midline ellipse method; B, Y-pattern method; C, Y-pattern variation method; D, lateral pattern method; E, U-pattern method; F, miscellaneous pattern method; and G, combined pattern method.

Scalp reduction is performed under local anesthesia. An estimate excision is drawn on the scalp, and one side is incised. Extensive undermining of the subgaleal region is performed, and the flaps are advanced. The maximum amount of scalp is excised to allow for approximation with some tension. If the scalp is not particularly flexible, a smaller than estimated amount of scalp is removed. A two-layer closure is advised, with the deep layer being a permanent or semipermanent suture to hold the galea without tension. A width of 2–5 cm is usually removed in one session. Repeated reductions may be attempted at 2- to 3-month intervals (as reviewed by Kabaker 1982).

Brandy (1986b) does more extensive undermining. With the "bilateral occipitoparietal (BOP) flap," the skin incision is made just behind the hairline of the temple region. Following this, the entire hair-bearing portion of the scalp is undermined. The hair-bearing portion of the scalp is then advanced anteriorly and medially as illustrated in Fig. 29.23b–e.

After an interval of 2–3 months, the "bilateral temporal (BT) flap" operation is performed.

According to Brandy (1986b), once the anesthesia is accomplished, the first incision is made along the line labelled 1 in Fig. 29.23c. One-half of the entire occipitoparietal scalp is then undermined past the galeal attachment, down to the hairline of the nape and the posterior rim of the ear (Fig. 29.23e). The occipital artery must be ligated before the next step is carried out (within about 2½ weeks). Upon completion of the undermining, the flap formed on that side is advanced upward and forward to meet line 2 (Fig. 29.23c). The bald scalp between lines 1 and 2 is then excised and discarded. The next incision is along line 3. After this incision is completed, the remainder of the scalp is undermined, again to the hairline of the nape, and the posterior, is undermined to the hairline of the nape and the posterior rim of the ear. Two test incisions are then made between lines 3 and 4 so that the operator can ensure that line 4 will be able to meet at the midline and temporal area. If it is decided that laxity is sufficient, an incision is made at line 4, and the bald skin is excised and discarded. The treatment of patients with bitemporal recessions and advanced midline balding can be accomplished in just one step (Brandy 1986b).

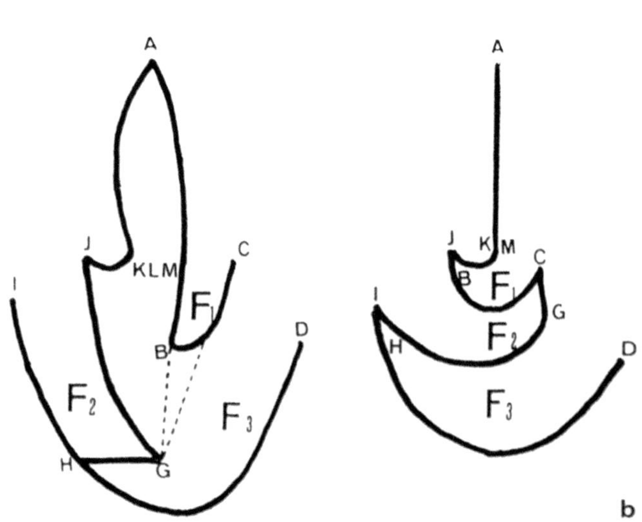

a b

Fig. 29.24. Incision lines of the three hair-bearing flaps **a** before and **b** after transposition. **c** A medial vertical scar or slot remains after using the Frechet Extender. **d** Design of incision lines. **e** Flap 2 (F2). **f** Flap 3 (F3). (Courtesy of Frechet 1994)

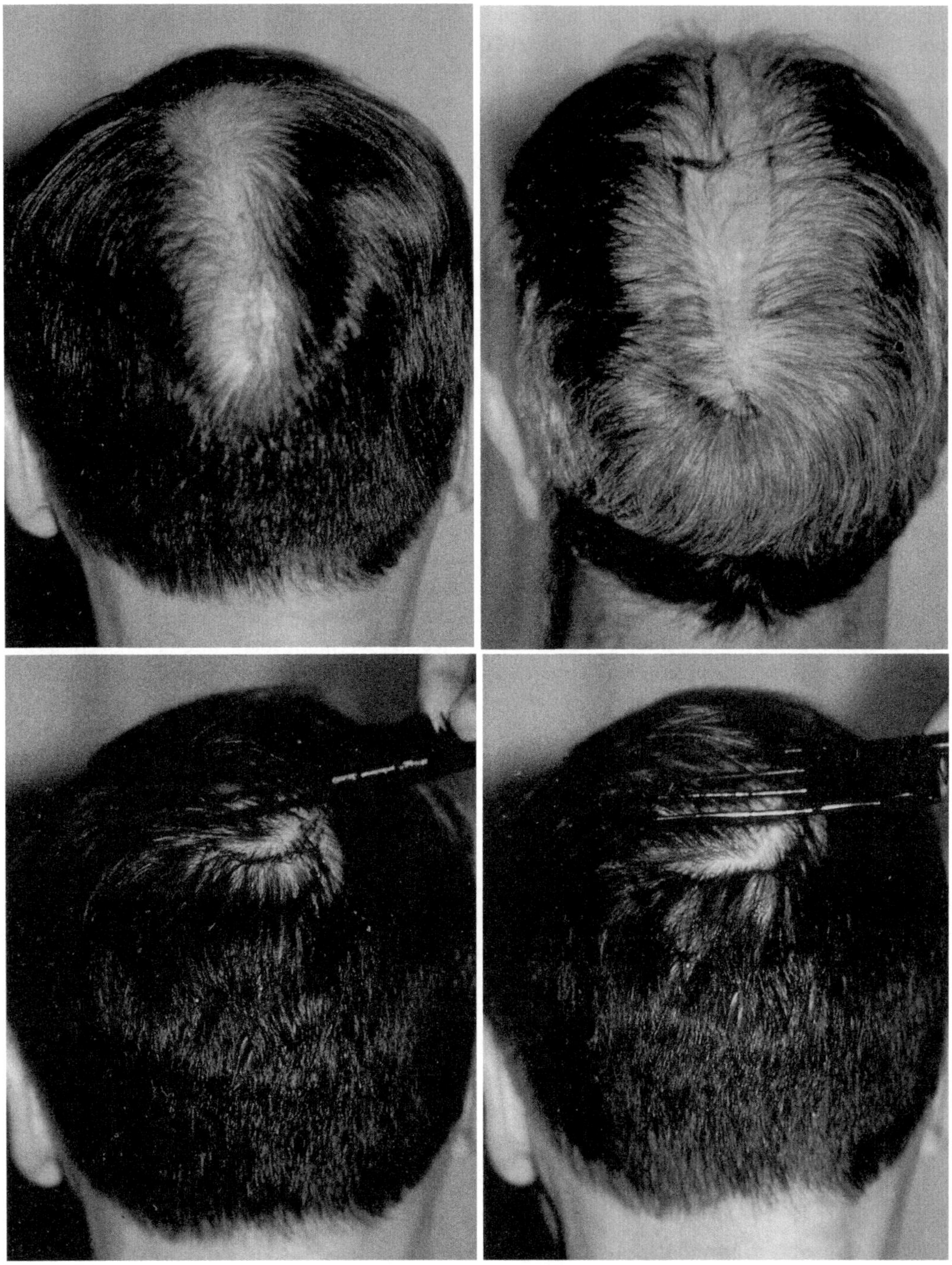

c d e f

Fig. 29.24. *Continued*

29.7.2 Scalp Reduction with a Random Flap

Frechet (1990, 1994) proposed a new technique for correction of the medial vertical scar of the scalp (or slot) after the extension flap method (Frechet 1993) using a three hair-bearing scalp-flap rotation procedure combined with scalp reduction. Incisions are made beginning in the most anterior area of the scalp reduction. Inferiorly, the undermining will reach the upper auricular sulcus, just above the ears, and posteriorly the limit of the undermining will be the nuchal ridge where the occipital muscles can be seen. No deeper undermining is necessary. This will avoid injury to occipital arteries which emerge at a lower level.

Then the surgeon proceeds to the scalp reduction per se, making sure that the right and left borders join without excess tension. Then the bald spot is eliminated and the tissues are brought closer together. This is done first by suturing together the galea at points K and M, followed by deep interrupted suture, along the anterior area of the scalp reduction (Fig. 29.24a,b). Rotation of the upper flap is then performed. This is started by suturing the galea of point B to point J. Subsequently, and in a similar fashion, the intermediate flap is rotated with deep suturing of points G to C and lastly that of the lower flap by bringing point H close to point I.

After this, suturing of the entire deep layer of flaps is performed using interrupted sutures, starting preferably at point D, gradually ascending to point I, then to points C, J and K. The procedure is completed by suturing the superficial layer with interrupted sutures or staples, preferably starting as previously from bottom to top, from D toward A.

The improvement in hair direction makes hair styling so much easier that even when there has been a temporary set-back due to telogen or necrosis, the patients have been able to appreciate the great advantages that this procedure offers.

29.8 Scalp Skin Elongation Method

Surgery to correct extensive alopecia requires increasing the surface of hair-bearing scalp and removing bald scalp. Two commonly used methods, scalp expansion and scalp extension, have advantages.

29.8.1 Expanded Scalp Flaps

Neumann published his original work on tissue expansion in 1957.

Radovan, in 1978 and 1984, helped usher in a new era of reconstructive surgery with his development of a completely contained subcutaneous prosthesis for tissue expansion. This work spurred future developments in tissue expansion. At approximately the same time, significant contributions to tissue expansion for reconstructive purposes were reported (Austad and Rose 1982; Argenta et al. 1983, 1985; Radovan 1984; Manders 1984; Kabaker et al. 1986; Nordström 1988b; Anderson 1987; Marks and Argenta 1988).

Tissue expanders are inflatable, strong silicon bags of various sizes that can be placed underneath tissue to be used for the flap reconstruction of an adjacent defect (Fig. 29.25). One or more expanders can be used, depending on the situation; they are placed under the hair-bearing scalp adjacent to the non-hair-bearing defect. Saline is injected percutaneously into an injection port placed at a slight distance from the expander. Injections are made at 3- to 5-day intervals, and when the increase in distance across the expanded tissues equals the distance across the defect, the expanders can be removed (reviewed from Kabaker et al. 1986).

However, two commonly used methods, scalp expansion and scalp reduction, have disadvantages. The major morphological modifications connected with the volumetric distension of the scalp make this exceptional procedure unpopular with patients, especially in the treatment of androgenetic alopecia.

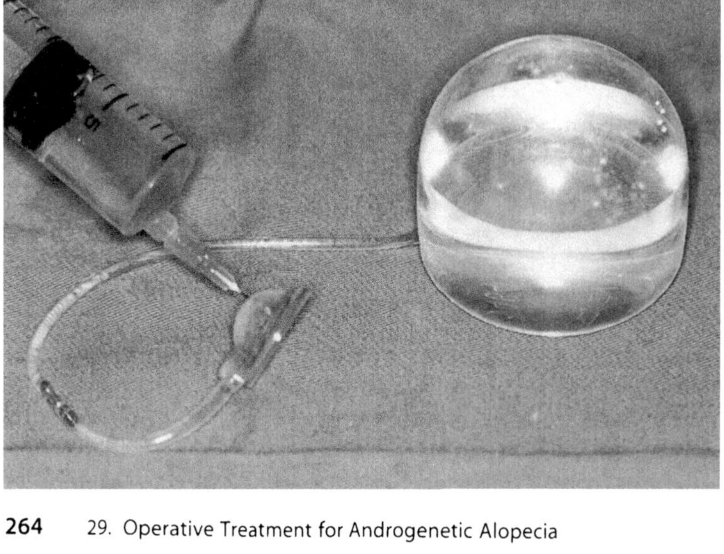

Fig. 29.25. Tissue expander apparatus

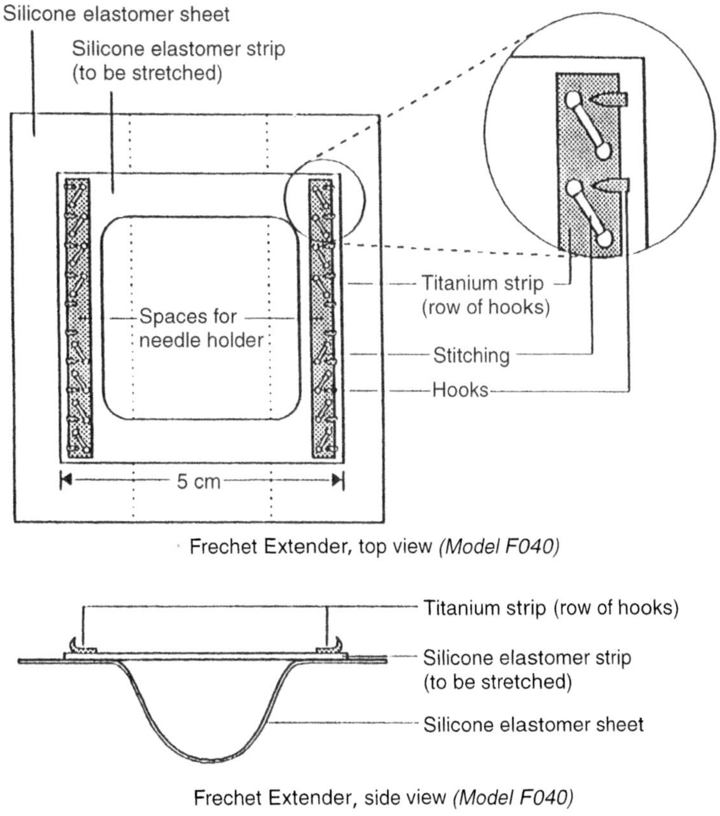

Available Models:

Model No.	*Width (unstretched)*	*Width at 100% extension (measured hooks to hooks)*
F040	5 cm	9 cm
F050	6 cm	11 cm
F060	7 cm	13 cm

a

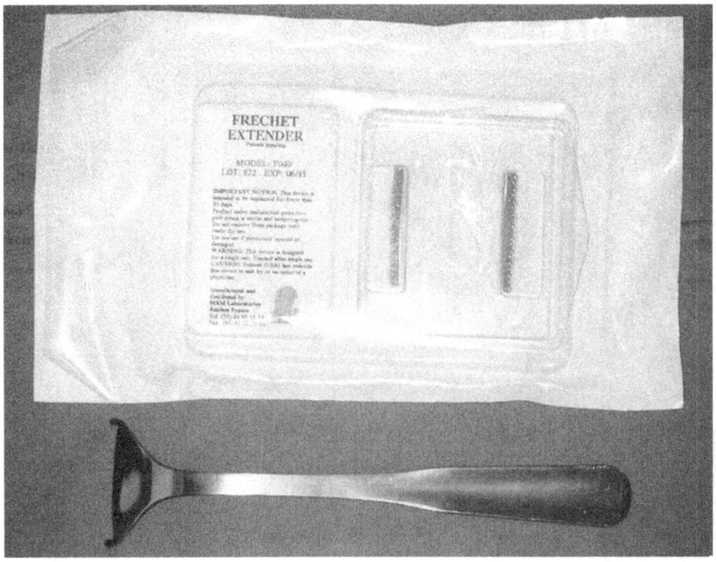

b

Fig. 29.26. a The Frechet Extender is available in three models, varying by extension width. **b** The forceps (*bottom*) are used to insert the Extender. **c** With the Frechet Extender, after incision the scalp is undermined laterally to the supra- and postauricular hair margin, then an elliptical excision can be made (*left*). Hooks on both sides of the Extender are attached to penetrate to the underside of the galea (*middle*). One month after the procedure a medial vertical scar, or slot, remains (*right*). The hair stream can be obtained only in the lateral direction. (**a, b** Courtesy of MXM Laboratories)

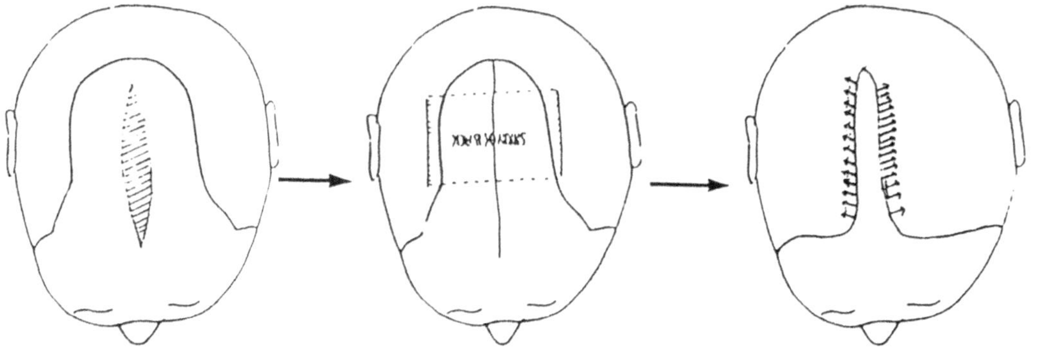

c

Fig. 29.26. *Continued*

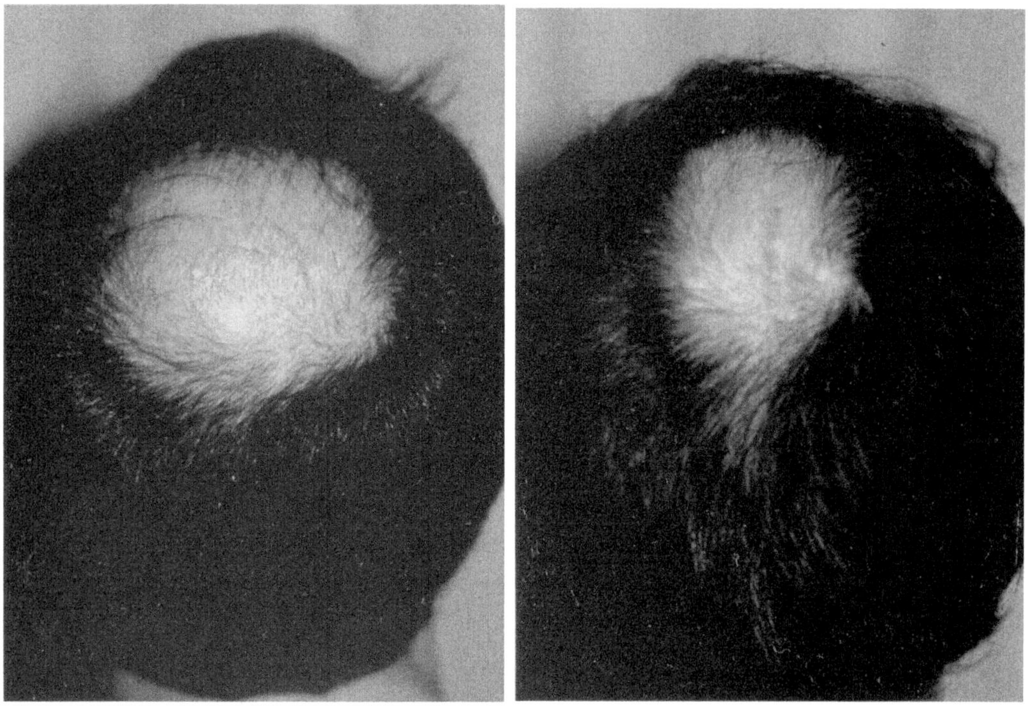

a

b

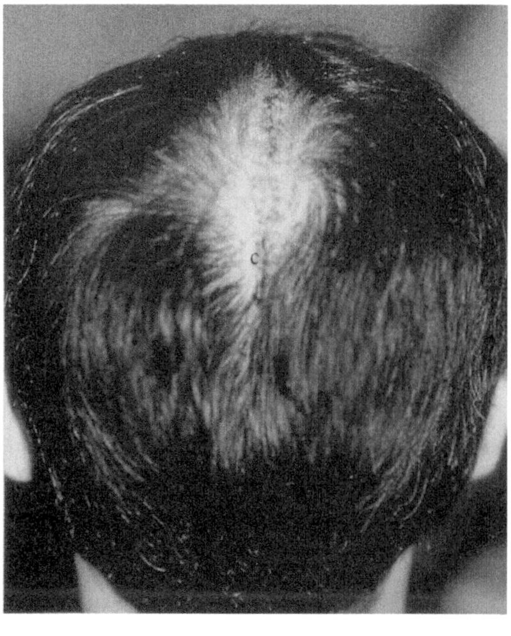

c

Fig. 29.27. **a** A typical manifestation of androgenetic alopecia. **b** After incising and undermining, the Frechet Extender is used. An elliptical excision can then be made, and the bald area is diminished. **c** One month after the procedure, a medial vertical slot remains. (Courtesy of Frechet 1993)

29.8.2 Extended Scalp Flaps (Frechet Extender Method)

Scalp extension was devised by Frechet (1993). Scalp extension consists of selective, constant tension on the hair-bearing scalp itself, employing a thin sheet of bioplastic (and extender) stretched and attached with hooks to the galea after scalp reduction (Fig. 29.26).

The basic extension is a thin sheet of silicone elastomer (silastic) produced by Dow Corning (Midland, MI, USA). The extender sheet is less than 1 mm thick and can vary in shape. In its simplest form, it is a rectangle of varying length (average 5 cm) with a row of titanium hooks on the two opposite ends. The sheet has elastic properties that enable it to stretch up to 200%, with a natural tendency to return to its original position. The Frechet Extender is manufactured by MXM Laboratories, Antibes, France.

After administering local anesthesia and undermining the scalp, laterally to the supra- and postauricular hair margin, the same width of bald scalp is excised as in the scalp reduction technique. However, during the initial procedures, the surgeon can excise a width of 0.5–1.0 cm or less as a precautionary measure. Before closure of the galea under moderate tension, one row of hooks is attached, using specially designed forceps, to the underside of the galea, with the hooks penetrating the deep adipose tissue. This row will be placed under the scalp about 1–2 cm inside the hair margin. The same procedure is repeated for the opposite side. The extender is left in place for 30 to 40 days (from Frechet 1993). Figure 29.27 shows a typical manifestation of androgenetic alopecia and the results of using the Frechet Extender.

29.9 Signs of Disturbed Circulation with Juri Flap Methods

When the flap is transposed into place (third phase), there are three possible options if the flap shows signs of disturbed circulation (Rabineau 1988):

a. If the most distant 3–4 cm does not bleed, do not perform the operation.
b. Cut off the most distant 3–4 cm and thus have a shorter, but surviving flap.
c. Do not try to avoid a dog-ear by flattening the flap. This dog-ear will disappear after a week, and if not, it will be easy to correct later.

29.10 Advantage and Disadvantages of Juri and Partial Flaps

The advantage and disadvantages of these flaps are:

(1) Advantage

They produce dense hair and hair growth immediately after the surgical procedure.

(2) Disadvantages (Unger 1990)

a. The direction of hair within the flaps is the opposite of that normally present in a hairline (hair is directed sharply posteriorly instead of anteriorly, as is usually found in men without androgenetic alopecia).
b. A less than ideal frontotemporal recession is formed.
c. Complications, both in the recipient and donor areas, can be considerably more serious than those which one may expect with punch transplantation.
d. This procedure needs much experience to be done skillfully. It is not at all unusual to see very wide and cosmetically embarrassing donor site scars because of the inadequate surgical skills of the operator (reviewed from Unger 1990).

29.11 Free Flaps

Harii et al. (1974) were the first to use free scalp flaps to repair cicatricial alopecia in the front of the temporal region.

Ohmori (1980, 1991) used microvascular surgical techniques under a microscope, and has described the use of free flaps to create a frontal hairline and hair growing anteriorly in the natural fashion. He used four methods: (a) free temporo-occipital flap, (b) free occipitotemporal flap, (c) free temporoparietal flap, and (d) free occipito-occipital flap (Fig. 29.28). However, microvascular surgical techniques must be mastered in order to carry out these procedures. They are therefore beyond the skill of most scalp surgeons.

The advantages of free flaps (Ohmori 1991; Unger and Marritt 1988) are:

1. They produce dense hair and hair growth immediately after the surgical procedure.
2. The procedure results in a grafted flap with a natural hair direction and density when a microsurgical free scalp flap transfer is used.
3. Minimal residual donor site deformity can be achieved without the dog-ear problem.

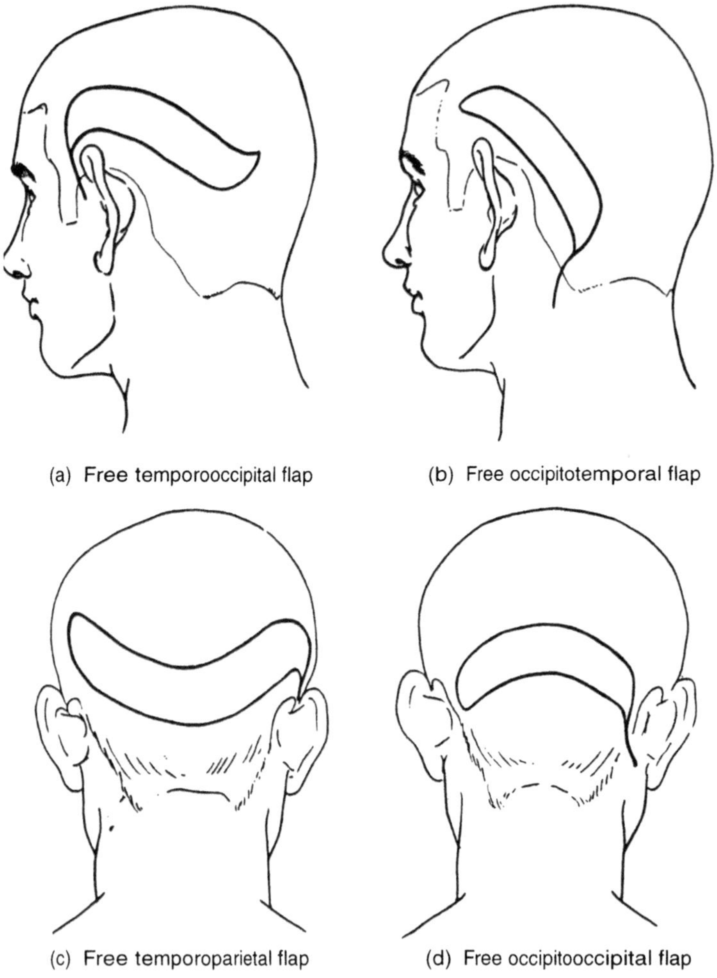

Fig. 29.28a–d. Free flaps. Ohmori has described the use of four kinds of free flaps to create a frontal hairline and to have the hair growing anteriorly in the natural fashion. (With permission from Ohmori 1988)

4. A flap of approximately 18 cm can restore the anterior hairline in one piece.

The disadvantages of free flaps are:

1. The surgeon must have a wide range of experience in microsurgical free flap transfers.
2. The operation itself requires more time than is required for the pedicle flap.
3. Since the hair grows anteriorly, it is difficult to conceal the bald crown area with the implanted hairs. For example, when it is windy, implanted hairs tend to hang down anteriorly if not fixed with a strong styling mousse.

29.12 Histological Study of Free Coarse Hair-Bearing Graft Transplantation

Hair-bearing graft transplantation is more difficult than an ordinary skin graft, since the hairs contained in the graft will frequently not survive. Of all free autogenous grafts, hair-bearing grafts have yielded some of the poorest results (Longacre et al. 1962). Meticulous surgical technique is a prerequisite, but even the most experienced of surgeons, practicing the best of techniques, fail to get optimum results in all hair patients (Norwood 1981).

In free coarse hair-bearing graft transplantation, we have transplanted the hair in the form of a composite flap according to the established practice. Hair matrix cells in the hair bulb were carefully preserved and it was anticipated that blood circulation would be resumed from the recipient site. However, hairs in the free coarse hair-bearing graft transplantation, specifically the peripheral region where the blood circulation is well facilitated, grew continuously without being lost, while in the case of a free coarse hair-bearing graft of more than 5 mm, hairs in the center of the graft fell out and were never regenerated. It can be presumed from these findings that for a free coarse hair-bearing graft to grow, resumption of blood circulation from the lateral face is essential.

We have already reported these findings to some extent in the *Japan Society of Aesthetic Surgery Journal* (in Japanese) (Inaba et al. 1981e; Inaba 1985; Inaba and Inaba 1990a), but we wish to explain the histological findings in detail.

29.12.1 Free Coarse Hair-Bearing Graft Transplantation

We will attempt to supplement the Inaba et al. (1981e) report on this subject.

29.12.1.1 Medium Split-Thickness Skin Graft in the Axillary Region

In the subcutaneous tissue-shaving method developed by Inaba, axillary hair regeneration is observed when the sebaceous gland and the upper isthmal portion of the hair follicle close to the secretory duct opening of the sebaceous gland are left intact. Hair germ is formed from the upper isthmal portion (sebaceous isthmus) when the subcutaneous tissue has been removed up to the medium split-thickness level, when blood circulation inhibitors such as subcutaneous fat tissue have been removed, and the sebaceous gland, as well as the isthmal portion, have been placed in contact with the basal lamina to facilitate a speedy resumption of blood circulation. As a result, while the sweat glands have been removed, the axillary hairs regenerate over a wide area (Fig. 29.29a).

The above finding supported the authors' hypothesis that the essential center of hair regeneration is sited at the upper isthmal portion of the hair follicle, in particular at the duct opening of the sebaceous gland (sebaceous isthmus) (Section 14.1.4).

29.12.1.2 Free Coarse Hair-Bearing Skin Graft Transplantation with a Width Exceeding 1 cm (Fig. 29.30)

In free coarse hair-bearing skin graft transplantation, only a few coarse hairs can be observed in the

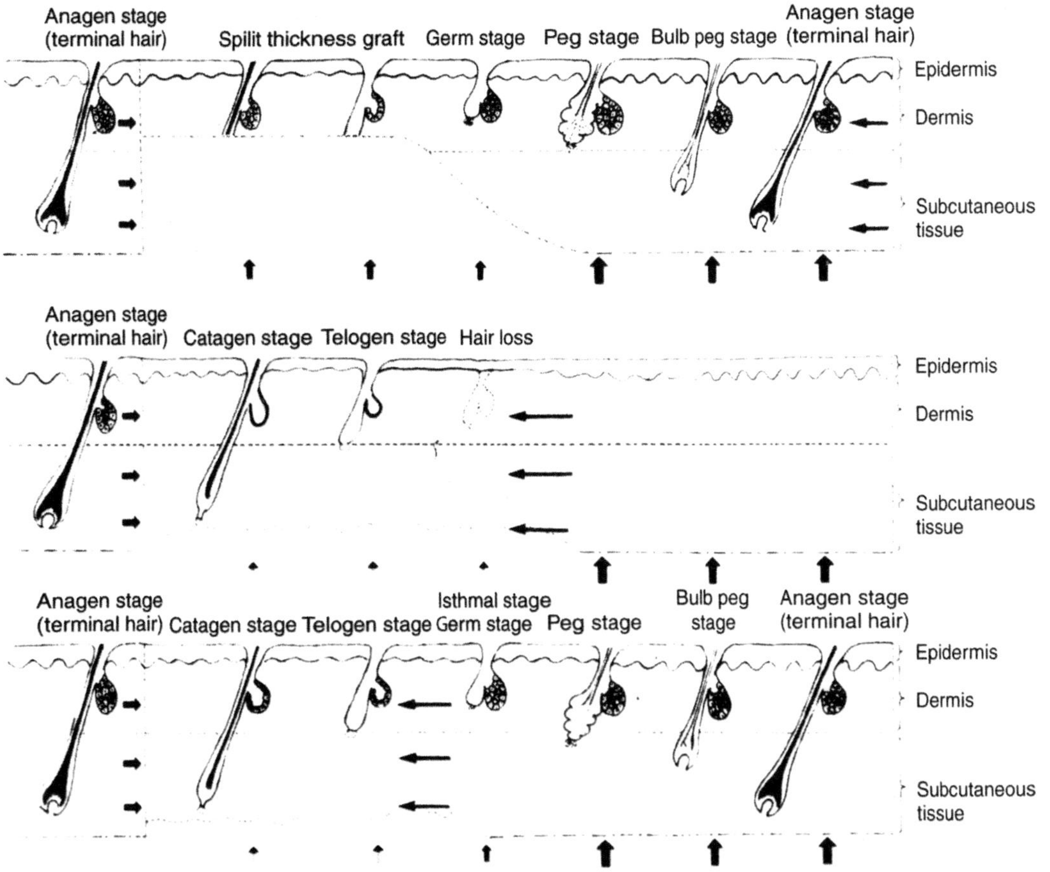

Fig. 29.29a–c. Dermo-appendage interaction in relation to hair regeneration. **a** Split-thickness graft more than 20 mm wide: When the sebaceous gland and upper isthmal portion of the hair follicles are left intact in the subcutaneous shaving method, axillary hairs regenerate over a wide area. **b** Wide hair-bearing skin graft (more than 10 mm wide). Coarse hairs in the center are permanently lost. **c** Narrow skin graft (less than 5 mm wide) Coarse hairs can be regenerated. (Inaba 1985)

a
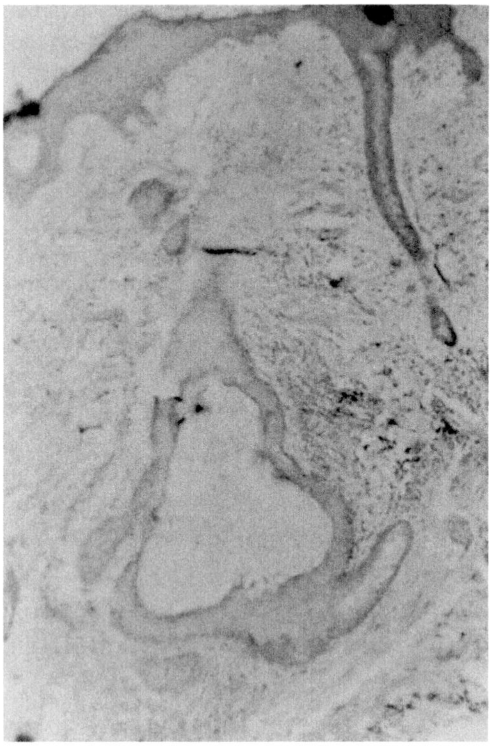

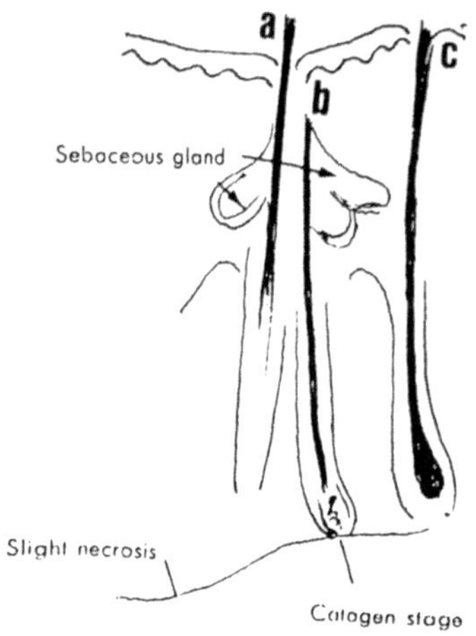

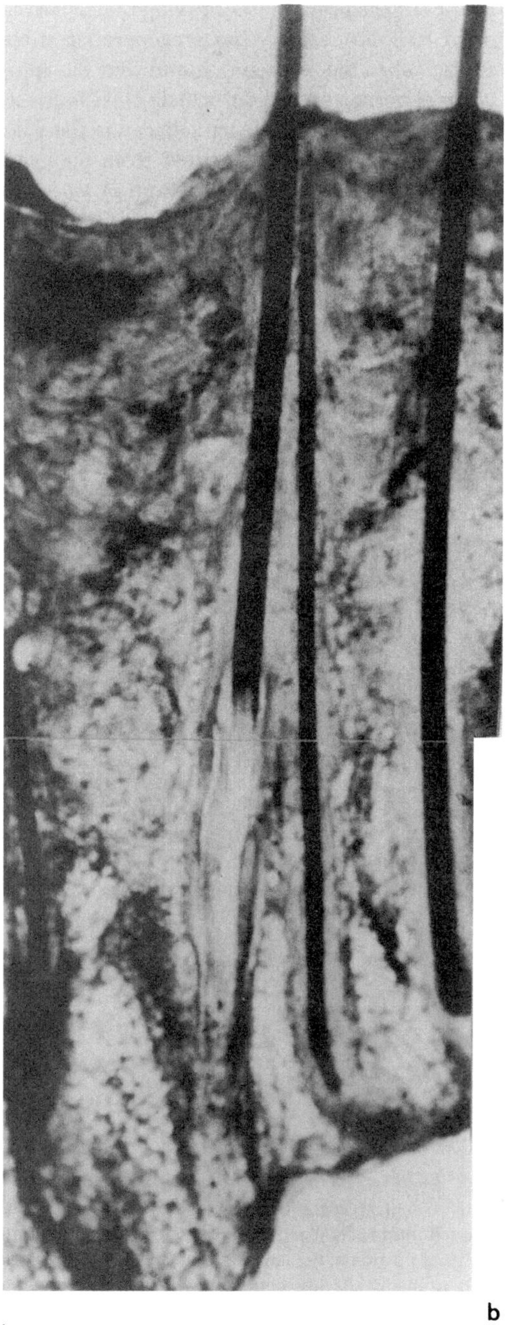
b

Fig. 29.30. **a** Free coarse hair-bearing skin graft transplantation with a width exceeding 1 cm (thin split-thickness specimen). Peripheral epithelial cells around the sebaceous gland have atrophied and disappeared. The acinous cells in the central area have dissolved and been excreted in the form of sebum. **b** Hair-bearing graft with a width exceeding 1 cm (thick split-thickness specimen). The transplanted hair follicle is in the phase of typical retrograde metamorphosis. *Above*: schematic illustration of same figure, showing hair follicles *a*, *b*, and *c*. **c** Sebaceous gland attached to hair follicle *a*. Peripheral epithelial cells around the sebaceous gland have atrophied and the nuclei of acinous cells have disappeared. **d** High-power view of hair follicle *b*. The hair bulb has atrophied and melanin granules are sporadically observed. **e** High-power view of the sebaceous gland attached to hair follicle *b*. Peripheral epithelial cells around the sebaceous gland have atrophied and the acinous cells inside have been excreted in the form of sebum. **f** Another case in which the sebaceous gland is attached to the hair follicle. Peripheral epithelial cells around the sebaceous gland have atrophied. **g** High-power view of the sebaceous gland attached to the follicle shown in **f**. Sebaceous glands have atrophied and the acinous cells inside have been excreted in the form of sebum

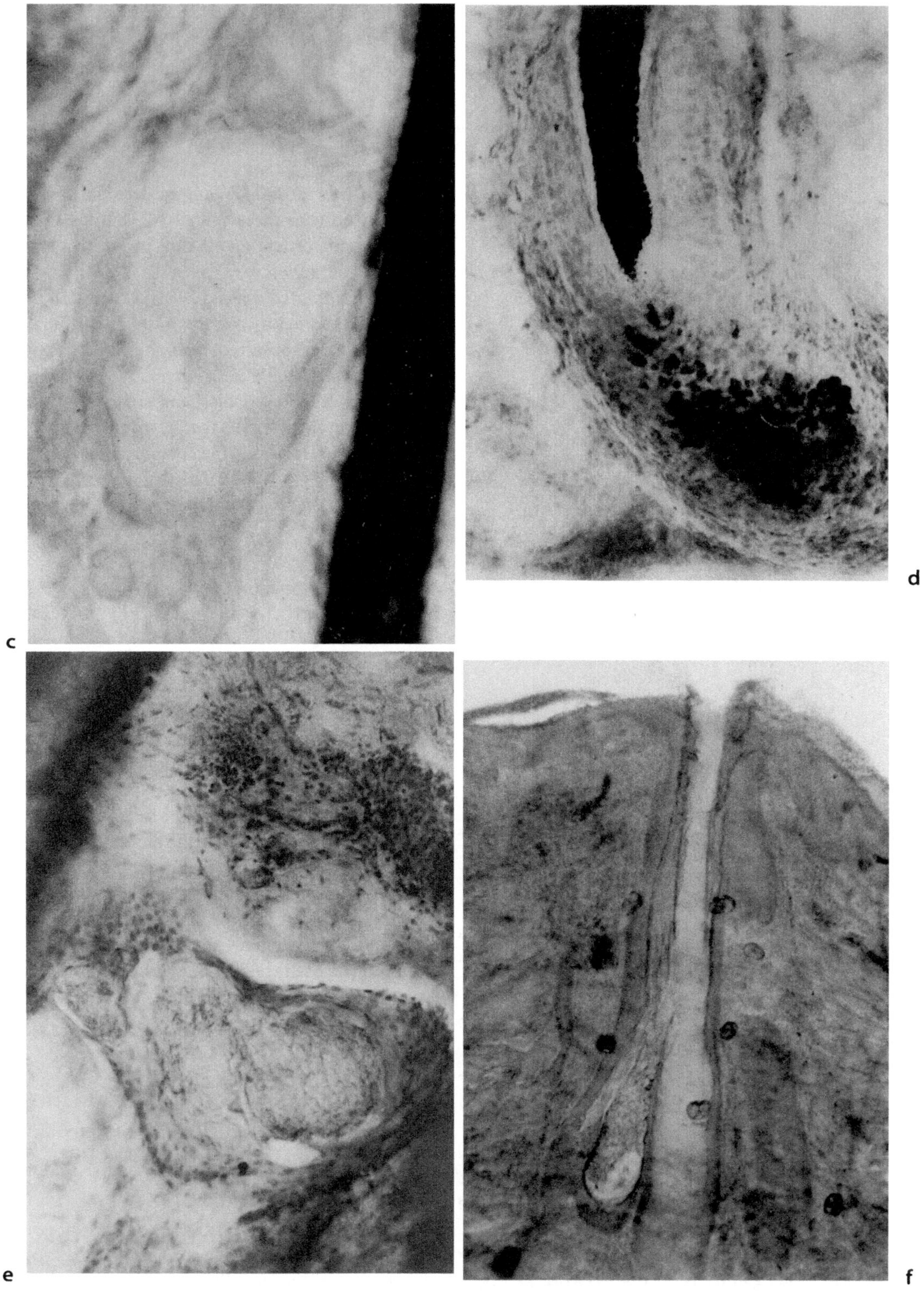

Fig. 29.30. *Continued*

g 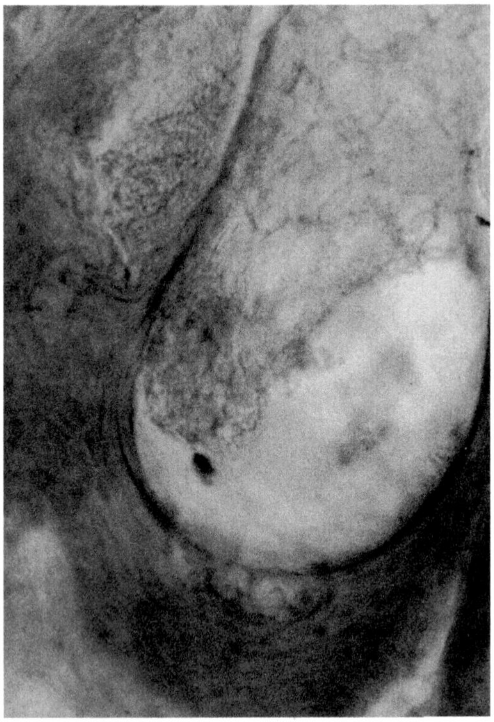

Fig. 29.30. *Continued*

peripheral region, and hairs in the center are permanently lost. The histological study of this phenomenon is summarized as follows:

(a) Thin Split-Thickness Tissue Specimen Observation (Fig. 29.30a). The skin graft with a width exceeding 1 cm takes well. The epithelial cells (germinal layer) in the sebaceous gland have atrophied and become flattened, while the acinous cells in the central area have dissolved and been excreted in the form of sebum.

(b) Thick Split-Thickness Tissue Specimen Observation (Fig. 29.30b). All the hair follicles are in retrograde metamorphosis. The lower hair follicle of the transplanted specimen is in the catagen stage, the hair matrix enveloping the dermal papilla has atrophied and become an epithelial cord, and a club hair is observed. The melanin granules in the lower hair follicle have disappeared. The sebaceous gland attached to it is shown in Fig. 29.30c; the glandular epithelial cells surrounding the sebaceous gland have atrophied and the nuclei of acinous cells have disappeared.

In the lower hair follicle (Fig. 29.30d), the hair bulb has atrophied and the melanin granule residue is scattered.

Figure 29.30e shows a high-power view of the sebaceous gland attached to hair follicle *b*. The acinous cells have been destroyed, the peripheral epithelial cell layer surrounding the sebaceous gland has disappeared, and the acinous cells in the sebaceous gland have been excreted in the form of sebum.

29.12.1.3 Punch Graft with a Width of Less Than 5 mm (Fig. 29.31)

Grafts with widths of 5 mm or less have been transplanted with success. Figure 29.31 a–c shows a punch graft of less than 5 mm in width on the 10th postoperative day.

The transplanted matrix cells (germinal layer) remain in satisfactory condition, no loss of melanin granules is observed, and the follicle is in anagen stage (Fig. 29.31a). The sebaceous gland attached to it has atrophied and shrunk, but the peripheral epithelial cell layer surrounding it has been well preserved, and the acinous cells can also be observed (Fig. 29.31b). The degree of destruction is less than that occurring with wider grafts (Fig. 29.31c).

29.12.1.4 Hair-Bearing Pedicle Flap Transplantation

In the hair-bearing pedicle flap (Juri flap, rotation flap, etc.), hair loss is less than in the free hair-bearing pedicle flap, and unlike the findings in the free hair-bearing pedicle flap, hairs regenerate well, because the blood circulation is maintained by preserving the pedicle of the flap. This can be attributed to the functions of the sebaceous gland being well preserved because the blood circulation is resumed in a satisfactory manner.

Temporary hair loss in the peripheral region of the flap occurs because the hairs in this region go through the phase of retrograde metamorphosis as the functions of the sebaceous gland are temporarily interrupted by the temporary impediment of the peripheral blood circulation.

29.12.1.5 Histological Findings After Hair-Bearing Skin Transplantation: Transplantation of Hairy Occipital Skin to Frontal Scalp in Macaques (Uno and Montagna 1982)

Uno and Montagna (1982) carried out autologous skin transplantation from the occipital to the frontal scalp in macaques. Full-thickness punch-biopsy specimens (9–6 mm) were taken from the occipital hairy scalp. In gross observations, the grafts were completely fused with the surrounding host skin after 2 months and new hair began to emerge on the surface of the grafts after 4 months. As the animals matured the frontal scalp became bald, but the long, thick hairs in the grafts continued to grow.

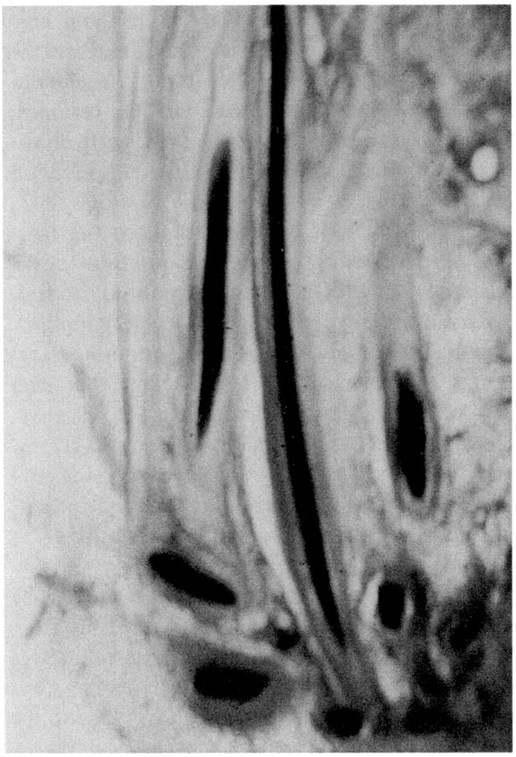

a

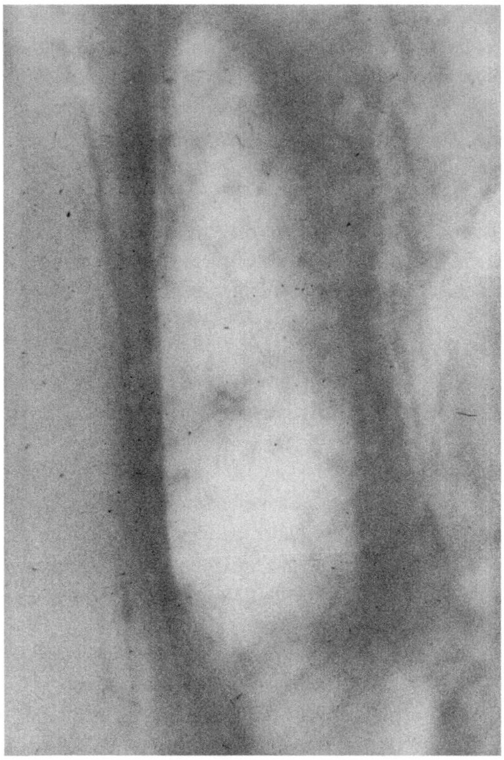

b

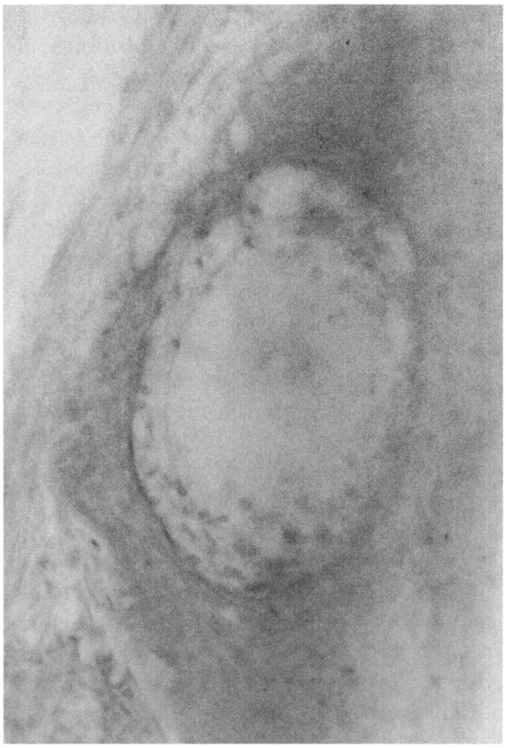

c

Fig. 29.31. a High-power view of punch graft with a width of less than 5 mm. Most of the hair follicles are in the anagen stage and no loss of melanin granules is observed. **b** Sebaceous gland attached to the hair follicle seen in the upper portion of **a**. The acinous cells inside the gland remain intact. **c** The sebaceous gland has now atrophied. The peripheral epithelial cells remain and the central portion has been excreted in the form of sebum

Histological observations 1 week after transplantation showed the graft skin fused with the surrounding host skin. The hair follicles, sebaceous glands, sweat glands, and piloarrector muscles of the graft skin displayed varying degrees of degeneration. Two weeks after transplantation, the dermal collagenous bundles and all the cutaneous appendages seemed to have disappeared. There were no traces of graft hair follicles or sebaceous glands. Four weeks after transplantation, a few hair follicles in early anagen seemed to be developing from the epidermis of the graft skin. Two months after transplantation, the epidermis and dermis of the graft skin were similar to those of the neighboring host skin. With the hair follicles were fully developed sebaceous glands and piloerector muscles. Graft and host tissues were indistinguishable, except that the graft had large terminal hair follicles.

However, Uno and Montagna cannot explain the mechanism responsible for the regeneration of hair follicles from transplanted skin.

29.12.2 General Concepts Underlying Hair-Bearing Skin Transplantation

The success rate of skin transplantation has become higher as grafts have become thinner, with transplantation of a full-thickness skin graft containing the subcutaneous fat layer generally being considered more difficult than the transplantation of thin split-thickness skin grafts.

It was believed that this was the case since, with the full-thickness skin graft, there is no appropriate connection between the transplanted graft and the mesenchymal tissue, and lymph or blood circulation is not sufficient for the graft. Coarse hair-bearing skin grafting was generally performed in the reconstruction of eyebrows and balding scalp; however, since the transplantation of grafts exceeding 4 mm in width was impossible, the arterial island flap method was adopted in the reconstruction of the eyebrow area (Ohmori 1981).

To date, no specific attention has been paid to the connective tissue sheath surrounding the pilosebaceous apparatus in hair-bearing skin transplantation. In this method, transplantation of wide grafts including coarse hairs results in impeding the communication between the epithelial cells in the hair follicles and the mesenchymal cells in the recipient site, due to the presence of the subcutaneous fat layer. The blood is thought to be supplied mainly through capillary networks from the surrounding recipient tissue and from the graft bed through the remaining fat layer. As a result, the peripheral epithelial cell layer surrounding the sebaceous glands and their secretory duct openings (sebaceous isthmal portion) is impeded, and the acinous cells inside the sebaceous gland are excreted in the form of sebum along with the hair canal, causing destruction of the germinal layer surrounding the sebaceous gland and then permanent hair loss (Inaba 1985) (Fig. 29.30c,g).

In the transplantation of narrower grafts, in contrast, the blood circulation of the adjacent region and the graft is resumed soon after the transplantation, and sufficient blood is supplied to the mesenchymal cells around the pilosebaceous apparatus, despite the insufficient blood supply to the dermal papilla. Thus, there is less and only partial destruction of the sebaceous gland and the sebaceous isthmal portion, enabling the hairs to regenerate when blood circulation has resumed. The transplanted hair-bearing skin graft shows temporary hair loss; later, hair regeneration occurs.

Hashimoto (1961) reported that, in the hair-bearing pedicle flap method, the functions of the sebaceous gland were resumed in about 10 days, while in the free hair-bearing pedicle flap method, it took about 3 months for these functions to return to the normal state. He also stated that, with the punch grafting, although the graft fits, it requires about 10–12 weeks for the hairs to regrow after temporary hair loss. His reference to the relation between hair regeneration and the functions of the sebaceous gland supports our findings.

We have developed our sebaceous gland hypothesis (essential hair cycle, Inaba and Inaba 1992a) that hair generation starts not only from the lower portion of the telogen hair follicle, as conventionally believed (common hair cycle), but also from the upper isthmal portion close to the secretory duct opening of the sebaceous gland, especially from the sebaceous isthmus. Our hypothesis has already gained substantial support both domestically and internationally (Inaba 1985; Inaba and Inaba 1989, 1990b, 1992a).

Inaba et al. (1987) also confirmed that, contrary to the belief that nutrition is supplied to the blood plexus of the pilosebaceous unit by the transverse branches of vessels in the dermal layer or by the candelabra vessels in the subcutaneous fat layer, there is a microcirculation between the papillary blood plexus beneath the epidermis and the pilosebaceous unit, with the enzymes and hormones from the sebaceous gland continuously controlling the dermal papilla and the hair matrix.

The above findings indicate that, as the width of the graft becomes narrower, speedy resumption of blood circulation between the graft tissue and the recipient tissue can be expected, and the hair regrows despite temporary hair loss.

As grafts become wider, it is less likely that blood circulation will start from the recipient site. Also, in wide grafts, because the resumption of blood circulation starting from the peripheral recipient site is delayed and the functions of the sebaceous gland are thus prevented, temporary hair loss occurs. Hairs start to regenerate as soon as blood circulation is resumed and the function of the sebaceous gland is improved.

In coarse hair-bearing graft transplantation covering a wide area, prevention of blood circulation and destruction of the sebaceous gland result in the destruction of the essential part of the hair, causing permanent hair loss.

It has been confirmed that the free single hair-bearing graft collected by the 1-mm punch method fits well and is superb from the esthetic standpoint. Furthermore, the hair starts to regrow immediately after transplantation. This finding indicates that the regrowth of the transplanted hair is influenced by whether or not the skin tissue attached to the hair-bearing graft specimen remains intact (see Section 29.5.1, Figs. 29.3b, 29.18a). In this single hair-bearing graft transplantation, no regeneration of hair immediately after transplantation can be expected unless the pilosebaceous unit containing the dermal tissue is transplanted in the recipient site, i.e., transplantation of only the lower hair follicle containing the hair matrix cells does not yield any hair (Section 29.5.2.3, Fig. 29.18b). However, Kim (1993) reported that the hair regrowth of the remaining stem cells in the hair bulb can occur from the hair matrix cells 8 months later. Because the dermal tissue of the free single hair-bearing graft fits with the peripheral recipient tissue, microcirculation is started between the subpapillary blood plexus below the epidermis and the pilosebaceous unit, and hair regeneration is enhanced without the hair matrix cell being atrophied. In turn, this dermal tissue contained in the coarse hair-bearing graft acts as a pump in the circulation. On the other hand, if the pilosebaceous unit is transplanted without epidermis, temporary hair loss may occur because blood circulation to the pilosebaceous unit may be diminished, causing atrophy of the sebaceous gland and the hair matrix.

The conclusion reached from such studies is that the differences experienced in hair regeneration between wide and narrow flaps depend on differences in blood circulation in these flaps. That is, given sufficient blood circulation throughout the flap, hair regeneration depends essentially on the survival of the sebaceous gland and duct (sebaceous isthmus).

29.13 Marechal Operation (Bilateral Ligation Method)

In 1977, Marechal proposed bilateral ligation of the superficial temporal and posterior auricular arteries for the treatment of male pattern baldness. The purpose of this operation was to decrease the normal blood flow and cause hypoxia, which would inactivate testosterone-dihydrotestosterone metabolism. A 3-cm vertical cutaneous incision is made in the temporal area above the zygomatic arch under local anesthesia. The temporoparietal and frontal branches are bound separately after locating them on the skin by palpation of the pulse and by the previous injection of a drop of blue dye through the skin. Although Marechal claimed that more than half of these patients were cured, his results were not reproducible by other surgeons, and this method was abandoned.

Artificial Hair Implantation

30

30.1 Artificial Hair Implantation

Various materials have been used unsuccessfully as implants for the treatment of male pattern baldness. Synthetic fibers have been the most commonly employed material and have caused serious complications in many patients. The complications have been reported in the medical literature, and include foreign-body granulomas, infection, pruritus, facial swelling, scarring, and permanent loss of natural scalp hair (Hanke 1979; Gonzalez and McBride 1979; Kuhn 1980).

The use of synthetic and wire implants to attach wigs to the scalp began more than a decade ago (Dick and Kurtin 1972).There is a 50%–70% risk of infection and rejection. Many studies on fiber implants have indicated that most fibers fell out spontaneously within 12 weeks or less after the procedure. The retained-implanted hair tends to fracture at the surface, leaving a coarse stubble (Hanke 1979).

Table 30.1. Various devices used for artifical hair implantation

Company	A	B	C	D	E	F	G[a]	H[a]	I[a]	J[a]	K	L
Fiber	PET	PET	Nylon	Processed human hair	Nylon	Nylon	Modacryl	Modacryl	PET	Modacryl	Modacryl	PET
Coloring	Pigment	Dye	Dye	Dye	Pigment	Dye	Dye	Dye	Dye	Dye	Dye	Dye
Shape and size of needle tip	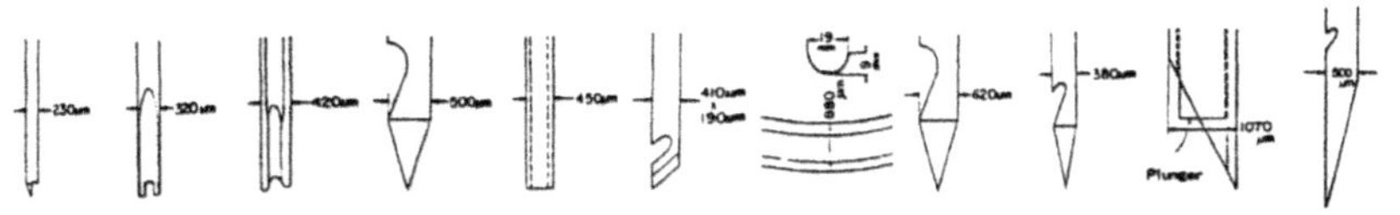											NA
Shape and size of artifical hair root	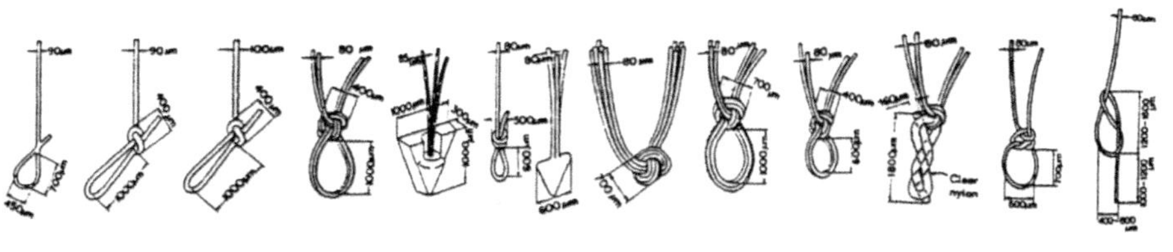											
Cross section of hair	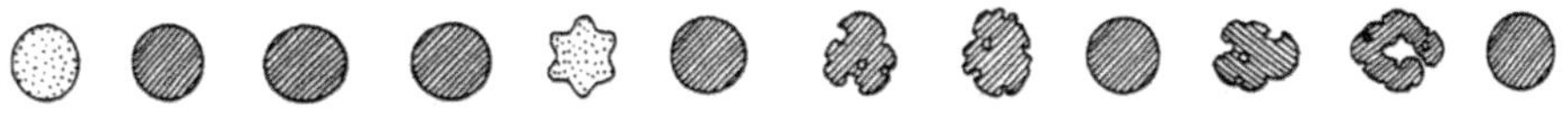											
Area of tissue destroyed (mm^2)	Approx. 0.05	0.20	0.30	0.40	0.40	0.20	0.70	0.70	0.30	0.90	0.33	NA

[a] American companies; other companies are Japanese.
PET, Polyethylene terephthalate; *NA*, not available.
(Reproduced with permission from Kobayashi 1984).

Fig. 30.1. One of the authors, with implanted artificial hairs (*AH*) in the receding frontal area (*arrows*). Hairs manufactured by Medical Hair Doctor Co. (Tokyo, Japan). Type E according to Kobayashi's classification (Table 30.1)

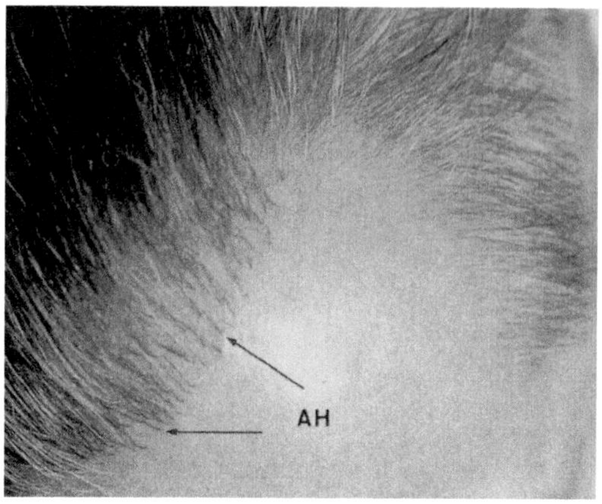

The implantation of artificial hairs was criticized several years ago because of complications such as post-implantation infection and rejection (Gonzalez and McBride 1979; Hanke 1979, 1981; De Gregorio and Rauscher 1981; Lepaw 1979, 1980b, 1982, 1983).

The FDA held public hearings three times in 1979 and listed prosthetic hair fibers as banned devices in the Code of Federal Regulations in 1982.

Following are the reasons why the ban on the manufacture of artificial hairs was announced:

1. The artificial hairs inserted may be regarded as an open foreign substance and infection from the outside world will persist.
2. Rejection reactions will occur against the inserted artificial hairs.
3. The Dacron dispersive dyes, red 73 and blue 79, revealed strong mutagenic response.
4. Artificial hairs will not survive for a long time.
5. Scar formation or other sequelae will occur.
6. Extraction of the remaining portion of the artificial hair is difficult.

Since 1976, experimental and clinical studies on synthetic hair have been reported in Japan (Fukuta et al. 1976; Taniguchi 1977, 1980, 1982, 1983, 1984; Kobayashi et al. 1979, 1981a). Kobayashi et al. (1981a) have carried out animal experiments, clinical and histological studies, and chemical and biological tests on a variety of synthetic hairs used in Japan and the United States. Table 30.1 shows Kobayashi's summary of the characteristics of these synthetic hairs .

30.2 Our Experience of Artificial Hair Implantation

One of the authors acted as a test subject for the research and development of artificial hair implantation, receiving a fiber implant produced at Medical Hair Doctor (Tokyo, Japan). In this implant of the E type artificial hair, as classified by Kobayashi et al. (1981a) (Table 30.1), three nylon fibers (85 μm) are fused electronically at the triangular portion of fixation. The first transplant of artificial hair to a bald site proved to be a pleasant surprise, since the hair stayed in place without

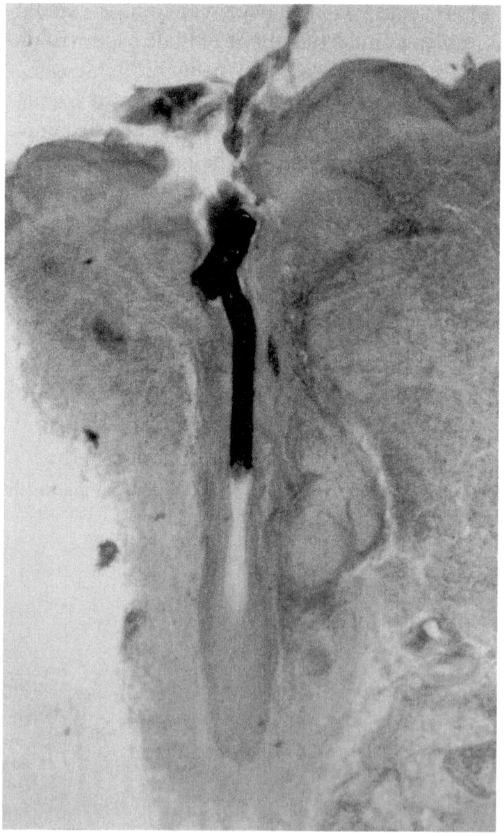

a

Fig. 30.2a Histological findings 6 months after implantation of MHD Co. artificial hair. Inverted depression is clearly visible. **b** High-power view of **a**. (*i*) Upper portion. Keratic substance adheres to the implant site. The epidermis of the artificial hair exposed externally is depressed. (*ii*) Middle portion. The artificial hair is enclosed by connective tissue and only slight inflamation is evident. (*iii*) Lower portion. Connective tissue is formed at the hair root portion and the peripheral area. The artificial hair seems to have fixed well

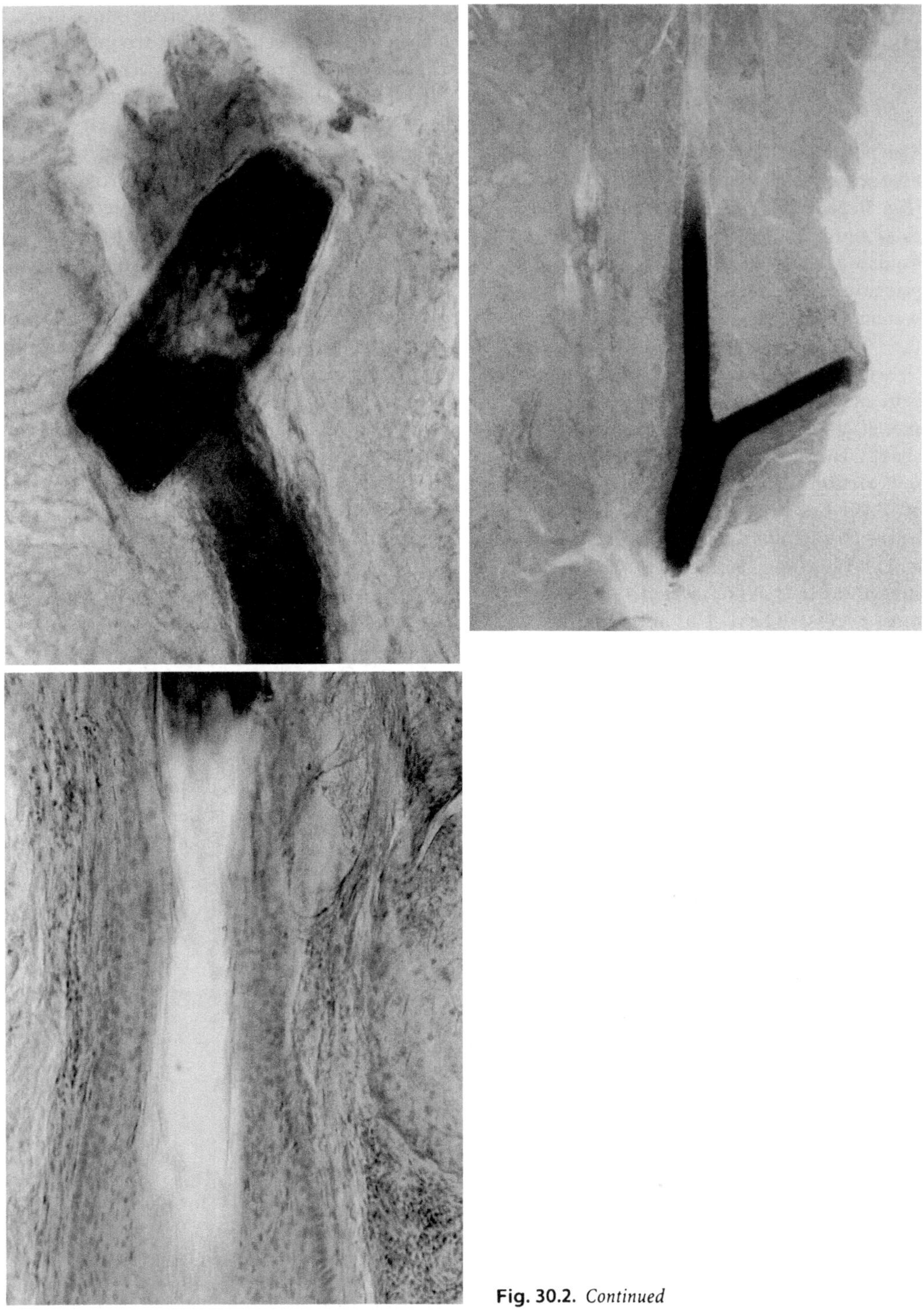

bi

bii

biii

Fig. 30.2. *Continued*

much pain. It was expected that rejection would occur and that the scalp would suffer from a serious inflammation or suppurative condition. However, inflammation was slight and soreness faded away within a few days (Fig. 30.1).

Six months after implantation, samples of skin tissue, taken by the punch method, were examined histologically (Fig. 30.2). Inverted depression was clearly seen. The artificial hairs were enclosed by connective tissue and only very slight inflammation was evident. Normal numbers of leukocytes and a small number of foreign body cells were observed, as is natural in the vicinity of a foreign body. Almost all inserted artificial hairs fell out within a period of 6 months to 1 year. The authors then began to question why these artificial hairs remained in place for such a long time despite the rejective mechanism.

30.3 Artificial Hair Newly Developed by Nido Ltd.

The polyester fibers and implantation needles used were all developed by Nido, Tokyo, Japan (Fig. 30.3a). This implantation method is efficacious and has almost no side effects. The average fixation rates were 88.7% at 6 months after implantation, 78% at 12 months, and 74.6% at 18 months (Taniguchi 1984). The authors have used these fibers only to conceal the scar remaining after refining of the hair-bearing flap. The synthetic hair, made from polyethylene terephthalate, is shown in Fig. 30.3b. The diameter of the fiber is about 90 μm and the cross section is round; the root portion is an α-shaped loop, the intersection of which has been electronically fused; and the tensile strength of the adhered joint is controlled at 110–120 g (the improved form has a tensile strength of 160 g.) If removal of a fiber should become necessary because of infection, this can be accomplished by a pulling force greater than 120 g, which will separate the joint section and allow removal of the entire fiber as a single filament. The tensile strength of the filament is 260–270 g.

This improved hair fiber has an amorphous silver coating of 40 Å thickness on the root area; and this coating has an antibacterial effect against infection due to invasion of exogenous bacteria. This fiber has great durability, surviving more than 1.2 million repeated bendings by a testing machine. The rate of hair breakage is thus very low.

However, when the tensile strength of the adhered joint is controlled at 120 g, hair loss will often be observed during implantation, shampooing, combing, or sleeping. As an improvement, an additional half twist has been applied to the α-shaped joint of this artificial hair to raise the tensile strength to 160 g; this resulted in an increased fixation rate.

Coloring of the polyester fiber with inorganic pigments (carbon, ferric oxide, ferrous oxide, and titanic oxide) is introduced inside the filament before melt-spinning; there is no surface coloring, so there is no danger of the chemical dyestuffs diffusing into the body (reviewed from Taniguchi 1984). The implantation needle is 230 μm and its cross-sectional area is 0.04 mm^2. It is the smallest of all the implantation needles and causes very little damage to the tissues at implantation. A device with an inner spring (Fig. 30.3a) is built into the implantation needle to automatically adjust implantation depth so that the root portion of the polyester fiber will be fixed and buried on the galeal aponeuroses without piercing it.

The device has been fashioned in such a way that the tip of the implantation needle taking the hair will not penetrate deeper than the galeal aponeuroses, which acts as the last barrier against infection.

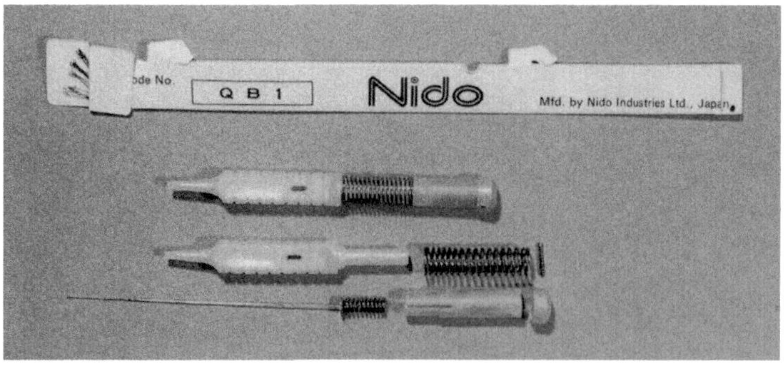

a

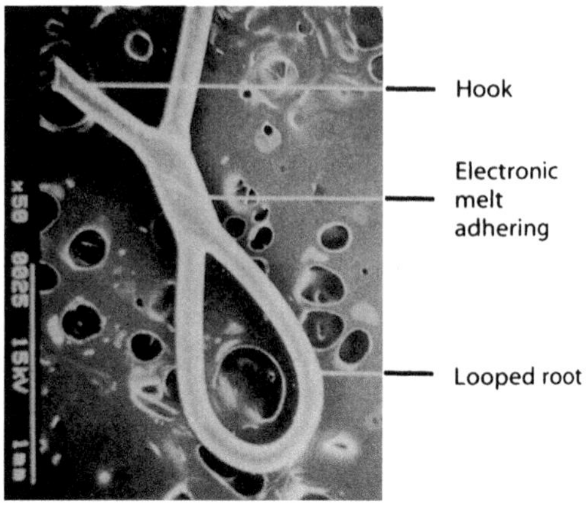

b

Fig. 30.3. **a** Polyester fibers (*above*) and implantation devices. **b** Lower portion of the polyester fiber. The root portion is an α-shaped loop. The tensile strength of the adhered joint is controlled at around 160 g. **c** One day after implantation, fibroblasts are seen in the area surrounding the fiber. Mild bleeding, neutrophil and lymphocyte infiltration can be seen. **d** One week after implantation, multinucleated giant cells are observed around fiber. **e** One month after implantation, fibroblasts and collagen fibers proliferate around the fiber. **f** Two months after implantation, small arteries have penetrated the fiber. **g** Twenty months after implantation, at shallow layer of the dermis. This figure shows less cell infiltration. **h** Twenty months after the implantation, at α-shaped loop. (Fig. 30.3a–h, courtesy of Nido Industries Ltd, Tokyo, Japan)

Fig. 30.3. *Continued*

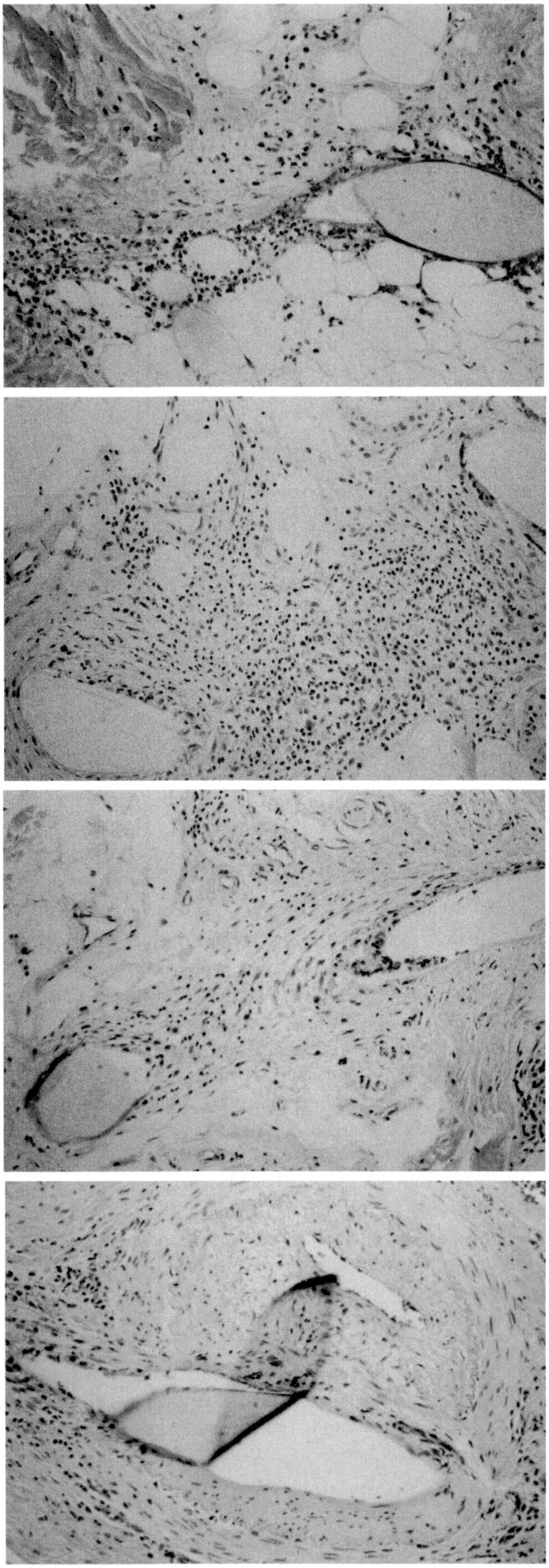

c

d

e

f

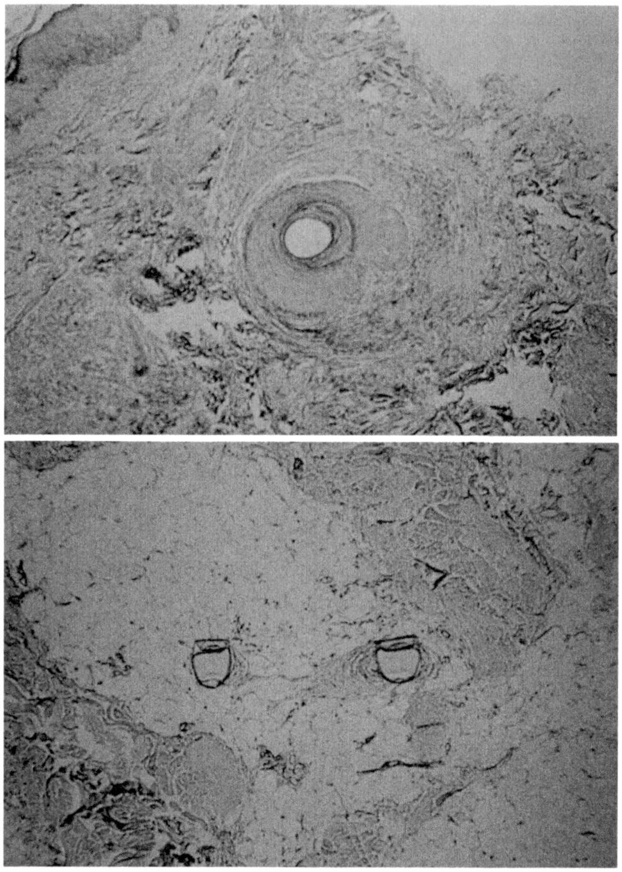

g

h

Fig. 30.3. *Continued*

30.4 Percutaneous Implantation

The loop portion is inserted into the area of the subcutaneous tissue in which fibrous tissue exists. If the root is inserted just above the galeal aponeuroses, fibrous connective tissue will be formed inside the α-shaped loop and around the fiber, anchoring it to the galeal aponeuroses. With the supplied implantation needle, the root portion will be placed immediately above the galeal aponeuroses.

It is impossible to avoid some histological damage to the tissue. Accordingly, if the polyester fibers are implanted too closely together, redness and swelling in the area will occur, so on the first day, polyester fibers should be spaced at least 4 mm apart. A final spacing of 1.5 mm can be achieved.

Following implantation, a cream (with or without antibiotics) is usually applied to the implantation site. The application of the cream makes the hair easier to comb.

30.5 Histological Findings

Taniguchi (1984) performed scalp biopsies of two bald patients 1 day; 1 and 2 weeks; and 1, 2, 5, and 20 months after implantation, and studied the histological changes. One day after implantation, there was mild bleeding and neutrophil and lymphocyte infiltration (Fig. 30.3c). One and 2 weeks after implantation, a major difference was observed. Fibroblasts in the loop formation of the fiber and histocytes in the area adjacent to the fiber were increased and there was an infiltration of a small number of neutrophils and lymphocytes. Multinucleated giant cells were observed around the fiber (Fig. 30.3d). One month after implantation, no significant histological changes were seen in comparison with the situation at 2 weeks (Fig. 30.3e). Two months after implantation, small arteries, of about 100 μm, had penetrated the fiber and a limited fibroblast and histocytes infiltration was recognized along the fiber. None of the changes were remarkable (Fig. 30.3f).

Fig. 30.5. **a** Alopecia cicatrisata after face-lift operation 2 years previously. **b** The scar area is camouflaged with artificial hairs

Twenty months after implantation, the epidermis had surrounded the fiber and entered the dermis. There was less cell infiltration at 20 months than at 5 months, although the cell infiltration was negligible in both specimens. There was little connective tissue inside and around the loop root in the 20-month specimen (Fig. 30.3g,h).

30.6 Case Reports

30.6.1 Case 1

A temporal-parietal flap operation was performed for the reduction of receding frontoparietal alopecia; unfortunately, necrosis occurred postoperatively (Fig. 30.4a). We first attempted to correct the region by the excision-suture (reduc-

a 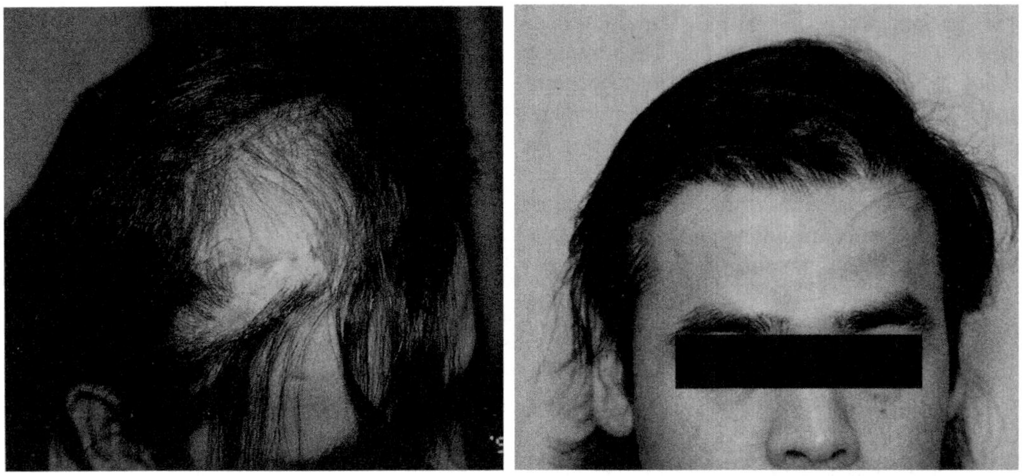 b

Fig. 30.4. a Temporal-parietal flap necrosis. Until scar formation occurred, the lower margin of the scar area was temporarily camouflaged with artificial hairs. **b** After implantation, the scar area is camouflaged; scar cannot be seen

a 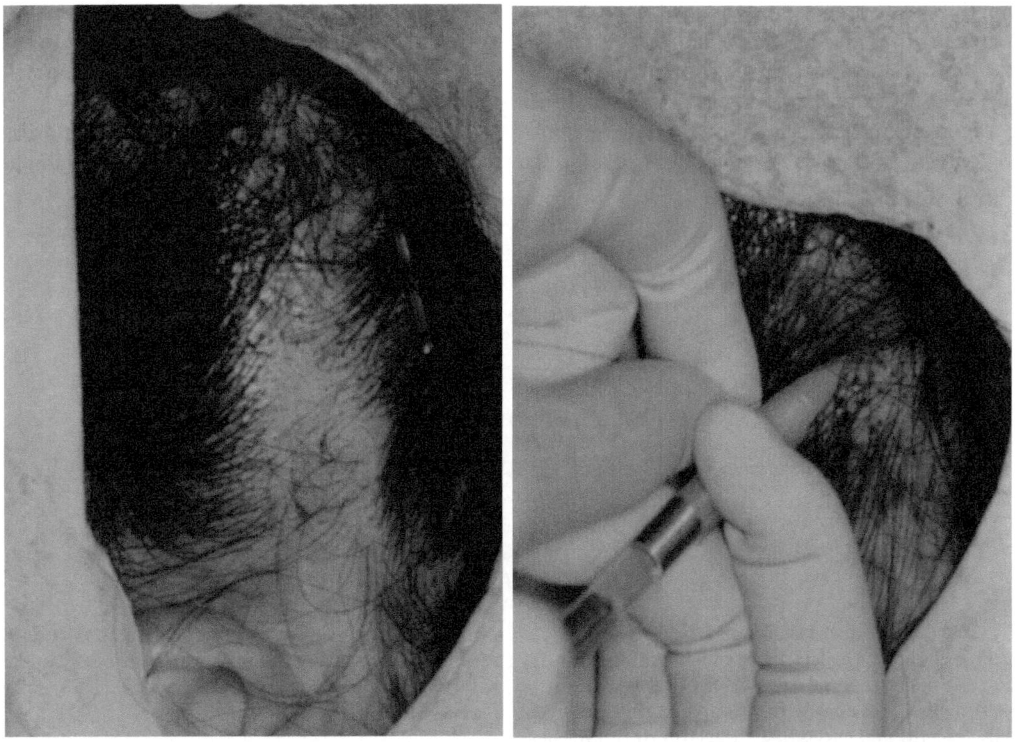 b tion) method, but were prevented by the presence of edema and inflammation. Then we decided to wait until a scar was formed to perform the reduction operation. To temporarily camouflage the necrosis, we used the Nido artificial hair under the margin of the scar area. After the implantation of these artificial hairs, the scar area was well camouflaged and was not visible (Fig. 30.4b).

30.6.2 Case 2

This patient was a 30-year-old female fashion model. She had undergone a face-lift operation about 2 years previously. Alopecia cicatrisata, about 2 cm in width, appeared in the temporal region, causing permanent hair loss (Fig. 30.5a). She was then suddenly scheduled to appear in a fashion show and wished to have the scar go unnoticed by her hairdresser. The authors decided to camouflage the scar area with Nido's artificial hair rather than performing a reduction operation (Fig. 30.5b). Follow-up results have not been obtained as the patient lives in a remote area.

30.7 Mechanism of Epilation After Implantation of Artificial Hair

Artificial hair is a substance foreign to the human body and its elimination is assumed to be inevitable. However, despite the comparatively rare occurrence of inflammation and the improved fixation, in particular the anchoring by the α-shaped loop with fibrous connective tissue, it was beyond our understanding why the hair remained for only a year or so. We therefore decided to pursue this question.

Progress on artificial hair implantation continues, and artificial hairs can last for as long as an average of 1 year at present if a superior technique is used. In an examination of postoperative specimens, we (Inaba 1985) found that the artificial hair was enclosed tightly by the epidermis and the corium layer, with only slight local inflammation being observed immediately after transplantation (Fig. 30.6*a*). With time, however, a keratic substance began to adhere to the implant site (Fig. 30.6*b*). The epidermal layer reacts to the production and adhesion of this keratic substance by descending along the artificial hair in a fashion that eventually encloses it (Fig. 30.6*c*). Later on, the production and adhesion of the keratic substance proceeds toward the root of the artificial hair, while, at the same time, the keratic substance enclosed by the epidermal layer reaches the lower surface of the dermal layer (Fig. 30.6*d*). This descending recipient epidermal cell activity forms a tube that encloses the keratic substance, separating the artificial hairs from the epidermis and dermal layer. As a result, the force which originally binds the artificial hair to the epidermis and dermal layer has no continuing effect, and eventually these artificial hairs fall out (Fig. 30.6*e*).

Of course, this keratic substance is also produced around natural hairs, but it is always pushed out of the epidermis by the growth of the natural hairs, this occurring at the rate of 0.35 mm/day; thus the substance neither adheres to nor extends along the hair. Since artificial hairs do not grow, the keratic substance extends downward once it begins to adhere. The keratic substance and epidermal cells loosen the binding site of the hair so that it is likely to fall out within around 6 months to 1 year on the average.

There are two requirements that will allow the success of long-term artificial hair implantation in the future. We need the development of:

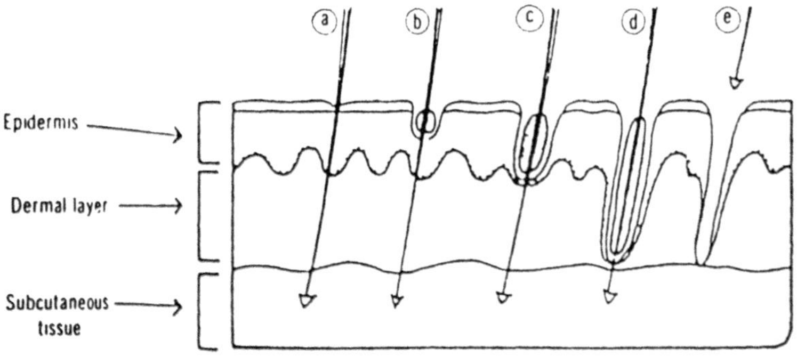

Fig. 30.6. Mechanism of epilation after implantation of artificial hair. The epilation is due to a local keratinizing process in the artificial hair implant (*a*). With time, a. keratic substance adheres to the implant (*b*). Epidermal cells descend and enclose the artificial hair in an isolating tube (*c*); this eventually causes the hair to fall out (*e*) when the process reaches the hair tip in the subcutaneous tissue (*d*). See text for explanation of *a*, *b*, *c*, *d*, and *e*. (Inaba 1985)

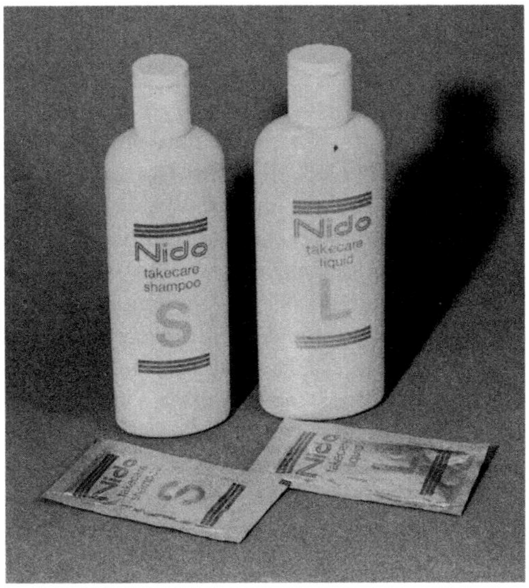

Fig. 30.7. Nido has developed this liquid and shampoo combination for preventing Keration adhesion (courtesy of Nido)

1. New artificial hairs that frustrate local keratin adhesion.
2. A cleansing agent that can prevent or remove that adhesion.

Nido Industries has developed a hair care liquid and shampoo for preventing keratin adhesion (Fig. 30.7).

30.8 Advantages of Artificial Hair Implantation

The artificial hairs developed by Nido reveal no side effects and seem to be close to perfection. However, they are, in any case, foreign to the human body and the mechanism of elimination is unavoidable. Because this artificial hair is exposed to the outside world, permanent fixation cannot be hoped for, although it is true that much improvement has been made to date. As stated above, Taniguchi found that the average fixation rates for the Nido artificial hair were 88.7% at 6 months after implantation, 78.7% at 12 months, and 74.6% at 18 months. The authors have confirmed that this product has a much higher fixation rate than other products. In this respect, Bouhanna (1989) experimentally implanted the Nido artificial hair for a period of 6 months and reported that hair loss was observed in about one-third of the 16 subjects after 180 days, while the hairs remained in the remaining two-thirds of the subjects.

The implantation of artificial hair is an ideal method for camouflaging the scar that remains after the performance of the flap methods. Since the artificial hair does not have permanent fixation, it will naturally fall out in time with the healing of the suture scar. If the scar is conspicuous after this method is used, single hair transplantation is more suitable.

However, with such surgical methods, there may be inconvenience, in that the patients cannot return to their normal social life immediately after operation. With artificial hair implantation, in contrast, there is no such inconvenience, since the patient can obtain a natural appearance immediately after operation by this very simple procedure. Artificial hair implantation also makes hair restoration possible for a patient who has insufficient hair-growing donor tissue.

a
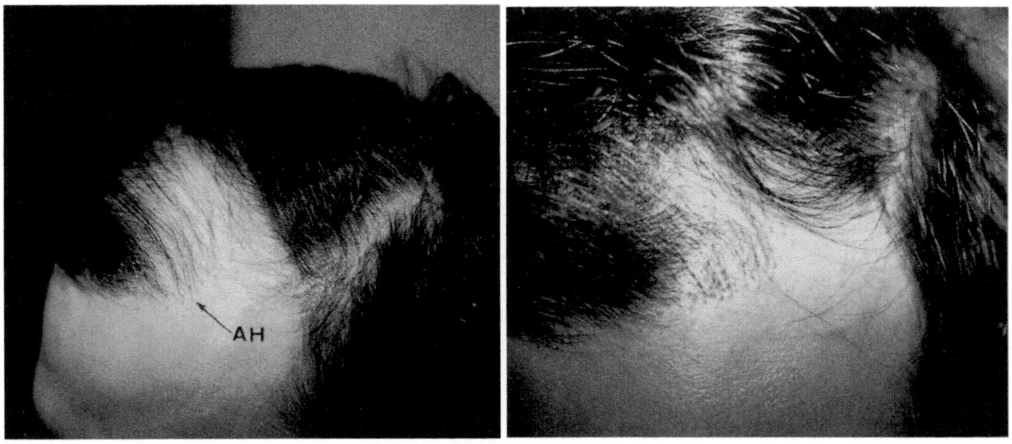

b

Fig. 30.8. **a** After artificial hair (*AH*) implantation. **b** Two months after procedure. Formation of ingrowing epidermis due to insufficient shampooing sometimes results in comedo-like appearance

30.9 Drawbacks of Artificial Hair

There are two drawbacks in the use of artificial hair:

1. The cost of implantation is extremely high. Additional implantation will be required, since permanent fixation cannot be expected. To take one example, implantation of 2000 hairs at the price of 250 yen per hair will cost 500 000 yen. In some cases of male pattern baldness, 5000–7000 hairs will be required and the patient's financial burden will be unbearably great in terms of the long-range maintenance of the treated area, including additional implantation.
2. If shampooing is insufficient after the insertion of the artificial hair, formation of ingrowing epidermis will result in a comedo-like appearance, as in acne vulgaris (Fig. 30.8b). Bouhanna (1989) observed seborrheic agglutination in the hair in 40% of his subjects, but observed no case of foreign granuloma.

To avoid this problem, the removal of the keratinized substance around the artificial hair will be required, much as removing deposits on the teeth is a requisite of dental care.

30.10 Other Problems Related to Artificial Hair

Various methods of artificial hair implantation have been attempted. However, the invasion of foreign bodies in the human body causes a rejection reaction to protect basic life functions. Therefore, these transplants do not "take" readily. Although the remarkable improvement in artificial fibers has lent confidence to researchers contending with artificial hair implantation, it is still the case that these transplants mostly fall out within 6 months to 2 years.

Artificial hairs can be dyed in two ways. One way is to mix facial paint coloring with the hair substance by fusion and spinning during the production process. The other way is to dye the sutured hairs with dispersion or acidic dyes after production. It is generally believed that the harmful influence which polymer compounds have on an organism is not due to the polymer compounds themselves but to residues from the monomers in the facial paint coloring, plastic agents, stabilizers, and so forth. Taking this into account, dyeing the hair material with facial paint color at the production stage is clearly better than dyeing later on. The artificial hairs used and described here were dyed by the former method. With these hairs, the extent of pain and inflammation was less than we expected. However, when we tested implants with artificial hairs that had been dyed after production, the postoperative skin reaction was strong. In the most serious case, the artificial coloring dissolved and was dispersed into the scalp, causing severe tissue reaction in the skin, with inflammatory symptoms accompanied by intense pain.

Another Solution: Hairpieces (Wigs)

31

31.1 Conventional Wig

The wig is said to have come into fashion well over 300 years ago. A portrait of King Louis the XIIIth painted in 1624 shows his head covered with abundant hair that is surely a wig.

Several autografting techniques are currently being used as treatments for baldness. However, these depend on the person's own hair, and, when the quantity of this is very small, the only alternative for the individual for whom the baldness is a problem is to wear a wig. The use of a wig leads to a sense of satisfaction and the individual may regard it almost as a part of the body.

However, wearing this sort of "stage wig" all the time is bothersome. The modern hairpiece for men is based on the attachment of an artificial scalp to a bald area, this being achieved with a special binding agent. The artificial scalp (wig) is made of polyurethane dotted with holes in which natural or artificial hairs are inserted. This type of hairpiece can be designed to fit over any shape or size of bald area. It takes a long time to produce and the cost would be quite high, but it is extremely natural in appearance (Fig. 31.1a–d).

However, from the medical and physiological standpoints, when a hairpiece (wig) is applied to a site where thin hairs remain, the binding agent (adherent tape) will strip off those remaining hairs whenever the hairpiece is removed. Also, the close adhesion of this artificial scalp to the true scalp can inhibit respiration in the true scalp or can over-

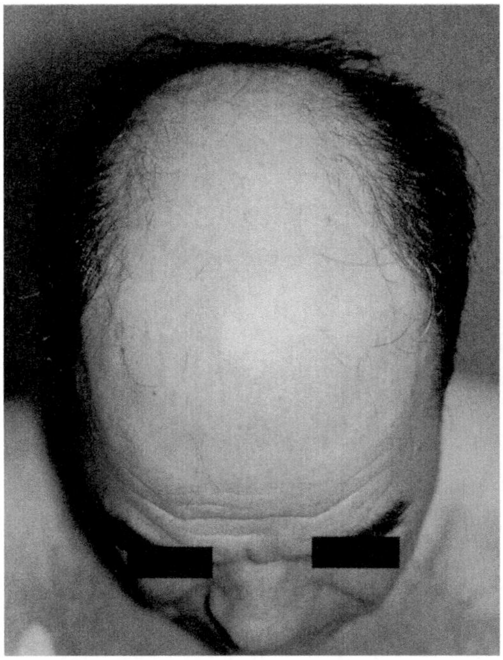

a

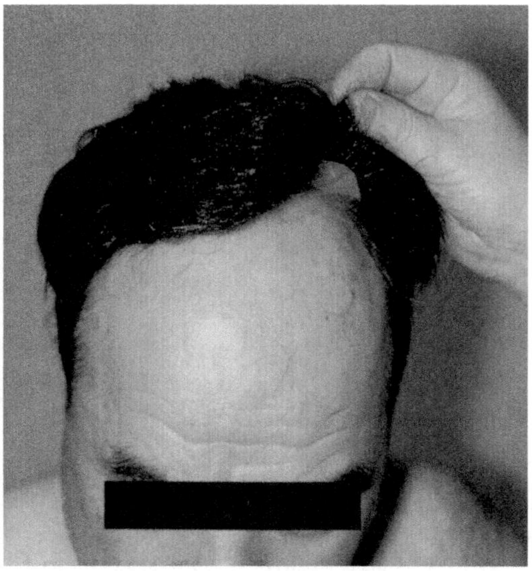

b

Fig. 31.1. **a** Bald area. **b** Fitting the wig. **c** Top view of the wig. **d** Reverse view

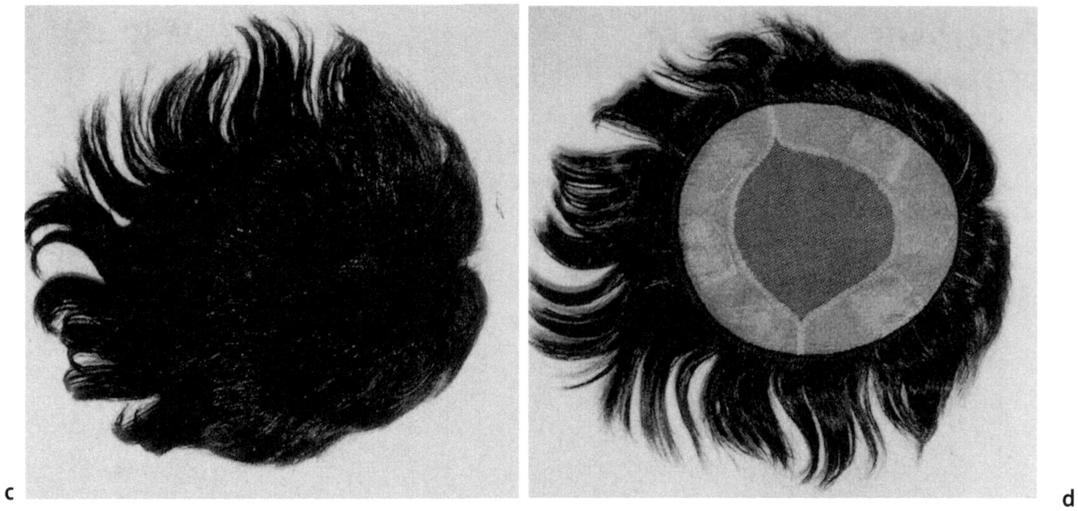

Fig. 31.1. *Continued*

heat the scalp, leading to physiological distress and discomfort.

The makers of these hairpieces conduct impressive, persuasive publicity campaigns on a large scale, and do seem to charm large numbers of customers.

Using clips to attach the hairpiece to residual hair is time-consuming. Fixation of a hairpiece by Teflon-coated sutures to the scalp provides initial security of attachment. Eventually, however, problems of infection and persistent draining sinuses develop at the sites of entry and exit of the Teflon-coated wire. This persistent infection and inflammation results in tissue absorption, and the sutures or anchor points come out. Bendl (1988) developed the tunnel-graft procedure in the parietal region for those who have decided to use a hairpiece; it is the most secure, most convenient, and safest of the available attachments and is free of many of the complications of other methods of attachment.

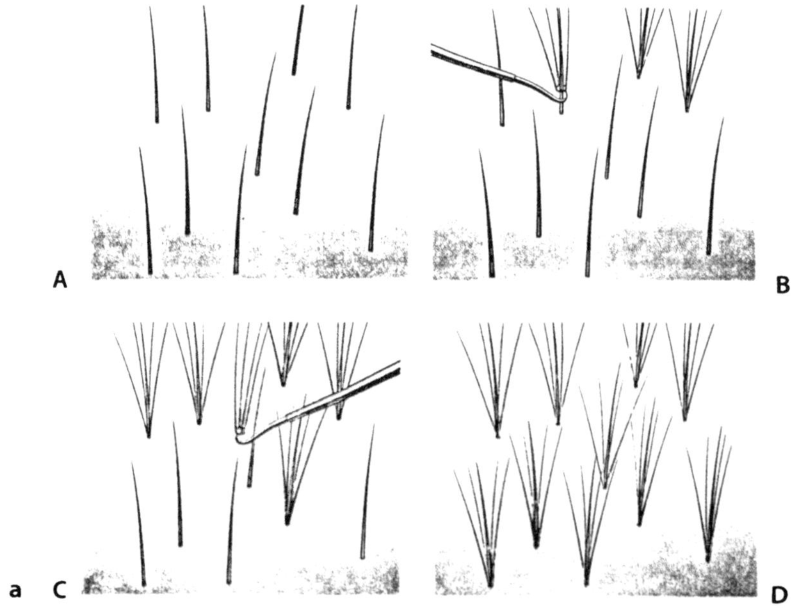

Fig. 31.2. **a** Pin-point hair increase method (Aderance, Tokyo, Japan). Several artificial hairs are directly conjoined with a natural hair. *A*, Analyze and study the bald area; *B*, determine the type and the number of artificial hairs to be used; *C*, conjoin several artificial hairs with each natural hair; *D*, the finished area looks as natural as it used to. **b** Cross-line hair increase method (Aderance, Tokyo, Japan). The natural hairs are combed out from the opening of the artificial hairs, which are planted in a cross-line pattern. *A*, Analyze the area of baldness and implant cyber hairs along the cross lines; *B*, attach cross lines over the scalp; *C*, comb out the natural hairs from the opening, using a hair brush; *D*, brush lightly for a perfect finish

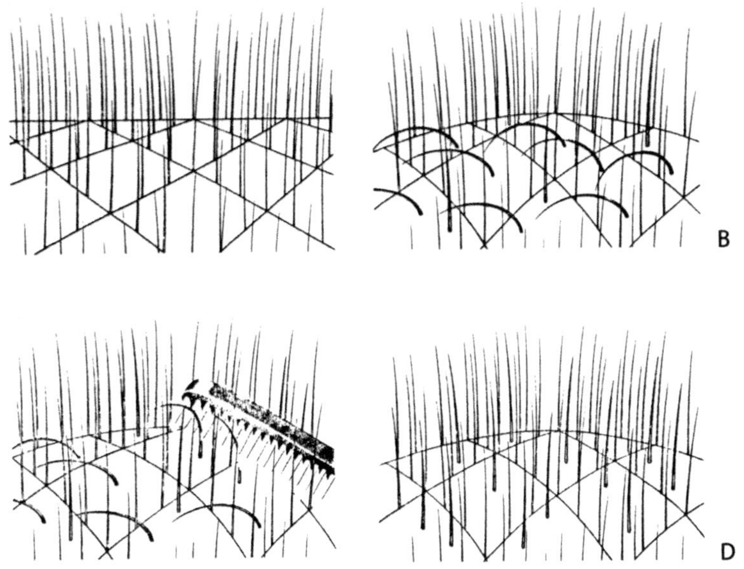

Fig. 31.2. *Continued*

31.2 New Wigs

Aderance (Tokyo, Japan) and Artnature (Tokyo, Japan) have developed new methods of adding artificial hairs to remaining natural hairs when wigs are used (Fig. 31.2).

With these new wigs, in the early stage of baldness, several artificial hairs are conjoined with a remaining hair to add volume (Fig. 31.2a). In a more advanced stage, transparent string lines with artificial hairs conjoined sporadically are used (Fig. 31.2b). In a further advanced stage, for the scalp with scarcely any hairs left, lines formed in a lattice-shape, with two to three artificial hairs conjoined with each line, are used.

The use of a comb specially made according to the shape of the scalp is recommended for fluffing out the remaining hairs to mix them with the artificial hairs to make them appear natural. The wig is then fixed to the scalp by clipping it to the remaining temporal hairs.

The advantages of these new wigs are:

1. Natural appearance. Artificial hairs conjoined with linear or lattice-shaped lines are mixed with the remaining natural hairs to give a natural appearance.
2. Sufficient aeration.
3. No need to remove the wig when participating in swimming and other sports.

Mechanism of Linear Scar Formation After Scalp Surgery: Preventive Measures

32

Various methods have been adopted for suturing incisions in hair-bearing scalp; the general suture method, the zigzag method, the skin flap method, and the tissue expander method.

With the simple suture method most commonly used, linear scar formation is inevitable (Fig. 32.1a). Satisfactory esthetic results with skin sutures have been obtained by using dense intradermic sutures. However, this method has not been employed in hair-bearing areas so as to avoid damage to the hair bulb, and a general suture method has been adopted instead, in which the galea aponeurotica is sutured; this often leaves a linear scar. It is not known why there is a linear scar although the hair bulb portion is left intact to avoid damage. A scar formed parallel to the hair stream appears conspicuous, and the patient obviously wishes to have such scars concealed.

To conceal any such linear scar, the zigzag (W-plasty) suturing method has been used; the pedicle flap method has been used to camouflage such a scar running along the hairstream. In the tissue expander method, a balloon-like silicone bag is inserted beneath the galea aponeurotica surrounding the scar, into which physiological saline is gradually injected. The flap will be expanded in about 3 months and an incision-suture operation will be performed to remove the redundant scalp containing the scar. However, its rather peculiar appearance, protruding in a tumor-like manner, is often a mental burden for the patient. The punch method has also been used, to transplant hairs in the scar region; however, the transplanted hairs failed to survive. Although these various methods have been used for the camouflage of postoperative scars, improvement of these scars is extremely difficult.

With the development of our radical treatment for bromidrosis, we proposed the hypothesis that contravenes the common hair cycle, in which hair regeneration is believed to start from the secondary hair germ located at the lower end of a telogen follicle. In our hypothesis, we have stated that, although hair regeneration does occur according the aforementioned mechanism, the essential hair center is located in the upper isthmal portion close to the secretory duct opening of the sebaceous gland. We named this the essential hair cycle and included an isthmal stage in the conventional concept of the hair cycle, which consists of three stages, anagen, catagen and telogen (see Chapter 13).

Based on our sebaceous gland hypothesis, we investigated methods for suturing the scalp, paying attention to avoiding atrophy of the sebaceous gland; we developed a deep wide (relaxation) suturing technique for tacking the incision, and observed no linear scar formation with the method (Fig. 32.1b). This successful result supports the validity of our hypothesis.

32.1 Case Studies

32.1.1 General Suturing

We were careful not to injure the hair bulb in the vicinity of the hair-bearing skin in a scar improvement operation. As shown in Fig. 32.2a, a cicatricial hair loss, 7 cm × 7 mm in size, was formed parallel to the hairstream. Because the scar was conspicuous, the patient returned to our clinic, wishing to undergo a scar improvement operation.

After excising the scar region, we undermined the loose connective layer above the galea aponeurotica to some extent, and sutured the incision, eliminating excessive tension, by three different methods, namely, a stapler suture (in the upper portion), a simple suture (in the middle portion),

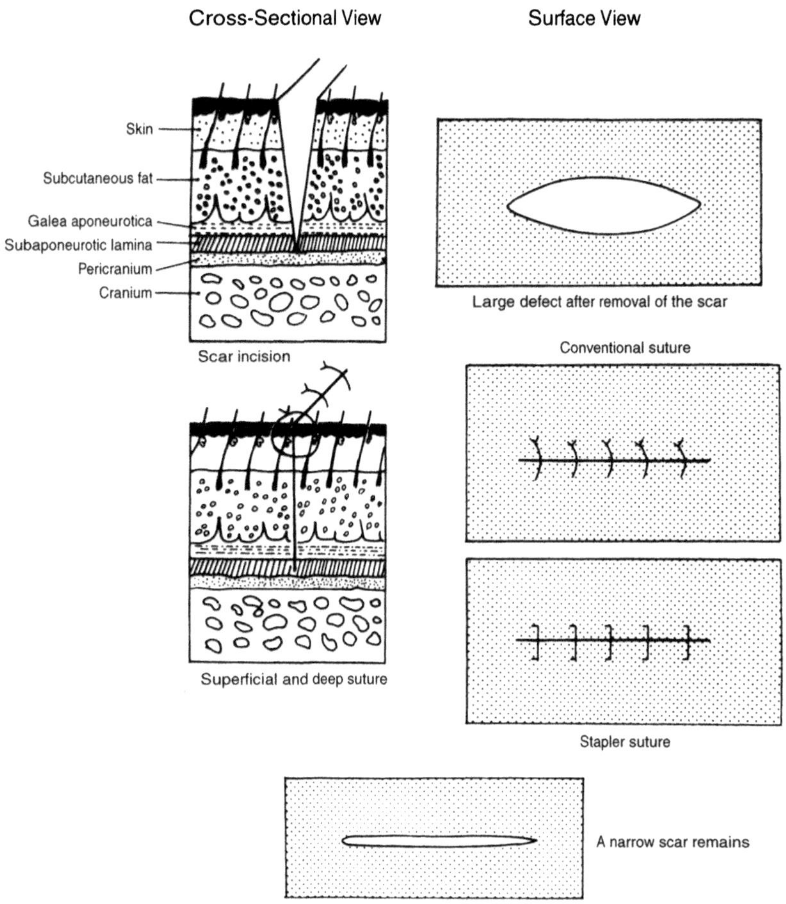

Cross-Sectional View
Surface View
Skin
Subcutaneous fat
Galea aponeurotica
Subaponeurotic lamina
Pericranium
Cranium
Scar incision
Large defect after removal of the scar
Conventional suture
Superficial and deep suture
Stapler suture
A narrow scar remains

a

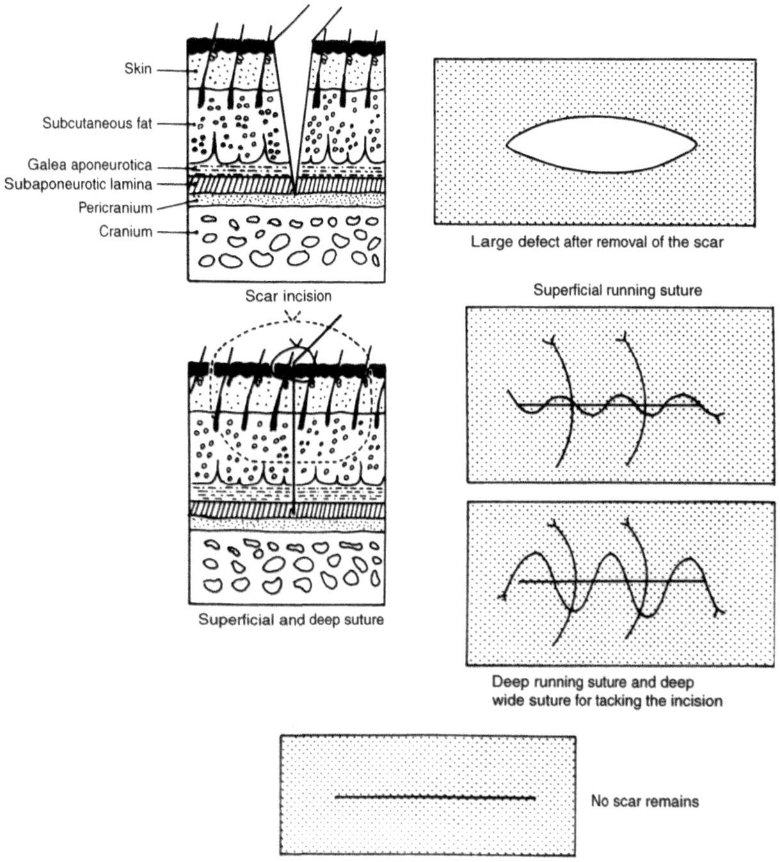

Skin
Subcutaneous fat
Galea aponeurotica
Subaponeurotic lamina
Pericranium
Cranium
Scar incision
Large defect after removal of the scar
Superficial running suture
Superficial and deep suture
Deep running suture and deep
wide suture for tacking the incision
No scar remains

b

Fig. 32.1. **a** Conventional suture method. **b** New suture method. Deep wide (relaxation) suture for tacking the incision does not leave a linear scar; the procedure is based on the sebaceous gland hypothesis

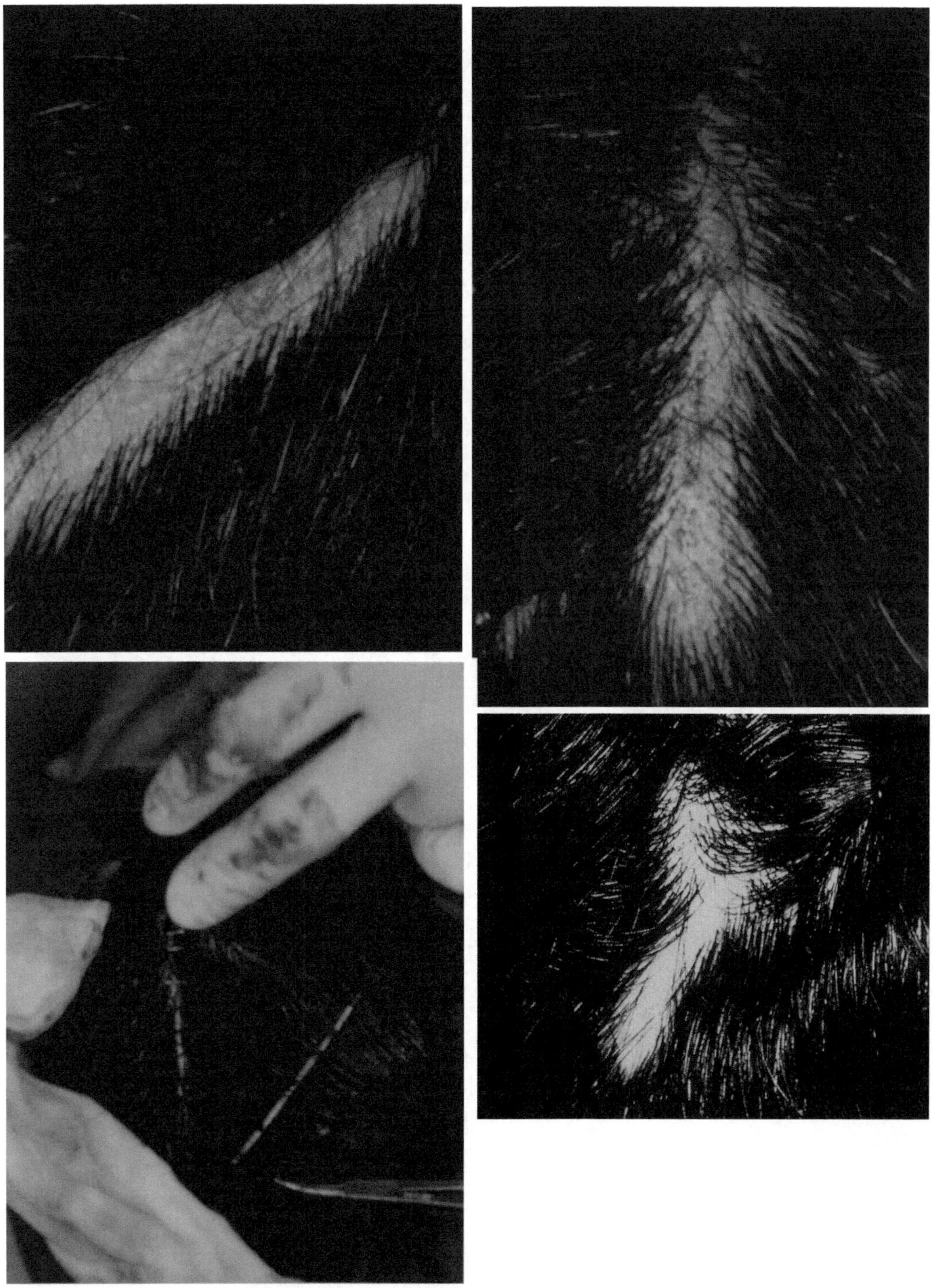

Fig. 32.2. **a** A cicatricial hair loss, 7 cm × 7 mm, is formed parallel to the hairstream. **b** After the scar was excised, the incision was sutured by three different methods; Stapler suture in the upper portion, a simple suture in the middle portion, and a continuous suture in the lower portion. **c** Follow-up result 1 month postoperatively reveals no improvement. However, hair regeneration was expected 10–12 weeks postoperatively. **d** Follow-up results after 1 year. In the lower two-thirds a scar can be seen clearly

and a continuous suture (in the lower portion) (Fig. 32.2b). We then compared the follow-up results.

One month postoperatively (Fig. 32.2c), no outstanding improvement was seen in the scar. However, regeneration was expected 10–12 weeks postoperatively, i.e., there was a period of several weeks before a result would be observed. The unevenness in the hair canal portion suggested that regeneration would occur.

At 1-year follow-up, we observed no linear scar formation in the upper one-third (stapler suture), whereas a linear scar remained in the lower two-thirds (Fig. 32.2d). Comparison of these three types of suture method thus showed that a stapler suture gave the best result in terms of hair regeneration.

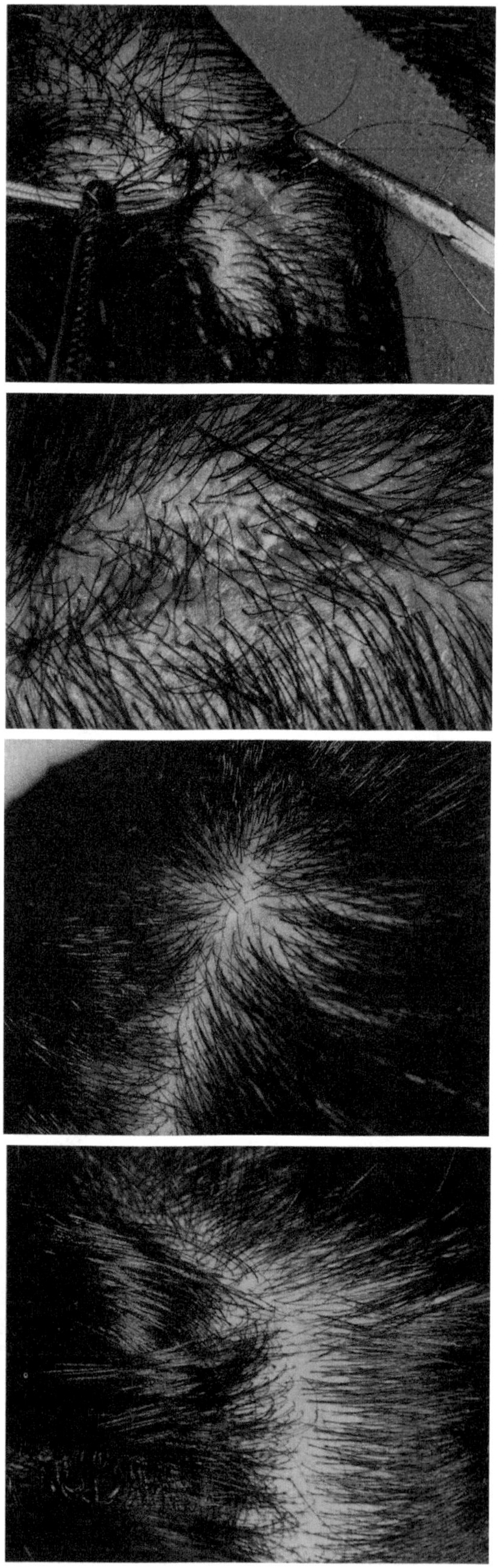

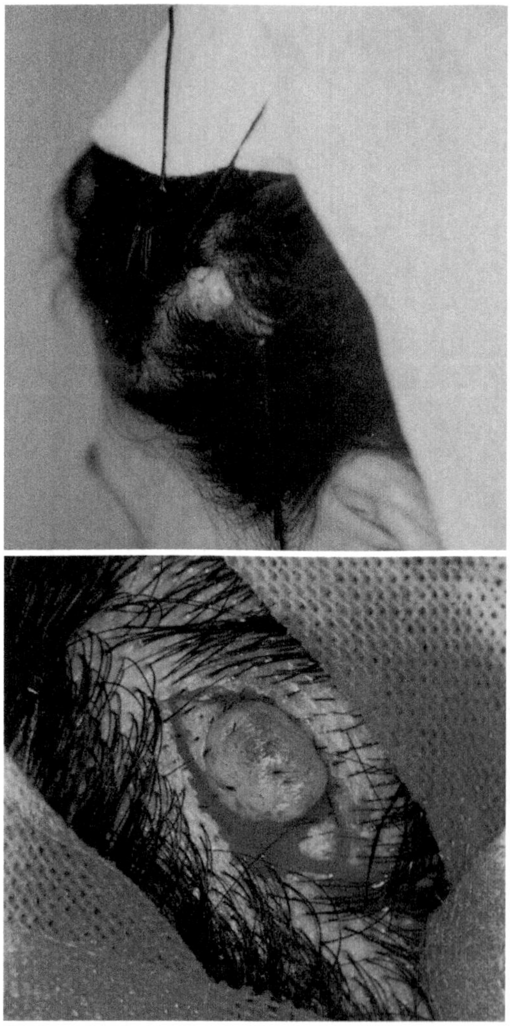

a b c d e f

Fig. 32.3a–f. Case 1. **a** A tumor was detected in the temporal region. **b** The excision is made. **c** Suturing was done with a thick nylon ligature at a distance of about 1 cm from the excisional margin, paying attention not to damage the sebaceous gland. **d** No hair loss was observed 1 month postoperatively. **e** Observation 6 months postoperatively revealed no typical linear scar. **f** Observation 1 year postoperatively. No visible scar

32.1.2 New Method (Inaba and Inaba 1992a, 1995)

32.1.2.1 Case 1

This patient, who was 30 years old, had a tumor in the scalp. A tumor 10 × 8 mm in size was detected in the temporal region (Fig. 32.3a). A fusiform excision was made, and dissection to a certain degree was employed above the galea aponeurotica to eliminate excessive tension in suturing (Fig. 32.3b). Suturing was done with a thick nylon ligature at a distance of about 1 cm from the excisional margin. Simple interrupted suture was not performed (Fig. 32.3c). However, those portions of the margin with different levels were continuously sutured with thin nylon ligatures for refinement, paying much attention not to damage the sebaceous gland. No hair loss was observed 1 month postoperatively (Fig. 32.3d). Observations 6 months postoperatively revealed no typical linear scar (Fig. 32.3e). One year postoperatively, the scar had completely vanished (Fig. 32.3f).

Histologically, the tumor showed a proliferation of nevus cells in the enlarged portion of the outer root sheath, due to nevus nevocellaris pattern lipomatosis. It was diagnosed as a nonmalignant tumor in which fat cells were present.

32.1.2.2 Case 2

In this patient, a tumor 7 × 7 mm in size, similar to that in case 1, was observed. There was virtually no hair loss on clinical observation about 2 weeks after enucleation and no formation of a linear scar was observed 3 months postoperatively.

a b c
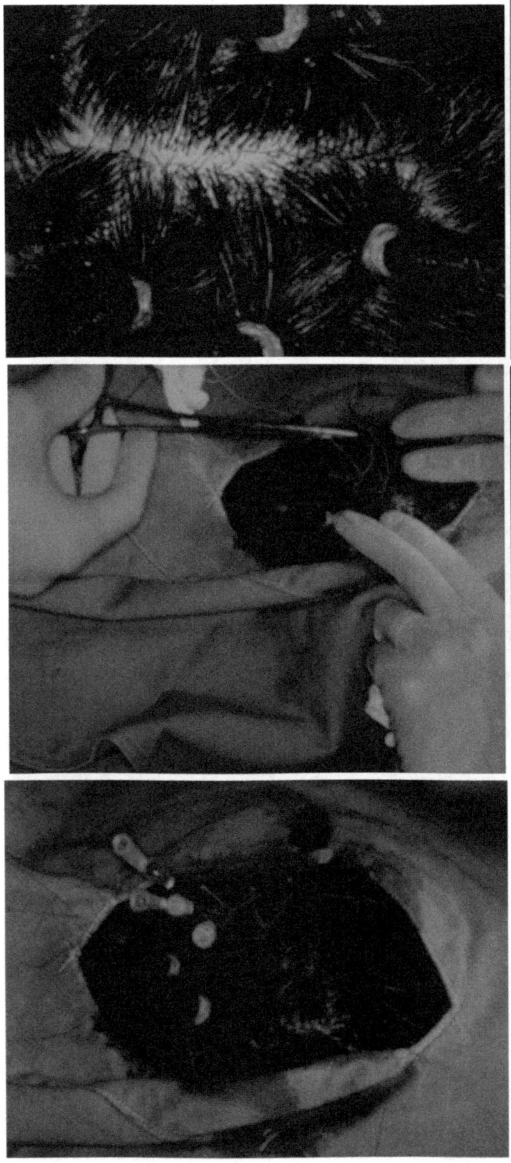

d e
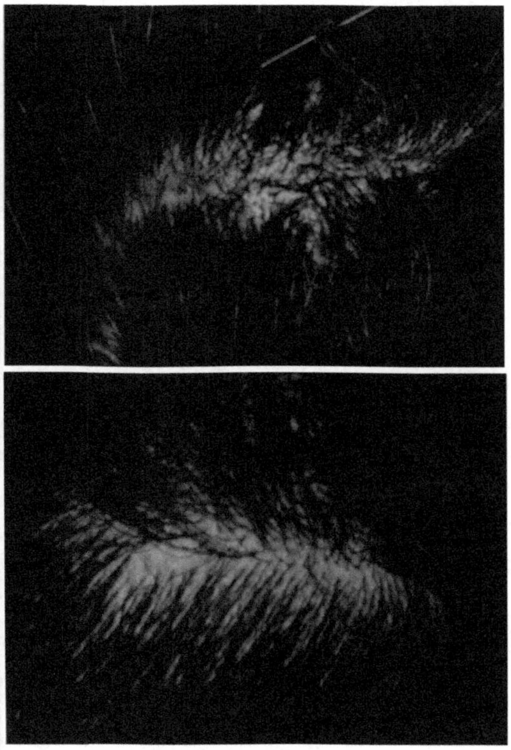

Fig. 32.4. **a** Case 3. A linear scar, about 3 cm long and 2 mm wide was observed in the left temporal region. **b** We experimentally excised half of the linear scar and sutured the incision as in cases 1 and 2. **c** We transplanted five single hair-bearing grafts in the remaining half portion of the scar, using the Marritt expansion method (Marritt 1988). **d** Observation 2 weeks postoperatively. Sutured area revealed scarcely any hair loss, and in the transplanted area five transplanted hairs could be seen. **e** Six months postoperatively, no linear scar was observed in the sutured area, and the transplanted hair had failed to survive on the left side with the remaining linear scar

32.1.2.3 Case 3

In this patient, a linear scar about 3 cm long and 2 mm wide was observed in the left temporal region (Fig. 32.4a). We performed single hair-bearing graft transplantation, using grafts collected by the 1-mm punch method. The results were not successful in terms of hair survival rate, suggesting that this method was not effective for the correction of linear scars.

We excised half of the linear scar and sutured the incision as in cases 1 and 2 (Fig. 32.4b), and transplanted five single hair-bearing grafts in the remaining half of the scar, using the Marritt expansion method (Marritt 1988) (Fig. 32.4c).

On extraction of the stitches 2 weeks postoperatively, there was scarcely any hair loss, and in the remaining scar area, five transplanted hairs could be seen (Fig. 32.4d). Six months postoperatively, no linear scar was observed in the su-

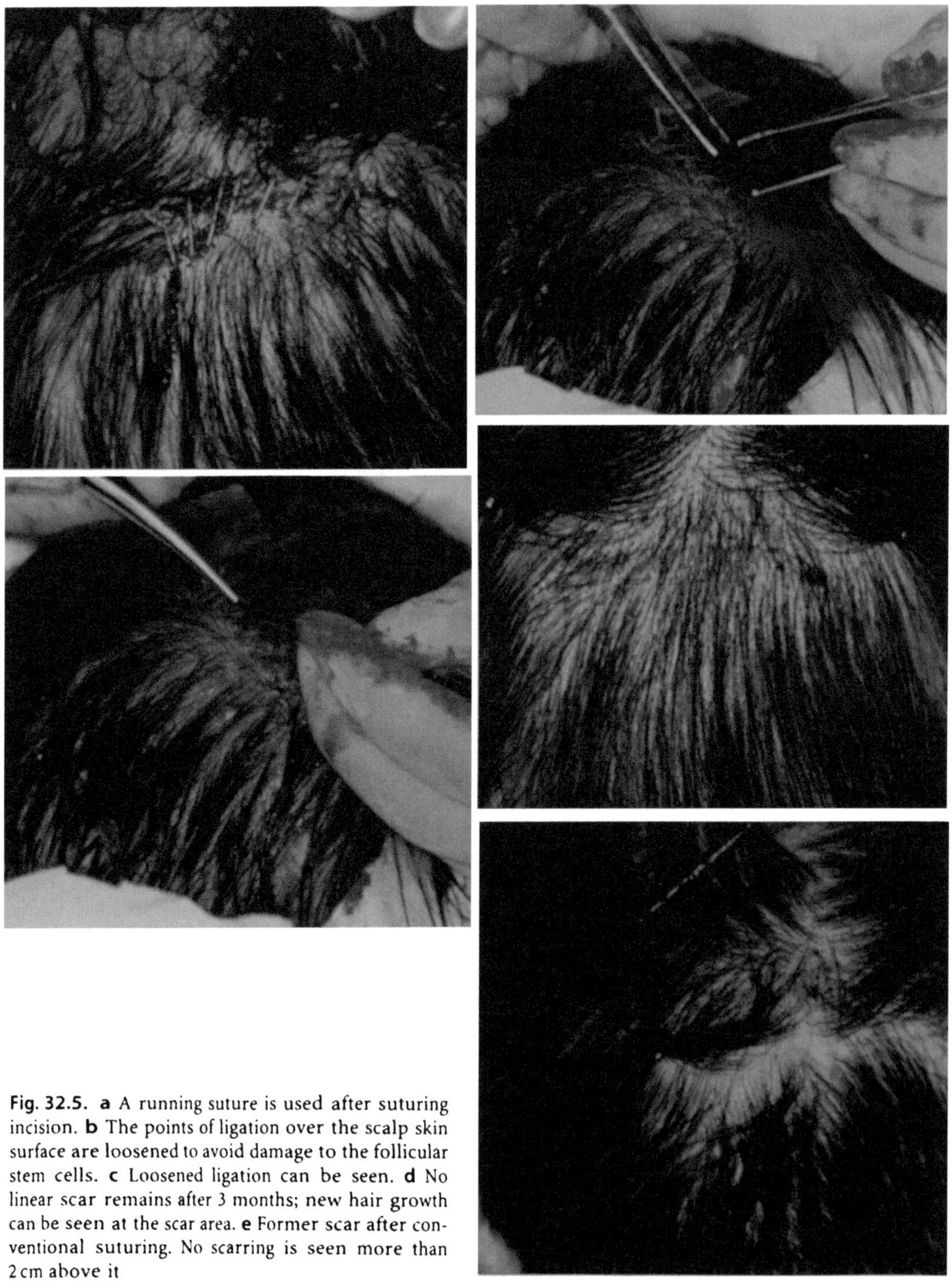

a b c d e

Fig. 32.5. **a** A running suture is used after suturing incision. **b** The points of ligation over the scalp skin surface are loosened to avoid damage to the follicular stem cells. **c** Loosened ligation can be seen. **d** No linear scar remains after 3 months; new hair growth can be seen at the scar area. **e** Former scar after conventional suturing. No scarring is seen more than 2 cm above it tured area (Fig. 32.4e), although the transplanted hairs had failed to survive in the latter half of that period. We recognize that hair transplantation cannot be used in the scar area, even if the scar tissue is expanded with an expanding device.

32.1.2.4 Case 4

We applied a running suture method in suturing incisions caused by collection of grafts in the occipital region. In performing this method, we pulled the points of ligation over the skin surface after suturing to loosen the sutured area so that damage to the stem cells could be avoided, leading to prevention of linear scar. Stough (1992) has also used this method experimentally but did not explain the causative mechanism.

32.1.2.5 Case 5

A scar formed in the occipital region after the punch operation. After removal of the punch graft, we applied a running suture method in suturing the incision caused by collection of grafts (Fig. 32.5a). In performing this method, we have pulled the points of ligation over the scalp skin surface after suturing to loosen the sutured area so that damage to the follicular stem cells (Fig. 32.5b) could be avoided, leading to prevention of linear scars. Stough (1992) has used this method experimentally but did not explain the causative mechanism. We cannot confirm this finding.

Figure 32.5e shows the scar after conventional suturing. The photograph shows that no scar has formed.

To date, linear scar formation after scalp suturing has been thought to be inevitable. Because, according to the conventional hair cycle theory, hair regeneration was believed to start from the secondary hair germ at the lower end of the telogen follicle, utmost attention was given to the protection of the hair bulb region. The authors found that stem cells reside not only in the lower end of the sebaceous gland but also in the upper portion, especially in the sebaceous isthmus. By placing a relaxation suture in scalp suturing to avoid tension to the upper stem cells, prevention as well as the surgical treatment of a linear scar can be done efficiently.

Afterword

Now that more than 20 years have passed since we developed the subcutaneous tissue shaving method as a radical treatment for bromidrosis, we feel convinced that no other method seems to be so effective as ours.

In this method, an incision about 1 cm in size is made over the axillary skin to remove the sweat glands and the hair root from the reverse side of the skin up to the level of a split-thickness skin graft, after which the upper and lower surfaces are pressed firmly together.

Since the eccrine sweat glands reside in the outer layer of the skin and the apocrine sweat glands regenerate from the region of the sebaceous gland, shaving has to be done up to the level of a medium split-thickness skin graft.

After performing our method on a great number of patients, we found that even when the telogen hair follicle, which is assumed to be the center of regeneration in the common hair cycle, is removed to the level of the sebaceous gland, regeneration of the axillary hair was observed, whereas, when the sebaceous gland was removed, no regeneration was observed. This phenomenon is obviously contradictory to the concept of the common hair cycle.

To confirm this phenomenon histologically, we prepared a thick tissue specimen, more than 50 times as thick as a conventional specimen, by using cellophane tape or sheet to enable easy histological observations.

To date, it has been impossible to elucidate the process of hair regeneration by using thin tissue specimens; however, with the development of the thick tissue specimen, three-dimensional observation has been made possible. As a result, we have been asserting for more than 10 years that the true center of hair regeneration seems to reside in the sebaceous gland, and that an isthmal stage should be added to the anagen, catagen, and telogen stages of the common hair cycle (essential hair cycle).

To our great regret, any research or study conducted by a non-academic or nonspecialist medical practitioner is likely to be disregarded, not only in Japan but also throughout the world. We decided to convince ourselves of the validity of our hypothesis, and we submitted our manuscript to Springer-Verlag, Tokyo. To our great pleasure, they published the book, *Human Body Odor*, in which we stated the hypothesis, in 1992. The publication of this book was a warning to the closed medical society of Japan, which tends to lay stress on one's academic clique or past career.

We have questioned the process of hair regeneration and have reviewed the pathogenesis and treatment of male pattern baldness on the basis of our hypothesis that the true center of hair regeneration resides in the sebaceous isthmal portion. We submitted our new manuscript on hair to the same publisher and it was again accepted for publication. It has been our great pleasure that Springer-Verlag, Tokyo made the publication of the two books possible, and we sincerely appreciate their broad vision in accepting our manuscripts.

Acknowledgments

The authors wish to acknowledge the warm support and advice given by Prof. Tai Ho Chung, M.D. (Biomedical Research Laboratory, Kyungpook National University, Dean) and Robert M. Nakamura, M.D. (Scripps Clinic, Chairman Emeritus of the Department of Pathology) during the preparation of the manuscript of this book.

The authors also wish to thank Prof. M. Niimura (Department of Dermatology, The Jikei University School of Medicine), Dr. I. Takashima (Former President of the Dermatology Department of Sapporo Railway Hospital), and Dr. T. Ezaki, who has worked in close cooperation with the authors mainly in surgical operations, for their kind collaboration and efforts.

Thanks are also due to Mr. William Dyne, Ms. Midori Nakagawa, and Ms. Chizu Sanjoba for the basic preparation of the English manuscript. Also, we would like to acknowledge the cooperation and support of Springer-Verlag, Tokyo and the assistance rendered by Ms. Yuko Murabayashi, President of M.H.R. Co., Ltd., and Ms. Mikiko Azuma, also of M.H.R. Co., Ltd.

References

Abe T (1983) Ideal diet for a long and healthy life (in Japanese). Mainichi Life 6:20–25

Abell E (1988) Histologic response to topically applied minoxidil in male pattern alopecia. Clin Dermatol 6:191–194

Adachi K (1973) The metabolism and control mechanism of human hair follicle. Curr Probl Dermatol 5:37–78

Adachi K (1974) Receptor proteins for androgen in hamster sebaceous gland. J Invest Dermatol 62:217–223

Adachi K, Kano M (1970) Adenylcyclase in human hair follicle: Its inhibition by dihydrotestosterone. Biochem Biophys Res Commun 41:884–890

Adachi K, Takayasu S, Takashima I, Kano N, Kondo S (1970) Human hair follicles: Metabolism and control mechanisms. J Soc Cosmet Chem 21:901–924

Agache P, Blanc D, Barrand C, Laurent R (1980) Sebum levels during the first year of life. Br J Dermatol 103:643–649

Aiman J, Griffin JE (1982) The frequency of androgen receptor deficiency in infertile men. J Clin Endocrinol Metab 54:725

Akamatsu H, Zouboulis CC, Orfanos CE (1992) Control of human sebocyte proliferation in vitro by testosterone and 5α-dihydrotestosterone is dependent on the localization of the sebaceous glands. J Invest Dermatol 99:509–511

Akhurst R, Fee F, Balmain A (1988) Localized production of TGF-β mRNA in tumour promoter-stimulated mouse epidermis. Nature 331:363–365

Al-Barwari SE, Potten CS (1976) Regeneration and dose-response characterization of irradiated mouse dorsal epidermal cells. Int J Radiat Biol 30:201–216

Alberts B, Bray D, Lewis J, Raff M, Roberts K, Watson JD (1989) In: Bloom W, Fawcett DW (eds) A textbook of histology, 10th edn. Saunders, Philadelphia, pp 372–395

Alfonsi M (1985) Composition of matter for improving hair growth. US Patent 4520012, May 28

Allegra F (1968) Histology and histochemical aspects of the hair follicles in pattern alopecia. In: Baccaredda-Boy A, Moretti G, Frey JR (eds) Biopathology of pattern alopecia. Karger, Basel, pp 107–128

Amer MA, El Garf A (1983) Photochemotherapy and alopecia areata. J Invest Dermatol 22:245–246

Anderson AS, Fulton JE (1973) Sebum: Analysis by infrared spectroscopy. J Invest Dermatol 60:115–120

Anderson NP (1950) Alopecia areata: A clinical study. Br Med J 4691:1250–1252

Anderson RD (1987) Expansion-assisted treatment of male pattern baldness. Clin Plast Surg 14(3):477

Andersson S, Bishop RW, Russell DW (1989) Expression cloning and regulation of steroid 5α-reductase, an enzyme essential for male sexual differentiation. J Biol Chem 264:16249–16255

Andersson S, Berman DMJ, Jenkins EP, Russell J (1991) Deletion of steroid 5α-reductase 2 gene in male pseudohermaphroditism. Nature 354:159–161

Ando Y (1978) Porphyrin compounds: for enzyme activity and the effect on hair growth (in Japanese). Jpn J Frag Journal 32:39–42

Andress KH (1966) Über die Feinstruktur der Rezeptoren an Sinushaaren. Z Zellforsch 75:339–365

Arai A, Nintzenstern JV, Kiesewetter F, Schell H, Hornstein OP (1990) In vitro effects of testosterone, dihydrotestosterone and estradiol on cell growth of human hair bulb papilla cells and hair root sheath fibroblasts. Acta Derm Venereol (Stockh) 70:338–341

Archibald A, Shuster S (1970) The measurement of sebum secretion in the rat. Br J Dermatol 82:146–151

Argenta LC, Watanabe MJ, Grabb WC (1983) The use of tissue expansion in head and neck reconstruction. Ann Plast Surg 11:31

Argenta LC, Marks MW, Pasyk KA (1985) Advances in tissue expansion. Clin Plast Surg 12:200

Ariga A (1989) Effect of strip scalp transplantation for extensive baldness after split-skin graft on the cranial periosteum (in Japanese). Jpn J Aesth Surg 11:53–59

Asada M, Kurokawa I, Nishijima S, Asada Y (1990) An immunohistochemical study on cell differentiation follicles with antikeratin monoclonal antibodies. Jpn J Invest Dermatol 100:1423–1430

Aso M, Hashimoto K, Hamzavi A (1985) Immunohistochemical studies on selected skin diseases and tumors using monoclonal antibodies to neurofilament and myelin proteins monoclonal antineural antibodies. J Am Acad Dermatol 13:37–42

Auber L (1952) The anatomy of follicles producing wool fibers with special reference to keratinization. Trans R Soc Edinb 62:191–254

Austad ED, Rose CI (1982) A self-inflating tissue

expander. Plast Reconst Surg 70:588
Axelrad H, Verley R, Farkas E (1976) Responses evoked in mouse and rat SI cortex by vibrissa stimulation. Neurosci Lett 3:265–274
Aydinlik S, lachnit-Fixson (1977) Diane-eine gestagen-ostrogen Kombination mit antiandrogenwirkung. Med Monatsschr Pharm 31:425–429
Ayres S (1964) Conservative surgical management of male pattern baldness. Arch Dermatol Syphilol 90:492–499
Bachelot I, Wolfsen AR, Odell WD (1977) Pituitary and plasma lipoproteins: Demonstration of the artificial nature of β-MSH. J Clin Endocrinol Metab 44:439
Baden HP (1987) Diseases of the hair and nails. Year Book Medical, Chicago
Baden HP, Kubilus J (1983) Effect of minoxidil on cultured keratinocytes. J Invest Dermatol 81:558–560
Baker CA, Uno H, Johnson GA (1991) Minoxidil sulfotransferase activity in hair follicles. J Invest Dermatol 96:576
Banfi A (1985) Compositions for stimulating keratin formation in hair bulbs employing horseradish and mustard seed extracts. United States Patent 4503047, March
Barber KA, Jackson R (1982) Basic principles of electrolysis. In: Epstein E (ed) Skin surgery, 5th edn. Thomas, Springfield, pp 428–429
Barman JH, Pecoraro V, Astore I (1964) Method technique and computations in the study of the trophic state of the human scalp hair. J Invest Dermatol 42:421–425
Barman JM, Astore I, Pecoraro V (1965) The normal trichogram of the adult. J Invest Dermatol 44:233–236
Barman JM, Pecoraro V, Astore I, Ferrer J (1967) The first stage in the natural history of the human scalp hair cycle. J Invest Dermatol 48:128–142
Barman JM, Astore IPL, Pecoraro V (1969) The normal trichogram of people over 50 years but apparently not bald. In: Montagna W, Dobson RL (eds) Hair growth. Pergamon, Oxford, pp 211–220 (Advances in biology of skin, vol 9)
Barth JH, Cherry CA, Wojnarowska F (1989) Spironolactone is an effective and tolerated systemic anti-androgen therapy for hirsute women. J Clin Endocrinol Metab 68:96–102
Bartosova L, Rebora A, Moretti G, Cipriani C (1971) Studies on rat hair culture. I. A reevaluation of technique. Arch Dermatol Forsch 240:95–106
Barnstable CJ, Bodmer WF, Brown G, Galfre G, Milstein C, Williams AF (1978) Production of monoclonal antibodies to group A erythrocytes, HLA and other human cell surface antigens—new tools for genetic analysis. Cell 14:9-20
Beek CH (1950) A study on extension and distribution of human body hair. Dermatologica 101:317–333
Bell M (1988) Complications of alopecia reduction and their management. In: Unger WP, Nordström REA (eds) Hair transplantation. Marcel Dekker, New York, pp 497–500
Bendl BJ (1988) Procedure for attachment of a hairpiece tunnel grafting. In: Unger WP, Nordstrom REA (eds) Hair transplantation. Marcel Dekker, New York, pp 563–567
Bernfield M, Banerjee SD, Koda JE, Rapraeger AC (1984) Remodelling of the basement membrane: Morphogenesis and maturation. Ciba Found Symp 108:179–192
Bhattacharya AK, Datta Chaudhari A, Bandyopadhyay D, Chatterjees Mandal AN (1977) Nutritional oedema in adults in clinical observation. Bull Calcutta Sch Trop Med 25:26
Bickenbach JR (1981) Identification and behavior of label-retaining cells in oral mucosa and skin. J Dent Res 60:611–620
Bickenbach JR, Mackenzie IC (1984) Identification and localization of label-retaining cells in hamster epithelia. J Invest Dermatol 82:618–622
Billingham RE (1958) The phenomenon of hair neogenesis. In: Montagna W, Ellis RA (eds) The biology of hair growth. Academic, New York, pp 451–468
Billingham RE, Mangold R, Silvers WK (1959) The neogenesis of skin in the antlers of deer. Ann NY Acad Sci 83:491–498
Bingham KD, Shaw DA (1973) The metabolism of testosterone by human male scalp skin. J Endocrinol 57:111–121
Birbeck MSC, Mercer EH (1957) The electron microscopy of the human hair follicle. Part 1. Introduction and the hair cortex. J Biophys Biochem Cytol 3:203–214
Biren CA, Barr RJ (1986) Dermatologic application of cyclosporine. Arch Dermatol 122:1028–1032
Blauer M, Vaalasti A, Pauli SL, Ylikomi T, Joensuu T, Tuohimaa P (1991) Location of androgen receptor in human skin. J Invest Dermatol 97:264–268
Bloom RE, Woods S, Nicoladies N (1955) Hair fat composition in early male pattern baldness. J Invest Dermatol 24:77
Bloom W, Fawcett DW (1975) Blood and lymph vascular system. In: Bloom W, Fawcett DW (eds) A textbook of histology, 10th edn. Saunders, Philadelphia, pp 372–395
Bonne C, Raynaud JP (1974) Activité anti-androgène du R2956 (17β-hydroxy-2,2,17α-trimethyl-estra-4,9,11-trien-3-one), II. Mécanisme d'action. J Pharmacol 4:521–532
Bonne C, Saurot JH, Chivot M (1977) Male pattern baldness and the metabolism of androgen by human scalp skin. J Soc Cosmet Chem 24:523–536
Bonne C, Saurot JH, Chivot M, Lehuchet D, Reynaud JB (1977) Androgen receptor in human skin. Br J Dermatol 97:501–503
Bouhanna P (1989) Clinical and macrophotographic study of the percutaneous implantation of synthetic hair (Nido SHI). In: Neste DV, Lachapelle JM, Antoine JL (eds) Trends in human hair growth and alopecia research. Kluwer Academic, Dordrecht, pp 257-265
Boulanger A, Bonne C, Secchi J (1974) Activité anti-androgène du R2956 (17β-hydroxy-2,2,17α-trimethyl-estra-4,9,11-trien-3-one), I. Profil endocrinien. J Pharmacol 5:509–520
Bradfield RB (1971) Protein deprivation—comparative response of hair roots, serum proteins, and urinary nitrogen. Am J Clin Nutr 24:405
Bradfield RB, Bailey MA, Margen S (1967) Morphological changes in human scalp hair roots during deprivation of protein. Science 157:438–439
Bradshaw RA (1988a) Micrografts. In: Unger WP, Nordström REA (eds) Hair transplantation. Marcel Dekker, New York
Bradshaw W (1988b) Quarter-grafts. A technique for minigrafts. In: Unger WP, Nordström REA (eds) Hair transplantation, 2nd edn. Marcel Dekker, New York,

pp 333–350
Brandy DA (1986a) The bilateral occipito-parietal flap. J Dermatol Surg Oncol 12(10):1062–1066
Brandy DA (1986b) The Brandy bitemporal flap. Am J Cosmet Surg 3:11–15
Brandy DA (1987) Conventional grafting combined with minigrafting: A new approach. J Dermatol Surg Oncol 13:60–63
Brasch SV, Amoore JA (1967) The effect of shampooing on solvent-extractable material on hair. J Soc Cosmet Chem 18:31–35
Bray PF (1959) Diphenylhydantoin (Dilantin) after 20 years. A review with re-emphasis by treatment of 84 patients. Pediatrics 23:151
Breathnach AC, Nazzaro-Porro M, Passi S (1984) Azelaic acid. Br J Dermatol 3:115–120
Breedis C (1954) Regeneration of hair follicles and sebaceous glands from the epithelium of scars in the rabbit. Cancer Res 14:575–579
Briggaman RA, Wheeler CE (1968) Epidermal-dermal interactions in adult human skin: Role of dermis in epidermal maintenance. J Invest Dermatol 51:454–465
Brooks JR, Baptista EM, Berman C (1981) Response of rat ventral prostate to a new and novel 5α-reductase inhibitor. Endocrinology 109:830–836
Brown AC, Rook AJ, Kubba RA (1980) Immunohistology and auto-antibody in alopecia areata. Br J Dermatol 102:609–610
Brown AC, Pollard ZF, Jarett WH (1982) Ocular and testicular abnormalities in alopecia areata. Arch Dermatol 118:546–554
Brown TR, Migeon CJ (1981) Cultured human skin fibroblasts: a model for the study of androgen action. Mol Cell Biochem 36:3
Bruchovsky N, Wilson JD (1968) The conversion of testosterone to 5α-androstane-17β-ol-3-one by rat prostate in vivo and in vitro. J Biochem 243:2012–2121
Buhl AE, Waldon DJ, Kawabe TT, Holland JM (1989) Minoxidil stimulates mouse vibrissae follicles in organ culture. J Invest Dermatol 92:315–320
Buhl AE, Waldon DJ, Miller BF, Branden MN (1990) Differences in activity of minoxidil and cyclosporin A on hair growth in nude and normal mice. Lab Invest 62:104–107
Buhl AE, Waldon DJ, Conrad WSJ, Mulholland MJ, Shull KL, Kubicek MF, Johnson GA, Brunden MN, Stefanski KJ, Stehle RG, Gadwood RC, Kamdar BV, Thomasco LM, Schostarez HJ, Schwartz TM, Diani AR (1992) Potassium channel conductance: A mechanism affecting hair growth both in vitro and in vivo. J Invest Dermatol 98:315–319
Bull RJ (1980) Health effects of alternate disinfectants and their reaction products. Research and Technology. JAWWA 72:299–303
Bullough WS (1946) Mitotic activity in the adult female mouse *Mus l.* A study of its relation to the oestrous cycle in normal and abnormal conditions. Philos Trans R Soc Lond [Biol] 231:435–517
Bullough WS (1955) Hormones and mitotic activity. Vitam Horm 13:261
Bullough WS (1975) Mitotic control in adult mammalian tissue. Biol Rev 50:99–127
Bullough WS, Laurence EB (1958) Mitotic activity of the follicle. In: Montagna W, Ellis RA (eds) The biology of hair growth. Academic, New York
Bullough WS, Laurence EB (1960) Experimental sebaceous gland suppression in the adult male mouse. J Invest Dermatol 35:37–42
Burk BM, Cunliffe WJ (1985) Oral spironolactone therapy for female patients with acne hirsutism or androgenic alopecia. Br J Dermatol 112:124–125
Burton JL, Marshall A (1979a) Male-pattern alopecia and masculinity. Br J Dermatol 100:567–571
Burton JL, Marshall A (1979b) Hypertrichosis due to minoxidil. Br J Dermatol 101:593–595
Burton JL, Libman LJ, Cunliffe WJ, Wilkinson R, Hall R, Shuster S (1972) Sebum excretion in acromegaly. Br Med J 1:406–408
Burton JL, Schutt WH, Caldwell IW (1975) Hypertrichosis due to diazoxide. Br J Dermatol 93:707–711
Butcher EO (1934) The hair cycles in the albino rat. Anat Rec 61:5
Butcher EO (1982) The specificity of the hair papilla in the rat. Anat Rec 151:231–238
Butcher RW, Robinson GA, Hardman JG, Sutherland EW (1968) The role of cyclic AMP in hormone action. In: Weber G (ed) Advances in enzyme regulation. Pergamon, Oxford, pp 357–389
Caballero MJ, Carreras E, Mallol J (1990) A possible specific receptor for 3-β-androstanediol in the human sebaceous gland. Rev Esp Fisiol 46:283–288
Cairns AB, Lala PK, Osmond DG (eds) (1976) Stem cells of renewing cell populations. Academic, New York
Calloway HD, Margen S (1966) Physiological evaluation of nutrient-defined diet for space flight metabolic studies. University of California Press, Berkeley
Calver NS, MacDonald HS, Parkin SM (1992) Autoantibodies in alopecia areata (abstract). Br J Dermatol 127:432
Cam C, Nigogosyan G (1963) Acquired toxic porphyria cutanea tarda due to hexachlorobenzene. J Am Med Assoc 183:88
Cameron EHD, Baillie AH, Grant JK, Mailne JA, Thomson J (1966) Transformation in vitro of (7α-3H)-dehydroepiandrosterone to (3H)-testosterone by skin from men (abstract). J Endocrinol 35:19–20
Cesarini JP (1990) Hair melanin and hair color. In: Orfanos CE, Happle R (eds) Hair and hair disease. Springer, Berlin Heidelberg New York, p 193
Chakrabarty K, Ferrari R, Dessingue OC (1980) Mechanism of action of 17α-propyltestosterone in inhibiting hamster flank organ development. J Invest Dermatol 74:5–8
Chang C, Kokontis J, Liao S (1988) Molecular cloning of human and rat complementary DNA encoding androgen receptors. Science 240:324–326
Chang C, Whelan CD, Popowich T, Kokontis J, Liao S (1989) Fusion proteins containing androgen receptor sequences and their use in the production of poly- and monoclonal anti-androgen receptor. Endocrinology 123:1097–1099
Chapman RE (1986) Hair, wool, quill, nail, claw, hoof and bone. In: Bereiter-Hahn I, Maltoltsy AG, Richards KS (eds) Biology of the integument, part 2, vertebrates. Springer, Berlin Heidelberg New York, pp 293–317
Chapman RE (1990) Non-human hair. In: Orfanos CE, Happle R (eds) Hair and hair disease. Springer, Berlin Heidelberg Tokyo, pp 199–236
Chase HB (1954) Growth of the hair. Physiol Rev 34:113–126
Chase HB (1955) The physiology and histochemistry of hair growth. J Soc Cosmet Chem 6:9–14

Chase HB (1958) Physical factors which influence the growth of hair. In: Montagna W, Ellis RA (eds) The biology of hair growth. Academic, New York, pp 435-459
Chase HB, Eaton GJ (1959) The growth of hair follicles in waves. Ann NY Acad Sci 83:365-368
Choi YC, Kim JC (1992) Transplantation using the Choi hair transplanter. J Dermatol Surg Oncol 18:945-948
Choi YC, Kim JC, Inaba M (1990a) Androgen metabolism in pilosebaceous apparatus. 49th Congress of the Japanese Association of Aesthetic Plastic Surgery, Tokyo, June 17, 1990
Choi YC, Choi KD, Kim JC (1990b) Single hair transplantation using Choi hair transplanter (in Japanese). J Jpn Aesth Plast Surg 27:76-80
Church RE (1965) Hypothyroid hair loss. Br J Dermatol 77:661-662
Cipriani R, Ruzza G, Foresta G (1983) Sex hormone binding globulin and saliva testosterone levels in men with androgenetic alopecia. Br J Dermatol 109:249-252
Clodius L, Smahel J (1979) Resurfacing denuded areas of the beard with full thickness scalp grafts. Br J Plast Surg 32:295-299
Cohen J (1961) The transplantation of individual rat and guinea pig whisker papillae. J Embryol Exp Morphol 9:117-127
Cohen J (1965) The dermal papilla. In: Lyne AG, Short BF (eds) Biology of skin and hair growth. Angus and Robertson, Sydney
Cohen J (1969) Dermis, epidermis and dermal papillae interacting. In: Montagna W, Dobson RL (eds) Advances in biology of skin and hair growth. Pergamon, Oxford, pp 1-17
Cohen RL, Alves MEAF, Weiss VC (1984) Direct effects of minoxidil on epidermal cells in culture. J Invest Dermatol 82:90-93
Coiffman F (1977) Use of square scalp grafts for male pattern baldness. Plast Reconstr Surg 60:228
Comaish JS (1981) Hair growth in disorders of metabolism. In: Orfanos CE, Montagna W (eds) Hair research. Springer, Berlin Heidelberg New York, p 267
Cook NS (1988) The pharmacology of potassium channels and their therapeutic potential. Trends Pharmacol Sci 9:21-28
Cooper MI, McGibbon D, Wilson PD, Shuster S (1979) Androgenic control of the human sebaceous gland. J Invest Dermatol 72:267
Cormack DH (1987) Ham's histology. Lippincott, Philadelphia
Cotsarelis G, Cheng SZ, Dong G, Sun TT, Lavker RM (1989) Existence of slow-cycling limbal epithelial basal cells that can be preferentially stimulated by proliferate: Implications in epithelial stem cells. Cell 57:201-209
Cotsarelis G, Sun TT, Lavker RM (1990) Label-retaining cells reside in the bulge area of pilosebaceous unit. Implications for follicular stem cells, hair cycle, and skin carcinogenesis. Cell 61:1329-1337
Couchman JR, King JL, McCarthy KJ (1990) Distribution of two basement membrane proteoglycans through hair follicle development and the hair growth cycle in the rat. J Invest Dermatol 94:65-70
Cronin E (1980) Cosmetics. In: Cronin E (ed) Contact dermatitis. Churchill Livingstone, Edinburgh, pp 93-170
Crounse RG, Stengl JM (1959) Influence of the dermal papilla on survival of isolated human scalp hairs in an heterologous host. J Invest Dermatol 32:477-479
Crounse RG, Bollet AJ, Owen S (1970) Quantitative tissue assay of human malnutrition using scalp hair roots. Nature 228:465-466
Crovato F, Moretti G, Bertamino R (1968) Histochemistry of dermis and blood vessels in male pattern alopecia. In: Baccaredda-Boy A, Moretti F, Frey JR (eds) Biopathology of pattern alopecia. Karger, Basel, pp 191-199
Crovato F, Moretti G, Bertamino R (1973) 17-β-hydroxysteroid dehydrogenases in hair follicles of normal and bald scalp: A histochemical study. J Invest Dermatol 60:126
Crovato F, Bertamino R, Moretti G (1975) Cutaneous hydroxysteroid dehydrogenases and rat hair-cycle. Arch Dermatol Forsch 251:325-328
Cunha GR, Taguchi O, Shannon JM, Cung LWK, Bigsby RM (1984) Sex differentiation disorders. In: Serio M, Motta M, Zanishi M, Martini L (eds) Sexual differentiation: Basic and clinical aspects. Raven, New York, pp 33-51
Cunliffe WJ, Cotterill JA (1975) The acnes. Clinical features, pathogenesis, and treatment. Saunders, Philadelphia
Daigie HJ, Dollery CT, Dandie LJ (1977) Minoxidil in resistant hypertension. Lancet II:515-518
Danforth CH (1925) Hair in its relation to questions of homology and phylogeny. Am J Anat 36:47-68
Daniel S (1985) Die pharmakokinetie von cyproteronacetat under der hochdosierten standard therapie bei androgenisierten frauen. Thesis, Freie Universitat, Berlin
Davidson P, Hardy MH (1952) The development of mouse vibrissae in vivo and in vitro. J Anat 86:342-356
Davidson S, Passmore R, Brook JK, Truswell AS (1975) Human nutrition and dietetics. Churchill Livingstone, Edinburgh, p 285
Davis JS (1911) Scalping accidents. Bull Johns Hopkins Hosp 16:257
Davis BP, Rampini E, Hsia SL (1972) 17β-Hydroxysteroid dehydrogenase of rat skin. J Biol Chem 247:1407-1413
Dawning DT, Strauss JS, Pochi PE (1970) Variability in the chemical composition of human surface lipids. J Invest Dermatol 53:322-327
de Meijere JCH (1894) Über die haare der saugetiere, besonders uber ihre andordung. Morphol Jahrb 21:333-411
De Gregorio VR, Rauscher G (1981) Experience with the complications of synthetic hair implantations. Plast Reconst Surg 68:498
De Peretti E, Forest MG (1976) Unconjugated dehydroepiandrosterone from birth to adolescence in humans; the use of a sensitive radioimmunoassay. J Clin Endocrinol Metab 43:982
Desai SC, Sheth RA, Udani PM (1981) Nutrition and hair anomalies. In: Orfanos CE, Montagna W, Stüttgen G (eds) Hair research. Springer, Berlin Heidelberg New York, pp 257-266
De Villez RL, Dunn J (1986) Female androgenic alopecia. Arch Dermatol 122:1011-1015
De Villez RLY (1990) The therapeutic use of topical minoxidil. Dermatol Clin 8:367-375
Devine BL, Fife R, Trust PM (1977) Minoxidil for severe hypertension after failure of other hypertensive drugs.

Br Med J 2:667–669

Dhouailly D (1977) Regional specification of cutaneous appendages in mammals. Wilhelm Roux Arch Entwicklungsmech Org 181:3–10

Diane regimen (1977) Ein gestagen-ostrogen-kombination mit anti-androgenwirkung. Med Mschr 31. Jahrgang Hept 9:425–429

Diani AR, Mills CJ (1994) Immunocytochemical localization of androgen receptors in the scalp of the stumptail macaque monkey, a model of androgenetic alopecia. J Invest Dermatol 102:511–514

Diani AR, Waldon DJ, Conrad SJ, Stenn KS (1990) The opening of potassium growth channels: a mechanism for hair. In: Messenger AG, Baden HP (eds) The molecular and structural biology of hair. Ann NY Acad Sci 642:504

Diani AR, Mulholland MJ, Shull KL, Kubicek MF, Johnson GA, Schostarez HJ, Brunden MN, Buhl AE (1992) Hair growth effects of oral administration of finasteride, a steroid 5α-reductase inhibitor, alone and in combination with topical minoxidil in the balding stumptail macaque. J Clin Endocrinol Metab 74:345–350

Dick LA, Kurtin SB (1972) Suture implantation for the correction of male pattern alopecia. Cutis 9:49–50

Dijkstra AC, Goos AA, Cunliffe WJ, Sultan C, Vermorken AM (1987) Is increased 5α-reductase activity a primary phenomenon in androgen-dependent skin disorders? J Invest Dermatol 89:87–92

Dillaha CJ, Rothman S (1952) Treatment of alopecia totalis and universalis with cortisone acetate. J Invest Dermatol 18:5–6

Dooms-Goossens A, Vandaele M, Bedert R (1989) Hexamidine isethionate, a sensitizer in topical pharmaceutical products and cosmetics. Contact Dermatitis 21:270

Dorfman RI, Dorfman AS (1962) Assay of subcutaneous administered androgens on the chick's comb. Acta Endocrinol (Copenh) 41:101–106

Downing DT, Strauss JS, Pochi PE (1972) Changes in skin surface lipid composition induced by severe caloric restriction in man. Am J Clin Nutr 25:365–367

Dry FW (1926) The coat of the mouse (*Mus musculus*). J Genet 16:287–340

Ducharme DW, Freyburger WA, Graham BE, Carlson RG (1973) Pharmacologic properties of minoxidil; a new hypotensive agent. J Pharmacol Exp Ther 184:662

Duggins OH, Trotter M (1951) Changes in morphology of hair during childhood. Ann NY Acad Sci 53:569

Durward A, Rundall KM (1958) The vascularity and pattern of growth of hair follicles. In: Montagna W, Ellis RA (eds) Biology of hair growth. Academic, New York

Eberhardt H (1978) MeB Methoden zur Prüfung der Wirkung von Antischuppenpräparaten. Vortrag DFG, Vortragstagung, Aachen, 11 October, 1978

Ebling FJ (1948) Sebaceous glands. I. The effect of sex hormones on the sebaceous glands of the female albino rat. J Endocrinol 5:297–302

Ebling FJ (1973) The effects of cyproterone acetate and oestradiol upon testosterone-stimulated sebaceous activity in the rat. Acta Endocrinol (Copenh) 72:361

Ebling FJ (1974) Hormonal control and methods of measuring sebaceous gland activity. J Invest Dermatol 62:161–171

Ebling FJG (1990) The hormonal control of hair growth. In: Hair and hair diseases. Springer, Berlin Heidelberg New York, pp 284

Ebling FJG, Cunliffe WJ (1986) Alopecia areata. In: Rook A, Wilkinson BR, Ebling FJG (eds) Textbook of dermatology: The hair. Blackwell Scientific, Oxford, pp 1985–1992

Ebling FJ, Hale PA (1983a) Hormones and hair growth. In: Goldsmith LA (ed) Biochemistry and physiology of the skin. Oxford University Press, New York, pp 522–552

Ebling FJ, Hale PA (1983b) The local effects of topically applied estradiol, cyproterone acetate, and ethanol on sebaceous secretion in intact male rats. J Invest Dermatol 81:448–451

Ebling FJ, Johnson E (1964) The action of hormones on spontaneous hair growth cycles in the rat. J Endocrinol 29:193–201

Ebling FJ, Rook A (1972) Cyclic activity of the follicle. In: Rook A, Wilkinson BR, Ebling FJG (eds) Textbook of dermatology II. Blackwell, Oxford, pp 1567–1573

Ebling FJ, Skinner J (1967) The measurement of sebum production in rats treated with testosterone and oestradiol. Br J Dermatol 79:386–393

Ebling FJ, Ebling E, McCaffery V, Skinner J (1971) The response of the sebaceous glands of the hypophysectomized-castrated male rat to 5α-dihydrotestosterone, androstenedione, dehydroepiandrosterone and androsterone. J Endocrinol 1:181–190

Ebling FJG, Randall VA, Sawers RS (1984) Interrelationships between body hair growth, sebum excretion and endocrine parameters. Prostate 5:347–348

Editorial (1984) Alopecia areata—an autoimmune disease? Lancet I:1335–1336

Eisen AZ, Holyske JB, Lobity WC (1955) Responses of the superficial portions of the human pilosebaceous apparatus to controlled injury. J Invest Dermatol 25:145–156

Ekoe JM, Burckhardt P, Ruedi B (1980) Treatment of hirsutism, acne and alopecia with cyproterone acetate. Dermatologica 160:338

Ellenberger W (1906) Handbuch der vergleichenden mikroskopischen Anatomie der Haustiere, vol 1. Parey, Berlin

Elliott RA (1979) Lateral scalp flaps. In: Vallis C (ed) The treatment of male pattern baldness. Thomas, Springfield

Ellis RA (1958) Aging of the human male scalp. In: Montagna W, Ellis RA (eds) Biology of hair growth. Academic, New York, pp 469–485

Ellis RA, Henrikson RC (1963) Eccrine sweat glands. In: Montagna W, Ellis RA, Silver AF (eds) Advances in biology of skin, vol 6. Pergamon, New York

Ellis RA, Montagna W, Fanger H (1957) Histology and cytochemistry of human skin. XIV. The blood supply of the cutaneous glands. J Invest Dermatol 30:137–145

Ellis S (1989) Looking young. Longevity 1:10

Emanuel SV (1936) Quantitative determination of the sebaceous glands function, with particular mention of the method employed. Acta Derm Venereol (Stockh) 17:444

Engstrand L (1965) Stop hair loss and grow more hair even in advanced cases of baldness. Health Plus, Phoenix

Eppenburger U, Hsia SL (1972) Binding of steroid hormones by the 105000 × g supernatant fraction from homogenates of rat skin and variations during their hair cycle. J Biol Chem 247:5463

Epstein EH (1983) Hormone receptors. In: Goldsmith

LA (ed) Biochemistry and physiology of the skin. Oxford University Press, New York, p 1200
Epstein W, Kligman AM (1956) The pathogenesis of milia and benign tumors of the skin. J Invest Dermatol 26:1–11
Epstein WL, Maibach HI (1969) Cell proliferation and movement in human hairbulbs. In: Montagna W, Dobson RL (eds) Hair growth. Pergamon, Oxford, pp 83–97
Evron S, Shapiro G, Diamant YZ (1981) Induction of ovulation with spironolactone aldactone in anovulatory oligomenorrheic and hyperandrogenic women. Fertil Steril 36:468
Ezaki T (1986) Temporal-parietal occipital pedicle flap method. Proceedings of the 33rd congress of the Japanese association of aesthetic plastic surgery, Tokyo, 28 June, 1986
Ezaki T (1990) Punch graft. In: Ohoura T (ed) Plastic reconstructive surgery, skin surface surgery (in Japanese). Kokuseido, Tokyo, p 132
Ezaki T (1993) An occipital parietal flap method. Proceedings of the 58th congress of the Japanese association of aesthetic plastic surgery, Tokyo, 21–23 October, 1993
Ezaki T, Kasori Y (1994) Bilateral temporal-parietal flaps in the treatment of male baldness (in Japanese). Jpn Aesth Plast Surg 19:41–47
Fair NB, Guptar BS (1987) The chlorine-hair interaction. I. Review of mechanisms and changes in properties of keratin fibers. J Soc Cosmet Chem 38:359–370
Fanta D (1978) Klinische und experimentelle Untersuchungen über die Wirkung von Benzoylperoxid in der Behandlung der Akne. Hautarzt 29:481–486
Farthing MJG, Mattei AM, Edwards CRW, Dawson AM (1982) Relationship between plasma testosterone and dihydrotestosterone concentrations and male facial hair growth. Br J Dermatol 107:559–564
Fazekas AG, Lanthier A (1971) Metabolism of androgen by isolated human beard hair follicles. Steroid 18(4):367–378
Fazekas AG, Sandor T (1972) Metabolism of androgens by isolated human hair follicles. J Steroid Biochem 3:485–491
Fazekas AG, Sandor T (1973) The metabolism of dehydroepiandrosterone by human scalp hair follicles. J Clin Endocrinol Metab 36:582–586
Fenton DA, Wilkinson JD (1983) Topical minoxidil in the treatment of alopecia areata. J Med 287:1015–1017
Ferrari R, Chakrabarty K, Beyler A, et al (1978) Suppression of sebaceous gland development in laboratory animals by 17α-propyltestosterone. J Invest Dermatol 71:320–323
Fiedler-Weiss VC (1987) Topical minoxidil solution (1% and 5%) in the treatment of alopecia areata. J Am Acad Dermatol 16:745–748
Finzi E, Harkins R, Horn T (1991) TGF-α is widely expressed in differentiated as well as hyper-proliferative skin epithelium. J Invest Dermatol 96:328–332
Fitzpatrick TB, Burnet P, Kukita A (1958) The nature of hair pigment. In: Montagna W, Ellis RA (eds) The biology of hair growth. Academic, New York, pp 255–303
Fleming RW, Mayer TG (1984) Scalp flaps in the treatment of male pattern baldness. In: Norwood OT, Sheill RC (eds) Hair transplant surgery. Thomas, Springfield, pp 278–314
Fono R (1950) Hypertrichosis during streptomycin therapy. Annal Poldia 174:389
Food and Drug Administration (FDA) (1979a) Proceedings of general and plastic surgery devices classification panel. Washington DC, October 18, 1979
Food and Drug Administration (FDA) (1979b) Proceedings of general and plastic surgery devices classification panel. January 18–19, 1979
Food and Drug Administration (FDA) (1980) Hair grower and hair-loss prevention drug products for over-the-counter human use. Fed Register 45:73955–73960
Food and Drug Administration (FDA) (1982) Listing of banned devices: prosthetic hair fibers. Code of Federal Regulation 21:895.101
Food and Drug Administration (FDA) (1985) Drug products containing active ingredients offered over-the-counter (OTC) for external use as hair growers or for hair-loss prevention. Fed Register 50:2190–2198
Fox CA (1985) Shampoo components. Cosmet Toiletries 100:31–46
Fox CY (1986) Technically speaking. Cosmet Toiletries 101:19–20
Frater R (1980) The effect of rat serum on the morphology of rat hair follicles in tissue culture. Arch Dermatol Res 269:13–20
Frater R, Whitmore PG (1973) In vitro growth of postembryonic hair. J Invest Dermatol 61:72–81
Frechet P (1990) A new method for correction of the vertical scar observed following scalp reduction for extensive alopecia. J Dermatol Surg Oncol 16:640–644
Frechet P (1993) Scalp extension. J Dermal Surg Oncol 19:616–620
Frechet P (1994) Slat correction by a three hair bearing transplantation flap in combination with scalp reduction. Int J Aesth Reconst Surg 2(1):27–32
Freinkel RK, Freinkel N (1972) Hair growth and alopecia in hypothyroidism. Arch Dermatol 160:349–352
Friederich HC (1970) Indikation und Technik der operativ-plastischen Behandlung des Haarverlustes. Hautarzt 21:197–202
Frost P, Gomez EC (1972) Inhibitors of sex hormone: Development of experimental models. In: Montagna W, Staughton RB, Van Scott EJ (eds) Advances in biology of skin, vol 12, Pharmacology and the skin. Appleton-Century-Crofts, New York, pp 403–420
Fuchs J, Nitschmann WH, Packer L (1990) The anti-psoriatic compound anthralin influences bioenergetic parameters and redox properties of energy transducing membranes. J Invest Dermatol 94:71–76
Fujita K (1953) Reconstruction of the eyebrow (in Japanese). La Lepro 22:364
Fujita K (1976) Hair transplantation in Japan. In: Kobori T, Montagna W (eds) Biology and disease of the hair. University Park Press, Baltimore, pp 519–527
Fujita K, Watanabe Y (1954) Punctiform homo-hair transplantation in humans (in Japanese). La Lepro 23:364
Fujita K, Ishiwara K, Takahashi M, Torashima Y (1960) Histological picture of rabbit hair autotransplanted after freezing (in Japanese). Jpn J Dermatol 70:713
Fujita K, Ishibashi A, Noritake M, Kikuya T (1984) Histologic studies on hair follicles. Japan Congress of Dermatology, Sapporo, 8–10 June, 1984
Fukuda O, Ezaki T (1975) Complications in reconstructive surgery for microtia. Jpn Plast

Reconstr Surg 18:109
Fukuta K, Narita I, Jodo T (1976) A new procedure of cosmetic prosthetic surgery. Jpn J Plast Reconstr Surg 19:613
Fukuzumi K (1986) Lipid peroxide and prevention of aging, rejuvenation of the skin, etc. (in Japanese). Fragrance J 76:35–40
Fulton JE, Farzad-Bakshanden A, Bradley S (1974) Studies on the mechanism of action of topical benzoyl peroxide and vitamin A acid in acne vulgaris. J Cutaneous Pathol 1:191–200
Funk CF (1951) Hormonale Haarwuchuchsstörung. Hautarzt 2:468
Galbraith GMP, Thiers BH, Jensen J, Hoehler F (1987) A randomized double-blind study of inosiplex therapy in patients with alopecia totalis. J Am Acad Dermatol 16:977–983
Gallegos AJ, Berliner DL (1967) Transformation and conjugation of dehydroepiandrosterone by human skin. J Clin Endocrinol Metab 27:1214–1218
Garn SM, Selby S, Young R (1954) Scalp thickness and the fat loss theory of balding. Arch Dermatol Syph 70:601
Geary JR (1952) Effect of roentgen rays during various phases of the hair cycle of the albino rat. Am J Anat 91:51–105
Georgala G, Papasotiriou V, Stavropoulos P (1986) Serum testosterone and sex hormone binding globulin levels in women with androgenetic alopecia. Acta Derm Venereol (Stockh) 66:532–534
Gerstein T (1986) Hair-growing innovations: An overview. Cosmet Toiletries 101:21–45
Giacometti L (1964) The anatomy of the human scalp. In: Montagna W (ed) Aging. Pergamon, Oxford, pp 97–120 (Advances in biology of skin, vol 6, Aging)
Giacometti L, Montagna W (1968) The nerve fibers in male pattern alopecia. In: Baccaredda-Boy A, Moretti F, Frey JR (eds) Biopathology of pattern alopecia. Karger, Basel, pp 208–215
Gianetti A, Disilveris A, Castellazzi AM, Maccatis R (1978) Evidence for defective T cell function in patients with alopecia areata. J Dermatol 98:361
Gibbs HF (1938) A study of development of the skin and hair of the Australian opossum *Trichosurus vulpecula*. Proc Zool Soc Lond 108:611–648
Giegel JL, Stolfi LM, Weinstein GD, Frost P (1971) Androgenic regulation of nucleic acid and protein synthesis in the hamster flank organ and other tissues. Endocrinology 89:904–909
Gilliland JM, Kirk J, Smeaton TC (1981) Normalized androgen ratio: Its application in clinical dermatology. Clin Exp Dermatol 6:349–353
Gloor M, Hubscher M, Friederich HC (1974) Untersuchungen zur externen Behandlung der Acne vulgalis mit Tetracyclin und Östrogen. Hautarzt 26:391–394
Gloor M, Klump H, Wirth H (1980) Cytokinetic studies on the sebo-suppressive effect of drugs using the example of benzoyl peroxide. Arch Dermatol Res 267:97–99
Goette DK, Odom RB (1976) Alopecia in crash dieters. JAMA 235:2622
Gollnick H, Orfanos CE (1990) Alopecia areata: Pathogenesis and clinical picture. In: Orfanos CE, Happle R (eds) Hair and hair diseases. Springer, Berlin Heidelberg Tokyo, pp 529–569
Goldsmith LA (1991) Summary of alopecia areata research workshop and future research directions. J Invest Dermatol 96:98–100
Gomez EC, Hsia SL (1968) Studies of in vitro metabolism of testosterone-4-14C Δ4-androstene-3, 17-dione-4-14C in human skin. Biochemistry 7:24–32
Gonzalez ER, McBride G (1979) Synthetic hair implantations continue; serious complications result. JAMA 241:2687–2689
Goolamali SK, Burton JL, Shuster S (1973) Sebum excretion in hypopituitarism. Br J Dermatol 89:21–25
Goolamali SK, Evered D, Shuster S (1976) Thyroid disease and sebaceous gland function. Br Med J 1:4321
Goos CMAA, Wirtz P, Vermorken AJM (1982) An improved method for the evaluation of anti-androgens. Arch Dermatol Res 273:333–341
Goth A (1978) Medical pharmacology, 9th edn. Mosby, St. Louis, pp 515–532
Grary JR Jr (1952) Effect of roentgen rays during various phases of the hair cycle of the albino rat. Am J Anat 91:51–106
Green MR, Couchman JR (1984) Distribution of epidermal growth factor receptors in rat tissue during embryonic skin development, hair formation and adult hair cycle. J Invest Dermatol 83:118–123
Green MR, Couchman JR (1985) Differences in human skin between the epidermal growth factor receptor distribution detected by EGF binding and monoclonal antibody recognition. J Invest Dermatol 85:239–241
Green MR, Clay CS, Gibson WT, Hughes TC, Smith CG, Westgate GE, Kealey T (1986) Rapid isolation in large numbers of intact, viable individual hair follicles from the skin: Biochemical and ultrastructural characterization. J Invest Dermatol 87:768–770
Greenberg SI (1955) Alopecia areata: A psychiatric survey. Arch Dermatol 72:454–457
Griffin JE, Wilson JD (1977) Studies on the pathogenesis of incomplete forms of androgen resistance in man. J Clin Endocrinol Metab 45:1137–1143
Griffin JE, Punyashthiti K, Wilson JD (1976) Dihydrotestosterone binding by cultured human fibroblasts: Comparison of cells from control subjects and from patients with hereditary male pseudohermaphroditism due to androgen resistance. J Clin Invest 57:1342–1351
Guin JD (1982) History manufacture and cutaneous reactions to perfumes. In: Frost P, Horwitz SN (eds) Principles of cosmetics for the dermatologist. Bosky, St. Louis, pp 111–129
Gummer CL (1985) Diet and hair loss. Semin Dermatol 4:35–39
Halata Z (1990) Specific nerve endings in vellus hair guard hair and sinus hair. In: Orfanos CE, Happle R (eds) Hair and hair disease. Springer, Berlin Heidelberg New York, pp 150–164
Hallmans G, Stenstrom S (1974) Regeneration of hair follicles from experimental wounds on the rabbit ear. Scand J Plast Reconstr Surg 8:207–210
Hamilton JB (1942) Male hormone stimulation is prerequisite and an incitant in common baldness. Am J Anat 71:451–480
Hamilton JB (1946) A secondary sexual character that develops in men but not in women upon aging of an organ present in both sexes. Anat Rec 94:466–467
Hamilton JB (1951a) Patterned loss of hair in man. Types and incidence. Ann NY Acad Sci 53:708
Hamilton JB (1951b) Quantitative measurement of a secondary sex character. Axillary hair. Ann NY Acad

Sci 53:585–599
Hamilton JB (1958) Age, sex, and genetic factors in the regulation of hair growth in man: A comparison of Caucasian and Japanese populations. In: Montagna W, Ellis RA (eds) The biology of hair growth. Academic, New York, pp 399–433
Hammerstein J, Cupceancu B (1969) Behandlung des Hirsutismus mit Cyproteronacetat. Dtsch Med Wochenschr 94:829
Hammerstein J, Meckies J, Leo-Robberg I, Moltz L, Zielske F (1975) Use of cyproterone acetate (CPA) in the treatment of acne, hirsutism and virilism. J Steroid Biochem 6:827–836
Hanke CW (1979) Fiber implantation for pattern baldness. FDA Consumer 13:18
Hanke CW (1981) Fiber implantation for pattern baldness—review of complications in 41 patients. J Am Acad Dermatol 4:278
Happle R (1979) DNCB-Therapie der Alopecia areata. Z Hautkr 54:426–429
Hara K (1987) Hair-growth promoter in the twenty-first century (in Japanese). Fragrance J 85:7–51
Harada T, Inaba M, Inaba Y (1984) Fine-detail electron microscope studies based on thick tissue section preparation (Cellophane tape method) (in Japanese). Jpn J Aesth Surg 23:31–35
Hardy MH (1947) The group arrangement of hair follicles in the mammalian skin. I. Notes on follicle group arrangement in thirteen Australian marsupials. Proc R Soc Queensl 58:125–148
Hardy MH (1949) The development of mouse hair in vitro with some observations on pigmentation. J Anat 83:364–384
Hardy MH, Goldberg EA (1983) Morphological changes at the basement membrane during some tissue interactions in the integument. Can J Biochem Cell Biol 61:957–966
Hardy MH, Lyne AG (1956a) The pre-natal development of wool follicles in merino sheep. Aust J Biol Sci 9:423–441
Hardy MH, Lyne AG (1956b) Studies on the development of wool follicles in tissue culture. Aust J Biol Sci 9:559–577
Harii K, Ohmori K, Ohmori S (1974) Hair transplantation with free scalp flaps. Plast Reconstr Surg 53:410–413
Harris H (1946) The inheritance of premature baldness in man. Ann Eugenics 13:172
Hashimoto K (1961) Action of physiological function of various auto-transplant grafts (in Japanese). Jpn J Plast Reconstr Surg 3:139–161
Hashimoto K (1970) The ultrastructure of the skin of human embryos. IX: Formation of the hair cone and intraepidermal hair canal. Arch Klin Exp Dermatol 238:333–345
Hashimoto K (1973) Fine structure of perifollicular nerve endings in human hair. J Invest Dermatol 59:432–441
Hashimoto Y (1976) Hair follicle, especially structure and differentiation of the outer root sheath (in Japanese). In: Sasagawa S, Morioka S (eds) Aspects on dermatology. Kanehara, Tokyo
Hashimoto K (1981) The environment of the hair follicles. In: Orfanos CE, Montagna W, Stuttgen G (eds) Hair research. Springer, Berlin Heidelberg New York, pp 172–182
Hashimoto Y, Iijima S, Mori W (1987) Diseases of the hair. In: Ishikawa H, Kageyama K, Shimamine T (eds) Current encyclopedia of pathology, vol 19, B. Nakayama, Tokyo, pp 227–232
Hashimoto K, Ito M, Suzuki Y (1990) Innervation and vasculature of the hair follicle. In: Orfanos CE, Happle R (eds) Hair and hair disease. Springer, Berlin Heidelberg New York, pp 117–147
Hasselquist MB, Goldberg N, Schroeter A, Spelsberg TC (1980) Isolation and characterization of the estrogen receptor in human skin. J Clin Endocrinol Metab 50:76–83
Hay JB, Hodgins MB (1973) Metabolism of androgens in vitro by human facial and axillary skin. J Endocrinol 59:475–486
Hay JB, Hodgins MB (1974) Metabolism of androgens by human skin in acne. Br J Dermatol 91:123–133
Hay JB, Hodgins MB (1978) Distribution of androgen metabolizing enzymes in isolated tissues of human forehead and axillary skin. J Endocrinol 79:29–39
Headington JT (1984) Transverse microscopic anatomy of the human scalp. Arch Dermatol 120:449–456
Heid HW, Moll I, Franke WW (1988) Patterns of expression of trichocytic and epithelial cytokeratins in mammalian tissues. J Differentiation 37:137–157
Herfert J, Wienker TF, Ropers HH (1980) The presence of androgen-binding receptors in genital and nongenital skin fibroblasts. Hum Genet 53:271–273
Hill PB, Wynder EL (1979) Effect of vegetarian diet and dexamethasone on plasma prolactin, testosterone, and dehydroepiandrosterone in men and women. Cancer Lett 7:273–282
Hinkel AR, Lind RW (eds) (1981) Electrolysis, thermolysis, and the blend. Arroway, Los Angeles, p 47
Holbrook KA (1983) Structure and physiology of the skin. In: Goldsmith LA (ed) Biochemistry and physiology of the skin. Oxford University Press, New York
Holbrook KA, Odland GF (1978) Structure of the human fetal hair canal and initial eruption. J Invest Dermatol 71:385–390
Holecek BU, Ackerman AB (1993) Bulge-activation hypothesis. Is it valid? Am J Dermatopathol 15:235–241
Hollis DE, Chapman RE (1987) Apoptosis in wool follicles during mouse epidermal growth factor (m EGF)-induced catagen regression. J Invest Dermatol 88:455–458
Hollis DE, Chapman RE, Panaretto BA, Moore GPM (1983) Morphological changes in the skin and wool fibres of the Merino sheep infused with epidermal growth factor. Aust J Biol Sci 36:419–434
Holt PJA, Marks R (1977) The epidermal response to change in thyroid status. J Invest Dermatol 68:299–301
Hori H, Moretti G, Rebora A, Crovato F (1972) The thickness of human scalp: Normal and bald. J Invest Dermatol 58:396–399
Horne KA, Jahoda CAB, Oliver RF (1986) Whisker growth induced by implantation of cultured vibrissa dermal papilla cells in the adult rat. J Embryol Exp Morphol 97:111–124
Houssay AB, Epper CE, Pazo JH (1965) Neurohormonal regulation of the hair cycles in rats and mice. In: Lyne AG, Short BF (eds) Biology of skin and hair growth. Angus and Robertson, Sydney, pp 641–654
Hsia SL, Mussallem AJ, Witten VH (1965) Further metabolic studies of hydrocortisone-4-14C in human

skin. J Invest Dermatol 45:384-390
Huang T, Larson DL, Lewis SR (1977) Burn alopecia. Plast Reconstr Surg 60:673
Huber E (1930) Evolution of facial musculature and cutaneous field of trigeminus. Q Rev Biol 5:133-188
Hume WJ, Potten CS (1980) Changes in proliferative activity as cells move along undulating basement membrane in stratified squamous epithelia. Br J Dermatol 103:499-504
Hümpel M, Dogs G, Wendt H, Speck U (1978) Plasmaspiegel und pharmakokinetic von cyproteronacetat nach oraler applikation als 50-mg-tablett bei 5 mannern. Arzneimittelforshung 28:319
Hunting ALL (1988) Can there be cleaning and conditioning in the same product? Cosmet Toiletries 103:73-82
Hurley HJ, Shelley WB (1960) The human apocrine sweat gland in health and disease. Thomas, Springfield
Ibrahim L, Wright EA (1975) The growth of rat and mouse vibrissae under normal and some abnormal conditions. J Embryol Exp Morphol 33:831-844
Ibrahim L, Wright EA (1977) Inductive capacity of irradiated dermal papillae. Nature 265:733-734
Ibrahim L, Wright EA (1978) The effect of a single plucking at different times in the hair cycle on the growth of individual mouse vibrissae. Br J Dermatol 99:365-370
Ibrahim L, Wright EA (1982) A quantitative study of hair growth using mouse and rat vibrissal follicles. I. Dermal papilla volume determines hair volume. J Embryol Exp Morphol 72:209-224
Igarashi R, Morohashi M, Takeuchi S, Sato Y (1980) Immunofluorescent studies of complement C3 in the hair follicles of normal scalps and of scalp affected by alopecia areata. Acta Derm Venereol (Stockh) 60:33
Ikoma E, Tsumoto S (1971) A study on the thickness of human parietal hair in reference to genetics (in Japanese). Wakayama Med Rep 15:65-74
Imada K (1983) Aspects of hair growth promoters (in Japanese). Fragrance J 58:24-27
Imai R, Miura Y, Mochida K, et al (1992) Organ culture conditions of human hair follicles. J Dermatol Sci 3:163-171
Imai R, Takamori K, Ogawa H (1994) Changes in populations of HLA-DR+CD3+ cells and CD57-CD16 cells in alopecia areata after corticoid therapy. Jpn Dermatol 188:103-107
Imura H (1982) Concept of neuroendocrinology. In: Nagatsu T, Matsuo T, Yuu M, Uwazima K (eds) Psychoneuroendocrinology. Nakyama, Tokyo
Inaba M (1976) Treatment of hircismus and hyperhidrosis of the axilla, 2nd edn (in Japanese). Kin-ensha, Tokyo
Inaba M (1981) How to regenerate the hair (in Japanese)? Jpn J Sci 1:106-116
Inaba M (ed) (1982a) Treatment of MPB (in Japanese). Mainichi Shimbun, Tokyo
Inaba M (1982b) The possible mechanism of severe alopecia areata and its treatment (in Japanese). Mainichi Life 11:74-80
Inaba M (1983a) Histologic study of the causative mechanism of alopecia areata (in Japanese). Jpn J Aesth Surg 21:90-95
Inaba M (1983b) Process of development of the fetal eyebrow (in Japanese). Jpn J Aesth Surg 21:127-137
Inaba M (1983c) Study on local anesthesia dilution (2nd report) (in Japanese). Jpn J Aesth Surg 21:122-126
Inaba M (1985) Can human hair grow again? Azabu, Tokyo
Inaba M, Ezaki T (1977) New instrument for hircismus and hyperhidrosis operation (subcutaneous shaver). Plast Reconstr Surg 59:864-866
Inaba M, Inaba Y (1984) Possible mechanism and treatment of male pattern baldness—with special reference to suppression of reductase enzyme activity (nonsteroidal anti-androgen). Int J Aesth Surg 2:112-120
Inaba M, Inaba Y (1986) Studies of human scalp hair leading to a new hypothesis of the human hair cycle. Int J Aesth Surg 3(2):83-95
Inaba M, Inaba Y (1989) Sebaceous gland hypothesis and male pattern baldness (in Japanese). Fragrance J 5:51-60
Inaba M, Inaba Y (1990a) Transitional observations of scalp hair in order of age (in Japanese). Proceedings of the 49th congress of Japan society of aesthetic surgery, Tokyo, June 17, 1990
Inaba M, Inaba Y (1990b) Male pattern baldness: Sebaceous gland hypothesis. Cosmet Toiletries 105:77-87
Inaba M, Inaba Y (1992a) The question of hair regeneration. In: Inaba M, Inaba Y (eds) Human body odor. Springer, Tokyo Berlin Heidelberg New York
Inaba M, Inaba Y (1992b) Basic principles of electrolysis and electrocoagulation. In: Inaba M, Inaba Y (eds) Human body odor. Springer, Tokyo Berlin Heidelberg New York, pp 142-146
Inaba M, Inaba Y (1993a) Single hair-bearing graft and minigraft transplantation and their histological findings. Proceedings of the congress of international society of hair surgeons, April 30-May 2, 1993. Dallas Hair Transplant Forum 3(3):12-13
Inaba M, Inaba Y (1994a) Follicular stem cell (abstract). In: Proceedings of the congress of the American academy of cosmetic surgeons 10th annual scientific meeting. Am J Cosmet Surg 11:64
Inaba M, Inaba Y (1994b) Epithelial-mesenchymal interaction especially on the process of formation of dermal papilla (in Japanese). Jpn J Aesth Surg 31:30-34
Inaba M, McKinstry CT (1982) Possible mechanism of male pattern baldness. Int J Aesth Surg 2:33-39
Inaba M, Anthony J, Ezaki T (1978a) Radical operation to stop axillary odor and hyperhidrosis. Plast Reconstr Surg 62:355-360
Inaba M, Anthony J, Ezaki T (1978b) A new "double tie-over mehod" and its applications. Aesth Plast Surg 2:277-284
Inaba M, Anthony J, Ezaki T (1978c) Regeneration of axillary hair and related phenomenon after removal of deep dermal and subcutaneous tissue by a special "shaving" technique. J Dermatol Surg Oncol 4:912
Inaba M, Anthony J, Ezaki T (1978d) Preparation of thick tissue sections using Cellophane tape (an improved method). Br J Dermatol 98:625-630
Inaba M, Anthony J, McKinstry CT (1979a) Histologic study of the regeneration of axillary hair after removal with subcutaneous tissue shaver. J Invest Dermatol 72:224-231
Inaba M, McKinstry CT, Anthony J, Ezaki T (1979b) Epilation by electrocoagulation: Factors that result in regrowth of hair. Jpn J Plast Reconstr Surg 22:29-35
Inaba M, McKinstry CT, Anthony J (1979c) The

development of the hair (in Japanese). IX World Congress of Gynecology and Obstetrics, Tokyo, October 25-31
Inaba M, McKinstry CT, Ezaki T (1980a) Studies of human scalp hair leading to a new theory of the human hair cycle (in Japanese). Jpn J Aesth Surg 19:16-31
Inaba M, McKinstry CT, Umezawa F (1980b) Histologic observation on the increase in density of axillary hair during adolescence (in Japanese). Jpn J Aesth Surg 19:7-15
Inaba M, McKinstry CT, Ezaki T (1981a) A study of free skin graft with hair, especially in connection with the sebaceous gland. J Int Soc Aesth Surg 1:88-94
Inaba M, McKinstry CT, Umezawa F (1981b) Clinical observations on the development and eventual character of hair in the axillae of human beings. J Dermatol Surg Oncol 7:340-341
Inaba M, McKinstry CT, Umezawa F (1981c) Regeneration of axillary hair after plucking. J Dermatol Surg Oncol 7:249-259
Inaba M, McKinstry CT, Ezaki T (1981d) The process of replacement of vellus hairs by coarse hairs. J Dermatol Surg Oncol 7:732-736
Inaba M, McKinstry CT, Ezaki T (1981e) A study of the free skin graft with hair, especially in connection with sebaceous glands. Int J Aesth Surg 1:88-94
Inaba M, McKinstry CT, Ezaki T (1982) Histologic observation on the increase in density of axillary hair during adolescence. J Dermatol Surg Oncol 8:59-66
Inaba M, Inaba Y, Choi YC (1987) The vascular system in hair follicles (in Japanese). Jpn J Aesth Surg 25:94-105
Inaba M, Inaba Y, Murakoshi S (1988a) Electro-coagulation in permanent epilation. Proceedings of the first international congress of cosmetic surgery, Oslo, October 10-13, 1988
Inaba M, Inaba Y, Choi YC, Tai HC, Song JY (1988b) Study of distribution of estrogen and progesterone receptors in scalp tissue (in Japanese). Jpn J Aesth Surg 25:175-180
Inaba M, Inaba Y, Choi YC (1989) Scalp hair transposition flap method. 46th Congress of J Soc Aesth Surg (J JSAS), 28 May
Inaba M, Inaba Y, Choi YC (1990b) Single hair graft transplantation (first series) (in Japanese). Jpn J Soc Aesth Surg 27:187-194
Inaba M, Inaba Y, Choi YC, Chung TH (1991) Effects of several anti-cancer agents on hair growth (first report) (in Japanese). Jpn J Soc Aesth Surg 28:89-99
Inaba M, Inaba Y, Inagaki H (1992) Hair cycles in the Japanese monkey, especially to hair regeneration. Proceedings of the 58th aesthetic surgeons congress, Tokyo, August 30, 1992
Inaba Y, Inaba M (1995) Prevention and treatment of linear scar formation in the scalp: basic principles of the mechanism of scar formation. Aesth Plast Surg 19:369-378
Inaba Y, Inaba M, Choi YC (1990a) Histological study of free coarse hair-bearing graft (second series) (in Japanese). Jpn J Soc Aesth Surg 27:195-205
Inaba Y, Inaba M, Mikami M (1993) Single hair-bearing graft transplantation: Inaba aesthetic surgery. Int J Aesth Restor Surg 1.2:137-144
Invernizzi G, Gala C, Russo R, Polenghi M, Manca G, Conte G (1987) Life events and personality factors in patients with alopecia areata. Med Sci Res 15:1219-1220
Ishibashi Y, Tsuru N (1976) Innervation of human hair follicles. In: Kobori T, Montagna W (eds) Biology and disease of the hair. Tokyo University Press, Tokyo, pp 73-85
Itami S (1993) The development of the hair and androgen (in Japanese). Mook, 23-30 Kanekara, Tokyo
Itami S, Takayasu S (1981) Activity of 17β-hydroxysteroid dehydrogenase in various tissues of human skin. Br J Dermatol 105:693-699
Itami S, Takayasu S (1982) Activity of 3β-hydroxysteroid dehydrogenase Δ4-5 isomerase in the human skin. Arch Dermatol Res 274:289-294
Itami S, Takayasu S (1983) An androgen-dependent pilosebaceous tumor spontaneously developed in the Japanese house musk shrew *Suncus murinus*. J Steroid Biochem 19:1141
Itami S, Kurata S, Sonoda T, Takayasu S (1991a) Mechanism of action of androgen in dermal papilla cells. Ann NY Acad Sci 642:385-395
Itami S, Kurata S, Sonoda T, Takayasu S (1991b) Characterization of 5α-reductase in cultured human dermal papilla cells from beard and occipital scalp hair. J Invest Dermatol 96:57-60
Itemize S, Kurata S, Takayasu S (1990) 5α-Reductase activity in cultured human dermal papilla cells from beard compared with reticular dermal fibroblasts. J Invest Dermatol 94:150-152
Ito M (1989) Biologic roles of the innermost cell layer of the outer root sheath in human anagen hair follicles. Further electron microscopic study. Arch Dermatol Res 281:254-259
Ito M, Sato Y (1986) The innermost cell layer of the outer root sheath in anagen hair follicle: Light and electron microscopic study. Arch Dermatol Res 279:112-119
Ito M, Sato Y (1987) Ultrastructure of the innermost cell layer of the outer root sheath in anagen hair follicles of animals. Jpn J Dermatol 97:1239-1246
Ito M, Sato Y (1990) Dynamic ultrastructural changes of the connective tissue sheath of human hair follicles during hair cycle. Arch Dermatol Res 282:434-441
Jackson D, Church RE, Ebling FJ (1972) Hair diameter in female baldness. Br J Dermatol 87:361-367
Jahoda CAB, Oliver RF (1981) The growth of vibrissa dermal papilla cells in vitro. Br J Dermatol 105:623-627
Jahoda CAB, Oliver RF (1984) Vibrissa dermal papilla cell aggregative behavior in vitro and in vivo. J Embryol Exp Morphol 79:211-224
Jahoda CAB, Oliver RF (1990) The dermal papilla and the growth of hair. In: Orfanos CE, Happle R (eds) Hair and hair disease. Springer, Berlin Heidelberg Tokyo, pp 19-44
Jahoda CAB, Horne KA, Oliver RF (1984) Induction of hair growth by implantation of cultured dermal papilla cells. Nature 311:560-562
Jakubovic HR, Ackerman AB (1985) Structure and function of skin: Development, morphology, and physiology. In: Moshlla SL, Hurley HJ (eds) Dermatology. WB Saunders, Philadelphia
Jarrett A (1955) The effects of stilbestrol on the surface sebum and upon acne vulgaris. Br J Dermatol 67:166-179
Jenkins JS, Ash S (1973) The metabolism of testosterone by human skin in disorders of hair growth. J Endocrinol 59:345-351
Jenkinson D, Moewan D, Elder HY, Montgomery I, Moss

VA (1985) Comparative studies of the ultrastructure of the sebaceous gland. Tissue Cell 17:683–698
Jensen EV, De Sombre ER (1972) Mechanism of action of the female sex hormones. Annu Rev Biochem 41:203
Jensen EV, De Sombre ER (1973) Estrogen receptor interaction. Estrogenic hormones effect transformation of specific receptor proteins to a biochemically functional form. Science 182:126
Jensen HA, Mikkelsen HI, Wadskov S, Sondergaard J (1976) Cutaneous reactions to propranolol (inderal). Acta Med Scand 199:363
Johnson E (1975) Epilation of growing hair follicles. J Exp Zool 192:259–263
Johnson MA, Latham MC, Roe D (1976) An evaluation of the use of changes in hair root morphology in the assessment of protein calorie malnutrition. Am J Clin Nutr 29:502
Johnson JI Jr (1977) Central nervous system. In: Hunsaker D II (ed) The biology of marsupials. Academic, New York, pp 157–278
Joseph J, Townsend FJ (1961) The healing of defects in immobile skin of rabbits. Br J Surg 48:557–564
Juri J (1975) Use of parieto-occipital flaps in surgical treatment of baldness. Plast Reconstr Surg 55:456
Kabaker S (1979) Juri flap procedure for the treatment of baldness. Arch Otolaryngol 105:509–514
Kabaker S (1982) Flap procedures in hair replacement surgery. In: Epstein E, Epstein E Jr (eds) Skin surgery, 5th edn, vol 1. Thomas, Springfield, pp 558–559
Kabaker S (1988) Lateral flaps in surgery for male pattern baldness. In: Unger WP, Nordstrom REA (eds) Hair transplantation. Marcel Dekker, New York
Kabaker S, Kridel RWH, Krugman ME, Swenson RW (1986) Tissue expansion in the treatment of alopecia. Arch Otolaryngol 112:720–725
Kahan BD (1982) Cyclosporin A: Selective anti-T cell agent. Clin Haematol 11:743–761
Kakizoe K (1969) Correlation between cancer of the stomach and alopecia (in Japanese). J Kurume Med 32:1540–1565
Kantouch A, Abdel-Fattah P (1972) Oxidation of wool with chlorine and some chlorinated compounds. Kolor Ertes 14:2-9
Katsuoka K (1991) Biological characteristics of cultured papilla cells—localization of androgen receptors and chemotactic factors for epithelial cells (in Japanese). Hum Cell 4(3):190–196
Katsuoka K, Schell H, Hornstein OP, Deinlein E, Wessel B (1986) Comparative morphological and growth kinetics studies of human hair bulb papilla cells and root sheath fibroblasts in vitro. Arch Dermatol Res 279:20–25
Katsuoka K, Inamura K, Nishioka K, Nishiyama S (1989) Effects of dihydrotestosterone on cultured hair papilla cells and localization of its receptors (in Japanese). Jpn J Dermatol 99:529–536
Kaufman JP (1976) Telogen effluvium secondary to starvation diet. Arch Dermatol 112:731
Kaufman M, Pinsky L, Simard L, Wong SC (1982) Defective activation of androgen receptor complexes: A marker of androgen insensitivity. Mol Cell Endrocrinol 25:151
Kealey I (1990) Isolated human skin glands and appendages. In: Kluwer JC (ed) Epithelia: Advances in cell physiology and cell culture. Academic, London
Keenan BS, Meyer WI, Hadjian AJ, Jonsett W, Migeon CJ (1974) Syndrome of androgen insensitivity in man: Absence of 5α-DHT binding protein in skin fibroblasts. J Clin Endocrinol Metab 38:1143–1146
Kessler EA (1963) Die Frontalotomie zur Behandlung der Glatzenbildung. Arztl Prax 14:2282–2284
Khoury EL, Price VH, Abdel-Salam MM, Stern M, Greenspan JS (1992) Topical minoxidil in alopecia areata: No effect on the perifollicular lymphoid infiltration. J Invest Dermatol 99:40–47
Kianto U, Rennala Y, Karvonen J (1977) HLA-B12 in alopecia areata. Arch Dermatol 113:1716–1717
Kiesewetter F (1992) Effect of androgens and antiandrogens on hair growth in vivo and in vitro. Science of Hair, 6th International Symposium, 18 November, Tokyo
Kiesewetter F, Schell H, Seidel C, Arai A, Hornstein OP (1989) Cell kinetics of anagen scalp hair bulbs in hirsutism analyzed by DNA flow cytometry. Arch Dermatol Res 281:507–509
Kiesewetter F, Schell H, Seidel C, Arai A, Hornstein OP (1990) Segmental cell kinetics of the human anagen hair: A DNA-flow cytometric analysis. J Invest Dermatol 94:456–460
Killackey HP, Belford G, Ryugo R, Ryugo DK (1976) Anomalous organization of thalamo-cortical projections consequent to vibrissae removal in the newborn rat and mouse. Brain Res 104:309–315
Kim JC (1993) Regrowth of grafted human scalp hair after removal of the bulb. Hair Transplant Forum 3:14–15
Kinebuchi S (1972) Undeveloped desmosome in the undifferentiated cells in the hair bulb (in Japanese). Jpn J Dermatol 82:1–17
Klaber MR, Munro DD (1978) Alopecia areata: immunofluorescence and other studies. Br J Dermatol 99:383–386
Klein-Szanto AJP (1977) Clear and dark basal keratinocytes in human epidermis. J Cutan Pathol 4:275–280
Klevar LM (1978) Hair as biopsy material—progress and prospects. Arch Intern Med 138:1127
Kligman AM (1961) Pathologic dynamics of human hair loss I. Telogen effluvium. Arch Dermatol 83:175–198
Kligman AM (1988) The comparative histopathology of male-pattern baldness and senescent baldness. Clin Dermatol 6:108–118
Kligman AM, Shelley WB (1958) An investigation of the biology of the human sebaceous gland. J Invest Dermatol 30:99–105
Kligman AM, Strauss JS (1956) The formation of vellus hair follicles from human adult epidermis. J Invest Dermatol 27:19–23
Kligman AM, McGinley KJ, Lyden JJ (1981a) Studies on the effect of shampoos on scalp lipids and bacteria. In: Orfanos CE, Montagna W, Stüttgen G (eds) Hair research. Springer, Berlin Heidelberg
Kligman AM, McGinley KJ, Lyden JJ (1981b) The nature of dandruff. J Soc Cosmet Chem 27:111
Knutson DD (1974) Ultrastructural observation in acne vulgaris. The normal sebaceous follicle and acne lesions. J Invest Dermatol 62:288–307
Kobayashi K (1987) Histological interaction in the morphological formation of hair. Bull Biosci Soc 1:4–16
Kobayashi K, Nishimura E (1991) Ectopic growth of mouse whiskers from implanted lengths of plucked vibrissa follicle. J Invest Dermatol 92:278–282
Kobayashi T (1984) Electrosurgery using double-coated

needles (in Japanese). 27th congress of the Japanese Society of Plastic and Reconstructive Surgeons, Tokyo, April 4-7
Kobayashi T (1985) Electroepilation using insulated needles: Epilation. J Dermatol Surg Oncol 11:993-1000
Kobayashi T, Kamiyama G, Akagawa T (1979) A study of synthetic fiber implantation for baldness (in Japanese). J Jpn Soc Aesth Plast Surg 1:132
Kobayashi T, Kamiyama G, Akagawa T (1981a) Research and study on artificial hair implantation (in Japanese). J Jpn Soc Aesth Plast Surg 3:12
Kobayashi T, Kamiyama G, Akagawa T, Akamatsu T (1981b) Research and investigation into synthetic fiber implantation for baldness. Transactions, 6th congress of international society of aesthetic and plastic surgery, Tokyo, September 22-29
Kobori T, Montagna W (eds) (1976) Medicine of hair (in Japanese). Bunkodo, Tokyo
Kollar EJ (1966) An in vitro study of hair and vibrissa development in embryonic mouse skin. J Invest Dermatol 46:254-262
Kollar EJ (1970) The induction of hair follicles by embryonic dermal papilla. J Invest Dermatol 55:374-378
Kondo S, Hozumi Y, Arno K (1990) Organ culture of human scalp hair follicles: Effect of testosterone and oestrogen on hair growth. Arch Dermatol Res 282:442-445
Koperski JA, Orenberg EK, Wilkinson DI (1987) Topical minoxidil therapy for androgenetic alopecia: A 30-month study. Arch Dermatol 123:1483-1487
Kropfi P (1976) Untersuchungen zur Wirkung der Vitamin-A-Säure bei experimentell ausgelöster Follikel-Keratase. Dermatologica 153:88-95
Krstic AV, Konstantinovic SV, Zunic MZ, Ilic-Krstic BJ (1981) Traction alopecia due to traditional hair styles. In: Orfanos CE, Montagna W, Stuttgen G (eds) Hair research. Springer, Berlin Heidelberg, pp 390-391
Kuchinska R (1973) Chemische Aspekte des Haarausfalls und ihre kosmetologische Bedeutung. Kosmetologie 5:177
Kuester W, Happle R (1984) The inheritance of common baldness: Two B or not two B? J Am Acad Dermatol 11:921-926
Kuhn SR (1980) Treatment of pattern baldness with fiber implantation. Arch Dermatol 116:21
Kukita A (1957) Changes in tyroninase activity during melanocyte proliferation. J Invest Dermatol 23:273-274
Kuntz BM, Selzle D, Braun-Falco O (1977) HLA antigens in alopecia areata. Arch Dermatol 113:1717
Kuroki T (1983) The birth of cancer cells (in Japanese). Asahi Shinbun, Tokyo
Kuttenn F, Mowszowicz I, Schaison IG, Mauvais-Jarvis P (1977) Androgen production and skin metabolism in hirsutism. J Endocrinol 75:83-91
Kuttenn F, Mowszowicz I, Wright F, Baudot N, Jaffiol C, Robin M, Mauvais-Jarvis P (1979) Male pseudohermaphroditism: A comparative study of one case of 5α-reductase deficiency with three complete forms of testicular feminization. J Clin Endocrinol Metab 49:861-865
Lajtha LG (1979) Stem cell concepts. Differentiation 14:23-24
Lajtha LG (1983) Stem cell concepts. In: Potten CS (ed) Stem cells: Their identification and characterization. Churchill Livingstone, New York, pp 1-11
Lajtha LG, Pozzi LV, Schofield R, Fox M (1969) Kinetic properties of haemopoietic stem cells. Cell Tissue Kinet 2:39-49
Lane EB, Wilson CA, Hughes BR, Leigh IM (1991) Stem cells in hair follicles. Ann NY Acad Sci 197-213
Lassus A, Kianto U, Johansson E (1980) PUVA treatment for alopecia areata. Dermatologica 161:298-304
Lattanand A, Johnson WC (1975) Male pattern alopecia. A histopathologic study. J Cutan Pathol 2:58-70
Lavker RM, Sun TT (1981) Heterogeneity in epidermal basal keratinocytes: Morphological and functional correlations. Science 215:1239-1241
Lavker RM, Cotsarelis G, Wei ZG, Sun T-T (1991) Stem cells of pelage, vibrissae, and eyelash follicles: The hair cycle and tumor formation. Ann NY Acad Sci 642:214-225
Lavker RM, Fryer E, Margolis-Fryer, Ostad M, Cotsarelis G, Sun TT (1992) Cells in the bulge region of mouse hair follicle undergo transient proliferation during onset of anagen and in response to physical and chemical stimuli (abstract). J Invest Dermatol 98:581a
Lavker RM, Miller S, Wilson C, Cotsarelis G, Wei ZG, Yand JS, Sun TT (1993) Hair follicle stem cells: Their location, role in hair cycle and involvement in skin tumor formation. J Invest Dermatol 101:16-26
Layne E (1957) Spectrophotonetric and turbidimetric methods for measuring proteins. Methods Enzymol 3:447-454
Lenoir MC, Bernard BA, Pautrat G, Darmon M, Shroot B (1988) Outer root sheath cells of human hair follicle are able to regenerate a fully differentiated epidermis in vitro. Dev Biol 130:610-620
Leonhardi G (1973) Biochemische Aspekte der Seborrhoe. Kosmetol Dermatol 10-13
Lepaw MI (1979) Complications of implantation of synthetic fibers into scalps for hair replacement. J Dermatol Surg Oncol 5:201
Lepaw MI (1980a) Scalp injuries from hair replacement. Consultant 149; February 20
Lepaw MI (1980b) Therapy and histopathology of complications from synthetic fiber implants for hair replacement. J Am Acad Dermatol 3:195
Lepaw MI (1982) Synthetic fibers and processed human hair implants for the correction of male pattern alopecia. In: Epstein E, Epstein E Jr (eds) Skin surgery, 5th edn. Thomas, Springfield, p 586
Lepaw MI (1983) Evaluation of various therapies for damaged scalps due to hair and fiber implants. J Dermatol Surg Oncol 9:460
Levy J, Burshell A, Marbach M, Ayllalo L, Glick JH (1980) Interaction of spinolactone with oestradial receptors in cytosol. J Endocrinol 84:371
Lewis LA (1979) Alternative techniques in punch transplanting. In: Unger WP (ed) Hair transplantation, 1st edn. Marcel Dekker, New York, pp 179-185
Liang T, Hoyer S, Yu R, Soltani K, Lorincz AL, Hiipakka RA, Liao S (1993) Immunocytochemical localization of androgen receptors in human skin using monoclonal antibodies against the androgen receptor. J Invest Dermatol 100:663-666
Li L, Margolis LB, Paus R, Hoffman RM (1992) Hair shaft elongation, follicle growth, and spontaneous regression in long-term, gelatin sponge-supported histoculture of human scalp skin. Proc Natl Acad Sci USA 89:8764-8768
Li ML, Aggeler J, Farson DA, Hatier C, Hassell J, Bissell

MJ (1987) Influence of a reconstituted basement membrane and its components on casein gene expression and secretion in mouse mammary epithelial cells. Proc Natl Acad Sci USA 84:136–140

Lille FR, Wang H (1941) Physiology of development of the feather. V. Experimental morphogenesis. Physiol Zool 14:103–133

Lille FR, Wang H (1994) Physiology of development of the feather. VII. An experimental study of induction. Physiol Zool 14:103–133

Lindberg K, Rheinwald JG (1989) Suprabasal 40kDa keratin (K19) expression as an immunohistologic marker of premalignancy in oral epithelium. Am J Pathol 134:189–198

Link RE, Paus R, Stenn KS, Kuklinska E, Moellmann G (1990) Epithelial growth by rat vibrissae follicles in vitro requires mesenchymal contact via native extracellular matrix. J Invest Dermatol 95:202–207

Longacre TJ, De Stefano GA, Halmstrand K (1962) Reconstruction of eyebrow: Graft versus flap Plast Reconstr Surg 30:638–648

Lookingbill DP, Egan N, Santen RJ, Dermers LM (1988) Correlation of serum 3α-androstanediol glucuronide with acne and chest hair density in men. J Clin Endocrinol Metab 986–991

Lookingbill DP, Dermers LM, Wang C (1991) Clinical and biological parameters of androgen action in healthy Caucasian versus Chinese subjects. J Clin Endocrinol Metab 72:1242–1248

Loriaux DL, Menard F, Taylor A (1976) Spironolactone and endocrine disfunction. Ann Intern Med 85:630–636

Lovell JE, Getty R (1957) The hair follicle epidermis, dermis and skin glands of the dog. Am J Vet Res 18:873–885

Lowry CH, Rosenbrough NJ, Farr AL, Randall F (1951) Protein measurement with the Folin phenal reagent. J Biol Chem 193:265–275

Lubahn DB, Joseph DR, Sar M, Tan J, Higgs HN, Larson RE, French FS, Wilson EM (1988) The human androgen receptor: Complementary deoxyribonucleic acid (DNA) cloning, sequence analysis and gene expression in prostate. Mol Cell Endocrinol 2:1265–1275

Lucky AW (1988) The paradox of androgens and balding: Where are we now? J Invest Dermatol 91:99–100

Lucky AW, McGuire J, Rosenfield RL, Lucky PA, Rich BH (1983) Plasma androgens in women with acne vulgaris. J Invest Dermatol 81:70–74

Lucky AW, Eisenfeld AJ, Visintin I (1985) Autoradiographic localization tritiated dihydrotestosterone in the flank organ of the albino hamster. J Invest Dermatol 84:122–125

Ludwig E (1962) Der heutige Stand des Wissens über die Glatze. Hautarzt 13:337–339

Ludwig E (1977) Classification of the types of androgenetic alopecia occurring in the female sex. Br J Dermatol 97:247–254

Luderschmidt C, Eirrmann W, Jawny J (1983) Steroid hormone receptors and their relevance for sebum production in the sebaceous gland ear model of the Syrian hamster. Arch Dermatol Res 275:175–180

Lutz G, Fritsche C, Kreyesel HW (1988) Zirkulierende T-lymphozytengruppen bei Alopecia areata. Aktuel Dermatol 14:222–226

Lyne AG (1957) The development and replacement of pelage hair in the bandicoot *Perameles nasuta* geoffroy (Marsupialia: Peramelidae). Aust J Biol Sci 10:197–216

Lyne AG (1959) The systematic and adaptive significance of the vibrissae. Proc Zool Soc Lond 133:79–132

Lyne AG (1966) The development of hair follicles. Aust J Biol Sci 28:374

Lyne AG (1970) The development of hair follicles in the marsupial *Trichosurus vulpecula*. Aust J Biol Sci 23:1241–1253

Lyne AG, Brook AH (1964) Neogenesis of wool follicles. Aust J Biol Sci 17:514–520

Lyne AG, Heideman MJ (1959) The pre-natal development of skin and hair in cattle (*Bos taurus* L). Aust J Biol Sci 12:72–95

Lyne AG, Heideman MJ (1960) The pre-natal development of skin and hair in cattle II. *Bos indicus* L, *B. taurus* L. Aust J Biol Sci 13:584–599

Lynfield VL (1960) Effect of pregnancy on the human hair cycle. J Invest Dermatol 55:323

Madsen A (1964) Studies on the "bulge" (wulst) in special basal cell epitheliomas. Arch Dermatol 89:698–708

Magara Y (1982) Stabilized chloride dioxide. (in Japanese) Jpn Med J 3059:152

Maibach HI, Feldmann R, Payne B, Hutshell T (1968) Scalp and forehead sebum production in male patterned alopecia. In: Baccaredda-Boy A, Moretti G, Frey JR (eds) Biopathology of pattern alopecia. Karger, Basel, pp 171–176

Mainwaring WIP (1977) The mechanism of action of androgens Monographs on endocrinology, vol 10. Springer, Berlin Heidelberg Tokyo

Malten KE, den Arend JACJ (1985) Irritant contact dermatitis. Traumiterative and cumulative impairment by cosmetics, climate, and other daily loads. Derm-Beruf Welt 33:125–132

Manders EK (1984) Skin expansion to eliminate large scalp defects. Ann Plast Surg 12:305–312

Manders EK, Au VK, Wong RKM (1987) Scalp expansion for male pattern baldness. Clin Plast Surg 14(3):469

Mann SJ (1968) The tylotrich (hair) follicle of the American opossum. Anat Rec 160:171–180

Marechal RE (1977) New treatment for seborrheic alopecia: The ligature of the arteries of the scalp. J Natl Med Assoc 69:709–711

Margot S (1980) Growing new hair! How to keep what you have and fill in where it's thin. Autumn, Brookline

Marks MW, Argenta LC (1988) Skin expansion in reconstructive surgery. Facial Plast Surg 5:301

Marritt E (1980) Transplantation of single hairs from the scalp as eyelashes. J Dermatol Surg Oncol 6:271–273

Marritt E (1988) Micrograft dilators: Pursuit of the undetectable hair line. J Dermatol Surg Oncol 14(3):268–275

Marrs JM, Voorhees JJ (1971) Preliminary characterization of an epidermal chalone-like inhibitor. J Invest Dermatol 56:353

Marton MH (1940) Treatment of hypertrichosis by improved apparatus and technique. Arch Phys Ther 21:678–683

Marzola M (1984) An alternative hair replacement method. In: Norwood OT, Shiell RC (eds) Hair transplant surgery, 2nd edn. Thomas, Springfield, pp 315–323

Mason P (1948) Pigment cells in man. In: Miner RW (ed) The biology of melanomas, vol 4. Special Publication of the New York Academy of Science, pp 15-52
Masters R (1984) Psychology and skin. In: Soter N, Baden HP (eds) Pathophysiology of dermatologic disease. McGraw-Hill, New York, pp 441-453
Matias JR, Orentreich N, Malloy V, DeFeo CP III, Matias L (1984) The lack of effect of 11α-hydroxyprogesterone on the flank-organ and ear sebaceous glands of adult male Syrian golden hamsters. Arch Dermatol Res 276:346-348
Maurer F (1895) Die Epidermis und ihre Abkömmlinge. Wilhelm Engelmann, Leipzig
Mauvais-Jarvis P, Bercovici JP, Crepy D, Gautheir F (1970) Studies on testosterone metabolism in subjects with testicular feminization syndrome. J Clin Invest 49:31-37
Mauvais-Jarvis P, Kutten F, Baudot N (1974) Inhibition of testosterone conversion to dihydrotestosterone in men treated percutaneously by progesterone. J Clin Endocrinol 38:142-147
Mauvais-Jarvis P, Kutten F, Wright F (1976) Testosterone 5α-reduction in human skin: An index of androgenecity. In: James VHT, Serio N, Giusti G (eds) The endocrine function of human ovary. Academic, New York, pp 481-494
McCarthy L (1940) Diagnosis and treatment of diseases of the hair. Mosby Yearbook, St. Louis
McKinstry CT (1979) Epilation by electrocoagulation: Factors that result in regrowth of hair. J Dermatol Surg Oncol 5:407-411
McLaren DS (1971) Nutritional disease. In: Fitzpatrick TB, Arndt KA, Clark WH Jr, Eisen AZ, Van Scott EJ, Vaughan JH (eds) Dermatology in general. McGraw-Hill, New York, p 1074
McPhaul MJ, Marcelli M (1992) Molecular defects in the androgen receptor causing androgen resistance. J Invest Dermatol 98:97S-99S
Mehta PK, Mamdani B, Sharsky RM (1975) Severe hypertension: Treatment with minoxidil. JAMA 233:249-252
Meiers HG, Grobbel B (1974) Das Kopfhaar im Alter. Z Geront 7:427-430
Meleney FL (1952) Present role of zinc peroxide in the treatment of surgical infections. JAMA 149:1450-1452
Merk HF (1990) Drugs affecting hair growth. In: Orfanos CE, Happle R (eds) Hair and hair diseases. Springer, Berlin Heidelberg New York
Messenger AG (1984) The culture of dermal papilla cells from human hair follicles. Br J Dermatol 110:685-689
Messenger AG (1989) Isolation, culture and in vitro behaviour of cells isolated from the papilla of human hair follicle. In: Van Neste D, Lachapelle JM, Antoine JL (eds) Trends in human hair growth and alopecia research. Kluwer, New York, pp 57-67
Messenger AG, Senior HJ, Bleehen SS (1986) The in vitro properties of dermal papilla cell lines established from human hair follicles. Br J Dermatol (Oxford) 114:425-430
Messenger AG, Elliott K, Temple A, Randall VA (1991) Expression of basement membrane proteins and interstitial collagens in dermal papillae of human hair follicles. J Invest Dermatol 96:93-97
Michel RH (1979) Inositol phospholipids in membrane function. Trends Biochem Sci 4:128
Miller JA, Darley CR, Karkavitsas, Carboy JD, Munro DD (1982) Low sex-hormone binding globulin levels in young women with diffuse hair loss. Br J Dermatol 106:331-336
Milne JA (1969) The metabolism of androgens by sebaceous glands. Br J Dermatol 81(suppl):23-28
Mishima Y (1964) Electron microscopic cytochemistry of melanosomes and mitochondria. J Histochem Cytochem 12:784-790
Mishima Y, Widlaw S (1966) Embryonic development of melanocytes in human hair and epidermis. J Invest Dermatol 46:263-277
Mitchell AJ, Krull EA (1984) Alopecia areata: Pathogenesis and treatment. J Am Acad Dermatol 11:763-775
Miyamoto J (1981) Powder grain and whole grain cultures (in Japanese). Shibata, Tokyo
Moll R, Franke WW, Schiller DL (1982) The catalogue of human cytokeratins: Patterns of expression in normal epithelia, tumors and cultured cells. Cell 31:11-24
Moll R, Moll L, Franke WW (1984) Differences of expression of cytokeratin polypeptides in various epithelial skin tumors. Arch Dermatol Res 276:349-363
Montagna W (1962) The structure and function of skin, 2nd edn. Academic, New York
Montagna W, Chase HB (1956) Histology and cytochemistry of human skin: X-irradiation of the scalp. Am J Anat 99:415-445
Montagna W, Ellis RA (1957) Histology and cytochemistry of human skin. XIII. The blood supply of the hair follicle. Natl Cancer Inst 19:451-463
Montagna W, Giacometti (1969) Histology and cytochemistry of human skin. XXXII. The external ear. Arch Dermatol 99:757-767
Montagna W, Parakkal PF (1974) The pilary apparatus in the structure and function of skin. In: Montagna W, Parakkal PF (eds) The structure and function of skin, 2nd edn. Academic, New York, pp 172-278
Montagna W, Van Scott EJ (1958) The anatomy of the hair follicle. In: Montagna W, Ellis RA (eds) The biology of hair growth. Academic, New York, pp 39-64
Montagna W, Chase HB, Malone JB, Melaragno HP (1952a) Cyclic changes in polysaccharides of the papilla of the hair follicle. Q J Microsc Soc 93:241-245
Montagna W, Chase HB, Melaragno HP (1952b) Skin of hairless mice. I. Formation of cysts and the distribution of lipids. J Invest Dermatol 19:83-94
Moore GPM, Panaretto BA, Robertson DJ (1981) Effects of epidermal growth factor on hair growth in the mouse. Endocrinology 88:293-299
Moore GPM, Panaretto BA, Carter NB (1985) Epidermal hyperplasia and wool follicle regression in sheep infused with epidermal growth factor. J Invest Dermatol 84:172-175
Moore GPM, Du Cross DL, Isaacs K, Pisansarakit P, Wynn PC (1991) Hair growth induction: Roles of growth factors. Ann NY Acad Sci 642:308-325
Moore PF (1968) The effects of diazoxide and benzothiadiazine diuretics upon phosphodiesterase. Ann NY Acad Sci 150:256
Moore RJ, Wilson D (1976) Steroid 5α-reductase in cultured human fibroblasts. Biochemical and genetic evidence for two distinct enzyme activities. J Biol Chem 251:5895-5900
Moore RJ, Griffin JE, Wilson JD (1975) Diminished 5α-reductase activity in extracts of fibroblasts cultured from patients with familial incomplete male

pseudohermaphroditism. J Biol Chem 250:7168–7172
Moretti G (1965) Das Haar. In: Stuttgen G (ed) Die normale und pathologische Physiologie der Haut. Gustav Fischer, Stuttgart, pp 506–553
Moretti G (1968) Das Haar. In: Jadassohn J (ed) Handbuch der Haut- und Geschlechts-krankheiten. Springer, Berlin Heidelberg, pp 491–623
Moretti G, Rebora A, Rampini E (1963) Il volume della ghiandola sebacea nell'alopecia areata. Minerva Dermatol 38:246
Morohashi M (1968) Electron microscopic study of sebaceous glands with special reference to effect of sexual hormones (in Japanese). Jpn J Dermatol Ser B 78:133–152
Mowszowicz I, Riahi M, Wright F, Bouchard P, Kuttenn F, Mauvais-Jarvis P (1981) Androgen receptor in human skin cytosol. J Clin Endocrinol Metab 52:338–344
Mowszowicz I, Wright F, Riahi M (1982) Androgen receptors in human skin cytosol: Physiological and pathological variations. Br J Dermatol 107 (suppl) 23:35–39
Moynahan EJ (1974) Acrodermatitis enteropathica: A lethal inherited human zinc deficiency disorder. Lancet II:339
Mulay S, Finkelberg R, Pinky L, Solomon S (1972) 4-14C testosterone by serially subcultured human skin fibroblasts. J Clin Endocrinol Metab 34:133
Muller SA, Winkelmann RK (1963) Alopecia areata: an evaluation of 736 patients. Arch Dermatol 88:20–297
Munro DD, Darley CR (1979) Hair. In: Fitzpatrick TB, Eisen AZ, Walff K, Freedberg IM, Austen KF (eds) Dermatology in general medicine. McGraw-Hill, New York
Muto Y (1986) Experience with artificial hair implantation (in Japanese). J Jpn Soc Aesth Plast Surg 8:8–11
Myers RT, Hamilton JB (1951) Regeneration and rate of growth of hair in man. Ann NY Acad Sci 53:562–568
Nanney LB, Magid M, Stoscheck M, King LE (1984) Comparision of epidermal growth factor binding and receptor distribution in normal human epidermis and epidermal appendage. J Invest Dermatol 83:385–393
Nataf J (1988) The long temporal vertical flap and various other scalp flaps. In: Unger W, Nordstrom RE (eds) Hair transplantation, 2nd edn. Marcel Dekker, New York, pp 675–690
Nataf J, Dardour JC (1988) The fusiform or navicular grafts. In: Unger WP, Nordstrom R (eds) Hair transplantation, 2nd edn. Marcel Dekker, New York, chap XXV
Nataf J, Elbaz JS, Pollet J (1976) Étude critique des transplantations de cuir chevelu et proposition d'une optique. Ann Chir Plast 21: 199–206
Nazzaro-Porro M, Passi S (1978) Identification of tyrosinase inhibitors in cultures of Pityrosporum. J Invest Dermatol 71:205–208
Nazzaro-Porro M, Passi S, Morpurgo G, Breathnach A (1979) Identification of tyrosinase inhibitors in cultures of *Pityrosporum* and their melanocytotoxic effect. In: Kalus NS (ed) Pigment cell 4: Biologic basis of pigmentation. Karger, Basel, p 234
Nazzaro-Porro MS, Boniforti SPL, Belsito F (1979) Effects of aging on fatty acids in skin surface lipids. J Invest Dermatol 73:112–117
Nazzaro-Porro M, Passi S, Picardo M, Breathnach A, Clayton R, Zina G (1983) Beneficial effect of 15% azelaic acid cream on acne vulgaris. Br J Dermatol 109:45–48
Neumann CG (1957) The expansion of an area of skin by progressive distension of a subcutaneous balloon. Plast Reconstr Surg 19:124
Neumann F (1977) Pharmacology and potential use of cyproterone acetate. Horm Metab Res 9:1–3
Nielsen PG (1982) Treatment of idiopathic hirsutism with spironolactone. Dermatologia 165:194–196
Nikkari TM, Valavaara (1969) The production of sebum in young rats. Effects of age, sex, hypophysectomy and treatment with somatotrophic hormone and sex hormones. J Endocrinol 43:113–18
Nikkari TM, Valavaara (1970) Effects of androgens and prolactin on the production and composition of sebum in hypophysectomized female rats. J Endocrinol 48:373–378
Nordström REA (1981) Micrografts for improvement of the frontal hairline after hair transplant. Aesthet Plast Surg 5:97
Nordström REA (1988a) Classification, anatomy, and instrumentation. In: Unger WP, Nordstrom REA (eds) Hair transplantation. Marcel Dekker, New York, pp 37–83
Nordström REA (1988b) Tissue expansion and flaps for surgical correction of male pattern baldness. Facial Plast Surg 5:347
Northcutt RC, Istand DP, Liddle GE (1969) An explanation for target organ unresponsiveness to testosterone in the testicular feminization syndrome. J Clin Endocrinol Metab 29:422
Norwood O'Tar T (1975) Male pattern baldness: Classification and incidence. South Med J 68:1359–1365
Norwood O'Tar T (1981) Predicting hair growth for hair transplantations. J Dermatol Surg Oncol 7:6
Norwood O'Tar T, Shiell RC (1984) Hair transplant surgery, 2nd edn. Thomas, Springfield
Novak E, Franz TJ, Headington JT, Wester RC (1985) Topically applied minoxidil in baldness. Int J Dermatol 24:83–87
Oba K (1988) Cosmetic products influencing hair growth. Cosmet Toiletries 103:69–79
Obermayer ME (1955) Psychocutaneous medicine. III. Thomas, Springfield
Ochi H (1989) Foods as viewed from the standpoint of control of aging (in Japanese). Fragrance J 1:76–81
Oericcochea M (1971) New three-flap scalp reconstruction technique. Br J Plast Surg 24:184
Ogata T (1953) Development of patterned alopecia (in Japanese). Sogo Rinsho (J Gen Clin Med) 2:101–106
O'Guin WM, Galvin S, Schermer A (1986) Patterns of keratin expression define distinct pathways of epithelial development and differentiation. In: Sawayer RH (ed) The molecular and developmental biology of keratins. Academic, New York, pp 97–125 (Current topics in developmental biology, vol 22)
Ohmori K (1980) Free scalp flap. Plast Reconstr Surg 65:42
Ohmori S (1981) Arterial island flap (in Japanese). In: Ohmori S (ed) Plastic surgery. Nanko-Do, Tokyo, p 52
Ohmori K (1988) Microsurgical free scalp flap and androgenic alopecia. In: Unger W, Nordström REA (eds) Hair transplantation, 2nd edn. Marcel Dekker, New York, pp 661–674
Ohmori K (1991) Microsurgical free temporoparietal flaps in surgery for male pattern baldness. Clin Plast

Surg 18:791–796
Ohmori K, Onizuka T (1965) Treatment of alopecia cicatricans using an artery flap. Plast Reconstr Surg 35:338–341
Okada T (1987) Wound healing and tissue transplantation: Mechanism of graft survival (in Japanese). In: Soeda S, Tsukada S, Ohoura T (eds) Color atlas of plastic and reconstructive surgery. Medical View, Tokyo, pp 70–73
Okochi T (1968) The study of interaction between secretion and perspiration in the disease region of 2-3 cases (in Japanese). Jpn J Dermatol 78:70
Okuda S (1939) Clinical and experimental studies on transplanting of living hair (in Japanese). Jpn J Dermatol 46:135–138
Oliver RF (1966a) Whisker growth after removal of the dermal papilla and lengths of the follicles in the hooded rat. J Embryol Exp Morphol 15:331–347
Oliver RF (1966b) Histological studies of whisker regeneration in the hooded rat. J Embryol Exp Morphol 16:231–244
Oliver RF (1967a) Ectopic regeneration of whiskers in the hooded rat from implanted lengths of vibrissa follicle wall. J Embryol Exp Morphol 17:27–34
Oliver RF (1967b) The experimental induction of whisker growth in the hooded rat by implantation of dermal papillae. J Embryol Exp Morphol 18:43–51
Oliver RF (1969) Regeneration of the dermal papilla and its influence on whisker growth. In: Montagna W, Dobson RL (eds) Advances in biology of skin, vol 9. Hair growth. Pergamon, Oxford
Oliver RF (1970) The induction of hair follicle formation in the adult hooded rat by vibrissa dermal papilla. J Embryol Exp Morphol 23:219–236
Oliver RF, Jahoda CAB (1981) Interfollicular interactions. In: Orfanos CE, Montagna W, Stüttgen G (eds) Hair research. Status and future aspects. Springer, Berlin Heidelberg Tokyo, pp 18–24
Oliver RF, Jahoda CAB (1988) Dermal-epidermal interactions. Clin Dermatol 6:74–82
Oliver RF, Jahoda CAB (1989) The dermal papilla and maintenance of hair growth. In: Rogers GE, Reis PR, Ward KA, Marshall RC (eds) The biology of wool and hair. Chapman and Hall, London, pp 51–67
Olsen EA, Delong E (1990) Transdermal viprostol in the treatment of male pattern baldness. J Am Acad Dermatol 23:470–472
Olsen EA, Weiner MS, Amara IA, DeLong ER (1990) Five-year follow up of men with androgenetic alopecia treated with topical minoxidil. J Am Acad Dermatol 22:643–646
Ono S (1980) The science of beard hair (in Japanese). University of Tamagawa Press, Tokyo
Orentreich D, Orentreich N (1988) Androgenetic alopecia and its treatment. In: Unger WP, Nordstrom REA (eds) Hair transplantation, 2nd edn. Marcel Dekker, New York, pp 18–20
Orentreich N (1959) Autografts in alopecia and other selected dermatological conditions. Ann NY Acad Sci 83:463–479
Orentreich N (1969) Scalp hair replacement in man. In: Montagna W, Dobson RL (eds) Advances in biology of skin, vol 9. Hair growth. Pergamon, Oxford, pp 99-108
Orentreich N (1978) Medical treatment of baldness. Ann Plast Surg 1:116–118
Orentreich N (1981) The problems of transplantation: In: Orfanos CE, Montagna W, Stüttgen G (eds) Hair research. Springer, Berlin Heidelberg Tokyo
Orfanos C (1967) Elektronenmikroskopischer Nachweis epithelioneuraler Verbindungen (Mechano-Rezeptoren) am Haarfollikelepithel des Menschen. Arch Klin Exp Dermatol 228:421–429
Orfanos CE (1990) Androgenetic alopecia: Clinical aspects and treatment. In: Orfanos CE, Happle R (eds) Hair and hair disease. Springer, Berlin Heidelberg Tokyo
Orfanos CE, Ruska H (1968) Die Feinstruktur des menschlichen Haares III. Das Haarpigment. Arch Klin Exp Dermatol 231:279–292
Orfanos CE, Vogels L (1980) Lokaltherapie der Alopecia androgenica mit 17α-oestradiol. Dermatologica 161:124–132
Osborn D (1916) Inheritance of baldness. J Hered 7:347
Otake K (1992) Reconstruction of hair-bearing skin in plastic surgery. 6th International Symposium, October 18–21, Prague, Czechoslovakia
Panaretto BA, Leish Z, Moore GPM, Robertson DH (1984) Inhibition of DNA synthesis in dermal tissue of merino sheep treated with depilatory doses of mouse epidermal growth factor. J Endocrinol 100:25–31
Parakkal PE (1967) The fine structure of anagen hair follicle of the mouse. Adv Biol Skin 9:441–469
Parakkal PE (1969) Morphogenesis of the hair follicle during catagen. Z Zellforsch Mikrosk Anat 107:174-186
Parnell JP (1949) Postnatal development and functional histology of the sebaceous glands in the rat. Am J Clin Anat 85:41–71
Pauss RJ, Stenn KS, Link RE (1989) The induction of anagen hair growth in telogen mouse skin by cyclosporin A administration. Lab Invest 60:365–369
Pauss RJ, Stenn KS, Link RE (1990) Telogen skin contains an inhibitor of hair growth. Br J Dermatol 122:777–784
Pecoraro V, Astrore I, Barman J, Aranjo CI (1964) The normal trichogram in the child before puberty. J Invest Dermatol 42:427
Peereboom-Wynia JDR, Bockhurst JC (1980) Effect of cyproterone acetate orally on hair density and diameter and endocrine factors in women with idiopathic hirsutism. Dermatologica 160:7
Pegun JS (1955) Dissociated depigmentation in vitiligo: Significance and therapeutic implications. Br J Dermatol 33:295–297
Perkins EM, Smith A, Fod DM (1967) A study of hair grouping in Primatus. Adv Biol Skin IX:357–367
Perret C, Happle R (1990) Treatment of alopecia areata. In: Orfanos CE, Happle R (eds) Hair and hair disease. Springer, Berlin Heidelberg Tokyo, pp 571–586
Peterson RE, Imperato-McGinley J, Gautier T, Sturla E (1977) Male pseudohermaphroditism due to steroid 5α-reductase deficiency. Am J Med 62:170–191
Philipou G, Kirk J (1981) Significance of steroid measurements in male pattern alopecia. Clin Exp Dermatol 6:53–56
Philpott MP, Green MR, Kealey T (1989) Studies in the biochemistry and morphology of freshly isolated and maintained rat hair follicles. J Cell Sci 93:409–418
Philpott MP, Green MR, Kealey T (1990) Human hair growth in vitro. J Cell Sci 97:463–471
Philpott MP, Westgate GE, Kealey T (1991) An in vitro model for the study of human hair growth. Ann NY Acad Sci 642:148–166

Philpott MP, Westgate GE, Kealey T (1992) The in vitro human hair growth model. Science of hair. Bioscience Conference in Artnature. 6th International Symposium, November 18, Tokyo, Japan, pp 3-22
Philpott MP, Green MR, Kealey T (1992) Rat hair follicle growth in vitro. Br J Dermatol 127:600-607
Phoades R, Pflanzer R (1989) The pituitary gland. In: Phoades R, Pflanzer R (eds) Human physiology. Saunders, Philadelphia, pp 403-410
Pierard GE, de la Brassinne M (1975) Cellular activity in the dermis surrounding the hair bulb in alopecia areata. J Cutan Pathol 2:240-245
Pierce CE (1985) Possible use of the Radovan tissue expander in hair replacement surgery. J Dermatol Surg Oncol 11:413
Pinkus F (1927) Die Normale anatomie der Haut. In: Jadassohns J (ed) Handbuch der Haut- und Geschlechtskrankheiten, I/1. Julius Springer, Berlin, pp 147-255
Pinkus H (1958) Embryology of hair. In: Montagna W, Ellis RA (eds) The biology of hair growth. Academic, New York, pp 1-32
Pinkus H (1969) Sebaceous cysts are trichilemmal cysts. Arch Dermatol 99:544-555
Pinkus H (1978) Epithelial mesodermal interaction in normal hair growth, alopecia, and neoplasia. J Dermatol (Tokyo) 5:93-101
Pinkus H (1981a) Outer keratinization in anagen and catagen of the mammalian hair follicle, a seventh distinct type of keratinization in the hair follicle, trichilemmal keratinization. J Anat 133:19-35
Pinkus H (1981b) Hair cycle. In: Pinkus H, Mehregan AH (eds) The guide to dermatohistopathology, 3rd edn. Appleton-Century-Crofts, New York, pp 30-32
Pinkus H, Mehregan AH (1981) The eccrine gland. In: Pinkus H, Mehregan AH (eds) The guide to Dermatohistopathology, 3rd edn. Appleton-Century-Crofts, New York, pp 32-33
Pinkus H, Steele CH (1955) Structure and dynamics of the human epidermis. AMA Scientific Exhibits, Grune and Stratton, New York, pp 46-53
Pisansarakit P, Moore GPM (1986) Induction of hair follicles in mouse skin by rat vibrissa dermal papillae. J Embryol Exp Morphol 94:113-119
Pitts RL (1987) Serum elevation of dehydroepiandrosterone sulfate associated with male pattern baldness in young men. JAMA 16:571-573
Plewig G, Luderschmidt C (1977) Hamster ear model for sebaceous gland. J Invest Dermatol 68:171-176
Pochi PE, Strauss JS (1965) The effect of aging on the activity of the sebaceous gland in man. In: Montagna W (ed) Advances in biology of skin, vol 6. Pergamon, Oxford, pp 121-127
Pochi PE, Strauss JS (1967) Effect of prednisone on sebaceous gland secretion. J Invest Dermatol 49:456-459
Pochi PE, Strauss JS (1969) Sebaceous gland response in man to the administration of testosterone delta 4-androstenedione and dehydroisoandrosterone. J Invest Dermatol 52:32-36
Pochi PE, Strauss JS (1974) Endocrinologic control of the development and activity of the human sebaceous gland. J Invest Dermatol 62:191-201
Pochi PE, Strauss JS (1977) Sebaceous gland studies in acne and endocrine disorders. Bull NY Acad Med 53:359-367
Pochi PE, Strauss JS, Mescon H (1962) Sebum excretion and urinary fractional 17-ketosteroid and total 17-hydroxycorticoid excretion in male castrates. J Invest Dermatol 39:475-483
Pochi PE, Strauss JS, Mescon H (1963) The role of adrenocortical steroids in the control of human sebaceous gland activity. J Invest Dermatol 41:391-399
Pochi PE, Downing DT, Strauss JS (1970) Sebaceous gland response in man to prolonged total caloric deprivation. J Invest Dermatol 55:303-309
Pochi PE, Strauss JS, Downing DT (1977) Skin surface lipid composition, acne, pubertal development, and urinary excretion of testosterone and 17-ketosteroids in children. J Invest Dermatol 69:485-489
Pochi PE, Strauss JS, Downing DT (1979) Age-related changes in sebaceous gland activity. J Invest Dermatol 73:108-111
Ponec M (1987) Hormone receptors in the skin. In: Fitzpatrick TB, Eisen AZ, Wolff K, Freedberg IM, Austen KF (eds) Dermatology in general medicine. McGraw-Hill, New York, pp 367-375
Pont A, Williams PL, Azhar S, Reitz RE, Bochra C, Smith ER, Stevens DA (1982) Ketoconazole blocks testosterone synthesis. Arch Intern Med 142:2137-2140
Ponten B (1963) The results of frontal galeotomies for loss of hair. Acta Chir Scand 126:406
Potten CS (1974) The epidermal proliferative unit: The possible role of the central basal cell. Cell Tissue Kinet 7:77-88
Potten CS, Merkow LP, Pondo M (1971) Ultrastructural changes in mouse hair follicle pigment cells after plucking, X-rays and actinomycin D treatments. Lab Invest 25:607-616
Potten CS, Hendrix JH, Moore JV (1987) Estimates of the number of clonogenic cells in the crypts of murine small intestine. Virchows Arch [Cell Pathol] 53:227-234
Powell B, Kuczek E, Crocker L, O'Donnell M, Rogers G (1989) Keratin gene expression in wool fibre development. In: Rogers GE, Reis PJ, Ward KA, Marshall RC (eds) The biology of wool and hair. Chapman and Hall, London, pp 325-335
Powell JA, Duell EA, Voorhees JJ (1971) Beta adrenergic stimulation of endogenous epidermal cyclic AMP formation. Arch Dermatol 104:359
Press M, Green GL (1984) Methods in laboratory investigation: An immunochemical method for demonstrating estrogen receptor in human uterus using monoclonal antibodies to human estrophilin. Lab Invest 50:480-486
Price VH (1975) Testosterone metabolism in the skin. A review of its function in androgenetic alopecia, acne vulgaris, and idiopathic hirsutism including recent studies with antiandrogens. Arch Dermatol 3:1496-1502
Price VH (1978) Topical minoxidil (3%) in extensive alopecia areata, including long-term efficacy. J Am Acad Dermatol 16:737-744
Puerto AM, Mallol J (1990) Regional scalp differences of the androgenic metabolic pattern in subjects affected by male pattern baldness. Rev Esp Fisiol 46:289-296
Punnonen R, Lovgren T, Kouvonen I (1980) Demonstration of estrogen receptors in the skin. J Endocrinol Invest 3:217
Rabineau P (1988) Complications of flaps in the treatment of baldness. In: Unger EP, Nordstrom REA

(eds) Hair and hair disease. Marcel Dekker, New York, p 657
Radovan C (1976) Adjacent flap development using expandable silastic implants. American Society of Plastic and Reconstructive Surgery Forum, Boston, September 30, 1976
Radovan C (1978) Reconstruction of the breast after radical mastectomy using a temporary expander. Plast Surg Forum 1:41
Radovan C (1984) Tissue expansion in soft tissue reconstruction. Plast Reconstr Surg 74:482
Ramastry P, Downing DT, Pochi PE, Strauss JS (1970) Chemical composition of human skin surface lipids from birth to puberty. J Invest Dermatol 54:139–144
Rampini E, Moretti G (1973) Cutaneous metabolism of estradiol and testosterone in the newborn rat till puberty. Minerva Dermatol 108:49
Rampini E, Bertamino R, Moretti G (1968) Size and shape of sebaceous glands in male pattern alopecia. In: Baccaredda-Boy A, Moretti G, Frey JR (eds) Biopathology of pattern alopecia. Karger, Basel, pp 155–165
Randall VA, Ebling FJ, Hargreaves G (1982) The in vivo uptake and metabolism of testosterone by the skin and other tissues of the rat. J Endocrinol 93:253–266
Randall VA, Thornton MJ, Hamada K, Messenger AG (1992) Mechanism of androgen action in cultured dermal papilla cells derived from human hair follicles with varying responses to androgens in vivo. J Invest Dermatol 98:865–915
Randall VA, Thornton MJ, Messenger AG, Hibberts NA, Laudon AS, Brinklow BR (1993) J Invest Dermatol 101 (suppl 1):1145–1205
Rando RR (1974) Chemistry and enzymology of K cat inhibitors. Science 185:320–324
Rassner B, Zaun H, Braun-Falco O (1963) Zum Pathomechanismus der männlichen Glatzenbildung. Arch Klin Exp Dermatol 216:307
Rawles ME (1947) Origin of pigment cells from the neural crest in the mouse embryo. Physiol Zool 20:248–266
Rawles ME (1965) Tissue interactions in the morphogenesis of the feather. In: Lyne AG, Short BF (eds) Biology of the skin and hair growth. Angus and Robertson, Sydney, pp 105–128
Raynaud JP, Boone C (1977) Antiandrogen devoid of systemic effects for topical treatment of seborrhea and acne. J Invest Dermatol 68:256
Razel AJ, Svensson J, Spelsberg TC, Coulam CB (1985) The androgen receptor in normal human foreskin I. Stabilization and identification of two receptor subunits. Am J Obstet Gynecol 153:410–416
Redmond GP, Gidwani GP, Gupta MK, Bedocs NM, Parker RN, Skibinsky MSC, Bergfeld WB (1990) Treatment of androgenic disorders with dexamethasone: Dose-response relationship for suppression of DHEAS. J Am Acad Dermatol 22:91–93
Remedco (1978) Minerals in hair and their major implications. Remedco Analytical Laboratory, Van Nuys, p 14
Reynolds AJ, Jahoda CAB (1990) Adult rat pelage dermal papilla cells induce type-specific follicle formation and hair growth in adult footpad skin. J Invest Dermatol 95:485
Reynolds AJ, Jahoda CAB (1991a) Hair follicle stem cells? A distinct germinative epidermal cell population is activated in vitro by the presence of hair dermal papilla cells. J Cell Sci 99:373–385
Reynolds AJ, Jahoda CAB (1991b) Inductive properties of hair follicle cells. Ann NY Acad Sci 642:226–242
Reynolds AJ, Oliver RF, Jahoda CAB (1991c) Dermal cell populations show variable competence in epidermal cell support: Stimulatory effects of hair papilla cells. J Cell Sci 98:75–83
Rheinwald JG, Green H (1975) Serial cultivation of stains of human epidermal keratinocytes. The formation of keratinizing colonies from single cells. Cell 6:331–344
Richter R (1963) Hormonale Einflüsse und Physiopathologie des Haarwachstums. In: Marchionini A, Spier HW (eds) Normale und pathologische Physiologie der Haut: I. Springer, Berlin Heidelberg New York, pp 359–372 (Handbuch der Haut-und Geschlechtskrankheiten, vol 1/3)
Rittmaster RS, Uno H, Povar ML, Mellin TN, Loriaux DL (1987) The effects of N,N-diethyl-4-methyl-3-oxo-4-aza-5α-androstane-17β-carboxamide, a 5α-reductase inhibitor and antiandrogen, on the development of baldness in stumptail macaque. J Clin Endocrinol Metab 65:188–193
Robaire B, Covey DF, Robinson CH, et al (1977) Selective inhibition of rat epididymal steroid 4-5α-reductase by conjugated allenic 3-oxo-5,10-secosteroids. J Steroid Biochem 8:307–310
Robertson DW, Steinberg MI (1990) Potassium channel modulators: Scientific applications and therapeutic promise. J Med Chem 33:1529–1541
Robins EJ, Breathnach AS (1969) Fine structure of the human foetal hair follicle at hair-peg and early bulbous-peg stages of development. J Anat 104:553–569
Robins EJ, Breathnach AS (1979) Fine structure of bulbar end of human foetal hair follicle at stage of differentiation of inner root sheath. J Anat 107:131–146
Rogers GE (1983) The occurrence of citrullin in structural proteins of the hair follicle. In: Goldsmith LA (ed) Biochemistry and physiology of the skin. Oxford University Press, New York, pp 511–521
Rogers GE, Roth SI (1967) Hair and nail. In: Zelickson AS (ed) Ultrastructure of normal and abnormal skin. Lea and Febiger, Malvern, p 105
Rogers G, Martinet N, Steinert P, Wynn P, Roop D, Kilkenny A, Morgan D, Yuspa SH (1987) Cultivation of murine hair follicles as organoids in a collagen matrix. J Invest Dermatol 89:369–379
Rollier R, Warcewski Z (1974) The treatment de la pelade par la Meladinine. Bull Soc Dermatol Syphiligr Fr 81:97
Ronchese E (1974) A comment on uneven whitening of senile hair. Int J Dermatol 13:84–85
Rook A (1972) The hair: alopecia areata. In: Rook A, Wilkinson DS, Ebling FJG (eds) Textbook of dermatology, 2nd edn. Blackwell Scientific, Oxford, pp 1985–1992
Rook AJ (1977) Common baldness and alopecia areata. In: Rook AJ (ed) Recent advances in dermatology. Blackwell Scientific, Oxford, pp 223–244
Roop DR, Huitfeldt H, Kilkenny A, Yupsa SH (1987) Regulated expression of differentiation-associated keratins in cultural epidermal cells detected by monospecific antibodies to unique peptides of mouse epidermal keratins. Differentiation 35:143–150
Rose LI, Underwood RH, Newmark SR (1977) Pathophysiology of spironolactone-induced

gynecomastia. Ann Intern Med 87:398–403
Rosen JF, Fleischman AR, Finberg L, et al (1979) Rickets with alopecia: An inborn error of vitamin D metabolism. J Pediatr 94:729–735
Ross RK, Bernstein L, Ludd M (1986) Serum testosterone levels in young blacks and white men. J Natl Cancer Inst 76:45–48
Ross RK, Bernstein L, Lobe RA, Shimiz H, Stanczyk FZ, Pike MC, Henderson BE (1992) 5α-Reductase activity and risk of prostate cancer among Japanese and U.S. white and black males. Lancet 339:887–889
Roth SI (1965) The cytology of the murine resting (telogen) hair follicle. In: Lyne AG, Short BF (eds) Biology of the skin and hair growth. Angus and Robertson, Sydney, pp 233–250
Rothman S (1958) Introduction. In: Montagna W, Ellis RA (eds) The biology of hair growth. Academic, New York
Rougeot J (1965) Thyroid hormones and the wool cuticle. In: Lyne AG, Short BF (eds) Biology of the skin and hair growth. Angus and Robertson, Sydney, p 625
Runne U, Martin H (1986) Veränderung von Telogenrate, Haardichte, Haardurchmesser und Wachstumsgeschwindigkeit bei der androgenetischen Alpezie des Mannes. Hautarzt 37:198–204
Rushton H, James KC, Mortimer CH (1993) The unit area trichogram in the assessment of androgen-dependent alopecia. Br J Dermatol 109:429–438
Ryan TJ (1973) The blood vessels of the skin. In: Jarrett A (ed) Physiology and pathophysiology of skin, vol 2. Academic, London, pp 577–801
Ryan KJ (1982) Biochemistry of aromatase; significance to female reproductive physiology. Cancer Res (suppl) 42:3342–3344
Sabourand R (1929) Pélades et Alopécies en aires. Masson, Paris, cited by Schweikert HU (1967) Arch Klin Exp Dermatol 230:96
Saito R, Hori Y, Kuribayashi T (1976) Alopecia in hyperthyroidism. In: Kobori, T, Montagna W (eds) Biology and diseases of the hair. University Park Press, Baltimore, pp 279–285
Salamon T (1966) Vererburg von Haar- und Nagelkrankheiten. In: Jadassohn J (ed) Handbuch der Haut- und Geschlechtskrankheiten. Ergänzungswerk, vol VII. Springer, Berlin Heidelberg New York, pp 364–439
Salamon T (1968) Genetic factors in male pattern alopecia. In: Baccaredda-Boy A, Moretti G, Frey JR (eds) Biopathology of pattern alopecia. Karger, Basel, p 39
Salamon T, Lazovic O, Nikulin A, Markovic A (1975) Histologische Untersuchungen an Scheitel und Hinterhaupt bei der Alopeica seborrhoica. Hautarzt 26:304–308
Sanford BH, Chase HB, Carroll SB, Arsennault CT (1965) The effects of grafting during various stages of the hair growth cycle. Anat Rec 152:17
Sansing J (1987) Bald truths, will science cure baldness? Can new drugs grow hair? The Washingtonian Magazine 22:103
Sansone-Bazzano G, Reisner RM (1971) Differential rates of conversion of testosterone to dihydrotestosterone in acne and in normal human skin. A possible pathogenic factor in acne. J Invest Dermatol 56:366–372
Sansone-Bazzano G, Reisner RM, Bazzano G (1972) Conversion of testosterone-1, 2-3H to androstenedione 3H in the isolated hair follicles of man. J Clin Endocrinol Metab 34:512–515
Sansone-Bazzano G, Reisner RM (1974) Steroid pathways in sebaceous glands. J Invest Dermatol 62:211–216
Sasagawa M (1930) Hair transplantation (in Japanese). Jpn J Dermatol 30:493
Sato Y (1976) The hair cycle and its control mechanism. In: Montagna W, Kobori T (eds) Biology and diseases of the hair. University of Tokyo Press, Tokyo, pp 3–13
Sato Y (1979) Mechanism of hair loss (in Japanese). Hifu Byo Shinryo (J Clin Dermatol) 1:891–896
Sato Y (1981) Alopecia areata—modern aspect. In: Orfanos CE, Montagna W, Stüttgen G (eds) Hair research—status and future aspects. Springer, Berlin Heidelberg Tokyo, pp 303–310
Sawada M, Terada N, Taniguchi H, Tateishi R, Mori Y (1987) Cyclosporin A stimulates hair growth in nude mice. Lab Invest 56:684–686
Sawaya ME (1991) Steroid chemistry and hormone control during the hair follicle cycle. Ann NY Acad Sci 642:376–384
Sawaya ME (1992) Purification of androgen receptors in human sebocyte and hair. J Invest Dermatol 98:92S–96S
Sawaya ME, Honig LS, Garland LD, Hsia SL (1988a) Delta-5-3β-hydroxy-steroid dehydrogenase activity in sebaceous glands of scalp in male pattern baldness. J Invest Dermatol 91:101–105
Sawaya ME, Honig LS, Hsia SL (1988b) Increased androgen binding capacity in sebaceous glands in scalp of male pattern baldness. J Invest Dermatol 92:91–95
Sawaya ME, Price VH, Harris KA, Kirsner RS, Hsia SL (1990) Human hair follicle aromatase activity in females with androgenetic alopecia (abstract). J Invest Dermatol 94:575
Schein M (1903) Über die Entstehung der Glatze. Klin Wochenschr 16:611–615
Schenk EA (1980) Autoantibodies in alopecia and vitiligo. In: Brow AC, Crounse RG (eds) Hair trace elements and human illness. Praeger, New York, p 334
Schmidt GH, Wilkinson MM, Ponder BAJ (1985) Cell migration pathway in the intestinal epithelium: An in situ marker system using mouse aggregation chimeras. Cell 40:425–429
Schweikert HU (1967) Quantitative Untersuchungen über die Talgdrüsenfunktion bei androgenetischer Alopecie. Arch Klin Exp Dermatol 231:200–206
Schweikert HU, Wilson JD (1974a) Regulation of human hair growth by steroid hormones. I. Testosterone metabolism in isolated hairs. J Clin Endocrinol Metab 38:811–819
Schweikert HU, Wilson JD (1974b) Regulation of human hair growth by steroid hormones. II. Androstenedione metabolism in isolated hairs. J Clin Endocrinol Metab 39:1012–1019
Schweikert HU, Wilson JD (1974c) Aromatization of androstenedione by isolated head hairs. J Clin Endocrinol Metab 40:413
Schweikert HU, Wilson JD (1981) Androgen metabolism in isolated human hair roots. In: Orfanos CE, Montagna W, Stuttgen G (eds) Hair research. Springer, Berlin Heidelberg Tokyo, pp 210–214
Schweizer J, Kinjo M, Furstenberger G, Winter H (1984) Sequential expression of mRNA-encoded keratin sets in neonatal mouse epidermis: Basal cells with

properties of terminally differentiating cells. Cell 37:159–170
Scott MJ, Seattle DO, Scott WAM, Washington RS (1992) Effects of anabolic-androgen steroids on the pilosebaceous unit. Cutis 50:113–116
Seidman M, Westfried M, Maxey R, Rao TKS, Friedman EA (1981) Reversal of male pattern baldness by minoxidil. Cutis 28:551–553
Segall A (1918) Über die entwicklung und den wechsel der haare meerschwinchen (Cavia Cobaya Schreb). Arch Mikrosk Anat Entwicklungsmech 91:1:218–291
Sengel P (1964) The determinism of the differentiation of the skin and the cutaneous appendage of the chick embryo. In: Montagna W, Lobitz WC (eds) The epidermis. Academic, New York, pp 15–34
Sengel P (1976) Morphogenesis of skin. Cambridge University Press, Cambridge
Sengel P (1984) Epidermal-dermal interaction. In: Bereiter-Hahn AG, Maltoltsy AG, Richards KS (eds) Biology of the integument, vol 2. Springer, Berlin Heidelberg Tokyo, pp 374–380
Serri F, Cerimele D (1990) Embryology of the hair follicle. In: Orfanos CE, Happle R (eds) Hair and hair disease. Springer, Berlin Heidelberg Tokyo, pp 1–17
Serri F, Huber W (1963) The development of sebaceous glands in man. In: Montagna W, Dobson RL (eds) The sebaceous glands. Pergamon, Oxford, pp 1–18 (Advances in biology of skin, vol 4)
Setala K, Heinonen H, Purola SI (1972) Safety and mode of effect of a hair preparation. Contributions from the first department of pathology and its radiologic laboratory of the University of Helsinki. Proc Eur Dial Transplant Assoc 9:514–520
Seto H (1963) Studies on sensory innervation (human sensibility) 2nd edn. Thomas, Springfield, pp 341–347
Settel E (1977) Control of excessive hair loss: Drug Cosm Industry. October
Setty LR (1970) Hair patterns of the scalp of white and negro males. Am J Phys Anthropol 33:49–55
Shansky A (1965) Comparative differences in formulations between professional products and consumer products. Am Perf Cosmet 80:39–41
Shapiro G, Evron S (1980) Novel use of spironolactone: Treatment of hirsutism. J Clin Endocrinol Metab 51:429–432
Sherad P, Marks R (1977) A pharmacological effect of oestrone on human epidermis. Br J Dermatol 97:383–386
Sherins RJ, Bardin CW (1971) Preputial gland growth and protein synthesis in the rat androgen-insensitive male pseudohermaphroditic rat. Endocrinology 89:835–841
Shiell RC (1972) Hair—facts and fallacies. Part 2. Baldness and its treatment. Austr Fam Physician 1:291
Shiell R, Norwood OT (1984) Micrografts and minigrafts. In: Norwood OT, Shiell RC (eds) Hair transplant surgery, 2nd edn. Thomas, Springfield, pp 107–110
Shuster A, Thody AJ (1974) The control and measurement of sebaceous secretion. J Invest Dermatol 62:172–190
Shuster S, Thody AJ, Goolamali SK, Burton JL, Plummer N, Bates D (1973) Melanocyte stimulating hormones and parkinsonism. Lancet I:463
Siiteri PK, Simberg NH (1986) Changing concepts of active androgens in blood. Clin Endocrinol Metab 15:247–258
Silman RE, Chard T, Lowry PJ, Smith I, Young IM (1976) Human foetal pituitary peptides and parturition. Nature 260:716–718
Silver AF, Chase HB (1967) Microcirculation of the mouse pinna. Physiol Zool 40:172–181
Silver AF, Chase HB (1970) DNA synthesis in the adult hair germ during dormancy (telogen) and activation (early anagen). Dev Biol 21:440–451
Silver AF, Chase HB (1977) The incorporation of tritiated urine in hair germ and dermal papilla during dormancy (telogen) and activation (early anagen). J Invest Dermatol 68:201–205
Silver AF, Chase HB, Potten CS (1968) Melanocyte precursor cells in the hair follicle germ during the dormant stage 8 telogen. Experientia 25:299–301
Simpson NB, Martin AR (1983) A more reliable photometric technique for the measurement of scalp sebum secretion. Br J Dermatol 109:647–652
Simpson NB, Cunliffe WJ, Hodgins MB (1983) The relationship between the in vitro activity of 3β-hydroxysteroid dehydrogenase isomerase in human sebaceous glands and their secretory activity in vivo. J Invest Dermatol 81:139–144
Singh F, Lal S (1966) Hypertrichosis and hyperpigmentation with systemic psoralen treatment. Br J Dermatol 79:501
Singh M, McKenzie J (1961) The histology and histochemistry of the disease of hairy and non-hairy parts of the human skin with special reference to baldness. J Anat 95:569
Skalli O, Pelte MF, Peclet MC, Gabbiani G, Gugliotta P, Bussolati G, Ravazzola M, Orci L (1989) α-Smooth muscle actin, a differentiation marker of smooth muscle cells, is present in microfilamentous bundles of pericytes. J Histochem Cytochem 37:315–321
Smith MA, Wells RS (1964) Male type alopecia, alopecia areata and normal hair in women: Family histories. Arch Dermatol 89:95–98
Smith QT, Allison DJ (1966) Studies on the uterus, skin and femur of rats treated with 17β-oestradiol benzoate for 1–21 days. Acta Endocrinol (Copenh) 53:598
Soler-Bechara J, Soscia JL (1963) Chronic hypervitaminosis A. Arch Intern Med 112:58–62
Solomon LM, Esterly NB (1970) Neonatal dermatology. I. The newborn skin. J Pediatr 77:888–894
Sorkin M, Shapiro B, Kass G (1966) The practical evaluation of shampoos. J Soc Cosmet Chem 17:539–551
Spencer LV, Callen JP (1987) Hair loss in systemic disease. Dermatol Clin 5:565–570
Sperling LC, Winton G (1990) The transverse anatomy of androgen alopecia. J Dermatol Surg Oncol 16:1127–1133
Spoor HJ, Linds SD (1973) Hair processing and conditioning. Cutis 14:689–694
Starico RG (1960) The melanocytes and the hair follicle. J Invest Dermatol 35:185–194
Starico RG (1961) Mechanism of migration of the melanocytes from the hair follicle into the epidermis following dermabrasion. J Invest Dermatol 36:99–104
Starico RG (1963) Amelanotic melanocytes in the outer sheath of the human hair follicle and their role in the repigmentation of regenerated epidermis. Ann NY Acad Sci 100:239–255
Stasiak PC, Purkis PE, Leigh IM, Lane EB (1989) Keratin

19: Predicted amino acid sequence and broad tissue distribution suggest it evolved from keratinocyte keratins. J Invest Dermatol 92:707–716
Static electricity (1992) In: The world book enclopedia, vol 6. Scott Fetzer, Chicago, p 167
Steggerda M (1940) Cross sections of human hair from four racial groups. J Heredity 31:474–476
Stenn KS (1988) The skin. In: Weiss L (ed) Cell and tissue biology. Urban Schwarzenberg, Baltimore, pp 539–572
Stenn KS, Bhawan J (1990) The normal histology of the skin. In: Farmer ER, Hood AF (eds) Pathology of the skin. Prentice-Hall International, London
Sterry W, Konrads A, Nase J (1980) Alopezie bei Schilddrüsenerkrankungen: Charakteristische Trichogramme. Hautarzt 31:308–314
Stewart ME, Pochi PE (1978) Antiandrogens and the skin. Int J Dermatol 17:167–179
Stewart ME, Pochi PE, Strauss JS, Wotiz HH, Clark SJ (1977) In vitro metabolism of (H3) testosterone by scalp and back skin: Conversion of testosterone into 5α-androstane-3β-diol. J Endocrinol 72:385–390
Stöhr P (1904) Entwicklungsgeschichte des menschlichen Wollhaares. Anat Hefte Abt 1:23:1–66
Stough DB (1992) Micrografts and minigrafts, vol 3. Hair Transplant Video Forum, Oklahoma City
Straile WE (1959) A study of the neoformation of mammalian hair follicles. Ann NY Acad Sci 83:499–506
Straile WE (1960) Sensory hair follicles in mammalian skin: The tylotrich follicle. Am J Anat 106:133–147
Straile WE (1965) Root sheath-dermal papilla relationships and the control of hair growth. In: Lyne AG, Short BF (eds) Biology of the skin and hair growth. Angus and Robertson, Sydney, pp 35–57
Straile WE, Chase HB, Arsenault C (1961) Growth and differentiation of hair follicles between periods of activity and quiescence. J Exp Zool 148:205–221
Strauss JB, Kligman AM (1959) The effect of ACTH and hydrocortisone on the human sebaceous gland. J Invest Dermatol 33:9
Strauss JS, Kligman AM (1961) The effect of progesterone and progesterone-like compounds on the human sebaceous gland. J Invest Dermatol 36:309–319
Strauss JS, Pochi PE (1961) The quantitative gravimetric determination of sebum production. J Invest Dermatol 36:293–298
Strauss JS, Pochi PE (1963) The hormonal control of sebaceous glands. In: Montagna W, Ellis RA, Silver AF (eds) Advances in biology of skin, vol 4, Sebaceous glands. Pergamon, Oxford, pp 220–254
Strauss JS, Pochi PE (1970) Assay of anti-androgens in man by the sebaceous gland response. Br J Dermatol 82 (suppl 6):33–42
Strauss JS, Kligman AM, Pochi PE (1962) The effect of androgens and estrogens on human sebaceous glands. J Invest Dermatol 39:139–155
Strauss JS, Downing DT, Ebling EJG (1991) Sebaceous glands. In: Goldsmith LA (ed) Biochemistry and physiology of the skin, 2nd edn. Oxford University Press, New York, chap 25
Strickland JH, Calhoun ML (1963) The integumentary system of the cat. Am J Vet Res 24:1018–1029
Stumpf WE, Sar M, Joshi SB (1974) Estrogen target cells in skin. J Experientia 30:196
Stumpf WE, Sar M (1976) Autoradiographic localisation of estrogen, androgen, progestin and glucocorticosteroid in "target tissues" and "non-target tissues." In: Pasqualini J (ed) Modern pharmacology-toxicology, vol 8. Marcel Dekker, New York, pp 41–84
Sudo K, Yoshida K, Kimura Y, et al (1979) Anti-androgen TSAA-291. V. Effects of the anti-androgen TSAA-291 on the androgen-receptor complex formation from [3H] testosterone in rat ventral prostates. Acta Endocrinol (Copenh) 92:67–81
Sudo T (1974) An illustrated book of the Japanese hair follicle (in Japanese), 8th edn. Japanese Association of Hair Science, Tokyo
Suga A, Hashimoto Y (1966) Microscopic study of the hair matrix. Hifuka Rinsho 8:90
Sugai T (1984) The causative mechanism of male pattern baldness (in Japanese). Jpn Med J 3163:151–152
Sugai T (1990) Recent medicated cosmetic products for prevention seen from the standpoint of dermatology (in Japanese). Fragrance J 11:31–36
Sugiyama S, Kukita A (1976) Melanocyte reservoir in the hair follicles during the hair growth cycle. Our electron microscopic study. In: Kobori T, Montagna W (eds) Biology and diseases of the hair. University Park Press, Baltimore, pp 181–200
Sugiyama S, Takahashi M, Kamimura M (1976) The ultrastructure of the hair follicles in early and late catagen, with special reference to the alteration of the junctional structure between the dermal papilla and epithelial component. J Ultrastruct Res 54:359–373
Sultan C, Bakkar K, Vermorken AJM (1989) The human hair follicle: A target for androgens. In: Van Neste D, Lachapelle JM, Antoine JL (eds) Trends in human hair growth and alopecia research. Kluwer Academic, Dordrecht, pp 89–98
Sulzberger MD, Witten VH (1952) The effect of topically applied compound F in selected dermatoses. J Invest Dermatol 19:101–102
Sun TT, Cotsarelis G, Lavker RM (1991) Hair follicular stem cells: The bulge-activation hypothesis. J Invest Dermatol 96:77–78S
Svensson J, Snockowski M (1979) Androgen receptor in preputial skin from boys with hypospadia. J Clin Endocrinol Metab 49:340–345
Sweet G (1907) The skin, hair, and reproductive organs of Notoryctes. Contribution to our knowledge of the anatomy of *Notoryctes typhlops* Stirling-Parts IV and V. Q J Microsc Sci 51:325–344
Szymonowicz L (1909) Über die Nervendigungen in den Haaren des Menschen. Arch Mikrosk Anat 74:622–635
Takashima I (1987) Development and alteration of human pelage. In: Kobori T, Montagna W (eds) Medicine of hair (in Japanese). Bunkodo, Tokyo, p 132
Takashima I (1990) Androgenetic alopecia: Pathophysiological aspects in man and animals. In: Orfanos CE, Happle R (eds) Hair and hair disease. Springer, Berlin Heidelberg New York
Takashima I, Kawagishi I (1975) Comparative study of hair growth in mammals, with special references to hair grouping and hair cycle, and hair growth rate in the juvenile stump-tailed macaque. In: Toda K, Ishibashi Y, Hari Y, Morikawa F (eds) Biology and diseases of the hair. University of Tokyo Press, pp 457–571
Takashima I, Montagna W (1974) Studies of common baldness of the stump-tailed macaque (*Macaca speciosa*) VI. The effect of testosterone on common

baldness. Arch Dermatol 103:527–534
Takashima I, Adachi K, Montagna W (1970) Studies of common baldness in the stump-tailed macaque. IV. In vitro metabolism of testosterone in the hair follicles. J Invest Dermatol 55:329–334
Takashima T, Iju M, Sudo M (1981) Alopecia androgenetica: Its incidence in Japanese and associated conditions. In: Orfanos CE, Montagna W, Stuttgen G (eds) Hair research. Springer, Heidelberg Berlin Tokyo, pp 287-293
Takayasu S (1978) Androgen binding to cytosol and nuclei of hamster sebaceous glands. J Steroid Biochem 9:181
Takayasu S (1979) Effect of antiandrogens on the binding of androgen to cytosol and nuclei of hamster sebaceous glands. Arch Dermatol Res 264:49–54
Takayasu S, Adachi K (1972a) The conversion of testosterone to 17β-hydroxy-5α-androstane-3-one (dihydrotestosterone) by human hair follicle. J Clin Endocrinol Metab 34:1098–1101
Takayasu S, Adachi K (1972b) The in vivo and in vitro conversion of testosterone to 17β-hydroxy-5α-androstane-3-one (dihydrotestosterone) by the sebaceous gland of hamsters. Endocrinology 90:73
Takayasu S, Itami S (1987) The hair follicle related to the secondary sexual character. In: Kobori T, Montagna W (eds) Medicine of hair. Bunkodo, Tokyo, pp 173-187
Takayasu S, Montagna W (1971) Studies of common baldness of the stump-tailed macaque (*Macaca speciosa*). VI. The effect of testosterone on common baldness. Arch Dermatol 103:527–534
Takayasu S, Wakimoto H, Itami S, Sano S (1980) Activity of testosterone 5α-reductase in various tissues of human skin. J Invest Dermatol 74:187–191
Tamm J, Volkwein U, Tresguerres JAF (1980) Plasma testosterone glucosiduronate: A reliable indicator of female hyperandrogenism. Clin Endocrinol 13:431-435
Tamm J, Seckelmann M, Volkwein U, Ludwig E (1982) The effect of the antiandrogen 11α-hydroxy-progesterone on sebum production and cholesterol concentration of sebum. Br J Dermatol 107:63–70
Tammi R (1982) Effects of sex steroids on human skin in organ culture. Acta Derm Venereol (Stockh) 62:107-112
Tamura H (1943) Pubic hair transplantation (in Japanese). Jpn J Dermatol 53:76
Tanaka H, Sato Y, Kato K (1965) Histological studies of the pilosebaceous system in the rat. I. Normal structure of the pilosebaceous system and relationship between the hair follicle and the sebaceous gland. Acta Med Biol 13:173–180
Taniguchi S (1977) Histological findings of the skin following transplantation of plastic hairs (in Japanese). Jpn J Plast Reconstr Surg 20(4):323
Taniguchi S (1980) Clinical and histological findings in synthetic hair implantation and investigation of its fixing rate (in Japanese). Jpn J Plast Reconstr Surg 2(4):25
Taniguchi S (1982) Artificial hair implantation-(2), fixation rate and the histological findings (in Japanese). Jpn J Plast Reconstr Surg 4(2):13
Taniguchi S (1983) A histopathological study of percutaneous implantation of artificial fibers. Transactions of the 8th International Congress of Plastic Surgery, Montreal

Taniguchi S (1984) A histopathological study of the percutaneous implantation of polyester fibers. Aesth Plast Surg 8:67–74
Tänzer (1926) Haut und haar beim karakul im rassenanalytishen vergleich. Thielle, Halle (Saale)
Tarnow G (1971) Disturbance of hair growth after severe cerebral damage (diffuse alopecia following a head injury). Neurovisc Relat Suppl X:549–556
Taylor AC (1949) Survival of rat skin and changes in hair pigmentation following freezing. J Exp Zool 110:77-111
Taylor M, Ashcroft ATJ, Messenger AG (1993) Cyclosporine A prolongs human hair growth in vitro. J Invest Dermatol 100:237–239
Tezuka M, Ito M, Ito K, Tazawa T, Sato Y (1991) Investigation of germinative cells in generating and renewed anagen hair apparatus in mice using anti-bromodeoxyuridine monoclonal antibody. J Dermatol Science 2:434–443
Thiele FDJ (1975) Chemical aspects of hair loss and its cosmetological significance. Br J Dermatol 92:355–358
Thody AJ, Shuster S (1971) Sebotrophic activity of β-lipotrophin. J Endocrinol 50:533–534
Thody AJ, Shuster S (1975) Control of sebaceous gland function in the rat by α-melanocyte stimulating hormone. J Endocrinol 64:504–510
Thody AJ, Shuster S (1989) Control and function of sebaceous glands. Physiol Rev 69:383–416
Thomas JP, Oake RJ (1974) Androgen metabolism in the skin of hirsutism in women. J Clin Endocrinol Metab 38:19–22
Thornton MJ, Messenger AG, Elliotte K, Randall VA (1991) Effect of androgens on the growth of cultured human dermal papilla cells derived from beard and scalp hair follicles. J Invest Dermatol 97:345–348
Toda K (1989) Modern concepts concerning the treatment of minoxidil (in Japanese). Fragrance J 17:110–115
Toshitani S (1989) Scalp tension theory and male pattern alopecia (in Japanese). Fragrance J 5:61–65
Trapman J, Klaassen P, Kuipen GGJM, van der Korput JAGM, Faber PW, van Rooij HCG, Geurts van Kessel A, Voorhorst MM, Mulder E, Brinkmann AO (1988) Cloning, structure and expression of a cDNA encoding the human androgen receptor. Biochem Biophys Res Commun 153:241–248
Tromovitch TA, Glogou RG, Stegman SJ (1985) Medical treatment of male pattern alopecia (androgenic alopecia). Head Neck Surg 7:336
Unger MG, Unger WP (1978) Management of the scalp by a combination of excisions and transplantations. J Dermatol Surg Oncol 4:670
Unger WP (1979) The hair line. In: Unger WP, Nordström REA (eds) Hair transplantation. Marcel Dekker, New York
Unger WP (1990) Surgical treatment of androgenetic alopecia. In: Orfanos CE, Happle R (eds) Hair and hair diseases. Springer, Berlin Heidelberg Tokyo, pp 1001-1030
Unger WP, Marritt E (1988) General principles of recipient site organization and planning. In: Unger WP, Nordström REA (eds) Hair transplantation. Marcel Dekker, New York
Unger WP, Nordström RE (1988) Advantages of punch graft. In: Unger WP, Nordström REA (eds) Hair transplantation. Marcel Dekker, New York
Unger WP, Schemmer RJ (1978) Corticosteroids in the

treatment of alopecia totalis. Arch Dermatol 114:1486-1490

Unna PG (1976) Beiträge zur Histologie und Entwicklungsgeschichte der menschlichen Oberhaut und ihrer Anhagsgebile. Arch Microskop Anat Entwicklungsmech 12:665-741

Uno H (1970) Studies of quantitative histochemistry of the hair follicle (in Japanese). Igaku no Ayumi (Progress of Medicine) 74:322-325

Uno H (1982) Nonhuman primate model of baldness. Int J Dermatol 21:21-23

Uno H, Montagna W (1982) Reinnervation of hair follicle end organs and meissner corpuscles in skin grafts of macaques. J Invest Dermatol 78:210-214

Uno H, Adachi K, Montagna W (1968) Glycogen contents of primate hair follicles. J Invest Dermatol 51:197-199

Uno H, Adachi K, Montagna W (1969) Morphological and biochemical studies of hair follicle in common baldness of stump-tailed macaque (*Macaca speciosa*). In: Montagna W, Dobson RL (eds) Advances in biology: Hair growth. Pergamon, Oxford, pp 221-245

Uno H, Adachi K, Allegra F, Montagna W (1978) Studies of common baldness of the stumptailed macaque. J Invest Dermatol 51:11-18

Uno H, Cappas A, Schlagel C (1985) Cyclic dynamics of hair follicle and the effect of minoxidil on the bald scalps of stump-tailed macaques. Am J Dermatol 7:283-297

Uno H, Cappas A, Brigham P (1987) Action of topical minoxidil in the bald stump-tailed macaque. J Am Acad Dermatol 16:657-668

Uno H, Kemnitz JW, Cappas A, Adachi K, Sakuma A, Kamoda H (1990) The effects of topical diazoxide on hair follicular growth and physiology of the stump-tailed macaque. J Dermatol Sci 1:183-194

Urabe A, Furumura M, Imayama S, Nakayama J, Hori Y (1992) Identification of a cell layer containing α-smooth muscle actin in the connective tissue sheath of human anagen hair. Arch Dermatol Res 284:246-249

Uzuka M, Takeshita C, Morikawa F (1977) In vitro growth of mouse hair root. Acta Dermatovenereol (Stockh) 57:217-219

Vallis CP (1964) Surgical treatment of receding hair line. Plast Reconstr Surg 33:247-252

Vallis CP (1969) Surgical treatment of receding hair line. Plast Reconstr Surg 44:271-278

Van Baar HMJ, Van Veijmen IMJJ, Ramaekers FCS (1994) Cyto keratin expression in alopecia areata hair follicles. Acta Derm-Venereol (Stockh) 74:28-32

Van der Loos H, Woolsey TA (1973) Somatosensory cortex: Structural alterations following early injury to sense organs. Science 179:395-398

Van Scott EJ (1958) Response of hair roots to chemical and physical influence. In: Montagna W, Ellis RA (eds) The biology of hair growth. Academic, New York, pp 441-449

Van Scott EJ, Ekel TM (1958) Geometric relationship between the matrix of the hair bulb and its dermal papilla in normal and alopecia scalp. J Invest Dermatol 31:281-287

Van Scott EJ, Reinertson RP, Steinmuller RJ (1957) The growing hair root of the human scalp and morphological changes therein following amethopterin therapy. J Invest Dermatol 29:197-204

Van Scott EJ, Ekel TM, Auerback R (1963) Determinants of rate and kinetics of cell division in scalp hair. J Invest Dermatol 41:269-273

Vath WR (1963) Man's oldest fallout problem. Baldness brochure of the American Medical Association, Chicago

Venning VA, Dawber RPR (1988) Patterned androgenic alopecia in women. J Am Acad Dermatol 18:1073-1077

Vexiau P, Husson C, Chivot M, Brerault J-L, Fiet J, Julien R, Villette J-M, Hardy N, Cathelineau G (1990) Androgen excess in women with acne alone compared with women with acne and/or hirsutism. J Invest Dermatol 94:279-283

Voigt W, Hsia SL (1973) Further studies on testosterone 5α-reductase of human skin: Structural features of steroid inhibitors. J Biol Chem 248:4280-4285

Voigt W, Castro A, Covey DF (1978) Inhibition of testosterone 5α-reductase by antiandrogenicity of allenic 3-keto-5,10-secosteroids. Acta Endocrinol (Copenh) 87:668-672

Wadel J (1933) Untersuchungen über den prämaturen chronischen Haarausfall. Wien Klin Wochenschr 46:1383

Wadel J (1935) Neue Untersuchungen über die Entstehung der prämaturen Alopecie. Arch Dermatol Syphil 172:128

Walsh PC, Madden JD, Harrod JL (1974) Familial incomplete male pseudohermaphroditism, type 2: Decreased dihydrotestosterone formation in pseudovaginal perineoscrotal hypospadias. N Engl J Med 291:944-948

Watanabe Y, Nagashima K (1984) Effectiveness of constituents contained in hair tonics (in Japanese). Hifu Rinsho (Jpn J Clin Dermatol) 24:877-883

Weinberg WC, Goodman LV, George C, Morgan DL, Ledbetter S, Yuspa SH, Lichti U (1993) Reconstitution of hair follicle development in vivo: Determination of follicle formation, hair growth, and hair quality by dermal cells. J Invest Dermatol 100:229-236

Weissmann GD, Roenig HH Jr, Maibach HI (1973) Psoriasis-liver-methotrexate interactions. Arch Dermatol 108:36-42

Weissmann I, Hofmann C, Wagner G, Plewig G (1978) PUVA-therapy for alopecia areata, an investigative study. Arch Dermatol Res 262:333-336

Weissmann I, Hofmann C, Wagner G (1981) PUVA-therapy for alopecia areata. Hair Research pp 336-340 Springer, Berlin Heidelberg Tokyo

Welker C (1971) Microelectrode delineation of fine grain somatotopic organization of 5 ml cerebral neocortex in albino rat. Brain Res 26:259-275

Weller WL (1972) Barrels in somatic sensory neocortex of the marsupial *Trichosurus vulpecula* (brush-tailed possum). Brain Res 43:11-24

Wester RC, Maibach HI, Guy RH, Novak E (1984) Minoxidil stimulates cutaneous blood flow in human balding scalps: Pharmacodynamics measured by laser Doppler velocimetry and photopulse plethysmography. J Invest Dermatol 82:515-517

Westgate GE, Craggs RI, Gibson WT (1991a) Immune privilege in hair growth. J Invest Dermatol 97:417-420

Westgate GE, Gibson WT, Kealey T, Philpott MP (1991b) Prolonged maintenance of human hair follicles in vitro in a serum-free medium. J Invest Dermatol 96:1001A

Weston AH, Longmore J, Newgreen DT, Edwards G, Bray KM, Duty S (1990) The potassium channel openers: A new class of vasorelaxants. Blood Vessels

27:306–313
Williams-Ashman HG (1975) Metabolic effects of testicular androgens. In: Greep RO, Astwood EB (eds) Handbook of physiology, vol 1, Sect 7, Endocrinology: Male reproductive system. American Physiological Society, Washington DC, pp 473–490
Wilson JD (1972) Recent studies on the mechanism of action of testosterone. N Engl J Med 287:1284-1291
Wilson JD, Walker JD (1969) The conversion of testosterone to 5α-DHT by skin slices of man. J Clin Invest 48:371-379
Winkelmann RK (1959) The innervation of a hair follicle. Ann NY Acad Sci 83:400–407
Winkelmann RK (1968) New methods for the study of nerve endings. In: Kenshalo DR (ed) The skin senses. Thomas, Springfield, pp 38-60
Wirth H, Neumahr W, Gloor M (1982) Über den Einfluß häufiger Haarwäschen auf die menschliche Talgdrüse. Dermatol Monatsschr 168:75-81
Wirth H, Spurgel D, Gloor M (1983) Untersuchungen zur Wirkung von Benzoylperoxyd auf die Talgdrusensekretion. Dermatol Monatsschr 169:289-293
Withers HR (1967) Recovery and repopulation in vivo by mouse skin epithelial cells during fractionated irradiation. Radiat Res 32:227-239
Wolback SB (1951) The hair cycle of the mouse and its importance in the study of sequence of experimental carcinogenesis. Ann NY Acad Sci 53:517-536
Woolsey TA, Van der Loos H (1970) The structural organization of layer IV in the somatosensory region (SI) of mouse cerebral cortex. The description of a cortical field composed of discrete cytoarchitectonic units. Brain Res 17:205-242
Wotiz HH (1956) The in vitro metabolism of testosterone by human skin. J Invest Dermatol 26:113–120
Wright F, Giacomini M (1980) Reduction of dihydrotestosterone to androstanediols by human female skin in vitro. J Steroid Biochem 13:639-643
Wright N, Alison M (1984) The biology of epithelial cell populations, vol 1. Clarendon, Oxford
Wüstner H, Orfanos CE (1974) Alopecia androgenetica und ihre Lokalbehandlung mit Östrogen- und corticosteroidhaltigen Externa. Z Hautkr 49:879-888
Wysiocki GP, Daley TD (1987) Hypertrichosis in patients receiving cyclosporine therapy. Clin Exp Dermatol 12:191-196
Yamada A, Uwanuma Y, Inaba M, Inaba Y (1992) Preparation of thick tissue sections using Cellophane sheet (in Japanese). Jpn J Aesth Surg 29:37–41
Yamada. S, Fukuta K (1995) Synthetic hair grafting. A study of a synthetic hair grafting and its safety and clinical results. In: Laiis ST (ed) Hair replacement: surgical and medical (3rd edn). Mosby Yearbook, New York, pp 345-358
Yamakado M, Yohro T (1979) Subdivision of mouse vibrissae on an embryological basis, with descriptions of variations in the number and arrangement of sinus hairs and cortical barrels in BALB/C and hairless strains. Am J Anat 155:153-174
Yamamoto T (1966) On the sensory innervation of the hair follicle in mice. In: Uyeda R (ed) Proceedings of 6th international congress of electron microscopy. Maruzen Tokyo, Singapore, pp 515–516
Yohro T (1969) The mitotic pattern of the embryonic epidermis during scale morphogenesis. J Embryol Exp Morphol 21:235-242
Yohro T (1977) Structure of the sinus hair follicle in the big-clawed shrew, *Sorex unguiculatus*. J Morphol 153:333–353
Yohro T (1985) Aspects of man (in Japanese). Chikuma, Tokyo, pp 114-134, 248-253
Yohro T (1988) A new aspect of the vibrissal pattern (in Japanese). J Jpn Dermatol 98:1301–1303
Young M (1947) Anatomical factors in senile alopecia; experimental production of baldness. Anat Rec 97:378
Young M (1980) Morphological and ultrastructural aspects of the dermal papilla during the growth cycle of the vibrissal follicle in rat. J Anat 121:355-365
Zarate A, Mahesh VB, Greenblatt RB (1966) Effects of an antiandrogen, 17α-β-nortestosterone, on acne and hirsutism. J Clin Endocrinol Metab 26:1394-1398
Zaun H (1986) Haarkrankheiten-Systematik, pathophysiologische Grundlagen, Differential-diagnose. Therapiewoche 36:2695-2700
Zelei BV, Walker CJ, Sawada GA, Kawabe TT, Knight KA, Buhl AE, Johnson GA, Diani AR (1990) Immunohistochemical and autoradiographic findings suggest that minoxidil is not localized in specific cells of vibrissa, pelage, or scalp follicles. Cell Tissue Res 262:407-413
Zimmermann AA, Becker SW (1959) Melanoblasts and melanocytes in fetal negro skin. III. Monogr Med Sci VI(3):1-59

Index

a
Acetylcholine 210, 232
Acid
  arachidate 203
  di-saturated lipid 203
  docosahexaenoic (DHEA) 202
  eicosapentaenoic (EPA) 202
  linoleic 202, 203
  linolic 203
  palmitic 202
  palmitolein 203
  salicylic 210
  saturated lipid 203
  stearic 202
Acinus
  cells 272
  sebaceous 6
Acne
  vulgaris 46, 147, 212, 213, 286
Adenyl cyclase
  activity 173, 175, 176
Adipose tissue 267
Adrenal
  androgens 144
  cortex 143, 155, 167
  cyclase activity 148
  gland 143, 146, 155
  origin 196
  steroid hormones 155
Adrenocorticotropic hormone (ACTH) 156
Aldosterone 213
Alopecia
  androgenetica 13, 14, 63, 146, 160–179, 185, 197, 201, 209, 211, 215, 226, 233
  see also Androgenetic alopecia
  aphiasis 191
  areata 7, 160, 161, 171, 191, 193, 194
  chignon 195
  cicatrisata 177, 195
  diffuse 161
  frontoparietal 283
  gradus 195, 196
  postpartum 196
  premature 161
  reduction 262
  seborrhoic scalp 145, 178
  totalis 191, 192
  traumatic 233
  universalis 191, 192
Amino acids 197, 210, 224, 230
Anagen
  early stage 7, 67, 121, 137–139
  follicle 1, 8, 9, 137–139, 173
  hair 5, 98, 166, 173
  stage 63–68, 77, 137, 165
  target tissue 10
Androgen 5, 10, 167
  active 10, 146, 212
  activity 145, 170, 172
  adrenal 156
  binding-globulin 152
  circulating 162, 172, 212
  -depeendent alopecia 162
  endogenous 197
  metabolic activity 146
  metabolism 45, 143, 144, 146
  metabolizing enzymes 144
  precursor 146, 172
  pretestosterone 144
  receptor 144, 146, 151, 212
  receptor protein (ARP) 148, 150
  stimulation 46, 145
  -transforming enzymes 145
Androgenetic alopecia
  definition of 161
  etiological mechanism of 173
  histological finding of 179
  hormonal factors 172
  in adult period 188
  in childhood period 186
  in complete baldness 189
  in neonatal period 185
  incidence of, in Japan 163
  nutritional factor 197
  occurrence and frequency 162
  solitary hair 167
Androstane
  5α-, 3β-17 β-diol 147, 149
Androstanediol 45, 147
  3α 148, 174

3β 145, 174, 178
Androstanedione
5α 147
Androstenediol
3β 149, 174
Androstenedione (ADION) 45, 145, 147–149, 152, 167, 173, 212
Δ^{4}- 10, 144, 146, 147, 177
5α- 149, 174
Androsterone (ARON) 45
epi- 144, 149
Anesthesia
local 16, 70, 233, 252, 255, 267
Anti-cancer agents 11, 109, 116, 129, 189
Apocrine
gland 2, 19, 21, 28, 59, 69, 71, 101, 200, 201
perspiration 200
Arrector pili muscle 1, 2, 5, 126
attachment of 5, 67, 68, 121
Arteriosclerosis 203
Artificial
hair 278–287, 289
implantation 277, 278
scalp 287
Atrophy 5, 169, 171, 179, 193–197, 205, 222, 272
Auber critical level (Auber's borderline) 2, 4, 35, 36, 96, 133, 134
Autografts 233
Axilla 69
Axillary
epidermis 47
hair 47, 49, 69, 73, 75, 82, 83, 85, 95, 96, 102, 107, 121, 139, 152
hair density 47
Azelaic acid 149, 150

b
Basal
cell 6, 123, 124, 126, 136, 140
daughter cell 123
lamina 5, 6, 8, 67, 269
layer 1, 2, 5, 83, 95, 123, 124
membrane 22
primary, cell 123
Basement membrane 5, 21, 22
Blood circulation 10, 15, 205, 209, 210, 242, 244, 251, 255, 268, 272, 274, 275
inhibitor 269
resumption 269
Blood plexus
cutaneous 39, 99
papillary 244, 251, 274
subpapillary 8, 39, 41, 44, 194, 275
Blood sinus
cavernous 140
ring 141
upper and lower 139
Blood vessels 2, 8, 43, 44
candelabra 39
papillary 8, 43
perifollicular network of 40
subpapillary 8, 43, 116
system 39
transverse branches of 39
Bromidrosis 11, 67, 69, 99, 175, 200
Bulb matrix 1
Bulbous peg stage 27-32, 44, 64, 66, 78, 80, 96, 107, 111, 119, 134
early 28, 30
late 30
Bulge
activation hypothesis 9, 67, 125, 126, 130
area 9, 75, 82, 119, 125–127, 129
cells 125, 126
region 9, 111, 119, 125, 126
Bundle hair 129, 187
compound 11, 12, 188

c
Candelabra vessels 39, 40, 99
Capillaries 5, 7
Capillary vessels 1, 2
peripheral 169
Carbohydrate 201, 202
food 199
Catagen
hair follicle 8, 65
stage 5, 7, 11, 63–68, 137
Cell division 1, 5, 63, 67, 90, 111, 176
see also Mitotic activity
Cellophane sheet method 18–20
Cellotape method 17, 109
Chlorine dioxide
staabilized 223–226
unstabilized 223
Cholesterol esters 6
Classification
Hamilton's 163–165, 255
Norwood's 163–165, 229
Ogata's 163
Takashima's 163
Clear layer 2
Club hair 9, 63, 66, 77, 110, 127, 138, 272
Coarse hairs 7, 47, 48, 50–52, 54, 59, 61, 95, 96, 129
solitary 187–189
Collagen
inner, layer 8
layer 5
middle, layer 8
outer, layer 8
Compound hair 129, 189
Connective tissue 1, 46, 85, 139, 279, 283
fibrous 282
layer 15
sheath 1, 7, 8, 22, 63, 251
Corium 1, 179
Corneal exfoliation 137
Cornified layer 1, 2, 136
Cortex 1, 2, 4, 5, 90, 91, 131
cuticle 2, 4, 77
hair 1, 3, 22, 30, 77, 80, 82, 91, 98, 103, 105, 107, 133, 135
Cortical barrel 141
Cranial bone 171
Cryostat technique 17
Cuticle 4, 5, 90
cell 4, 131
hair 1, 80, 82, 90, 91, 96, 98, 133, 135
sheath 77, 80, 133, 135

Cyclic adenosine monophophate (c-AMP) 45, 148, 173
Cyclosporin 194
A (CsA) 218
Cyoctol 213, 217
Cyproterone
acetate (CPA) 210–213
Cyst
epidermoid 98
formation 32
keratinous 96
-like bulge 90
pilar 98
trichilemmal 96, 98
Cytosol 144
protein 154
receptor 173

d
Dandruff 169
Dehydroepiandrostenedione (DHEA) 145, 146, 148, 172–174, 186
Dehydroepiandrosterone (DHA) 143, 144, 172, 177, 178
sulphate (DHEAS) 212, 155
Deoxycorticosterone 212
Dermal
cells 9, 10
component 1, 9, 10
future, papilla 26, 77
layer 1, 10, 75, 90, 251, 284
papilla 1, 2, 4, 5, 8–12, 28, 39, 40, 44, 63, 67, 80–82, 85, 99, 107, 119, 124–127, 133–135, 139, 176, 249, 272
papilla cells 8–10, 22, 67, 121, 125, 126, 145, 150
rat vibrissa, papilla 9
remmnant, papilla 11, 68, 109–111, 117, 129, 139
sheath 9
tissue 155, 244, 251, 275
Dermis 1, 2, 3, 5, 11, 13, 15, 19
culture of 10
Diazepam 233, 237, 255
Diazoxide 216, 217
Dietary factors 169
Dihydrotestosterone (DHT) 45, 46, 145–150, 173, 174, 189, 211, 212, 225
activated 10
5α- 45, 144–148, 151, 167, 173–177, 221, 222
formation 147, 173, 185
receptor 148
Dog ear 254
portion 252
skin 257
Dominant gene 170
Donor
area 234, 252
dominance 235
graft 234, 242
plug 234
punches 234
scalp plugs 234
site 234, 242, 252, 257
Doppler flow meter 251, 255
Double-tie over dressing 70

e
Eccrine
duct 19
gland 1, 2, 19, 21, 71
perspiration 200
Edema 197, 215, 284
Electrocoagulation 69, 99–101
Electrolysis 69, 99, 102
Electron microscopic
examination 98
observation 22
specimen 20–22
study 22
view 21, 22
Embryogenesis 8
Embryonic
follicles 95
hair 34, 125
stage 46
Endocrine
abnormalities 196
diseases 191
disorder 162, 172
organs 156, 201
Enzyme
activity 7, 34, 41, 160, 183, 232
5α-reductase 176, 205, 221, 222
keratinolytic 96
systems 146
tyrosinase 33
Epi-Aron 144, 149
see also Androsterone
Epidermal
cell 5, 8, 10, 135, 140, 217
component 10
growth factor (EGF) 67, 131, 217
keratinocyte 9, 98, 126
layer 8, 284
melanosome 33
populations 9
repigmentation 83
skin 244
structure 10
thickness 1
Epidermis 1, 2, 5, 6, 9, 11, 13, 15, 19, 62, 95, 116, 123, 124, 130, 251, 274, 275, 284
culture of 10
glabrous 8
primitive 136
undifferentiated 23
Epinephrine 233, 234, 255
Epithelial
bud 11-13, 75, 110, 112, 113, 116
bulb 8
cell 10, 22, 43, 54, 80, 90, 103, 107, 109, 111, 112, 118, 119, 126, 130, 133, 135, 141, 272
cell buds 12
cell layer 12, 113
collar 82, 123
column 9, 63, 64, 77, 78, 82, 126
component 1, 8, 126
differentiation 145
follicle 10
follicular, cells 145
germ 133
growth 10

layer 85, 90, 119
matrix cell 37, 80, 91, 107
portion 5
sac 12, 24, 25, 77, 85, 90, 96, 103, 105, 107, 111, 131–133
sebaceous, cells 109
sheath 63
structures 10
tissue 10, 12, 129, 139
Epithelium
cells 10
follicular 7, 159
keratinized 7
keratotic 129
stratified squamous 7
trichilemmal 77, 98, 105
Estradiol 231, 148, 152
17α- 211
17β- 144, 152
Estrogen 210, 231
-binding protein 152
receptor 152–155
Excision suture method 283, 284
Excretory organ 69
Exocrine organ 46

f
Fat
animal 197–203
animal, consumption 198
cells 8
intake 199
tissue 15
vegetable 199
Fatty acids
esterified 169
free 6, 169
saponified 206
saturated 198, 202
unsaturated 169, 202
Fetal
hair 47
life 6, 11, 23, 50, 81
period 47, 50, 185, 186
Fibers
sensory 160
Fibril 132, 133
Fibroblast 8, 282
cells 8
Fibrous
protein 1
tissue 15
Filamentous structure 4, 54, 77, 88, 90, 103, 132, 133, 137, 138
5α-reductase 146, 148-152, 173, 175, 201, 211, 212
activity 10, 46, 144-147, 151, 170, 173, 174, 177
enzymes 176, 205, 221, 222
inhibitor 218, 226
Flap
bilateral 255–257
bitemporal 237, 262
composite pedicle, method 238
free 267, 268
hair-bearing pedicle 272
initial 255
lateral 255
method 13
occipital-parietal long, method 257
parietal 255
pedicle 237, 254, 291
post-auricular 257
pre-auricular 257
skin flap 291
temporal-parietal 283
temporal-parietal-occipital pedicle 237, 251
Follicular
appendix 8, 41
canal 5, 6, 46
nerve plexus 1
orifice 248
Frontal
area 16
hairline 13, 148, 234, 238, 251, 255, 257, 267
muscle 15

g
Galea
aponeurotica 15, 16, 171, 252, 280, 282, 291, 295
Generation
hair 11, 23, 116
of hair follicle 129, 139
of the mass of mesenchymal cells 113
Genetic inheritance 170
Genotypes
BB 170
Bb 170
bb 170
Germ cell 23, 24, 85
layers 25, 26, 126
Germ sac 126
Glandular epitheelial cells 272
Glucide 202
Glucocorticoids 155, 156, 212
Glucose
−6-phosphate-dehydrogenase (G6PDH) 45, 173, 174
Glycerin 201, 224
Glycogen 5
productivity 232
Gonadotropin
facilitate 143
Graft
Choi's single hair 246–248
coarse hair-bearing 238, 251
elliptical 246
free coarse hair-bearing 268, 269
free punch 233
free skin 233
hair-bearing 275
single hair-bearing, transplantation 238–240, 244, 275, 296
skin 272, 273
Granular
layer cells 1, 2, 96, 136
Gynecomastia 213

h
Hair bud 64, 96, 98, 110, 114, 121

Hair bulb 1, 2, 7–9, 11, 20–22, 50, 63, 64, 69, 75, 77, 78, 80, 82, 85, 96, 99, 107, 124, 126, 133–135, 291
portion 4, 5, 20–22, 148, 149, 244, 248, 291
Hair bundling 50, 59, 62
Hair canal 3, 6, 27–30, 32, 50, 99
Hair cone 26, 43, 64, 77, 95, 135, 136
Hair cuticle 1, 2, 80, 82, 90, 91, 96, 98, 133
Hair cycle 7, 9, 32, 63, 64, 165
common 9, 63, 64, 66, 69, 103, 130, 139, 291
common, theory 73, 109, 113, 117, 119, 121, 129
conventional 64, 67, 68, 139
essential 9, 64, 103, 121, 130, 139, 291
Hair fiber 64, 96, 105, 133, 135, 194, 248
Hair follicle 1–3, 5, 7, 10–12, 18, 21, 130
buds 8, 9
bundle 12, 13, 61, 117, 129
cells 135
compound 12, 113, 117, 129
embryonic 34, 95
epithelial components of 8
epithelium 10
groups 62
infundibular portion of 8
primary 50, 55, 188
primary central coarse (PCO) 50–62
secondary 50, 55, 187, 188
secondary lateral (SL) 50–62
secondary lateral derived 57–62
single 117
terminal 165
see also Terminal
Hair germ 62, 67, 68, 111, 117, 119, 127, 129–132
cells 43, 77, 133
ellipsoid 25
primary 11, 24, 25
primitive 23, 24
secondary 11, 64–66, 109, 111, 113, 117, 121, 127, 128, 139, 189
stage 23-26, 30, 64, 74, 75, 96, 103, 104, 133, 136
Hair grouping 55, 59, 61
Hair peg 6, 96
early, stage 77
late, stage 77, 78
stage 26, 27, 32, 64, 75, 76, 78, 82, 103, 110, 111, 119, 132, 133, 136
Hair roots 1, 81, 90, 93, 99, 103, 133, 175
accessory 82, 123
Hair shaft 4, 191
Hair tissue 2, 78
Hair transplantation 195
Hairline
frontal 13, 148, 234, 238, 251, 255, 257, 267
refinement 237, 238, 243
temporal 13, 255
transplanted 238
Henle's layer 2, 4, 5, 22, 77, 80, 98, 133, 135
keratinization of 105, 133
Heterogenous
syndrome 192, 194
Hirsismus 200, 201
Hirsutism 45, 147, 148, 212
Hormone
active 143
activities 41, 160, 167, 172, 225
adrenal cortex 143
adrenocortical 143
androgenic 174
circulating 172
female 143
female, receptor 175
growth 156, 157
imbalance 172, 175, 176
male 10, 129, 143, 147, 167, 169, 172, 175, 176, 205, 211
male, receptor 151, 155, 175
melanocyte-stimulating 156
non-steroid 143
pituitary 143, 231
sex 45, 143, 150, 155
steroid 67, 143, 150
thyroid 143, 156
Huxley's layer 2, 4, 5, 22, 77, 80, 98, 133, 135
Hydrocortisone 155, 156
Hydroxysteroid
3β-oxoreductase 174
17β-oxydoreductase 174
Hyperandrogenemia 155
Hyperkeratinization 7, 129
Hyperkeratosis 201
Hypernutrition 167, 169
Hypertrichosis 215, 216

i

Infundibulum 7, 30, 69, 75
follicular 6
Inner endocuticle 4
Inner root sheath 2–5, 9, 22, 26, 28–32, 63, 64, 75, 77, 78, 80, 82, 90, 91, 94, 95–98, 105, 107, 119, 131–135
Interlocking fusion 30, 32, 77, 80, 90, 96, 105, 133
Intermediate
cells 136
layer 136
Interrelation
mesenchymal-epithelial 139
Isthmal
portion 5, 54, 99, 102, 112, 148
stage 64, 67
upper 2, 6, 12, 50, 54, 57, 61, 68, 75, 96, 97, 99–103, 110, 111, 113, 116, 139
upper, close to the duct opening of the sebaceous gland 4, 64, 95, 96, 113, 116, 119, 121, 127, 129
upper, portion of hair follicle 4, 5, 46, 64, 68
Isthmus 73, 75, 82

j

Juri
flap 251
flap method 263
method 237

k

Keratin 1, 6, 124, 126
antibodies 126
fibers 202, 224
hair 221
Keratinase 96

Keratinization 4, 5, 7, 32, 74, 75, 96, 98, 133
follicular 136, 137
of epidermis 1, 5, 135, 136
of Henle's layer 105, 133, 137
stratified 85
trichilemmal 96–98
Keratinized
cell 4, 134
fiber 135
hair 1, 4, 132
rootlets 77, 137, 138
Keratinocytes 21, 33, 34, 124, 194
basal 136
follicular matrix 46
Keratinolytic enzyme (keratinase) 96
Keratohyalin
granules 6, 7, 9, 96, 98, 135
Ketosteroids (KS)
17- 170, 172
17, metabolites 174
Kwashiorkor 197

l
Lamellar granules 7
Lanugo hair 47, 48, 50, 185–188
Leydig cells 143
Lidocaine 233
Lipid
animal 198
droplets 6
excretion of 201
formation 7
hair 169
intake 201, 203
membrane 205, 207
peroxide 203
-producing cell 6
products 6
vacuoles 7
Lipocytes
sebaceous 116
Lipofuscin 203
Lymph duct 1
Lymphocytes 191, 282

m
Male pattern baldness 147, 161, 165, 169–173, 175–179, 189, 209, 211
classification of 13, 163, 164
infant 185
Marasmus 197
Maritt expansion method 241, 296
Matrix 1, 2, 5, 80, 82, 96, 131
cell 4, 5, 63, 85, 134, 248
ectodermal 10
epidermal 8
epithelial, cell 37, 80, 91, 107
extracellular 8
geminative 10
hair 4, 5, 22, 30, 91, 96, 98, 111, 119, 133–135, 175, 176, 244, 248, 249, 272
hair, activity 222
hair bulb, cells 8, 50
hair, cell 10, 22, 109, 133, 191, 217, 268, 275
Medulla 1, 2, 4, 77
hair, cells 98, 133, 135, 136
Melanin
formation 36, 232
granule 22, 30, 34, 37, 40, 51, 55, 57, 77, 80, 85, 90, 91, 103, 107, 139, 244, 272
pigmentation 34–37
synthesis 33–35
Melanocytes 2, 9, 21, 33–37, 63, 80, 83, 91, 107, 194
amelanotic 83, 123
dendric 80
Melanosome 33, 34, 136
Membrane coating granules 7
Merkel
cells 159
Mesenchyma 141
Mesenchymal
cell 10–13, 23, 24, 26, 28, 51, 75, 76, 107, 109, 118, 119, 130, 139, 274
component 145
ectodermal-, relationship 10
-epithelial tissue interaction 10–12, 109, 142
layer 9
mass of, cells 26, 54, 80, 82, 90, 104, 109, 110, 112, 113, 116, 117, 119, 129, 131, 135, 189
mass of, tissue 24, 43, 44, 50, 91, 96, 107, 137
structures 10
tissue 10, 11, 25, 26, 29, 77
Mesoblast 141
Metabolic
activity 143, 193, 201
Metabolites
5α-reduced 173, 174
17 ketosteroid 173
Methotrexate 109, 129, 189
Microcirculation 8, 39, 41, 44, 194, 244, 251, 274, 275
Microcirculatory system 8, 41, 43, 44
Micrografts 238–240, 244
Micropunch
1 mm 238
Microtome 17, 18
Migration 123
downward 131
Minigrafts 237, 238, 241–243
Minoxidil 216, 217
topical 194, 215
Mitosis 25, 26, 119
cell 152
Mitotic activity 1, 10, 25–26, 30, 46, 64, 75, 77, 80, 90, 91, 96, 132, 133
of cells 6
see also Cell division
Mucopolysaccharides 8, 183, 218, 231
Multilobular 50, 54, 55, 57, 61, 62, 75, 90, 180
configuration 103, 104, 137, 138
hair follicle 93, 96

n
Necrosis 235, 237, 264, 283, 284
Nerve
autonomic 193
autonomic, fibers 160
cell 141
endings 159

fibers 159
myelinated somatic sensory 159
perifollicular 159
plexus 183, 193, 194
sensory 160, 193
sensory, plexus 160
Neuroblast 141
Neurofibra
multiple 141
Nevus cells 295
Niconinamide adenine dinucleotide phosphate (NADPH) 146, 148, 212
Nuclei
crowiding of 10–12
Nutritive elements
essential 199

o
Occipital
area 13, 16, 148, 234, 238, 257
artery 13, 15, 16, 262
muscle 15, 16, 263
nerve 16
scalp 248, 252, 272
Ostium 61, 187, 188
Outer exocuticle 4
Outer root sheath 1–3, 5, 9, 22, 28, 30, 55, 67, 73, 75, 78, 80, 82, 83, 85, 91, 95, 98, 107, 119, 126, 133, 140
cells 22, 123–125, 127, 131, 132
Oxidizing agent 216, 217, 221, 223, 229

p
Papillary cells
dermal 8
Paraffin-embedded specimen 17, 18
Parietal region 167
Pattern alopecia 7
Pelage
hair follicles 82, 139–142
Periderm 136
Permanent poriton 82, 121
of hair follicle 68, 71, 72
Physical therapy 99
Physiological saline 237, 291
Pigmentation 77
epidermal, re- 83
hair 33, 34
melanin 34, 35
Pilary canal 7
Pilosebaceous
apparatus 5, 148, 172, 244, 248, 274
complexes 73, 74, 76
unit 2, 5, 8, 39–41, 45, 109, 121, 145, 146, 150, 251, 274, 275
Pituitary
anteerrior, gland 156
gland 160
Plugs
hair 242, 244
Premature baldness 171, 177, 194, 205
Proandrogens 143
Progesterone 211, 212
receptors 153–155
Prostaglandin 203, 217
Prostate
gland 146
Protein 197, 201, 202
animal 198, 199, 202
hard 221
intake 199, 200
kinase system 173
source 200
synthesis 146, 173
Protoplasm 155
Pseudohermaphroditism 144
incomplete 151
Psychosomatic
stress 191, 193
tension 193
Pubic hair 50, 151, 152, 233
Punch
graft 238, 240, 272, 274
graft method 233–235, 237
hair grafting 233
method 13, 242, 291, 296
1 mm, method 242
transplanting 234
PUVA therapy 194

r
Recipient
area 234, 237, 252, 255
holes 233–235
plug 234
site 233, 237, 238, 241, 251, 257, 275
skin 234
tissue 244, 251, 274, 275
Regeneration
center of 139
epidermal 123, 127
from bundle telogen hair 113
of dermal papillae and whiskers 9
of hair 63–67, 117, 121, 123, 175, 194, 211, 221, 225, 275, 291
of hair follicle 64, 109–112, 129, 139, 180–182
of hair germ 109, 115

s
Scalp 5
disease 193
excision 242
expansion 264
extension 264, 267
frontal 257, 272
hair 13, 82, 103, 107, 121, 163, 165–167, 171, 185–187
parietal 252, 257
plugs 234
reduction 257, 262–264, 267
skin 171, 254
tension 171, 188
Scar
formation 238, 278
linear 195, 291, 294–297
linear, formation 291, 294
region 244
tissue 177, 297

Sebaceous duct 3, 82, 85, 95
cells 7
keratinization 7
Sebaceous gland 1, 2, 5-7, 18, 19, 21, 30, 32, 44-47, 50, 55, 62, 69, 73, 75, 77, 81-83, 85, 99-102, 116, 118, 129, 139, 175-177, 179, 180, 272, 274
activity 47, 48, 145, 193, 156
anlagen of 6
attachment of 7
cell receptors 177
cells 7, 102, 109
duct opening of 11, 12, 46, 61, 62, 75, 90, 127, 175, 193, 194, 269
enlargement of 150, 186, 189, 198, 201, 205
function 48, 145, 156, 205
hypertrophy of 50, 119, 187, 201
hypothesis 10, 12, 67, 139, 175-177, 205
lobes of 54-57, 68, 78, 121
multilobular 103, 104, 187
primordial 24, 26
secretion 152, 156, 207, 212
size of 81-83, 145
Sebaceous isthmus 13, 50, 51, 121, 127, 130
close to the duct opening of the sebaceous gland 9, 11, 12, 129, 175
Sebaceous lobule 6
Sebocytes 46, 146, 151
facial 145
non-facial 145
Seborrhea
theory 205, 206
Sebum 30, 32, 46, 167
excretion 46, 69, 186
production 6, 150, 156, 169
secretion 145, 152, 153, 155, 157, 168, 169, 174, 193, 194, 200, 205, 207
Secretory
activity 207
cells 46
duct 6
duct opening of sebaceous gland 46, 68, 69, 90, 112, 139
organ 143
Sensory
nerve ends 141, 194
organ 139, 141
17β-hydroxysteroid
dehydrogenase (17β-HSD) 146-149
17-ketosteroids (17 KS) 170, 172
Sheath cuticula 2, 77, 80, 131
Sinus hair 82, 141
Smooth muscle cells 8
Solitary (single) hairs 50, 59, 189
Spinous
cells 136
layer 1, 2, 5
Spironolactone 210
Split-thickness graft
medium 73
thick 69
Squalene 6
Stem cell 7, 11, 67, 119, 125, 129, 130, 194
bulge 126
epidermal 133
follicular 9, 111, 123-125, 139, 297
primary 123, 130
secondary 130
upper 100, 194
Steroids
adrenal 143, 155
adrenocortical 172
androgenic 143, 144
C_{19} 173
natural 211
19-carbon 143
ovarian 143
Stratum
corneum 7
granulosum 7
Subcutaneous
adipose tissue 40
fat layer 15, 274
fatty tissue 47, 269
layer 15, 16, 19
level 71
tissue 1, 2, 15, 73, 90, 139, 175, 282
tissue shaving method 11, 37, 67, 69, 70, 71, 96, 175
Suture
running 297
simple 294
stapler 291, 294
Sweat glands 18, 22, 69, 175
apocrine 21, 200
eccrine 21, 200
Syphilis
secondary 196

t
Target
cells 146, 147
organ 212
tissue 10, 145, 147, 150, 151, 217
Telogen
bundle, hair follicle 11, 117
effluvium 191, 196, 237
hair follicle 11, 12, 65-68, 103, 109-113, 116, 119, 121, 129
late 9
lower end of, follicle 127, 129, 130
stage 5, 7, 11, 63-68, 99, 109, 113, 117, 129, 137-139, 165, 248
Temporal
hairs 289
-parietal flap 283
-parietal-occipital pedicle flap 237, 251
region 16, 145, 167, 191, 196, 255, 295, 296
superficial, artery 15, 16
Terminal
follicle 5
hair 8, 47, 50, 57, 65, 80, 96, 119, 127, 136, 145, 188
hair stage 30, 55, 107
Teste 143, 152
Testosterone 10, 143-149, 151, 152, 167, 170, 172, 173, 175, 176, 211, 212
action 212
estradiol binding globulin 150
free 146, 167, 212
labeled 45, 173
metabolism of 144, 148, 172
metabolite 146
metabolite of 45, 145

methyl 145
secretion 167
3H 149, 173
Thick tissue 85
preparation method 18, 91, 137
sections 18, 20, 21
specimen 11, 17–22, 109, 127, 244
Thin tissue
sections 17, 22
specimen 21, 22
3β-hydrosteroid dehydrogenase (HSD) 146
Three dimentional
clarity 18
observations 18–20, 91
sections 17
view 21, 55
Thyroid
disease 191, 196
function 201
hormone 20
-stimulating hormone 156
Thyroxine 201, 210
Tissue
expander method 291
expansion 264
soft 243, 262
thick split-thickness, observation 272
thin split-thickness, observation 272
Tonofibrils 7
Tonofilaments 7
Transient amplifying cells 125
Transient portion 82, 121
of hair follicle 68, 71–75
Transplantation
coarse hair-bearing graft 251
hair 241, 243, 244
hair-bearing skin 272, 274
Inaba's single hair-bearing graft 238, 242, 244
single hair 8, 238, 242, 251
Transverse
branch vessels 39, 40, 99
collagenous fibers 8
Trichilemma 5, 55–57, 75, 85, 90, 96
Trichogenous
agent 229, 232
effects 221, 222, 232
Trichohyalin granules 22, 135
Trigeminal ganglion 141
Trio group 57, 59, 62
Tyrosinase 33–35, 225
enzyme 33

u
Undifferentiated
cell 6
matrix 133
region 134

v
Vascular
system 8, 39–44, 99, 116–118, 121
tissue 15
Vascularization
of hair follicle 112, 129
Vellus
follicle 5, 183
hairs 5, 7, 47, 48, 50, 52, 54, 59, 61, 62, 81, 95, 96, 129, 145, 183, 188
transformation 179
Vibrissa
follicle 9, 10, 82, 139–142
mammalian 139, 140
Vitreous membrane 5, 8, 63, 65

w
Wax esters 6, 186
W-plasty method 291

z
Zigzag method 291

GPSR Compliance

The European Union's (EU) General Product Safety Regulation (GPSR) is a set of rules that requires consumer products to be safe and our obligations to ensure this.

If you have any concerns about our products, you can contact us on ProductSafety@springernature.com

In case Publisher is established outside the EU, the EU authorized representative is:

Springer Nature Customer Service Center GmbH
Europaplatz 3
69115 Heidelberg, Germany

Batch number: 10845121

Printed by Printforce, the Netherlands